The Complete Home Medical Encyclopedia

by Elizabeth E. Elias

Consulting Editor: Vincent L. Guandolo, M.D.

Westport Corporation • New York, N.Y. 10010

a

abacterial — without or free from bacteria.

abdomen — the space between the diaphragm at the top and the pelvic basin at the bottom. It is the lower portion of the trunk, plus the lower portion of the backbone and back muscles in the back, and the four lower ribs and abdominal muscles on the sides and front.

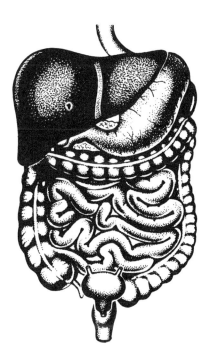

ABDOMEN

The abdomen contains many important organs: the liver in the upper right, entirely under the ribs; the stomach in the upper left; the small and large intestines in the lower portion of the abdominal cavity; the kidneys, one on each side, high up in the back; and the urinary bladder just back of the front of the pelvis where it is frequently injured from a fractured pelvis. Also included are the pancreas, duodenum, gallbladder, and spleen. There are also large blood vessels and other organs in the abdominal cavity.

The abdomen is lined with a smooth, transparent membrane called the peritoneum.

abdominal wall — the muscles in front of and along the sides of the abdomen. The muscles can be stretched in pregnancy.

abnormal — not normal.

abortion — an unnatural termination of a pregnancy. The termination takes place at a time when the fetus has not developed enough to live in the outside world.

There are three types of abortions. An accidental abortion, usually referred to as a miscarriage, may be due to abnormalities of the egg or infant, glandular or nutritional problems in the mother, as well as other internal problems.

Severe bleeding and cramps usually indicate that a miscarriage is in progress. An accidental abortion is just that — an accident.

On the other hand, a therapeutic abortion is a deliberate step, taken for medical reasons, to stop a pregnancy. Therapeutic abortions are gener-

3

ally performed when the life or the health of the mother is threatened by the pregnancy. In this type of abortion, the decision to end the pregnancy is made and carried out by a doctor.

The third type of abortion, deliberate abortion, is performed when the mother decides that she does not wish to continue the pregnancy. When abortion on demand is illegal, a woman who is pregnant may try to find a doctor who will do an illegal abortion, or she may try to abort herself. Self-induced abortions caused by entrance of unsterile instruments or other unclean objects into the uterus can lead to serious consequences such as shock, infection, abscesses, loss of the ability to bear children, and even death.

When abortions are performed by qualified personnel under sterile conditions, they are relatively safe. However, when the person performing the abortion is not qualified, or when the instruments or surroundings are not sterile, an abortion can be a grave risk to the woman involved.

See miscarriage.

abrasions — wounds caused by rubbing or scraping. These wounds are seldom deep, but a portion of the skin has been removed, leaving a raw, bleeding surface. Abrasions become infected quite easily because of the amount of underskin surface exposed, and because dirt and germs are usually ground into the tissues. "Rope burns," "floor burns," and "skinned" knees or elbows are common examples of abrasions.

abreaction — a method employed in psychoanalysis to relieve a patient's feelings of guilt or hostility by reenacting the experience which brought on the feelings.

abscess — a collection of pus in a localized area. An abscess is formed when foreign organisms destroy tissue. The defense mechanisms of the body keep the infection localized but sometimes are not, of themselves, strong enough to destroy the foreign organisms. When they fail to destroy the foreign organisms, a doctor may operate to remove the pus, or he may prescribe antibiotics to aid the body's defense mechanisms in destroying the cause of the infection.

An abscess can form in any part of the body.

See pus.

abstinence syndrome — *See addiction, withdrawal symptoms.*

abuse — excessive use, or misuse. The term is frequently used in connection with drugs, such as in "drug abuse."

abused child syndrome — *See child abuse.*

accidents — an unplanned happening leading to or causing an injury or death. Over 45 million people are injured each year as a result of accidents. Accidents kill approximately 93,000 people every year and are the first cause of death from age one to thirty-four, although the ratio is two males for every one female killed in accidents.

Many, if not most, accidents can be prevented. Prevention might include more care in handling tools and machinery when in use, and careful storage when not in use. Keeping chemicals (including drugs and household supplies) out of a child's reach is important. Careful maintenance of automobiles and equipment can prevent many accidents. Homes should be equipped with a fire extinguisher, and quick access to outside safety should be included in every room. Firearms should never be stored with ammunition in them. Seat belts should be worn in cars and extra care taken when driving conditions are poor.

accoucheur — an obstetrician or person trained as a midwife.

See obstetrician.

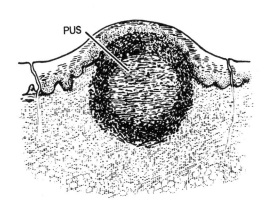

PUS

ABSCESS

4

acetabulum — the socket (one on each side of the pelvis) into which the femur or thigh bone fits.

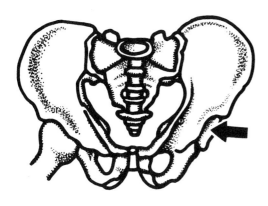

ACETABULUM

acetarsone — a drug derivative of arsenic used in the treatment of amebiasis.

acetone — a liquid substance found in the urine. It has a distinct odor and is found in excess in cases of diabetes.

acetylcholine — an acid found in the body. It plays an important part in nerve impulse transmissions. It was synthesized in 1867 by Baeyer and is used as a drug to stimulate the parasympathetic nerves.
See parasympathetic nervous system.

acetylsalicylic acid — a drug, commonly known as aspirin. It was first made in 1899 by Dresser and since that time has gained enormous popularity. Acetylsalicylic acid or aspirin is one of the most widely used drugs known to man. It is an analgesic (pain reliever) and an antipyretic (fever reducer). The body does not develop a tolerance for it, which means that its effects are the same no matter how long it is used.

Achilles tendon — a large, powerful tendon situated just above the heel. It connects the muscles of the calf to the heel bone. A torn Achilles tendon is usually the result of an athletic accident and must be repaired surgically.
The name refers to the only spot on Achilles' body which was vulnerable. His mother had held him by the ankle when she dipped him in the protective water of the river Styx.

achlorhydria — the absence or lack of hydrochloric acid in the digestive juice of the stomach. This acid plays a vital role in reducing food to usable protein.

acholic — without bile.

achondroplasia — an inherited congenital condition in which the bones of the limbs and head are affected. People with achondroplasia are dwarfs with enlarged foreheads. The condition is restricted to bones.

acid — a sour substance. In the body acids are balanced by bases or alkalis. Acids turn blue litmus paper red.

acid burns — burns caused by acids. Acid burns should be washed immediately to remove the acid. Treatment then consists of applying a solution of sodium bicarbonate (baking soda) or some other mild alkali to neutralize any chemical which remains on the skin. (An exception is an acid burn from carbolic acid which should be treated by washing the skin with alcohol.) The affected area is then washed with fresh water and gently dried. At this point it is treated as though it were a true burn.
See burn.

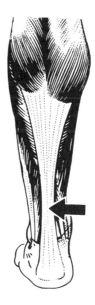

ACHILLES TENDON

acidosis — a condition in which the chemical balance of the body is lost by having too much acid or not enough base. Acidosis can be caused by disease of or failure of the lungs or kidneys (the two body organs which help regulate acids and bases). It can also be caused by dehydration (including severe diarrhea), diabetes, and acid poisoning.

acid poisoning — poisoning by acid taken by mouth. The antidote for acid poisoning is usually an alkali diluted in water which is swallowed to neutralize the acid.
See poison.

acme — *See crisis.*

acne — a common skin condition among teenagers who have reached puberty. Acne usually appears on the face, although it can also appear on the chest and back. It is characterized by comedos (blackheads) and small skin elevations (with or without pus). Acne is caused by excessive secretions of grease from the sebaceous glands. The grease dries and blocks pore openings (blackheads) and sometimes becomes infected (skin elevations with pus, usually referred to as pimples). Treatment of acne includes a diet low in greasy foods. The diet will often prohibit chocolates and carbonated beverages. The use of astringents can be helpful. Acne will normally subside in the late teens when puberty is completed.

Acne is not serious in a physical sense, although severe cases can leave scars. More importantly, acne can lead to psychological problems because of the unpleasant appearance of the face.

acquired — any disease or condition which is caused or produced by an agent outside the body. A disease or condition which is not congenital, that is, not present at birth.

acrid — a term used to denote pungency.

acro — a prefix used to denote the hands or feet.

acrodolichomelia — hands or feet which are abnormally long.

acromegaly — a condition in which there is excessive or abnormal growth of normal tissue, particularly in the areas of the face, fingers, and toes. It is caused by an excess of secretions of hormone from the pituitary gland.
See pituitary gland.

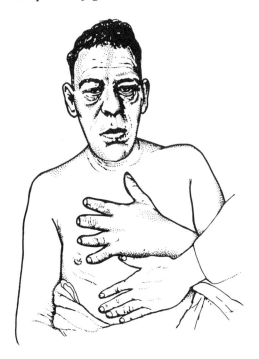

ACROMEGALY

acromion — the highest and outermost extension of the shoulder.
See scapula.

ACTH — abbr. for adrenocorticotropic hormone.
See adrenocorticotropic hormone.

actinomycosis — a disease usually found in cattle but sometimes passed on to man. It is caused by the microorganism *Actinomyces bovis.* The infection forms abscesses in the neck, chest, and abdomen. It is treated with antibiotics such as penicillin.

activated charcoal — *See charcoal.*

acupuncture — one of the methods of treatment used by the Chinese for a variety of conditions, diseases, and disorders. The treatment is based on inserting needles into various specified points on the body. Each point relates to a different area of the body.

Acupuncture is also used in place of an anesthetic.

acute — a term used to denote a disease or condition which is short but severe, as opposed to the term chronic, which implies a disease or condition that is of longer duration.

acute abdomen — medical slang used to indicate a serious undiagnosed problem in the abdominal region needing immediate exploratory surgery.

acute rheumatism — *See rheumatic fever.*

addict — a person suffering from addiction. The term usually refers to people who are physically or psychologically dependent on drugs or alcohol. *See addiction.*

addiction — the condition of being physically or psychologically dependent on some foreign matter.

In the United States, addiction is usually to drugs or alcohol. Drug addiction has become one of the most serious problems facing society.

Addiction frequently leads to antisocial behavior because the cost of supporting the addiction is so high. Most authorities agree that the involvement with crime of a narcotics (specifically heroin) addict is not a direct effect of the drug itself, but turning to crime is usually the only method the addict has of getting the large amounts of money needed. Many addicts who are desperate due to withdrawal sickness will resort to violence.

See alcoholism, heroin addiction, and different types of abused drugs.

Addison, Thomas — London physician (1793-1860) whose chief contribution was in the study of various types of anemia.

Addison's disease — a disorder of the adrenal glands in which there is a shortage or lack of hormones. It is characterized by a deficiency of blood sugar, low blood pressure, and low temperature.

Addison's disease is a result of disease or malfunction of the adrenal cortex and causes progressive anemia, diarrhea, low blood pressure, and a bronze skin coloration. The disease can be fatal.

adenoid — a small, spongy mass of tissue at the back of the nose which is similar in its function to other glands in the body, particularly those at the side of the neck, in the armpit and groin. Like those other glands, adenoids combat germs; they become involved when a cold or throat infection is present. After repeated respiratory troubles, they may remain so swollen that they interfere with breathing. If the situation becomes urgent, the physician may feel that they should be removed.

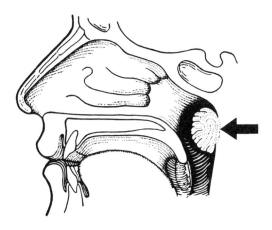

ADENOIDS

In years past, adenoids were removed whenever tonsils were removed; that is no longer the general rule. Today, the operation is never done routinely in a general attempt to improve health in some vague way.

Problems with tonsils and adenoids are frequently encountered in childhood.

adenoidectomy — surgical removal of the adenoids.

adenopathy — general term for any disease of the glands, particularly of the lymph glands.

adenosine triphosphate — a compound found in muscles which is the storage place for extra muscular energy (abbreviated ATP).

adenovirus — a virus which is responsible for many common upper respiratory diseases.

ADH — abbr. for antidiuretic hormone.

adhesion — sticking together. The term is also used to indicate an abnormal joining together of two or more body parts. This may happen as a result of the body's defense mechanisms, such as inflammation and clotting.

adipose tissue — fatty connective tissue found under the skin and surrounding various body organs. Adipose tissue is the soft layer between skin and bones. It protects against bumps and jars and against sudden external temperature changes. It is also a storage area for fat and energy.

adiposis — obesity resulting from an excess of fat or adipose tissue.
See obesity.

Adler's theory — theory postulated by Alfred Adler (1870-1937), a Viennese psychiatrist. The theory states that people develop neuroses to compensate for some inferiority.

adnexa — appendages.

adolescence — the period of life from the onset to the conclusion of puberty.

adrenal cortex — the outer layer of an adrenal gland.
See adrenal glands.

adrenal glands — a pair of glands, one situated on top of each kidney. Each gland is approximately the size of a pea. Each gland is made up of two distinct parts, and each part has different functions. The outer layer, or adrenal cortex, is essential to life and life processes; the inner part, or adrenal medulla, while important, is not essential.

ADRENAL CORTEX

When the adrenal cortex is stimulated by ACTH (adrenocorticotropic hormone), it in turn secretes cortisone, thus helping to regulate the metabolism of both sugar and protein. Other hormones secreted by the adrenal cortex are aldosterone, which regulates the amount of salt that is excreted by the kidneys, and a sex hormone.

If the adrenal cortex is not secreting enough hormones, there is a marked loss of certain functions. One of the most important of these is salt retention. When the body does not retain enough salt, it can not retain enough water. Another serious problem can be low blood sugar and low blood pressure, causing weakness and fainting.

On the other hand, an excess of hormones from the adrenal cortex can cause puberty praecox (weight gain due to excessive retention of salt and hence excessive retention of water) and in females secondary masculine sex characteristics. The bearded lady in the circus is usually troubled by an excess of hormones from the adrenal cortex.

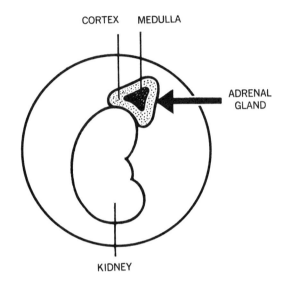

ADRENAL GLAND

ADRENAL MEDULLA

The adrenal medulla, the second part of the adrenal gland, is surrounded by the adrenal cortex. It is an extension of the sympathetic nervous system. The adrenal medulla secretes epinephrine and norepinephrine. Norepinephrine is concerned with regulating a normal blood pressure. Epinephrine is the hormone the adrenal glands secrete when in danger or when an extra push is needed. Epinephrine is often referred to as the "flight or fight" hormone because the body's reactions to it are those normally associated with emergencies: increased heart rate, rise in blood pressure and blood sugar level, and dilation of the pupils of the eyes. Epinephrine also stimulates an increase of blood flow through the muscles.

The adrenal glands are also known as the suprarenal glands.

adrenaline — *See epinephrine.*

adrenal medulla — the inner portion of an adrenal gland.
See adrenal glands.

adrenocorticotropic hormone — a hormone secreted by the anterior pituitary. Adrenocorticotropic hormone (abbreviated ACTH) stimulates the adrenal cortex of the adrenal glands to secrete hormones. ACTH has been synthesized and has been used to replace secreted ACTH. More frequently, however, it is used as a diagnostic tool.
See adrenal glands.

Aedes — a genus of mosquitoes. Different types transmit yellow fever, encephalitis, and dengue.

aeration — the process of giving off carbon dioxide and taking on oxygen, which occurs to blood in the lungs.

aerobic — a term applied to any living organism which can live in an oxygen atmosphere. The direct opposite of an anaerobic, which only lives in an oxygen-free atmosphere.

aerophagy — air-swallowing spasms.

aerosols — a solution suspended in gas which comes out of a container as a fine mist.
The propellants in many household and commercial aerosol sprays produce an intoxicated state when inhaled and are used by adolescents as a means of distorting consciousness. The propellants in these sprays are gases containing chlorinated or fluorinated hydrocarbons. Aerosols which have been abused include insecticides, deodorants, glass chillers, and hair sprays. Abuse of aerosols from spray cans appears to be increasing.

after-birth — *See placenta.*

after-pains — the contractions of the uterus after delivery. They are very much like menstrual cramps. Sometimes they are more uncomfortable with a second or third baby than with a first one. They usually stop in a few days.

agar — a culture media.

age-adjusted death rate — death rates that have been standardized by age for the purpose of making comparisons between different populations or within the same population at various intervals of time. Also called age-adjusted mortality rate.

aged — elderly.
See aging.

agent — something which acts upon or against something else.

age-specific death rate — the ratio of deaths in a specific age group to the population of the same age group during a given period of time, such as a year. It is calculated by dividing the deaths that occurred among the specific age group during the year, by the mid-year population in the same group of the same year.

agglutination — the part of the healing process in which the wound closes by adhesion.

aggregation — clumping together.

aging — the process of growing old.
Everyone is subject to aging, starting from the moment of conception. Aging is part of the growing process. As the individual matures, there takes place a constant and simultaneous tearing down of old tissue and a building up of new tissue. In children, the building up process is more rapid than the tearing down process. When the child becomes an adult, the tearing down process begins to catch up with the building up process. Throughout an individual's lifetime, he is subject to this simultaneous dual process.
Due to the progress made by scientists, medical researchers, and public health officials during the past few decades, most people can count on living longer than their grandparents did. In 1900 the life expectancy of a newborn baby was forty-nine years. A person of sixty could expect to live to the age of seventy-four. Today, an average infant can be expected to live about sixty-nine years and the sixty year old to age seventy-seven. Thus, practically within a lifetime, twenty years have been added to the infant's life expectancy, and the average person of sixty can count on living three years longer than his 1900 counterpart.
Most doctors believe there is a good possibility that the lifespan of older persons can be increased considerably. Most animals live to an age about seven times their age at maturity. Only the human animal falls short of that mark. The average

man lives to be only about three times his age at maturity. Since he stops growing at about the age of twenty-five, perhaps his average lifespan someday will carry him to an average age of 150 or 175.

Many people feel that they would not want to live to be 150 years old, but it is highly possible that the 150 year old man of the future will be the equivalent of today's seventy-five year old man. It is important to remember that a person of any age today is "younger" than a person of the same age in 1900. Then, a man of fifty was old; today, a man of fifty is in the prime of life. The average person today cannot even begin to be considered old until he is in his seventies or eighties.

CHANGES

With age, a number of changes take place in the body. These changes are very evident. Take the eye and the ear, for example. Most children are able to adjust their eyes automatically, and equally well, to distant objects and to close objects. But as they grow older their ability to make this automatic adjustment decreases. Eventually, they may have to rely on glasses. Today there is no stigma attached to wearing glasses so most people are able to adjust to this physical impairment very well. The ears are similarly affected, for hearing ability, too, decreases gradually. Today, people are able to adjust to not hearing as well as they used to, even to the point of relying on hearing aids if their hearing is seriously impaired.

A decrease in agility, in muscular coordination and stamina is a natural byproduct of aging and must be accepted and adjusted to. Normally, these are not serious impairments. Of course they may affect one's ability to play baseball but, except in extreme cases, they are not disabling for the average person.

TYPES

There is not just one kind of age. A person may be a number of different ages at the same time. There is, of course, chronological age, that is, the actual number of years a person has lived. Most often compulsory retirement is based on this chronological age. But there are also other ages which must be taken into consideration. A person who has had seventy birthdays may have the physical condition of the average fifty year old. He may have the philosophy and the temperament usually found in a much younger person, he may be "young at heart," as the saying

goes. In that case his outlook on life may be that of a person of thirty or forty. He may also have the quickness and keenness of intellect more often found in a much younger person, so that his intellectual age is much lower than his chronological age of seventy.

The rate of advance in chronological age is, of course, the same for everyone; every twelve months adds one year. But the rate of advance in other kinds of age may be very different in different people, and the rates of physical, emotional, and intellectual development may be quite different in the same person. Some people develop physically very rapidly, others very slowly; some develop emotionally or intellectually very rapidly, others very slowly. And some people develop at one pace physically, at another pace emotionally, and still another pace intellectually. Even within the process of physical aging, an individual may be subject to different rates of aging; for example, a man of any chronological age may have the sight of a man of twenty, the hearing of a man of fifty, and the liver of a man of eighty.

As a rule, the rate of physical growth is most rapid before the person is actually born. After birth, although the baby and the child grow rapidly, the rate of growth gradually decreases. Related to this change in rate of growth is the fact that the older a person becomes, the longer it takes for him to recover from an injury. The damaged tissues just do not repair themselves as rapidly in an older person as in a younger one.

Most of a person's capacities (strength, muscular coordination, agility, learning ability, reasoning ability, etc.) increase very rapidly during childhood and early adulthood and most reach a peak in the individual's twenties or thirties. Then some of them, particularly the physical capacities, start to decline. Intellectual abilities usually decline much later and much more slowly. Sometimes they do not begin to decline at all until the person is quite advanced in age, if then. Emotional stability also may not decline at all and may even continue to advance into very old age; a person may become increasingly better able to accept whatever comes along as he advances in years and experience.

HEALTH

Heart disease, cancer, and stroke take the heaviest toll of life among the older segments of the population.

Many of the deaths that occur in middle life or later are not preventable in view of our limited knowledge about some degenerative diseases.

On the other hand, many premature deaths could be averted with preventive and therapeutic measures. Immunization against influenza would reduce fatalities among the aged and chronically ill. Incipient cancer sometimes develops slowly in older persons, allowing time for diagnosis and treatment.

Many elderly people suffer from problems caused by poor nutritional habits. Usually less physical work is performed in advanced age and therefore the body's requirement for calories is lower. Dietary calories which are not used are stored in the form of body fat and many persons who continue the richer diet of their physically more active days may become too heavy. This is the main reason why fewer carbohydrates and less fat are needed in the food of the aged.

Since the total amount of food eaten may be smaller, the diet should contain in proportion at least as much protein, vitamins, and minerals. The requirements for these essential nutrients must continue to be met, especially since there is a possibility that in advanced age the body may absorb and utilize some of these food elements less efficiently.

An ample fluid intake is important, particularly in warm weather. A liberal consumption of fluids such as water, milk, juices, coffee, and tea spaced throughout the day helps to maintain regular bowel habits and normal kidney function.

agnail — a hangnail.

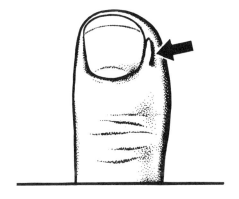

AGNAIL

agony — extreme physical pain or suffering.

ague — a severe chill resulting in violent shaking as in malarial fever.

aid — assistance given to a person in need of help. *See first aid.*

air embolism — the blockage of any blood vessel by a bubble of air. *See embolism.*

air pollution — fouling the air with man-made or man-caused pollutants.

Air pollution is a serious and difficult problem which affects everybody in the United States. Factories, furnaces, autos, burning dumps, power generating stations and many daily activities create air pollution.

When air pollution is severe, it triggers illness and may bring premature death to thousands of people. Even "ordinary" levels of air pollution can cause coughing, sneezing, and wheezing. Short-range discomfort may be followed by long-range disease. Both emphysema and lung cancer are more prevalent in areas of high air contamination.

Air pollution costs the country billions of dollars a year. The economic loss is enormous: crop damage, corrosion, cleaning bills, wasted fuel, accidents from reduced visibility. The health costs are serious; they cannot be measured in dollars alone.

Ironically enough, air pollution goes with economic progress. It is a "mix" compounded from the exhausts of millions of automobiles, emissions from power plants and industries, emissions from incinerators and heating plants, smoke from backyard trash fires and municipal rubbish dumps.

The insistence of aroused citizens has demonstrated that smoke can be eliminated, auto exhaust can be controlled, waste disposal can be clean, factories can make things without belching soot and gases.

There are now ways of controlling most forms of air pollution, and people can insist that these means be used.

Federal aid helps with research, training of control officers and research workers, enforcement and abatement programs, technical and financial assistance.

States and cities, as well as agencies of the federal government, are moving in the direction of improved control regulations and more funds for enforcement of these regulations.

Progressive industries are developing better control techniques.

air sickness — *See motion sickness.*

alastrim — variola minor, a mild type of smallpox. The major difference between smallpox and alastrim is that alastrim has a significantly lower mortality factor.
See smallpox.

albino — an inherited condition in which there is a lack of normal pigmentation, usually affecting the skin, hair, and eyes. The lack of normal pigmentation causes the skin and hair to be white and the eyes to be pink. Albinos must be careful of the amount of sun to which they are exposed.

albumin — a protein found in the body. The presence of albumin (which is not usually excreted) in the urine may indicate kidney damage, toxemia, or other problems.

alcohol — a colorless liquid which can be used as an astringent or antiseptic. One type of alcohol, ethyl alcohol, is the major ingredient in wines, beers, and distilled beverages. In this form, alcohol is a colorless inflammable liquid which has intoxicating effects. It is important to note that the type of alcohol in beverages should only be ethyl alcohol. Other types, such as isopropyl alcohol, are poisonous if taken internally.

By strict definition, ethyl alcohol is classified as a food because it contains calories. However, it has no nutritional value. Ethyl alcohol could also be classified as a drug because it dramatically affects the central nervous system. However, it should never be used as a drug (nor used at all) in cases of shock or suspected shock.

Twenty percent of the alcohol in an alcoholic beverage is absorbed directly and immediately into the bloodstream through the stomach walls. It does not have to be digested. The blood carries it directly to the brain where the alcohol acts on the brain's central control areas, slowing down or depressing activity. The other eighty percent of alcohol is processed only slightly slower through the gastrointestinal tract and into the bloodstream. Minutes after it is consumed it can be found in all tissues, organs, and secretions of the body.

EFFECTS

A low level of alcohol in the blood, such as would result from taking one drink an hour, has a mild tranquilizing effect, since alcohol is a central nervous system depressant. At first, however, it may seem to be a stimulant. Alcohol's first effects are exerted on the upper parts of the brain where learned patterns such as self-control are stored. After a drink or two, this learned behavior may temporarily disappear, causing talkativeness, aggressiveness, depression, and a general loss of inhibitions.

Higher blood alcohol levels depress brain activity further to a point where memory, as well as muscular coordination and balance, may be temporarily impaired. Still larger alcohol intake within a relatively short period of time depresses deeper parts of the brain, producing a state of loss of control in which judgment is severely affected, and sensory perceptions are dulled.

If steady, heavy drinking continues, the alcohol will anesthetize the deepest levels of the brain, and may result in coma or death.

The rapidity with which alcohol enters the bloodstream and exerts its effect on the brain and body depend on the following:

1. How fast the alcohol is consumed. A half ounce of alcohol can be burned up (oxidized) in the body in about an hour. Imbibed at this rate, the alcohol will not jolt the brain. However, more **rapid** consumption will produce immediate intoxicating effects and depression of deeper brain centers.

2. Whether the stomach is empty or full. Eating, especially before drinking as well as while drinking, will slow down the absorption rate of alcohol into the bloodstream.

3. What type of drink is consumed. Wine and beer are absorbed less rapidly than hard liquors because they contain small amounts of non-alcoholic substances that slow down the absorption process. These substances have been removed from liquor in the distillation process. Diluting an alcoholic beverage with another liquid, such as water, slows down absorption, but mixing with carbonated beverages can increase the rate of absorption.

4. Body weight. The same amount of alcohol can have a greater effect on a person weighing

120 pounds than on a person weighing 180 pounds. Alcohol is quickly distributed uniformly throughout the circulatory system. Therefore, the heavier person will have smaller concentrations throughout the bloodstream and body than the lighter person.

5. Individual mood. A person who is emotionally upset, under stress, or tired while drinking will find that alcohol has a stronger impact than normal.

See alcoholism, hangover, alcoholic poisoning.

alcoholic poisoning — poisoning from alcohol. Alcoholic beverages taken in excess act as depressant poisons. The patient has the odor of alcohol on his breath. He is partly or completely unconscious, although usually he can be aroused temporarily but soon relapses into a stupor. He often mutters in delirium. In the early stages his face is moist and flushed, his pulse strong, and his breathing deep. Later his face becomes dry and bloated, with a bluish cast, his pulse becomes weak and rapid and his breathing is shallow. His eyes are bloodshot and his pupils natural or large but of equal size.

It is important to keep the patient warm to avoid shock. The patient should be given salt water, mustard water, or soapy water to promote vomiting.

See poison.

alcoholism — an addictive disease characterized by a craving for alcohol and its effect in relieving psychic and physical pain, and which brings about, for the drinker or the people around him, serious problems in physical, mental, family, social, or economic areas.

PROGRESSIVE STAGES

There are a number of symptoms in the way people drink that can indicate the onset of alcoholism. There may be indications from the very start that they are using alcohol to help themselves over rough spots and that this habit is growing on them.

1. One of the more obvious early signs of a predisposition to alcoholism is that the individual drinks more than is customary among his associates and makes excuses to drink more often. This is an indication that he is developing an insistent need, or a psychological dependence, on alcohol to help him escape from unpleasant worries or tensions.

2. As the condition progresses he begins to experience "blackouts." He does not "pass out" or become unconscious, but the morning after a drinking bout he cannot remember what happened after a certain point. If this happens repeatedly or after taking only a moderate amount of alcohol, it is a strong indication of developing alcoholism.

3. As his desire for alcohol becomes stronger, the alcoholic gulps, rather than drinks, his beverage. He senses that his drinking is getting out of hand and he starts drinking surreptitiously so that others will not know how much he is consuming.

4. Finally he loses control of his drinking. After one drink, he feels a physical demand for the drug so strong that he cannot stop short of intoxication. Suffering from remorse, but not wanting to show it, he strikes out unreasonably at others. As he realizes that he is losing the respect of his associates and hurting his loved ones, he tries to stop or to drink moderately, but he can't. He becomes filled with discouragement and self-pity and tries to "drown his troubles" in more liquor. But his drinking has passed beyond the point where he can use it as a way of coping with his problems, and he is faced with the disease of alcoholism.

5. When the illness becomes chronic the alcoholic starts going on binges for days at a time, developing physical tremors, hallucinations, and terrible fears.

6. The late effects of alcoholism are painful neuritis of the extremities, liver disease, delirium and hallucinations, loss of memory, diminution of intellect, depression; and personality, vocational, and moral deterioration.

CAUSES

The cause of alcoholism is still obscure. Prolonged and heavy drinking does not always produce alcoholism. Character defects have been thought to underlie the compulsion to drink. The heavy drinker is often insecure, self-centered, immature, and intolerant of frustration. Some people need no alcoholic support in facing difficulty. Some turn to alcohol only occasionally. Others find their situation so intolerable that they drink to excess in an attempt to suppress painful emotional conflicts.

Some think that emotional problems instigate the chain of events. It is likely that the burden of psychic and physical living, borne readily by most, is too heavy for some, and they seek escape from their worries and anxieties. Viewed from a psychological standpoint, the alcoholic is considered immature, since he has not developed the capacity to cope successfully with his problems. He depends on alcohol and uses it again and again to escape from uncomfortable situations.

It is believed chemical alterations take place which create physiological and biological need and dependence—in short, "addiction." A change in metabolism and body chemistry may then occur and lead to a loss of tolerance and to pathological intoxication whenever alcohol is consumed.

Some scientists believe that alcoholism may have a physical or biological cause: a defect in the body chemistry or some nutritional deficiency. Another theory is that the craving for alcohol is brought on by its effect on the adrenal glands, which regulate the production of chemical energy in the body.

In summary, no conclusive evidence is yet available on the causes of alcoholism. It is a medical-social problem far too complicated for simple answers.

TREATMENT

The idea that anything could, or should, be done for alcoholics is comparatively new in our society. Until recently, alcoholics were generally considered perverse, weak-willed, and deserving of punishment rather than help. Only within the past two decades has alcoholism come to be accepted as a medical problem. Even with this recognition, a small number of physicians still believe that little can be done to help the alcoholic because his condition is so difficult and unmanageable.

This attitude is rapidly changing, however, and interested persons have demonstrated, through new therapeutic approaches, that alcoholics can recover. This does not mean that a cure for alcoholism has been found; no method known today can free the alcoholic from the chronic disorder which makes it impossible for him to control his drinking. What it does mean is that through medical, psychological, and spiritual help, many alcoholics can be helped to stop drinking and resume normal living without substituting other injurious practices. However, the alcoholic can maintain his recovery only by leaving alcohol strictly alone.

The primary goal of treatment, then, is to help the patient remain sober and to handle his problems constructively so that staying sober will not be too difficult. Various forms of treatment are in use and each has met with some success; but none of them is effective with all alcoholics. Some respond to one treatment program and some to another; unfortunately, many alcoholics are unwilling to accept or unable to profit from any therapy offered today. Increasing numbers are seeking treatment, however, and with beneficial results, often to the point of recovery.

1. Medical treatment

Medical treatment is often required during the period of acute intoxication and is used to some extent in dealing with chronic alcoholism. For some patients, doctors have prescribed drugs which are helpful as deterrents to drinking. Persons taking these drugs become violently ill if they drink alcohol while the anti-alcoholic medication is in their system. But such drugs have no effect whatever on the alcoholism itself. Unless the patient is helped to overcome his compulsion through some other therapy, he faces the same problems when the drugs are withdrawn.

Some of the tranquilizing drugs have proven useful in treating alcoholism by temporarily quieting the anxieties that induce drinking. Drugs also can be used to build up physical stamina and to overcome vitamin deficiencies which are common in alcoholics. But overcoming alcoholism usually calls for some form of psychotherapy in addition to whatever medication is used.

2. Psychotherapy

It is almost impossible for a person who has become dependent on alcohol to break away from it completely unless he receives emotional support and guidance. Psychotherapy can furnish the alcoholic with the psychological help he needs to work out his problems constructively and be comfortable without drinking. The purpose of psychotherapy is to help the patient understand his problems, realize his potentialities, and establish a better way of life.

Alcoholics can receive psychiatric help on an individual basis or they can be treated in groups. Group psychotherapy has proven very effective in the treatment of alcoholism. Some alcoholics, however, respond better to individual therapy.

A new approach has been developed recently in which the alcoholic is helped through his family. In group psychotherapy, the husbands and wives of alcoholics are aided in overcoming emotional difficulties that may have a bearing on the drinking of their marriage partners. Such treatment helps to create a more favorable environment for the patient's recovery.

3. Alcoholics Anonymous

Remarkable success in helping alcoholics has been achieved by Alcoholics Anonymous. This is a loosely knit organization of alcoholics who have banded together to help themselves and others to stay sober. While AA is not usually classified as "treatment," the method its members employ for overcoming alcoholism has resulted in recovery or relief for thousands of people. AA meetings have some of the advantages of group therapy. They provide an opportunity for group discussion of common problems and give members a chance to unload their personal anxieties before a group of understanding, noncritical peers. As a fellowship of individuals devoted to a common purpose, AA gives emotional support to its members. The social activities do a great deal to ease the loneliness that an alcoholic always feels. The AA program helps the members to rely on "a Power greater than ourselves" for strength in overcoming their difficulties. This approach has the psychological effect of releasing tension and replacing despair with hope.

AA is not a complete therapy and AA members often take other forms of treatment. In turn, many doctors who work with alcoholics refer them to Alcoholics Anonymous for the psychological help it offers. In general, alcoholics who join AA respond favorably to its program, but there are some alcoholics who are unable to enter into this type of group association.

Not until they reach the point of desperation do most alcoholics seek help; many never do. But if they can be brought to recognize their illness and accept treatment at an early stage, they can often save themselves and their families much suffering.

aldosterone — a hormone secreted by the adrenal cortex of the adrenal glands which regulates the amount of salt that is excreted by the kidneys.

alignment — the act of straightening or placing in a line a body part which is out of shape or place.

alimentary canal — officially that part of the digestive system consisting of the esophagus, stomach, and intestines. However, the term is occasionally used to indicate the entire digestive system.

alkali — a base substance. In the body, alkalis are balanced by acids. Alkalis will turn red litmus paper blue. Lye, ammonia, and potash are alkalis.

alkali burns — burns caused by alkalis. Alkali burns should be washed immediately to remove the alkali. Treatment then consists of applying vinegar, lemon juice or some other mild acid to neutralize any chemical remaining on the skin. The affected area is then washed with fresh water and gently dried. At this stage it can be treated as though it were a regular burn.
See burn.

alkali poisoning — poisoning by an alkali taken by mouth. The antidote for alkali poisoning is usually an acid diluted in water which is swallowed to neutralize the alkali.
See poison.

alkalosis — a condition in which the chemical balance of the body is lost by having too much alkali or not enough acid. Alkalosis can be caused by lack of carbon dioxide from excessive breathing, vomiting, and by overdoses of alkalis.

allergen — any substance which causes allergic reactions.

allergist — a doctor whose specialty is treating allergies.

allergy — a sensitivity to a normally harmless substance. An allergic person who receives more of the irritant than he can tolerate will show an allergic reaction. An allergic reaction may resemble a cold, an upset stomach, a skin disease, a sinus disorder, or a number of other disorders.

CAUSES

If a person is sensitive to certain materials such as the pollens of plants, trees or grass, he may develop antibodies to them. After that, if one of these substances (called antigens) gets into the body again, it may cause an antigen-antibody reaction or allergic attack. The reaction between the antigen and antibody may slightly damage tissues, thus causing the release of histamine, which in turn causes some of the symptoms of an allergic attack.

Heredity is believed to play a part in the development of allergic diseases. Many people with allergies have come from families where the parents or other close relatives have had some form of allergic manifestation. Although people do not inherit a specific disease such as hay fever, they do inherit the tendency to become sensitive to certain things. Members of the same family who have inherited such a tendency may develop altogether different allergic diseases, or they may go through life without a symptom.

It is also possible to develop an allergy without an inherited tendency. A person can suddenly develop an allergy to something which has previously been harmless to him.

The allergic reaction itself is the body's abnormal reaction to a substance to which it has become sensitized. Why the body becomes sensitized is not completely understood. However, it is known that worry and other forms of emotional stress have caused allergies to flare up. In some cases, the appearance of an allergic illness is due to disturbances inside the body rather than to outside irritants such as pollens. The sensitivity may be associated with bacterial infection, especially of the sinuses, nose, or throat.

Climate, season, degree of exposure, state of mind, and other factors seem to contribute to the frequency and intensity of reactions.

REACTIONS

A person may be allergic to certain foods (such as eggs, chocolate, strawberries, milk, fish); to fine particles which are breathed (dust, pollen, feathers); to irritants which he touches (poison ivy, dog or cat hair, wool, glue, soap, detergent); to drugs which are taken by mouth or injections (sedatives, antibiotics, antitoxins); or to germs which are released in the body by an infection.

People vary in their reactions to allergens. For instance, a person who is allergic to eggs may be slightly upset by eating one as frequently as every day; another might become violently ill from the amount of egg he would get in a trace of mayonnaise dressing.

Some of the common allergic reactions are: asthma, hay fever, eczema, sinus irritations, and hives.

TREATMENT

Sometimes it is relatively easy to find the cause of an allergy and to eliminate it from the person's life so that he gets complete relief. In other cases, the person is sensitive to so many things or to such widely present substances that the particular offenders cannot be eliminated.

Often, an allergist (a doctor specializing in allergies) will have to be consulted and a battery of diagnostic tests made to determine the particular substances to which the person is reacting. When the substances cannot be avoided, an allergist will attempt to desensitize the person by means of a series of injections.

During an actual attack, physicians often prescribe an antihistamine to help counteract the effects of histamine.

See asthma, hay fever, eczema, hives.

allopathy — the method of treating diseases and conditions by using drugs which produce effects opposite those from which the patient is suffering. For example, a person suffering from a fever would be given an antipyretic or fever-reducer. Allopathy is the normal method of treatment. The term is only used to indicate the opposite of homeopathy.

allopurinol — a drug used in the treatment of gout and some other diseases resulting from high concentrations of uric acid. It works by sharply reducing the body's production of uric acid.

See gout, uric acid.

aloe — a cathartic obtained from the juice of the leaves of the aloe plant. It is not used very much because it is very irritating. It was once thought to help cause abortions, but this is not true.

alopecia — baldness, or lack of hair in normally hairy body areas.

See baldness.

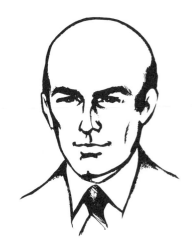

ALOPECIA

alveoli — tiny air sacs. These sacs are found at the end of bronchioles in the lung. In these sacs, the oxygen from the air is picked up by the blood, to be pumped through the entire body. At the same time, the waste product, carbon dioxide, is removed from the blood and breathed out.

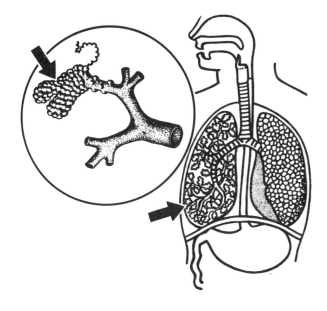

ALVEOLI

alveolus — a general term indicating a small sac, cavity, or socket.

Alzheimer's disease — a rare disease in which there is mental deterioration similar to senility, but the disease occurs in middle age.

Amanita — a genus of mushrooms. Some are very poisonous, but others are edible.

ambivalence — a term used in psychology to indicate a patient's opposite feelings of like and dislike, or love and hate, towards a person, object, or goal.

amblyopia — dimness or loss of sight for which no organic reason can be found in the eye.

amblyopia ex anopsia — a condition of reduced or dim vision in an eye which appears to be normal. It sometimes is called "lazy eye." It occurs when the two eyes do not see the same thing with the same degree of clarity, and the poorer eye is not stimulated to develop or maintain clearness of vision. An example is when the eyes are not straight or have grossly unequal vision. Amblyopia ex anopsia usually is not caused by a disease process and it can generally be corrected if discovered early enough. The condition usually begins in children during preschool years and may go undiagnosed into adulthood. It is estimated that two to four percent of the population of the United States is affected. It is a common cause of blindness throughout the world.

If a person with an amblyopic eye should injure his good eye, he might well find himself without useful vision. Therefore, it is important to find and correct eye defects which lead to amblyopia. If amblyopia is already present, the eye must be retrained, if possible, to focus properly for central vision and to work as a team with the other eye.

DEVELOPMENT

In normal vision the back of each eye receives a picture and the two pictures are blended by the brain into a single image. However, if one eye is turned and does not look straight at what is being observed by the other (as in crossed eyes), or if the two eyes have different refractive errors (one eye may be nearsighted and the other farsighted, or one may be more nearsighted than the other), the two pictures will be so different that they will not fuse into a single image. This causes "confused" or "double" vision. The brain will not tolerate such double or confused vision and it ignores, or suppresses, one of the pictures. Thus, the eye which transmits the distorted image cannot develop its ability to see clearly and the vision steadily declines.

Authorities disagree about where the actual suppression of the image takes place. Most of them believe it occurs in that area of the brain in which nerve impulses from the eye are interpreted as vision. Others think that suppression takes place within the sensitive retina of the eye. All the experts, however, recognize the fact that amblyopia ex anopsia requires early attention, because the amblyopic person often is unaware that anything is wrong with his vision. The reason for this is that image suppression beginning early in childhood interrupts normal development of vision, and the person, therefore, has no normal visual standard with which to compare his ability to see properly.

TREATMENT

There are three main methods of treating am-

17

blyopia. By far the most widely used is "patching," or covering, the good eye to force the patient to use the amblyopic eye. Patching alone is often successful with children. In some instances, eyeglasses are prescribed to correct refractive errors. In others, muscle surgery sometimes is used to correct the out-of-line amblyopic eye.

When amblyopia has progressed beyond a certain stage, or when the routine treatments do not work, there is pleoptic-orthoptic therapy as a method of treatment. The principle of pleoptic therapy is to retrain the eye, with partially screened light flashes, to use its most sensitive areas in vision.

Pleoptic therapy usually is followed by orthoptic therapy (which retrains the eyes to work together as a team). Some authorities believe there is no age limit for pleoptic-orthoptic treatment. Therapy has been reported to be successful with patients over age fifty who have lost the sight of their better eye and are forced to use the amblyopic eye. However, the therapy is most successful when the patient is treated at the earliest age possible.

PREVENTION

Amblyopia ex anopsia is preventable. Abnormal conditions of the eyes that may lead to it often can be detected easily and corrected.

Ideally, every child should have a thorough eye examination for visual acuity prior to the fifth birthday. The acuity test can be done easily by the pediatrician or family doctor during the routine office examination of the child, or the test can be performed at a well-baby clinic. A parent cannot always tell if there is something wrong with a child's eyesight, but a simple vision acuity test often can indicate whether there is any need to take the child to an eye specialist.

There are many characteristic actions that may indicate that a child has a vision problem. It could be a warning of such problems if a child:

1. Rubs his eyes excessively, closes or covers one eye when looking at an object.

2. Tilts his head forward when focusing his eyes, or has difficulty reading or in other efforts requiring close use of the eyes.

3. Blinks more than is usual or is irritable when doing close work.

Parents should also notice if the child:

4. Trips over small objects.

5. Holds books close to his eyes.

6. Cannot participate in games requiring distance vision.

7. Squints or frowns excessively.

An involuntary turning in or out of one or both eyes at any age is an immediate problem urgently needing attention. A child will not outgrow crossed eyes.

ameba — a simple single cell protozoan. Some types cause diseases in man. Alternate spelling — amoeba.

See amebiasis.

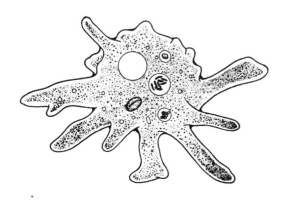

AMEBA

amebiasis — an infection of the bowel caused by a microscopic ameba whose technical name is *Entamoeba histolytica.* The infection can occur in mild or severe forms. In its severe form, amebiasis is known as amebic dysentery. More rarely, the infection may spread to the liver or other parts of the body.

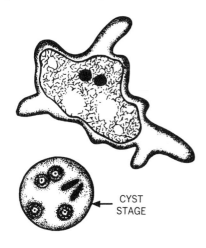

CYST STAGE

ENTAMOEBA HISTOLYTICA

Although severe cases of amebic dysentery are more common in the tropics than in temperate zones, the disease does occur occasionally in the United States. No statistics are currently available to show the exact number of persons stricken with acute amebiasis. In its milder or chronic form (which generally has no serious ill effects) the infection is believed to be carried by three to five percent of the population as a whole. The distribution of infections is spotty.

CAUSES

Amebiasis is contracted by swallowing parasites in polluted food or drinking water. The infective stage consists of a round, nonmoving cyst with a fairly resistant cell wall. Once inside the body, the parasite comes out of the cyst and develops into an active form called the trophozoite which multiplies and may invade the tissues. In chronic amebiasis some trophozoites continue to multiply in the body, whereas others revert to cyst stages which are passed out in the stools and may infect other individuals. In amebic dysentery, cysts are not formed and only the relatively fragile active stages are found in the stools.

The infection may be spread through drinking water contaminated by sewage, and for this reason, amebiasis is more often associated with poor sanitation. Particularly dangerous is the water of shallow wells or streams in badly drained areas where cysts often live for a month in ideal conditions of coolness and moisture. They resist sterilizing agents better than most bacteria but are unable to live at temperatures of 160° F or more, dying quickly once they are dried.

Food can be contaminated by flies or other insects which enter the home after they have fed on human waste matter outdoors or in poorly constructed privies. Leafy vegetables become carriers of the disease if they are harvested where human waste is used as fertilizer or when they are washed in polluted water. Careless practices of infected food handlers, some of whom may carry ameba without suffering from the disease, may also be responsible for spread of the parasite.

SYMPTOMS

Symptoms of the mild form of amebiasis are often similar to symptoms which occur in entirely different diseases. The person may be underweight and show a sallow skin. Headache, fatigue, flatulence, nausea, tenderness of the abdomen, and bowel irregularity may be reported. Although chronic amebiasis may result in intermittent symptoms which do not grow worse over a period of years, it may also develop into acute amebic dysentery or into an amebic abscess of the liver in a small percentage of cases.

Amebic dysentery varies greatly in severity. Usually, but not always, the beginning signs are abdominal pains and diarrhea with stools often streaked with small amounts of blood and mucus. Fever and chills are present in more acute cases. Relief may come as a result of spontaneous recovery, but this can be followed in turn by repeated attacks.

Amebic abscess of the liver may develop in individuals who have had no previous indications of infection in the bowel. The patient may develop a low grade fever, the abdomen may become tender over the area of the liver, and chills and sweats may occur. Distinct jaundice is rare. However, as in the case of the chronic and acute intestinal forms of the disease, no single symptom occurs so regularly that it proves the existence of amebiasis.

DIAGNOSIS

Examination of the stools under a microscope is the way in which a definitive diagnosis of amebiasis is made. Several specimens may need to be examined in chronic cases because the number of amebae present changes from day to day.

TREATMENT

Amebiasis can usually be treated with some success through the use of drugs chosen by a physician. Favorable reports have been received on the use of compounds of iodine and arsenic, quinolines, and some of the antibiotics. The drugs differ in their effectiveness depending on where the amebas are located in the body.

PREVENTION

Prevention of amebiasis is both a community and a personal matter. The community can prevent the disease by taking proper sanitary precautions with regard to food and water. Settling and sand filtration procedures in the water supply system of cities have almost always effectively eliminated the cysts. On the other hand, the common public health measure of water chlorination is inadequate protection against amebiasis because the cysts are able to withstand larger dosages of chlorine than those used in the chlorination procedure.

Persons living or visiting in areas where sanitary conditions are poor can take a few simple precautions. They can boil their drinking water or, if they prefer, add tablets available from drug stores which contain large enough amounts of chlorine or iodine to kill the cysts. In general, all foods should be thoroughly cooked, unless they are non-leafy vegetables or fruits, which can be safely eaten once they have been scraped and peeled. Raw, leafy vegetables should be avoided. Since flies and insects are known to be carriers of the disease, the use of proper screening in infected areas is still another important safety measure.

amebic dysentery — the severe form of amebiasis.
See amebiasis.

amenorrhea — the absence or the abnormal stopping of the menstrual periods. There are four main categories of amenorrhea:

1. Amenorrhea in young girls prior to the age of puberty.

2. Amenorrhea due to pregnancy.

3. Amenorrhea during and following menopause.

4. Amenorrhea which is a symptom of illness or disorder.

See menstruation.

amine — an organic compound that may be derived from ammonia by the replacement of one or more of the hydrogen atoms by hydrocarbon radicals.

amino acids — the chief chemical components of proteins.

During the process of digestion, food proteins are broken down into simple components called amino acids, which are reassembled into other proteins needed by the human body. The proteins in food are usually made up of eighteen or more amino acids. The body can make its own supply of more than half of these, but eight of them are called "essential" since body tissues cannot manufacture them and they must come ready-made from food.

Proteins differ in their essential amino acid content. Those proteins which contain a large amount of the essential amino acids are said to have a high nutritional value; those that are lacking in any of the essential amino acids or have insignificant amounts of one or more of these amino acids, have a low or poor nutritional value. In general, foods of animal origin such as eggs, meats, fish, poultry and milk contain proteins of better nutritional value than foods of plant origin. However, a diet containing both animal and plant proteins is nutritionally acceptable and economically more practical. By consuming a mixture of foods containing both animal and plant proteins at each meal, one is more likely to secure all the essential amino acids.

See nutrition, proteins.

aminophylline — synthesized white or slightly yellowish granules or powder used as a drug to relax spasms associated with asthma.

aminopyrine — a synthetic drug which relieves pain and reduces fevers and has been used in the treatment of rheumatic fever. However, it is used infrequently at present due to the possibility of dangerous side effects.

ammonia — a colorless gas which is soluble in water. Different compounds containing ammonia are used as diuretics, expectorants, and stimulants.

When inhaled, ammonia gas can be very irritating; and, if inhaled in high concentrations, it may be fatal.

See spirit of ammonia.

amnesia — loss of memory or inability to remember past events. Amnesia may be caused by a mental trauma so great that the brain doesn't want to remember, or it may be caused by a blow to the head. Diseases may also cause amnesia. When the cause is mental, a psychiatrist's help may be needed to ease the pain of remembering. Injury to the brain can cause an actual loss of memory which may never return.

There are two general types of amnesia, anterograde and retrograde. In anterograde, the patient cannot recall events following the injury or mental trauma. Retrograde amnesia is an inability to remember events before the injury or mental trauma.

amniotic fluid — the fluid in which the fetus lives until birth. It is clear at the beginning of pregnancy, but cloudy by the end of pregnancy. The fluid serves to protect the baby against shocks and bumps.

amoeba — *See ameba.*

amphetamines — drugs which stimulate the central nervous system. They induce a transient sense of well-being, self-confidence, and alertness. They are used to combat fatigue, curb appetite, and reduce mild depression. In general, they are classified as stimulants.

Amphetamines resemble the natural body hormones, epinephrine and norepinephrine. As a result of this similarity, these drugs can act directly, by mimicking the natural hormones, in their effect on nerve endings and/or indirectly by causing increased release of the natural hormone. Whichever the case, amphetamines stimulate certain areas of the nervous system which control blood pressure, heart, respiratory, and metabolic rates, all of which are increased. Appetite is markedly decreased and the senses are hyper-alert. The body is in a general state of stress, as if it were extremely threatened or expecting a violent fight. Amphetamines artificially intensify and prolong such stimulation, keeping the body in a state of tension for prolonged periods of time.

LEGITIMATE USES

Amphetamines were synthesized for medical purposes in the 1920's in a search for chemicals that would constrict blood vessels. They were first used to treat colds because they shrink the nasal membranes and give temporary relief to "stuffy" nasal passages. More effective drugs with fewer side effects are now used for this purpose. Amphetamines are now mainly prescribed for narcolepsy (overwhelming episodes of sleep during normal waking hours), depression, and to control appetite. Physicians also prescribe them to ward off fatigue during dangerous and prolonged tasks. Paradoxically, these drugs are sometimes used in the treatment of hyperactive children with certain behavioral disorders.

EXTENT OF USE

Amphetamines are available in all countries where Western medicine is practiced. In the United States, approximately one-fourth of all medical prescriptions for mood-altering drugs are for stimulants, mainly amphetamines.

Half of the legally manufactured supply of amphetamines is estimated to find its way into illegal channels for non-prescribed use. Amphetamines are also produced in black-market laboratories. Although the exact number of amphetamine abusers is not known, the use of enormous quantities of amphetamines has drastically increased. Quantities of amphetamines are also used without supervision for weight reduction, or to keep awake over prolonged periods.

ABUSE

Overuse of amphetamines may start in the physician's office, where doses are prescribed for depression, lethargy, or obesity, and subsequent supervision is inadequate. Most cases, however, originate in illicit channels where drugs are sold indiscriminately to such customers as truck drivers who want to stay awake during long hauls, or teenagers and young adults looking for "kicks."

Amphetamines were in widespread use long before their abuse potential was recognized. Limiting them to use only by prescription did not end their misuse. Today their abuse is a major medical and social problem.

Until recently there have been chiefly two types of abusers. One includes the sporadic user who occasionally takes the drug to exert himself beyond his physiological limits. He may want to stay awake, to drive, excel in an athletic contest, or cram for an examination. This type of abuse rarely leads to difficulties, but it may. Instances of death during athletic contests have been traced to amphetamine use.

A second type of abuse is taking moderate amounts to "keep going," to "feel high," or to counteract the depression that occurs when an attempt is made to stop the drug. "Spree" or "binge" abusers use the drug in social settings for "kicks." Heavy users of this type may use seventy-five to one hundred mg. per day (the average is fifteen to thirty mg.) for long periods. These individuals are likely to become drug dependent.

Since 1967, a new type of abuse has developed which involves repeated injections of massive doses intravenously. This type of amphetamine use produces practically the same effect as cocaine. Such users are called "speedfreaks" or "methheads."

In ordinary amounts the amphetamines provide a transient sense of alertness, wakefulness, well-being, and mental clarity. Hunger is diminished, and short-term performance may be enhanced in the fatigued person. The drugs may increase the heart rate, raise the blood pressure, produce palpitation (throbbing heart) and rapid breathing, dilate the pupils, and cause dry mouth, sweating, and headache.

But these drugs create a dependence upon them, as tolerance increases rapidly, requiring higher and higher doses to obtain the original effect. Usually, if the drug is stopped for a week or so, the body becomes sensitive to amphetamines as before. If use continues, however, a person can become psychologically dependent on the drug in a few weeks. The sense of power, self-confidence, and exhilaration artificially created by amphetamine use is so pleasant, and the fatique and depression that follow discontinuance are so severe, that the user is heavily tempted to revert to the drug.

When amphetamines are taken intravenously in large amounts, an ecstatic "high" occurs which ebbs in a few hours. To regain the high, reinjection is necessary. This cycle can go on for days until the user is physically exhausted. Shakiness, itching, and muscle pains are common. A person on amphetamines has a tendency to talk rapidly and volubly, and to pace around or perform other stereotyped acts. He appears oversensitive to stimuli and may be jumpy and anxious. A mood of apprehension or panic may develop.

Heavy amphetamine users and "speedfreaks" become physically debilitated and suffer from malnutrition. With no desire for food or sleep, they lose weight and become careless about personal hygiene. They become susceptible to infections, such as viral hepatitis, caused by a dirty needle. There is evidence of liver damage from high doses. Brain cell damage has also been reported.

Social and moral deterioration also occur with heavy users. They tend to become impulsive, irritable, unreliable, and unstable. Behavior may become assaultive and unpredictable. Of all drug abusers, "speedfreaks" most resemble the cocaine user, whose behavior was largely responsible for the term "dope fiend." "Speedfreaks" invariably become suspicious of those around them, and in extreme cases suffer from paranoid delusions of being threatened or the object of a plot. Schizophrenia-like disturbances resulting from prolonged, heavy use may last for several months after the drugs are discontinued. The depression into which heavy amphetamine abusers fall when they come down from their high ("crash") is extremely severe. Suicide during such moods is known. Lethargy, fatigue, muscle pains, ravenous hunger, and mental depression are the chief symptoms when the drugs

are discontinued. Some scientists regard these as stimulant withdrawal symptoms indicating a true physical dependence.

"Speed" can occasionally kill, from accidents resulting during paranoid delusions, homicidal rages, or through injections with contaminated substances. Death from overdose in the tolerant individual, however, is uncommon. Most frequently, the deterioration of personality, judgment, and health resulting from continued use of "speed" leaves the "speedfreak" in a limbo, neither physically dead nor physically alive.

Medical experts believe that heavy amphetamine abusers usually suffer from some form of psychic instability which existed before the drug was tried. Such persons use stimulants to help them deal with problems of living and their emotional inadequacies.

TREATMENT FOR ABUSE

Because compulsive drug abuse, particularly the intravenous injection of speed, is a comparatively recent phenomenon, few appropriate treatment and rehabilitation services exist. Most formal drug treatment programs in the U.S. are designed primarily for narcotic addicts. However, today informal drug treatment clinics are springing up in communities where the drug problem is particularly acute, and community mental health centers are beginning to develop services for the young drug abuser.

Treatment of the "speedfreak" is very difficult. Like heroin users, persons who have broken the habit often relapse. Both medical and psychiatric help may be needed. Because compulsive drug abuse is usually related to a breakdown in human relationships, a considerable amount of social and psychological support is required.

One of the more effective treatment approaches is group therapy, in which recovered ex-users interact with users. Those who have come through the speed scene are trusted, and their counsel is likely to be accepted by those who wish to stop the destructive use of drugs. Such groups provide a substitute for the drug-using groups to which these persons formerly related, and provide supportive help. Such groups also open up opportunities for self-exploration and learning to trust and relate to others, which is important in personality reconstruction.

ampicillin — a semisynthetic penicillin derivative. Because penicillin has several drawbacks, scientists have developed a new group of antibiotics with properties quite similar to penicillin, but without many of the drawbacks. Ampicillin is one of these.

See penicillin.

amputation — the surgical removal or loss through accident of a part or all of a limb.

The primary reasons for amputations are trauma, death of tissues due to inadequate circulation, malignant tumors, chronic infections of bone or tissue, heat or cold injuries, uselessness in a limb, and congenital deformities.

The application of principles of industrial and highway safety, vigorous and adequate treatment of infections, early diagnosis and treatment of degenerative diseases, such as diabetes, arteriosclerosis, and cancer, can reduce the incidence of amputations. It is essential for the patient with diabetes that careful pedicure be maintained, since this is often a source of infection, gangrene, and ultimate amputation.

After surgery, the patient's medical condition is stabilized and his other systemic conditions are brought under control. Patients who are suitable candidates for a prosthesis become involved in a program of physical conditioning, use of parallel bars, learning to walk on crutches, shaping and conditioning the stump, ordering the prosthesis, and the beginning of ambulation training.

REHABILITATION

Rehabilitation of the amputee begins immediately. Adjusting to a prosthesis and achieving maximum independence is the goal, but it can not always be attained. Each patient's rehabilitation program must be worked out individually because of the number of variables in his physical condition, his personality, and his environment.

After he learns the mechanics of walking, the patient must build up increasing tolerance for the prosthesis. In older persons, tolerance takes longer to achieve. When a reasonably good level of function is attained, training includes activities required to live independently. Each goal is determined individually, usually consisting of learning to walk up and down stairs, to travel alone, to board buses and trains or climb into a car, and to stand for long periods of time.

Complete rehabilitation programs have been worked out scientifically for all amputees, with a high degree of accuracy in predicting outcome. These range in classification from full restora-

tion to usual activities, to self-care independence. For others, use of cosmetic devices is a realistic goal. Some cases are appropriately classified as not amenable to a prosthesis.

It is estimated that one out of every 400 persons in the United States has a major amputation. Each year 35,000 amputations are performed. The ratio of amputation is three in the upper extremities for every ten in the lower extremities. Amputation of an upper extremity is more common among young people because of industrial or automobile accidents. The most common type of amputation is one leg, above the knee. More than seventy-five percent of amputations performed on the lower extremities are on people over sixty years of age, as a result of chronic degenerative disease.

amyl nitrite — a drug that has the primary purpose of relaxing smooth muscles. As such it is frequently used in the treatment of angina pectoris. Amyl nitrite is inhaled as a vapor.

See angina pectoris.

amylo — a prefix meaning starch.

amylopsin — an enzyme secreted from the pancreas. Amylopsin converts partially digested starches into simple sugars such as maltose.

anabolism — any body process that builds complex compounds from simple compounds.

anaerobic — a term applied to any living organism that cannot live in an oxygen atmosphere. This is the direct opposite of an aerobic organism which can only live in an oxygen atmosphere.

anal — *See anus.*

analeptic — any drug that stimulates the central nervous system.

analgesic — any agent, but usually a drug, that relieves pain without causing unconsciousness. Analgesics relieve minor aches and pains and act as antipyretics (fever reducers). Some also have anti-inflammatory properties.

How analgesics reduce pain is not completely understood — except that analgesics work on the central nervous system. The antipyretic effect is achieved by releasing sweat and increasing the flow of blood.

In the United States analgesics such as aspirin (acetylsalicylic acid) can be obtained without a doctor's prescription. They are among the most widely used drugs.

analogous — a term used to indicate a similarity in function but a difference in origin or development.

analysis — an examination of the different parts or elements that make up the whole.

anaphase stage — the stage in cell division (mitosis) during which the chromosomes are pulled or drawn toward the two poles. The anaphase stage follows the metaphase stage and precedes the telophase stage (the last step in cell division).
See mitosis.

anaplasia — a phenomenon of tumors (benign or malignant) in which the cells composing the tumor revert to simple, unspecific cells incapable of performing the highly developed, very specific functions associated with the tumor area.

anatomist — a specialist in anatomy.

anatomy — the study of the structure and organization of the human body, based on dissection.

The body is composed of solids (bones and tissues) and fluids (blood and secretions of various organs and membranes).

The human body is divided into three parts:

1. The head, made up of the skull (a bony case that encloses and protects the brain) and the face.

2. The trunk (the main part of the body) is divided into two parts by a muscular partition known as the diaphragm. The upper portion of the trunk is the chest, its cavity and organs. The lower portion is the abdomen, its cavity and organs.

3. The extremities. The upper extremity on each side consists of the shoulder joint, the arm, the forearm, the wrist, and the hand. The lower extremity on each side consists of the hip joint, the thigh, the leg, the ankle, and the foot.

There has been considerable interest in anatomy for thousands of years; however, studying human anatomy was very difficult until the sixteenth century. Prior to that time, dissection was usually forbidden by religion and custom. Until then, there was a tendency to accept the teachings of the past regardless of how that knowledge had been gained.

Andreas Vesalius (1514-1564), a Flemish physician, is considered by many to be the father of modern anatomy.

ancillary — anything that plays a secondary or supportive role.

Ancylostoma — a genus of hookworms causing ancylostomiasis (hookworm disease).
See hookworm disease.

ancylostomiasis — *See hookworm disease.*

Anderson and Goldberger's test — a test for typhus fever involving the injection of the patient's blood into a guinea pig.
See typhus fever.

androgen — any substance or hormone causing masculine characteristics.

androsterone — an important male sex hormone.
See hormone.

anemia — a condition of the blood resulting from a reduction either in the number of red blood cells or in the amount of hemoglobin. Hemoglobin is the red-colored substance in the red blood cells; it carries oxygen to the body tissues. If the amount of hemoglobin is below normal, or if there are too few red blood cells, not enough oxygen will get to the tissues.

CAUSES

1. Improper diet

The marrow of the bones manufactures the blood cells and puts the red coloring into them. Protein and iron, derived from certain foods, go into the making of hemoglobin. Many other dietary substances, including vitamins, minerals, and energy foods, are needed to build red cells. Because cells keep wearing out and must be replaced by new ones, the daily diet should always include all the necessary building materials. Normally it is possible to prevent the anemias that result from nutritional deficiency by eating a variety of nourishing foods.

Foods rich in iron include meat (especially liver), eggs, dried peas, and beans, nuts, dried fruits, green leafy vegetables, and whole-grain or enriched cereals and cereal products. An expectant mother needs additional iron to build extra blood cells for herself and the baby.

2. Faulty absorption of food
The intestines of certain persons do not readily absorb iron or certain necessary vitamins from food. Much of the iron passes through their bodies unused instead of being used to manufacture hemoglobin.

3. Loss of blood
Heavy bleeding from a wound may cause anemia. Anemia can also develop from continued unseen or unnoticed loss of blood, as from hemorrhoids (piles), immoderate flow at or between menstrual periods, tumor tissue or ulcerations of the stomach and intestines.

4. Injury to bone marrow
If healthy bones marrow is injured, it can no longer manufacture enough blood, and anemia results.

Used without proper safeguards, certain chemicals and X-rays in industry can damage the bone marrow of workers exposed to them.

The blood-building marrow can also be injured by certain drugs contained in some patent headache remedies and other commercial "pain killers." Tumor tissue in the body also can damage bone marrow.

5. Infections and parasites
Some diseases such as malaria or bacterial infections may affect the blood and cause anemia. A person whose intestines are infected with hookworms or tapeworms generally is anemic.

SYMPTOMS
Typical symptoms are fatigue, lack of pep, a washed-out feeling, and shortness of breath.

TREATMENT
The exact treatment for anemia depends upon the cause. For example, anemia caused by excessive blood loss may be partially treated by a blood transfusion, while anemia resulting from parasites usually necessitates removal of the parasites. The object of any and all treatment is to restore the correct level of red blood cells and the proper amount of hemoglobin.
See pernicious anemia.

anencephalia — an abnormality of the embryo in which the brain is absent or does not fully develop.

aneroid — devoid of liquid.

anesthesia — a loss of sensation that can be local or body-wide. Defects in the central nervous system can result in anesthesia, but as the term is generally used, it means an artificially induced inability to perceive pain (particularly during surgical procedures).

Narcotics, alcohol, and ether are different types of substances that produce a degree of anesthesia in the entire body. On the other hand, drugs such as novocaine produce anesthesia in a local area of the body.
See anesthetics.

anesthetics — the general term for a substance that artificially produces complete or partial lack of feeling. There are two types of anesthetics: local anesthetics and general anesthetics.

LOCAL ANESTHETICS
Local anesthetics include drugs such as novocaine which are injected into the area to be numbed. They can also be applied onto the surface of the skin. Local anesthetics are used frequently by dentists in performing minor surgery (such as pulling a tooth), and by dermatologists in removing moles. Local anesthetics have the advantage of removing pain without causing unconsciousness.

GENERAL ANESTHETICS
General anesthetics are used during major surgery. The history of the use of general anesthetics is quite interesting. For centuries, physicians used narcotics or alcohol to help relieve pain during operations and to keep the patient from screaming and jumping around on the operating table. These substances usually proved to be less than satisfactory, and the lack of a good general anesthetic forced surgeons to operate as quickly as possible. The speed with which operations were accomplished killed many patients whose insides had not been carefully stitched. The shock of unanesthetized surgery killed many others.

The first major breakthrough came in 1776, although it wasn't recognized as a breakthrough at the time. In 1776, nitrous oxide, the first inhaled anesthetic, was discovered by Priestley. Nitrous oxide is more commonly known as laughing gas.

During the 1840's, the real work on anesthetics began. Ether, which had been discovered before 1795, was first demonstrated on a human in 1846; chloroform, discovered in 1831, was first used on a human in 1847.

The first public demonstration of the use of ether as a general anesthesia was made by Morton at the Massachusetts General Hospital in Boston. Under the watchful eyes of a group of very skeptical doctors, Morton succeeded in anesthetizing the patient. The observers were properly amazed but could not deny what their eyes had recorded.

aneurysm — a spindle-shaped or sac-like bulging of the wall of a vein or artery, due to weakening of the wall by disease or an abnormality at birth.

When there is a danger of the aneurysm bursting, surgery must be performed. If the aneurysm occurs in the aorta, it can be especially dangerous.

Surgery on an aneurysm generally involves the removal of the aneurysm and the damaged areas around it. The length of artery or vein that is removed is replaced by a section of vein from another part of the patient's body or by a synthetic section of tube.

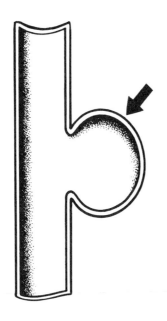

ANEURYSM

angina — a choking, suffocating sense of pain. *See angina pectoris.*

angina pectoris — literally, a chest pain. A condition in which the heart muscle receives an insuf-

ficient blood supply, causing pain in the chest and often in the left arm and shoulder. It commonly results when the arteries supplying the heart muscle are narrowed by atherosclerosis. Angina pectoris affects five times more men than women.

The heart has great strength and works twenty-four hours a day. Even when fatty deposits have narrowed one or more of the coronary arteries, the blood supply reaching the heart muscle may still be adequate to fill the need for food and oxygen which this steady work load imposes.

These same arteries, however, may not be capable of furnishing the extra blood the heart demands when a person exerts himself more than usual, such as in dashing to catch a bus, or when he becomes overexcited by some especially good or bad news.

At such times "angina," as angina pectoris is often called, may be felt in the chest. This severe pain, often accompanied by a sense of pressure or suffocation under the breastbone, normally subsides within a few (three to five) minutes after the added exertion is over. It sometimes extends into the left shoulder, arm, and hand.

Angina pectoris is not a disease itself, but a symptom of a disease. Chest pains may be the result of many conditions other than an insufficient flow of blood to the heart muscle.

The symptoms appear with exertion, emotion, exposure to cold, or overeating, and can be relieved by rest or nitroglycerine. To prevent attacks, treatment consists of counseling the patient to limit exertion and to avoid strenuous activity. Medications to dilate the coronary arteries and emotional tranquilizers are used. Dieting for overweight is important. In specialized cases, surgical procedures are used.

The patient with angina must determine the level of activity he can maintain without precipitating an attack and must learn to live within these limits. He must also learn to live with the ever-present possibility of an attack. The fear and apprehension regarding the next attack may pose some difficulties for the patient. He must strike a reasonable compromise between the one extreme of giving up all activity and the other extreme of refusing to place any limits on the amount of exertion he can safely undertake.

angiocardiography — a method of examining the heart and great blood vessels. This is done by

X-raying the area to follow the course of an opaque fluid which has been injected into the blood stream.

angiocarditis — an inflammation of the heart and/or great blood vessels.

angiogram — an examination of a blood vessel by means of X-rays.

angioma — any tumor that is made up of blood vessels or lymph vessels.

angiotensin — a substance found in the blood. Angiotensin is a blood vessel constrictor.

aniline — a poisonous substance which is the base for both phenacetin and acetanilid, two drugs used as analgesics and antipyretics.

animal bites — any break of the skin caused by the bite of an animal. Any animal may suffer from rabies. When a rabid animal bites, the saliva enters the wound and the disease is transmitted to the person who has been bitten. A person who has been bitten by an animal should always suspect the animal to be rabid until proved otherwise.
See rabies, insect bites, snake bites.

ankle — the joint of the leg and foot. The ankle permits movement of the foot up and down. When the ankle turns to the side (as may happen when a person trips), it is said to be strained.

Because of the amount of use the ankle is subjected to, it is frequently strained, sprained, and occasionally broken.

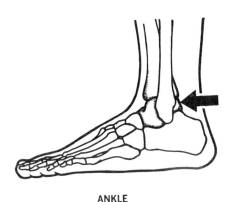

ANKLE

ankylosing spondylitis — immobility of the vertebrae similar to rheumatoid arthritis.

ankylosis — loss of mobility in a joint. This can be caused by several factors. A joint that has been in a cast for too long may develop this problem.

anodmia — absence of the sense of smell.

Anopheles — a genus of mosquitoes that transmits malaria to humans.

anopsia — *See amblyopia ex anopsia.*

anorexia — the lack or loss of appetite for food. Anorexia can be caused by a nervous condition. It is more of a symptom than a disease. People with high fevers often exhibit anorexia. Certain drugs will also induce it. Among those are drugs prescribed as diet aids for people who are overweight.

anoxia — literally, no oxygen. This condition most frequently occurs when the blood supply to a part of the body is completely cut off. This results in the death of the affected tissue. For example, a specific area of the heart muscle may die when the blood supply (and hence the oxygen supply) has been blocked, as by a clot in the artery supplying that area.

However, anoxia may also occur when the entire body is lacking in oxygen as a result of breathing air with a low percentage of oxygen.
See asphyxia.

antacid — a substance that restores the acid-base chemical balance in the body by correcting acidity. In the United States, antacids are usually available without prescription. They are most frequently used to relieve discomfort in the stomach caused by excess acid.

antepartum — an event, disease, etc., happening or occurring before childbirth.

anterograde amnesia — *See amnesia.*

anthracosis — a type of pneumoconiosis caused by inhaling particles of coal dust into the lungs.
See pneumoconiosis.

anthrax — a disease of cattle; it can attack man. Anthrax is infectious, and it used to cause epidemic disease and death in cattle. In the United States it has almost entirely disappeared. In the infrequent occurrences of anthrax in this country, the source can usually be identified as being imported.

In man, anthrax appears as a carbuncle and occasionally as an infection of the lungs. Antibiotics are used to treat both types, but pulmonary anthrax (also called woolsorter's disease) can be extremely serious.

antibiotic — a substance that is antibacterial. Antibiotics started with living organisms; however, several have now been synthesized.

The discovery of antibiotics ranks as a landmark in the field of medicine. The number of people who owe their lives to antibiotics is incalculable. Similarly, the number of people who died prior to the discovery and use of antibiotics is staggering.

Antibiotics are either bacteriostatic or bactericidal. That is, they inhibit growth of bacteria (bacteriostats) or they destroy them (bactericides). In either case, they work with the body's own defense system to cure the illness.

The first group of antibiotics to be used was the sulfonamide group. This was the antibiotic used during World War II. The sulfonamides are generally bacteriostatic.

Although Fleming discovered penicillin in 1928, it was not until the 1940's that it was tried and tested. The pencillin group (which is bactericide in action) is one of the most potent groups in the antibiotic family.

Despite the remarkable effectiveness of antibiotics against a wide range of diseases caused by bacteria, antibiotics do have drawbacks. Some people are hypersensitive, or allergic, to antibiotics. Penicillin is the one antibiotic to which people seem to react most frequently.

The use of antibiotics may also lead to superinfections. These are infections caused by bacteria that normally live in the body without causing illness. The action of an antibiotic may upset the natural bacterial balance within the body, causing usually harmless bacteria to multiply into infections.

One of the problems that has arisen following the widespread use of antibiotics is the appearance of strains of bacteria that are resistant to antibiotics that once destroyed them. This problem is being overcome by using different antibiotics and by restricting the use of antibiotics to cases in which they are known to be effective.
See penicillin.

antibodies — substances developed in the plasma of the blood when a foreign material enters the blood stream. When the body is invaded by disease-producing organisms, two protective mechanisms are activated. One is the action of white cells, and the other is the development of antibodies. These antibodies begin at once to protect the body from the invading organism. They accomplish this by dissolving them or causing them to clump so that they cannot circulate freely through the blood stream. Sometimes antibodies simply inactivate the organisms so that the white cells can destroy them. Antibodies develop against each type of disease-causing invader to which the body is exposed. They may remain in the blood stream for a long time after the body has recovered, and, as long as they remain, the body is immune to that specific disease.
See antigen, Rh factor, immunity.

anticarcinogen — an environmental agent offering some protection against a carcinogen which is similar in chemical construction.

anticoagulant — a drug that delays or prevents clotting of the blood. When given in cases of a blood vessel plugged up by a clot, it tends to prevent new clots from forming and prevents the existing clots from enlarging, but it does not dissolve an existing clot. Examples are heparin and coumarin derivatives.
See clotting, coagulation.

antidote — a substance that neutralizes or counteracts a poison. Each type of poison has a different antidote.
See universal antidote, poison.

antiemetic — a general term for a drug or substance used to stop or prevent nausea and/or vomiting.

antigen — any foreign matter that causes antibodies to develop. In an allergic attack, the antigen is the substance against which the body is reacting.
See antibodies, allergy.

antihemorragic — a general term for any drug or substance that helps slow, stop, or prevent hemorrhaging. This type of agent is particularly important in treating people with hemophilia.
See clotting, hemorrhage, hemophilia.

antihistamine — any drug or agent that counteracts or prevents the effects of histamine. Antihistamines have two major uses. The first is in the treatment of allergies and allergic reactions; the second is the prevention of motion sickness.

One of the side effects of antihistamines is drowsiness; at the same time, the patient may experience difficulty in falling asleep.

See histamine.

antihypertensive agents — drugs that are used to lower blood pressure, such as reserpine, hydralazine, and many others.

See blood pressure.

antimetabolite — a substance closely similar to an essential cell-building material. An antimetabolite will tend to replace the essential material.

antipyretic — any drug or agent that helps reduce fevers. Most antipyretics have no effect on the body temperature when it is normal.

antiseptic — a fluid containing chemicals that kill germs. Antiseptics are used on the skin only. They are similar to disinfectants in that both kill germs, but disinfectants are too strong to apply to the human body.

The discovery of the importance of antiseptics and antiseptic (or clean) conditions in relation to surgery has greatly reduced the number of patients who become infected during and after surgery.

antiserum — a serum that contains antibodies. It is obtained by withdrawing blood from an animal that has manufactured the antibodies as a result of exposure to antigens.

antitoxin — an antibody to a specific toxin (or poison) released by bacteria within the body. The body will form these, but they can also be obtained from an animal and injected into the patient.

antitussive — any drug or agent which relieves or prevents coughing.

antivenom — a general term for any antitoxin administered to neutralize or counteract snake venom. There is a specific antivenom for all common poisonous snakes.

See snake bite.

antivivisectionist — a person opposed to surgical experimentation (for research purposes) that is performed on animals.

Anton's symptom — the failure or inability of a person who is blind to recognize or accept the fact of his blindness. Named for Gabriel Anton, a German psychiatrist.

antrostomy — a surgical procedure that opens an antrum and allows it to drain.

antrum — a natural cavity within the body, usually a cavity in a bone. The maxillary antrum is a pair of sinuses located in the cheekbone on either side.

See sinus.

antuitary — a term referring to the anterior lobe of the pituitary gland.

anuresis — failure of the bladder to empty, leaving urine in it.

anus — the external opening of the rectum. Solid wastes are held there by a powerful muscle (shaped like a ring) which can be voluntarily opened or shut. When a colostomy is performed, an artificial anus is made.

See colostomy, hemorrhoids.

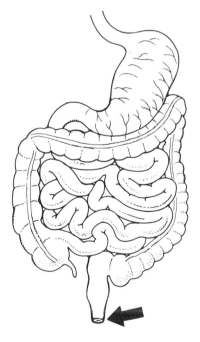

ANUS

anvil — the small bone located in the middle ear. It is situated between the stirrup and the hammer. Also called the incus.

See ear.

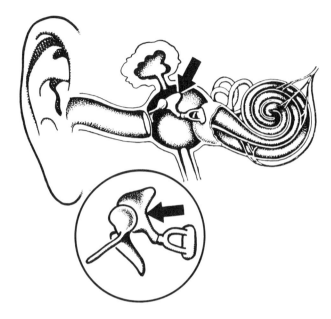

ANVIL

anxiety — a psychological term indicating uneasiness, apprehension, and similar emotions and feelings. Anxiety is a result of fear, but usually the person is bothered by what might happen, or a reoccurrence of something unpleasant, rather than a fear of danger.

Everyone experiences some anxiety. The difference between normal anxiety and anxiety indicating some form of mental illness has to do with the cause of the anxiety, the degree of anxiety, and the way in which the anxiety is handled.

Many people will feel anxiety when confronted with situations that have been unpleasant in the past. For example, a child who has had a tooth pulled may have some anxiety when told that he is going to see the dentist again. On the other hand, an adult in that same situation will experience much less anxiety.

A person may experience anxiety about something which has never happened (such as the death of a loved one) and which may never happen (such as the loss of a job). It is also possible to have anxiety and yet to be unaware of the reason or cause.

When a person is suffering from anxiety, his thinking is usually in terms of "what if," as opposed to "that or it is going to happen unless I," which characterizes fear from explicit present danger. Anxiety is a reaction to a possibility; fear is a reaction to a clear and present danger.

The reaction of the body to anxiety is similar to its reaction to fear: there is an increase in blood pressure and a surge of epinephrine.

A certain amount of anxiety helps keep a person "on his toes" and allows him to function at his best. An excess of anxiety has just the opposite result. The person becomes so involved with his anxieties that he is not capable of constructive thought or action, and his awareness of this leads him to further anxieties.

aorta — the largest artery in the body. It carries the full load of blood away from the heart to begin its distribution to many lesser arteries, which then conduct the blood to all parts of the body except the lungs.

The aorta receives blood from the lower left chamber of the heart. It originates from the base of the heart, arches up over the heart like a cane handle, and passes down through the chest and abdomen in front of the spine.

Any damage to the aorta can have grave consequences, because all blood must pass through it on the way to other parts of the body. For example, an aneurysm occurring in the aorta can be compared with a blowout in an automobile tire. Just as the blowout allows all of the air to escape, an aneurysm in the aorta can allow large quantities of blood to escape the circulatory system.

See heart.

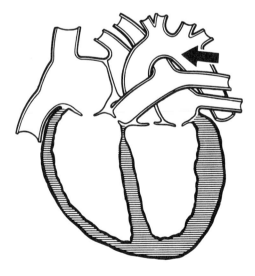

AORTA

aortic arch — a part of the aorta or large artery leaving the heart; it curves up like the handle of a cane over the top of the heart.

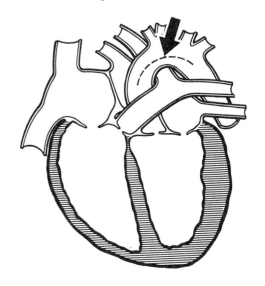

AORTIC ARCH

aortic insufficiency — a condition in which there is an improper closing of the valve between the aorta and the lower left chamber of the heart. This allows a backflow of blood.

aortic stenosis — a narrowing of the valve opening between the lower left chamber of the heart and the large artery called the aorta. The narrowing may occur at the valve itself or slightly above or below the valve. Aortic stenosis may be the result of scar tissue forming after a rheumatic fever infection, or it may have other causes.

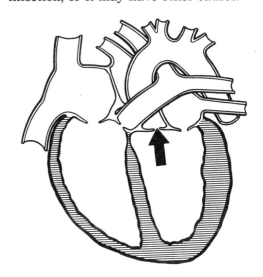

AORTIC VALVE

aortic valve — the valve at the junction of the aorta, or large artery, and the lower left chamber of the heart. Formed by three cup-shaped membranes called semilunar valves, it allows the blood to flow from the heart into the artery and prevents a backflow.

When the aortic valve does not close properly, and there is a backflow of blood, the condition is called aortic insufficiency.

aortography — an examination by X-ray of the aorta and its main branches. This is made possible by the injection of a dye which is opaque to X-rays.

apex — a term used to indicate the top or uppermost part of a body organ.

The blunt, rounded end of the heart, directed downward, forward, and to the left is also referred to as the apex.

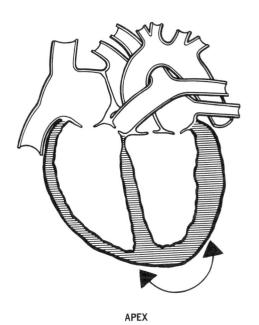

APEX

aphthous stomatitis — a disease that causes recurring outbreaks of blister-like sores inside the mouth and on the lips. The sores are called canker sores.

Like herpes simplex, aphthous stomatitis is a common infection. It has been estimated that anywhere from twenty to over fifty percent of the population suffer from canker sores. Women seem to be more susceptible than men.

The disease usually begins to show itself in both men and women when they are in their twenties. The incidence among women is highest between the ages of twenty and eighty, while men experience the disease most frequently in the forties, and seldom after seventy.

There is some evidence that canker sores "run" in families. Thus, a youngster developing these sores may very likely have brothers or sisters, or one or both parents, suffering from the same illness.

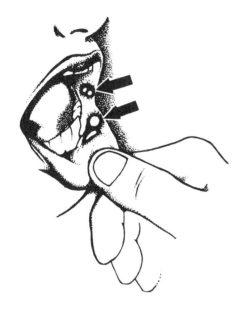

APHTHOUS STOMATITIS

SYMPTOMS

These sores appear on the lining of the cheeks, the edge of the tongue, floor of the mouth, and the palate. The sores on the lip develop only on the red part, in contrast to the sore of herpes simplex, which always erupts near the lip, on the adjoining skin. Pain and a burning sensation accompany the development of the canker sores. Occasionally other parts of the body may be affected, such as the conjunctiva, genital, or anal membranes. Some arthritic pain also may be felt in severe cases.

In the early stages of the disease, a small blister forms, but it often goes unnoticed. Symptoms do not occur until the blister breaks and the typical sore or canker forms. This is a small oval, light yellow or yellow in color, surrounded by a red margin.

The number of recurrences of canker sores and the severity of each attack varies from person to person. Some may have only an occasional single canker. At the other extreme, the victim may

literally have a mouthful of painful sores which rarely have time to heal before the next crop appears.

The patient is often debilitated by the disease, for eating and drinking are quite difficult. The repeated outbreaks also have a demoralizing effect on the patient with a severe case.

CAUSES

Science has not yet determined the exact causes of aphthous stomatitis. It was once thought that eating chocolate or some varieties of fruit caused the canker sores to develop. More recently the herpes simplex virus was named the culprit. However, repeated attempts in the laboratory to induce canker sores using the herpes virus have been unsuccessful, thus ruling out this theory.

Recent investigations have shown an L-form of streptococcus in the sores and blood stream of aphthous patients. This bacterial lead may give scientists a clue to the cause and the mechanism of recurrence of the disease.

Whatever the cause may be, canker sores tend to appear when the patient has experienced some physical or emotional stress. Indeed, one of the earliest medical reports of this type of infection, in 1889, involved three women who were all having financial difficulties. A modern-day study of a group of university students revealed that canker sores were more likely to develop during examination period than during vacation.

A slight injury while brushing the teeth, eating harsh foods, and possibly some allergies are also factors that tend to produce canker sores. The endocrine system may be involved in some way, since women patients have reported appearance of sores in relation to menstruation. Other women have experienced complete absence of cankers during pregancy.

TREATMENT

The aphthous sores tend to heal spontaneously in about ten to fourteen days. Various agents, such as cortisone, vitamin C in high dosages, antimicrobial drugs, gamma globulin, iodines, gentian violet, and various mouthwashes have been used with limited success to reduce the duration of the canker sores. No effective treatment is yet available.

aphthous ulcers — general name for canker sores.

apnea — a momentary loss of the impulse to breathe. It often follows forced breathing.

apomorphine — an opium derivative that causes nausea and vomiting very rapidly after it has been injected.

The primary use for apomorphine is to induce vomiting when the patient has swallowed a poisonous substance.

It has also been used to help alcoholics and drug abusers. The person involved in the treatment is given a shot of apomorphine and is then given an alcoholic drink (or, in the case of a drug abuser, the drug he usually takes). The person will begin to feel nauseous almost immediately and will then begin to vomit. After this procedure has been employed a number of times, the patient begins to associate the alcohol (or drug) with nausea and vomiting. This technique is called conditioned aversion.

apoplexy — frequently called an apoplectic stroke or simply a stroke.
See stroke.

appendectomy — a surgical operation to remove the appendix.

appendicitis — an inflammation of the appendix. Doctors usually recommend the removal of the appendix during attacks of appendicitis. An inflamed and infected appendix that is not removed may rupture, spilling pus into the rest of the body. Since there is no way of predicting when an appendix will rupture, an attack of appendicitis usually means that an emergency operation should be performed without delay. Operations performed for this reason account for a large percentage of emergency operations.

Symptoms of an attack of appendicitis include abdominal pain, elevated temperature, and

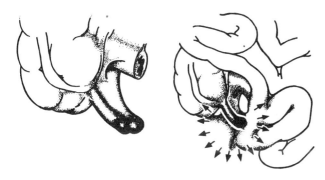

APPENDICITIS

frequently a fast or increased pulse. Patients suffering these symptoms should not use a heating pad or take any kind of laxative.

appendix — a three- to six-inch-long slender tube attached to the intestines. In man, no detectable function has been found for the appendix. It is assumed that it once served a purpose but that during the course of man's evolution, the function was no longer needed or that the function was assumed by some other body organ. Despite its lack of functional importance, the appendix can cause serious problems when it becomes inflamed or infected (appendicitis), and in these cases it must often be removed (appendectomy).
See appendicitis, appendectomy.

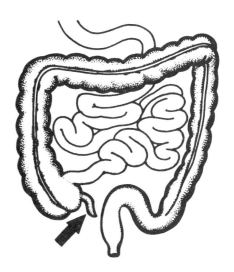

APPENDIX

appestat — a part of the hypothalamus which regulates hunger.

appetite — a natural craving. Appetite is usually a desire for food. Everyone has a different appetite. Some people like only certain foods; others like any and all food. Some people have large appetites; others have small appetites.

The size of a person's appetite depends on his metabolism, the amount of physical exercise he gets, and his general health.

apprehension — a psychological term indicating a feeling of uneasiness about future events.

apsithyria — a nonphysical condition in which the

patient is unable to speak. Apsithyria is caused by hysteria.

arachnidism — poisoning by a spider bite.
   See insect bites.

arachnoid — a very thin membrane of the brain. One of the layers of the meninges.
   See meninges.

arbor urinae — a burning sensation experienced during urination.

areola — the dark, circular area surrounding the nipple of the breast.

arhigosis — an inability to feel cold.

arm — the area of the body from the shoulder to the hand. It can also mean the area from the shoulder to the elbow, with the area from the elbow to the hand referred to as the forearm.

   The arm is composed of three large bones: the humerus, the ulna, and the radius. The humerus extends from the shoulder to the elbow, where it meets the ulna and the radius. The ulna and radius extend from the elbow to the wrist.

aromatic ammonia spirit — *See spirits of ammonia.*

armpit — the area under the arm where it joins the shoulder. The armpit is a small, hollow area. Its proper name is axilla.

aroma — an odor or scent.

arrest — to stop, as in cardiac arrest, a condition in which the action of the heart stops.

arrhythmia — an abnormal rhythm of the heartbeat.
   See heart.

arsenic — a poisonous nonmetal with many properties similar to the heavy metals.

   Arsenic has been used for centuries. It has always been known to be poisonous, but at times it has been used in small doses as a medicine and even as a tonic.

   Arsenic can be lethal in large doses, and repeated small doses can have the same effect. Chronic arsenic poisoning can result from repeated skin contact with arsenic.

   Arsenic attacks the intestinal tract, the blood, the skin, the central nervous system, etc.

arterial — of or pertaining to one or more arteries.

arterial blood — oxygenated blood. The blood is oxygenated in the lungs, then passes from the lungs to the left side of the heart via the pulmonary veins. It is then pumped by the left side of the heart into the arteries, which carry it to all parts of the body.

   Arterial blood is bright red in color.
   See venous blood.

arteries — *See artery.*

arterioles — the smallest arterial vessels (about 0.2 mm. or 1/125 inch in diameter), resulting from repeated branching of the arteries. They conduct the blood from the arteries to the capillaries.

arteriosclerosis — a generic term that includes a variety of conditions that cause the artery walls to become thick and hard and to lose their elasticity. Arteriosclerosis is frequently called hardening of the arteries.

   The most common form of arteriosclerosis is atherosclerosis, which is caused by deposits of a fatty substance.

   Hardening of the arteries is a major health problem in the United States today. It has been on the increase in recent decades. This may be simply because more people live longer and thus have more chance of developing hardened arteries. But more and more scientific evidence indicates that many other complex and interwoven factors may be involved, too. Our modern way of life may be responsible for some of the suspected factors, such as a high-calorie diet with an abundance of fats, too little exercise, and heavy cigarette smoking.

   Hardening of the arteries strikes young people as well as old. A few years ago this disease was generally considered to be associated only with old age, but today it is known to affect seriously the health of many people who are much younger, especially men. To be sure, hardening of the arteries is still by far most common in middle and old age. But it is also the underlying reason for the growing number of heart attacks suffered today by men in their thirties, or even younger.

   Hardening of the arteries may actually begin in early youth, perhaps even at birth. How troublesome it eventually becomes varies with each individual who has it. Some escape any consequence of the condition whatsoever. Others develop some symptoms, but with proper medical care they continue normal and productive lives. Many people, however, suffer death or disability as a result of hardening of the arteries.

The exact way an artery "hardens" is one of the major unsolved problems of medical science and the subject of hundreds of research studies. For some reason still not clearly understood, fat-like substances build up on the inside walls of the arteries. They gradually accumulate and form thick deposits called plaques. These deposits both roughen the artery's normally smooth inner lining and narrow the channel for blood flow, making it more difficult for enough blood to get through. Making matters worse, the artery also loses elasticity with age and loses its flexibility.

Every artery throughout the body is subject to hardening, but the most often and most seriously affected vessels are the largest arteries, such as the aorta, the coronary arteries, and the arteries that feed the brain and kidneys. Arteries may harden in one part of the body more rapidly then in other areas.

It is believed that some, but probably not all, of the fatty substances that build up on the artery wall come from the blood fats. People with high concentrations of fat in their blood develop hardening of the arteries earlier and are more likely to suffer serious consequences in later years.

Just what starts the process of hardening of the arteries is not known.

More than half of all deaths from various kinds of heart disease are the consequence of hardening of the arteries. It is the culprit behind several of the most familiar afflictions of the cardiovascular system. For instance, hardening of the arteries sets the stage for many strokes by clogging arteries that carry blood to the brain. The damaged artery or arteries may be located either inside the brain itself or in the neck.

When kidney arteries harden, one type of hypertension, or high blood pressure, may develop. In turn, hypertension may aggravate hardening of the arteries in other parts of the body. Although hypertension and hardening of the arteries often go hand in hand, each intensifying the other, they are separate diseases.

Hardening of the leg arteries may cause off-and-on weakness and pain in the legs when taking a walk. These symptoms grow worse until walking is no longer possible, but they disappear after a period of rest.

Another site of hardening, and by far the most frequent trouble spot, is the coronary arteries, the network of vessels that bring the heart muscle its own blood supply. Gradual reduction in blood flow in a coronary artery because of hardening may cause heart pain, known as angina pectoris. When more drastic or sudden restriction in the flow of food- and oxygen-laden blood occurs anywhere in the coronary artery network, starving a part of the heart muscle, a heart attack may result. This is often precipitated by the formation of a clot at an area affected by hardening.

Nature has her own remarkable way of averting disaster even through the coronary arteries have started to harden. It is called collateral circulation. Neighboring arteries carry more blood than formerly to compensate for a narrowed vessel, and new arterial branches open up to help transport blood to where it is needed. This partly explains why many people even with severe hardening of the coronary arteries do not suffer heart attacks and why some do not even experience the pains of angina pectoris.

CAUSES

Many things influence the development of hardening of the arteries. Unlike some illnesses, this one is not the result of a single identifiable cause. What all the factors are, how important each individual factor is, and how each contributes over a long period of time to hardened arteries (and the troubles that result, such as heart attack and stroke) are issues that still require broad study.

However, there are some factors that scientists today believe may be involved to a greater or lesser extent.

1. Age

The bulk of heart attacks from hardening of the arteries occurs in the middle and later years of life. Nothing can be done to keep anyone from growing older, of course. But scientists are urgently seeking knowledge that will enable them to reduce the high number of heart attacks suffered by middle-aged men and to halt the trend toward big heart attack tolls in younger age groups as well.

2. Sex

Women, apparently just because they are

women, have an advantage over men in respect to the risks of getting hardening of the arteries and having heart attacks. Symptoms of hardening of the arteries show up in women ten to twenty years later than in men, and women generally have a less serious form of trouble.

Medical research has attributed the years of extra protection enjoyed by women at least in part to the female sex hormones, called estrogens. As their estrogen production diminishes during menopause, women begin to have more heart attacks, although these attacks continue to be milder than those striking husbands or brothers. Scientists have given the estrogens to men to test this as a potential means of shielding men from so many heart attacks, but undesirable side effects result.

3. Heredity

Another factor over which a person or his physician has no control, besides age and sex, is heredity. If a person's family history includes a record of frequent heart trouble, however, he can and should give extra attention to other factors about which something can possibly be done.

4. Cholesterol

There is scientific evidence that the more cholesterol, a fatty substance, a person has in his blood, the greater are his chances of hardening of the arteries causing a heart attack or some other cardiovascular affliction. Indeed, to date it seems that the primary factor in causing hardened arteries may be a failure in the body's metabolism of fatty materials, that is, the way the body regulates the blood concentration of cholesterol and related substances.

Whether or not cholesterol (which is found in most animal fats we eat, as well as manufactured within the body itself) is the guilty party, or even the most guilty, has still not been proven. Persons with normal amounts of cholesterol in their blood sometimes develop hardening of the arteries. Some other factor or condition, as yet unrecognized as the real culprit, may therefore be responsible both for the large amounts of cholesterol in the blood and for the sequence of events that hardens arteries and leads to heart attacks. High blood concentrations of other fats, the neutral fats or triglycerides, also seem to entail greater risks from hardening of the arteries.

5. Diet

In general, diets high in fat content, especially animal and dairy fats, tend to raise the level of cholesterol in the blood. Many doctors and scientists feel that dietary changes that reduce the total intake of fat and substitute polyunsaturated fats for animal and dairy fats can have a beneficial effect.

6. High blood pressure

Hypertension, or high blood pressure, accelerates hardening of the arteries, and vice versa. The higher an individual's blood pressure goes, and the longer it remains elevated, the greater is his risk of suffering a heart attack. Most cases of high blood pressure, even severe cases, can be effectively treated today with modern drugs.

7. Cigarette smoking

A man who smokes cigarettes is twice as likely to have a heart attack as is a nonsmoker. Although so far there is no proof of how smoking is related to heart attacks, or to the hardened arteries that underlie the attack, it is known that the person who stops smoking cigarettes greatly reduces his heart attack risk. This is true no matter how long he has been smoking. On the other hand, the more cigarettes a person smokes, the greater are his chances of suffering a heart attack.

8. Other factors

A host of additional factors may also be involved in causing hardening of the arteries and other heart disease. Four of these possible factors are discussed briefly below.

Obesity often contributes to high blood pressure and may or may not make a significant contribution by itself to the development of heart troubles, including hardening of the arteries.

Stress and strain, especially of an emotional nature or for prolonged periods of time, may play a part in some heart attacks. Many medical men think, however, that the role of such pressures probably becomes important only after already hardened arteries have created the setting for an attack.

Physical activity and hard work are not the same thing as stress. Vigorous work and play on a regular basis are recognized as good for most people and are a part of any lifelong formula for the best heart health.

Environmental conditions such as air pollution, climate, and altitude are also under some suspicion. They are undergoing scientific scrutiny to determine the effect of these and other facets of our living habitat on the development of heart disease and other illnesses.

See angina pectoris, atherosclerosis, heart attack.

arteritis — an inflammation of one or more arteries.

artery — any of the blood vessels that carry blood away from the heart to the various parts of the body. They usually carry oxygenated blood, except for the pulmonary artery, which carries unoxygenated blood from the heart to the lungs for oxygenation.

The main artery is the aorta. The aorta receives blood directly from the heart and passes the blood along to many lesser arteries. The smaller arteries pass the blood on to the arterioles, which in turn pass the blood on to the capillaries.

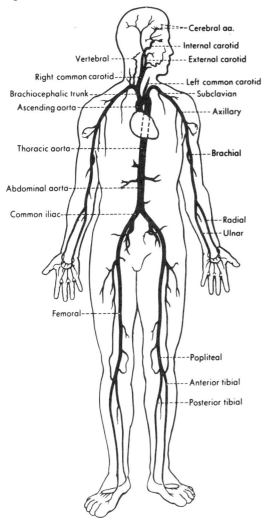

Labels on the figure:
- Cerebral aa.
- Internal carotid
- Vertebral
- External carotid
- Right common carotid
- Left common carotid
- Brachiocephalic trunk
- Subclavian
- Ascending aorta
- Axillary
- Thoracic aorta
- Brachial
- Abdominal aorta
- Common iliac
- Radial
- Ulnar
- Femoral
- Popliteal
- Anterior tibial
- Posterior tibial

ARTERIES

Blood moves through the arteries in spurts corresponding to the contractions of the heart muscle, which is forcing blood throughout the body.

When a large artery is cut, the wound will literally spurt blood. Because the bleeding is very rapid, death may result almost immediately. For example, rupture of the main arteries of the chest and abdomen may cause fatal hemorrhage in less than half a minute.

A spurting stream of blood will not clot. For that reason, any arterial bleeding is extremely dangerous. To promote formation of a clot in arterial bleeding, the flow of blood must be slowed to a comparative stop. In the case of limb arteries, a tourniquet is used. It should always be placed above the wound, thus restricting the flow of arterial blood to the wound. In an emergency, extreme pressure should be applied to the wound immediately. A fist covered with any clean cloth can be used for this purpose until a tourniquet can be applied.

athral — of or pertaining to a joint.

arthritic — a person suffering from arthritis or gout.

arthritis — an inflammation of the joints, and a disease that damages the ligaments and covering of the joints.

Arthritis, the commonest rheumatic disease, is man's oldest known chronic illness. The bones of the Java Ape Man and the mummies of Egypt show signs of arthritic damage. The ancient Greeks and Romans often were victims. Throughout the ages this disease has tormented mankind.

Rheumatic disease is called arthritis when it attacks the joints. Other types, such as those that involve the muscular tendons, ligaments, bursae, etc., are grouped under the term rheumatism. The effects of rheumatic disease may vary from a slight pain, stiffness, or swelling, to crippling and total disability.

Arthritis is the nation's number one crippler. About 13 million Americans suffer from its effects. About 3,300,000 Americans are limited in their activities in some way due to arthritis, with 700,000 in this group unable to work, keep house, or carry on a major activity.

The socioeconomic cost of this disease is beyond measure. Annually, it accounts for 186 million days of restricted activity and 12 million days lost from work. It affects more people than any other chronic ailment; it costs the nation over a billion dollars a year in medical expenses, relief, and lost wages.

Rheumatoid arthritis affects three times as many women as men, sometimes runs in families, and usually starts between the ages of twenty-five and fifty.

The disease causes inflammation and thickening of the lining of the joints. This lining may grow into the joint space and fill it. Meanwhile, the cartilage that covers the ends of the bones may become eroded; often small bony spurs form. Finally, the bones may grow together, and the joint becomes permanently fused.

SYMPTOMS

Often the first signs of rheumatoid arthritis are fatigue, muscular stiffness, and a loss of appetite and weight. Painful swelling then begins at one or more joints; nodules, from the size of a pea to a walnut, may appear under the skin; muscular wasting and spasm frequently occur. The disease may affect various organs and is sometimes accompanied by fever. Most frequently the small joints in the hands and the feet become involved. Other joints involved may be the knees, elbows, and ankles. They may become stiff, warm, red, and swollen.

CAUSE

The exact cause is unknown. There are two main theories: infection, and that the body's own defenses go awry and attack its own tissues. Emotional stress is believed to play an important role.

TREATMENT

At present, although there is no known cure for rheumatoid arthritis, proper medical treatment early in the course of the disease can prevent severe crippling in seventy percent of the cases. In some patients, despite treatment, the disease leads to chronic disability, sometimes to complete crippling.

The established forms for the treatment of rheumatoid arthritis are:

1. Physical and emotional rest.
2. Physical therapy, such as heat and corrective exercises.
3. Aspirin in adequate amounts.
4. Gold salt treatment.
5. Antimalarials.
6. Phenylbutazone.
7. Steroid hormones.
8. Corrective surgery.

The physician's choice of treatment depends largely on the location and stage of the disease.

In 1949, the symptoms of rheumatoid arthritis were found to respond dramatically to two steroid hormones: corticotropin (ACTH) and cortisone. For a time, it was thought that these drugs might be the long-awaited cure for rheumatoid arthritis, and a sharp swing to this therapy took place. Later experience showed that cortisone and ACTH were not curative and, in addition, had certain undesirable side effects. At present, physicians confine themselves to using these drugs on those cases that do not respond to other measures. In certain instances, it has been shown that injection of a cortisone-type drug directly into the affected joint is helpful.

Disillusionment with the steroid hormones has led to a reassessment of the known benefits of aspirin and gold salts and to the use of new drugs such as the antimalarials and phenylbutazone. Aspirin is the most reliable and least toxic of all arthritic drugs. It is the one that is most likely to provide sustained control of symptoms. Gold salts and antimalarials may bring about remissions of the disease, but treatment of several months duration is required. Phenylbutazone is especially useful in controlling the discomfort of ankylosing spondylitis (a form of arthritis that chiefly affects the hips and spine) and in certain cases of gout.

See fibrositis, gout, osteoarthritis.

arthrodesis — a surgical procedure to put a joint in a fixed, rigid position. This operation is performed occasionally on patients suffering from severe forms of arthritis. The patient loses any remaining mobility in the joint but also loses most of the pain.

artificial pacemaker — *See pacemaker.*

artificial respiration — a method by which normal respiration is imitated by manual movements to induce breathing in persons whose respiration has stopped. Because there are no means of influencing muscular action in an unconscious person to produce normal inspiration, it is necessary to depend on manual means of forcing air from the lungs by compression and to depend on the natural elasticity of the walls of the chest cavity plus the drop of the arch of the diaphragm to draw fresh air into the lungs when the compression is released, as in the prone-pressure method; also, by pressure on the back or chest, to force air out of the lungs and induce it into the lungs by raising the arms to move the muscles of the chest walls.

Where breathing has stopped or is very irregular and feeble, artificial respiration is usually required. The most frequent conditions under which artificial respiration is required are electric shock, gas poisoning, drowning, and suffocation from various causes.

In many conditions where breathing has ceased, or apparently ceased, the heart action continues for a limited time. If fresh air is brought into the lungs, so that the blood can obtain the needed oxygen from the air, life can be sustained. This can be accomplished in many instances by artificial respiration.

Certain general principles must always be kept in mind in applying any method of artificial respiration.

Time is of prime importance; even seconds count. Do not take time to move the victim to a more satisfactory place unless the place is unsafe for victim or rescuer; begin at once. Do not delay resuscitation to loosen the victim's clothes, warm him, apply stimulants, etc. These are secondary to the main purpose of getting air into the victim's lungs.

If at all possible, incline his body slightly to permit better drainage of fluid from the respiratory passage.

As soon as artificial respiration has been started and while it is being continued, an assistant should remove from the victim's mouth all foreign bodies, such as false teeth, tobacco, gum, and any loose material; see that the tongue is forward and not over the windpipe; and loosen any tight clothing about the victim's neck, chest, or waist.

Keep the victim warm by covering him with blankets, clothing, or other material; if possible, his underside should also be covered. Place hot-water bottles, hot bricks, or other heated objects, well-wrapped in cloth or paper and tested to prevent burning the victim, about him.

Continue artificial respiration rhythmically and uninterruptedly until spontaneous breathing starts or a doctor pronounces the patient dead.

If the victim begins to breathe of his own accord, adjust your timing to his. Do not fight his attempt to breathe.

A brief return of natural respiration is not a signal for stopping the resuscitation treatment.

Not infrequently a patient, after a temporary recovery of respiration, stops breathing again. He must be watched; if natural breathing stops, resume artificial respiration at once.

Always treat the victim for shock during resuscitation, and continue such treatment after breathing has started. Do not give any liquids whatever by mouth until a patient is fully conscious.

If it is necessary (due to extreme weather or other conditions) to move a patient before he is breathing normally, continue artificial respiration while he is being moved.

METHODS

The standard methods of artificial respiration are the mouth-to-mouth method (with variations) and several manual methods (back-pressure, arm-lift; chest-pressure, arm-lift; back-pressure, hip-lift). Of these the mouth-to-mouth method is considered the best. Although first advocated for infants and children, it is now the recognized method of choice.

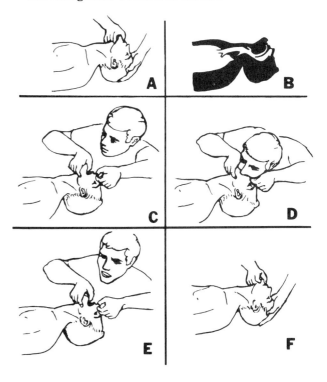

ARTIFICIAL RESPIRATION

When administering mouth-to-mouth artificial respiration, use the following procedures:

1. Place the victim on his back immediately. Don't waste time moving to a better place, loosening clothing, or draining water from lungs.

2. Quickly clear his mouth and throat. Remove any dentures, mucus, food, and other obstructions.

3. Tilt the victim's head as far back as possible. His head should be in a "chin-up" position and his neck stretched to ensure an open airway.

4. Lift his lower jaw forward. Grasp the jaw by placing your thumb into the corner of his mouth. Do not hold or depress his tongue.

5. Pinch his nose shut (or seal his mouth). Prevent any air leakage.

6. Open your mouth wide and blow. Take a deep breath and blow forcefully (except for babies) into his mouth or nose until you see his chest rise.

7. Quickly remove your mouth when his chest rises. Listen for exhalation — if the victim makes snoring or gurgling sounds, his jaw is not high enough.

8. Repeat fifteen to twenty times per minute. Continue until the victim begins to breathe normally.

9. Remove air blown into the victim's stomach. Periodically, between breaths, if the stomach is distended, place your hand on his upper abdomen and gently but firmly press the air out of his stomach.

10. For infants, seal both mouth and nose with your mouth. Blow with small puffs of air from your cheeks.

GENERAL RULES

1. Do not attempt to remove water from the victim's lungs or stomatch.

2. Keep the victim sufficiently covered so that he will not suffer from exposure.

3. Do not allow bystanders to crowd around the victim and interfere with the first-aid treatment.

4. Do not attempt to give the victim anything to drink while he is unconscious or you may cause him to choke.

5. Artificial respiration must be continued for at least four hours unless the natural breathing is restored before that time or a medical officer declares the person dead. Some people have been saved after as much as eight hours of artificial respiration.

6. Do not give up in less than four hours, even if the victim appears to be dead. All persons who have suffered an interruption of breathing do not have the same appearance. In some cases, the face is bluish-black. In other cases it is pale and white. In cases of carbon monoxide poisoning the skin is often (although not always) a peculiar cherry-red in color. In many cases of suspended breathing the pulse is so weak that it cannot be detected. Sometimes after electric shock the entire body becomes stiff and rigid — a condition that is occasionally mistaken for the rigidity of death. It is difficult to judge whether a person in this condition is dead or alive, and the usual indications of death cannot be trusted in cases of asphyxiation.

TREATMENT AFTER RECOVERY

To avoid strain on his heart, keep the patient prone, and do not allow him to sit up or stand after he revives. If he must be moved, carry him on a stretcher. To avoid additional strain on the heart, turn him over on his back when breathing becomes regular.

After the victim is revived and conscious, slowly give him a stimulant, such as one teaspoon of aromatic spirits of ammonia in half a glass of water or a hot drink of coffee, tea, or water.

Keep the patient warm, and continue to treat him for shock.

asab — a venereal disease found in Africa.

asbestosis — a disease of the lungs resulting from the inhalation of particles of asbestos or asbestos dust. Asbestosis is a form of pneumoconiosis. *See pneumoconiosis.*

ascaris — *See worms.*

ascending paths — term used for the paths nerve impulses take on their way to the brain.

Aschheim-Zondek test — a test to determine if a woman is pregnant. Urine from the woman is injected into a young female mouse.

Aschoff bodies — spindle-shaped nodules, occurring most frequently in the tissue of the heart, often formed during an attack of rheumatic fever. Named after Ludwig Aschoff (1866-1942), a German pathologist, who described them.

ascorbic acid — *See vitamin C.*

asepsis — a state in which there are no infections or bacteria. The term is usually used to describe conditions in an operating room when surgery is being performed. The discovery of the importance of asepsis and the development of techniques to insure asepsis during operations are landmarks in medical history.

See Lister.

asomnia — *See insomnia.*

asphyxia — suffocation. A person who has stopped breathing but who is still alive is said to be in a state of asphyxia.

A person who has stopped breathing is not necessarily dead, but he is in immediate, critical danger. Life is dependent upon oxygen, which is breathed into the lungs and then carried by the blood to every body cell. Since body cells cannot store oxygen, and since the blood can hold only a limited amount (and that only for a short time), death will result from continued lack of breathing.

However, the heart may continue to beat for some time after breathing has stopped, and the blood may still be circulated to the body cells. Since the blood will, for a short time, contain a small supply of oxygen, the body cells will not die immediately. Thus, for a very few minutes, there is some chance that the person's life may be saved.

CAUSES

Drowning, electric shock, and gas poisoning are the three most common accidents likely to result in asphyxiation. Asphyxiation also occurs from such accidents as choking, hanging, and burial in materials like grain, sand, or gravel. Excessive use of alcohol or drugs may also cause breathing to stop. Also, some illnesses, such as poliomyelitis (sometimes called polio or infantile paralysis), may result in asphyxiation.

In general, cases of asphyxiation may be classified as being caused by one or more of the following:

1. Blocked air passages

Blocked air passages cause asphyxiation in cases of drowning, choking, and suffocation. In drowning, the air passages are blocked by water. In choking, they may be blocked by bones, large pieces of food, false teeth, chewing gum, or any other foreign object that becomes caught in the throat and cuts off the supply of air.

2. Insufficient oxygen in the air

Even if the air passages are not blocked, asphyxia may occur because of insufficient oxygen in the air. For example, aviators and mountain climbers are sometimes asphyxiated because there is not enough oxygen in the air at high altitudes.

3. Inability of the blood to carry oxygen

Carbon monoxide poisoning is the primary example of asphyxiation due to an inability of the blood to carry oxygen. Carbon monoxide combines with certain blood cells very rapidly, in such a way as to prevent the blood from carrying oxygen. Thus the body cells (especially in the brain) suffer a lack of oxygen which causes death.

4. Paralysis of the breathing center in the brain

Breathing can also be stopped by paralysis of the breathing center in the brain. The most frequent causes of paralysis of the breathing center are electric shock; excessive amounts of alcohol, drugs, or anesthetics; and breathing too much carbon dioxide.

5. Compression of the body

Since breathing movements cannot be made against any great amount of pressure, compression of the body can easily stop a person's breathing. Accidental burial in dirt, sand, gravel, coal, cinders, or similar material is likely to cause asphyxiation because of body compression. In such cases death may occur even though the nose and mouth are uncovered.

TREATMENT

Artificial respiration must begin at once, and the cause of the patient's condition should be removed as quickly as possible.

See artificial respiration.

aspirin — an analgesic and one of the most widely used of all drugs.

See acetylsalicylic acid.

asthenia — lack of strength, weakness.

asthma — a chronic noncontagious disease of the lungs. The asthma sufferer has periodic attacks of difficulty in breathing, which may be mild or severe. Asthma may start in childhood or may appear at any age. Asthma sometimes disappears in children, as well as in adults. But this is probably because, by accident, the agent responsible for the asthma has been removed from the patient's environment. It is much more likely that untreated childhood asthma will grow worse rather than go away.

In the healthy lung, large bronchial tubes (bronchi) leading from the windpipe (trachea) carry the air that has been breathed in through the mouth and nose. These large tubes divide into smaller and smaller ones (bronchioles) until they are the size of fine threads. At the end of each small tube there is a cluster of tiny air sacs (alveoli). In these sacs, the oxygen from the air is picked up by the blood, to be pumped through the entire body. At the same time, the waste product, carbon dioxide, is removed from the blood and breathed out. This process is repeated about sixteen times every minute.

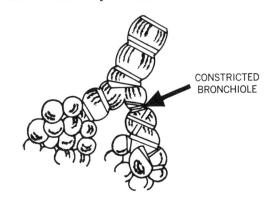

CONSTRICTED BRONCHIOLE

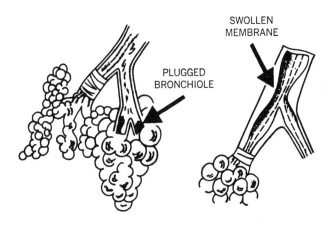

SWOLLEN MEMBRANE

PLUGGED BRONCHIOLE

ASTHMA

SYMPTOMS

The choked breathing of the asthma sufferer is caused by a narrowing of the small bronchial tubes during the asthma attack. This may be due to swelling of the membrane that lines the tubes, to spasm of the tubes, or to mucus plugging the tubes. Whatever the cause, breathing becomes like trying to force air through a clamped tube. If the attack is severe, the patient seems to be suffocating. He turns pale and bluish, sweats, and appears to be using all his strength to draw his breath in and force it out.

Fortunately, most attacks of asthma are mild. They are more distressing than dangerous and can be relieved by modern medical treatments. However, with repeated attacks, the forced breathing stretches the lung tissue and may damage it permanently. When this happens, the person no longer breathes out completely, and a condition known as emphysema results. He then has less endurance and may be short of breath after slight exertion. An extra load is placed on the heart, which must work harder to force blood through the damaged lungs. The better the asthma attacks are controlled, the less permanent damage will be done to the lungs.

There are several illnesses that cause wheezy, difficult breathing. Two illnesses that mimic bronchial asthma are heart disease and obstructions in the bronchial tubes. Only a medical doctor can tell the patient which one he has.

CAUSES

There appear to be many causes of bronchial asthma, among which allergic reactions are prominent. About seventy-five percent of the people who have asthma are allergic to one or more substances which they breathe in, eat, or have injected. Foods, drugs, feathers, fur, animal danders, face powder, and pollens are among the numerous possible causes. Ragweed pollen can cause hay fever and asthma at the same time. Some people have asthma only during the ragweed season.

Many cases of asthma are associated with bacterial infections, especially of the sinuses, throat, and nose. Most of these people improve if the infection clears up. Some feel better in a climate where they have little or no trouble with infections of the respiratory tract.

In some asthmatic patients, attacks are brought on or made worse by emotional stress. This type of asthma improves when the stress is lowered.

There is growing evidence that air pollution plays an important part in causing asthma. Some patients suffer attacks after exposure to smoggy air. People who live in communities with smog problems are generally in poorer health than those who live where the air is cleaner.

TREATMENT

Asthma due to an allergy can't really be cured, since the person remains allergic. The person must recognize that since asthma is a chronic disease, it will require treatment over a long period of time. But if the patient cooperates with his doctor, asthma can be treated successfully in many cases.

A physician can show the patient how to avoid many attacks and how to relieve those that come on. The substance causing the allergy can be avoided; or in some cases, the patient can be desensitized to it by a series of injections.

A few asthma patients need a change of climate. They are usually people who have severe asthma that has not improved with ordinary treatment, or their asthma may be directly related to colds, sinusitis, and other respiratory infections.

RESEARCH

Scientists in many research laboratories and hospitals across the country receive funds from the National Institute of Allergy and Infectious Diseases, PHS, to look for ways to prevent or treat asthma. Drugs for treating the allergies that cause asthma are being improved. Materials used for desensitization are being standardized. The relationship of asthma to other diseases of the respiratory tract is under study; so is the effect of emotional stress on asthma. Basic studies are going on to determine how allergies develop and why some people get them while most people do not. Much remains to be learned, but research is constantly paving the way to better methods of controlling asthma.

astigmatism — the faulty vision that results from irregularity in the curvature of one or more refractive surfaces (the fault is usually in the cornea) of the eye. When such a condition occurs, rays emanating from a point are not brought into focus at a point on the retina but appear to spread as a line in various directions, depending on the curvature.

Astigmatism can occur in one eye or in both eyes and can be corrected by eyeglasses whose lenses compensate for the irregularity.

astragalus — *See talus.*

astringent — liquids applied to the skin (usually for cleansing purposes) which tend to shrink or contract the surface layer of the skin, thus helping to stop or slow discharges from below the skin.

ataxia — inability to coordinate muscular actions. The problem can be a result of disease, brain malfunction, etc. Ataxia is dangerous in that the patient's lack of coordination may lead to serious falls.

atelectasis — noninflation or incomplete inflation of a lung or lungs at birth, and, in adults, collapse of a lung.

athermic — a term used to indicate a condition in which the patient does not experience a rise in temperature.

atheroma — a deposit of fatty (and other) substances in the inner lining of the artery wall, characteristic of atherosclerosis. Plural form of the word is atheromata.
See atherosclerosis.

atherosclerosis — a kind of arteriosclerosis in which the inner layer of the artery wall is made thick and irregular by deposits of a fatty substance. These deposits (called atheromata) project above the surface of the inner layer of the artery and thus decrease the diameter of the internal channel of the vessel.

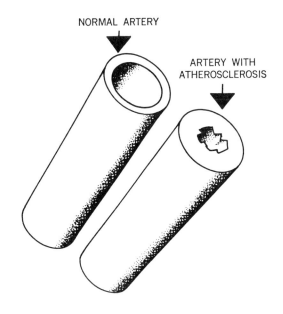

NORMAL ARTERY

ARTERY WITH ATHEROSCLEROSIS

ATHEROSCLEROSIS

Just how and why the complex fatty substances are deposited in the blood vessels and why they collect in different parts of the body in different people are unanswered questions. It is known that cholesterol, normally present in everyone's blood, makes up a large part of the deposit. But the relationship between circulating blood cholesterol and these deposits is not yet fully known.

Nevertheless, several studies have indicated that the incidence of coronary heart disease is greater among men with cholesterol levels above the average range. Thus, some physicians will prescribe treatment to decrease the amount of blood cholesterol if it is considered abnormally high.

In addition to diet, other influences may also play an important role in raising the levels of blood cholesterol. They include smoking, lack of exercise, and emotional tension.

Moreover, even if blood cholesterol is successfully lowered, there is no final evidence that such a change will delay or prevent atherosclerosis. High blood cholesterol is only one factor that has been found to be associated with the condition. Other factors are overweight, high blood pressure, and a family history of coronary heart disease.

Atherosclerosis is the most common form of arteriosclerosis and it affects primarily the larger arteries of the body. The complications of atherosclerosis, such as heart attacks, are the most common immediate causes of adult death in the United States today.

See arteriosclerosis, cholesterol.

athetoid — a type of cystic fibrosis in which the patient shows constant uncontrolled motion.

athlete's foot — a ringworm of the feet, the most common of the fungus diseases that attack the skin. Athelete's foot, which is a communicable disease, develops on a person's feet when the fungus, which may be present but causes no trouble on some feet, begins to grow and multiply. This fungus grows best in moist, warm, poorly ventilated places such as on skin between toes that stay damp with perspiration.

The symptoms of infection are: itching, cracking or scaling of the skin, and sometimes small blisters that contain a watery fluid. If the disease continues without treatment, there can be large blisters and raw places on the skin that resemble the effects of poison ivy.

Athlete's foot can be prevented by keeping the feet clean and dry; by wearing a clean pair of socks every day; by dusting the feet frequently with a fungicidal powder; and by using only gymnasium, swimming pool, and clubhouse locker rooms that are cleaned and disinfected daily. It is also important to wear shoes and socks that are comfortably roomy, so that air can get to the feet. Athlete's foot is most stubborn and prevalent in the summer.

atlas — the first cervical vertebra.
  See vertebra.

atomizer — an instrument used to apply liquids in a fine spray or mist. Atomizers are frequently used to apply liquids to the back of the throat.

atopy — hypersensitivity or allergy, usually inherited, such as hay fever and asthma. An atopic reaction is a displaced reaction; that is, the reaction takes place at a site other than the one where the allergen came in contact with the body.

ATP — abbreviation for adenosine triphosphate.

atrial septum — the muscular wall that divides the left and right upper chambers of the heart which are called atria. The atrial septum is sometimes referred to as the interatrial septum or the interauricular septum.
  See septum.

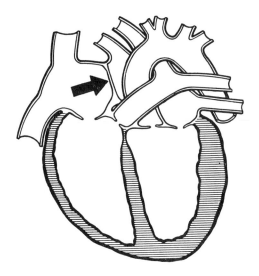

ATRIAL SEPTUM

atrioventricular bundle — a bundle of specialized muscle fibers running from a small mass of muscular fibers (atrioventricular node) between the upper chambers of the heart, down to the lower chambers. It is the only known direct muscular connection between the upper and lower heart chambers, and it serves to conduct impulses for the rhythmic heartbeat from the atrioventricular node to the heart muscle. The atrioventricular bundle is also called the bundle of His, auriculoventricular bundle, or A-V bundle.

atrioventricular node — a small mass of special fibers at the base of the wall between the two upper chambers of the heart. It forms the beginning of the bundle of His (atrioventricular bundle), which is the only known direct muscular connection between the upper and the lower chambers of the heart. The electrical impulses controlling the rhythm of the heart are generated by the pacemaker, conducted through the muscle fibers of the right upper chamber of the heart to the atrioventricular node, and then conducted to the lower chambers of the heart by the bundle of His.

atrioventricular valves — the two valves, one in each side of the heart, between the upper and lower chamber. The one in the right side of the heart is called the tricuspid valve, and the one on the left side is called the mitral valve. These valves keep the blood from flowing in the wrong direction.
See mitral valve, tricuspid valve.

atrium — one of the two upper chambers of the heart.

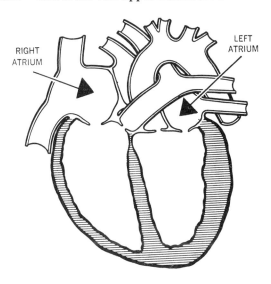

ATRIUM

An atrium is also called an auricle, although that term is now generally used to describe only the very tip of the atrium. The right atrium receives unoxygenated blood from the body. The left atrium receives freshly oxygenated blood from the lungs. In a healthy adult, the normal capacity of an atrium is about fifty-seven cubic centimeters.

atrophy — a shrinking or wasting away of body tissue. There are several different causes of atrophy. The two most common are atrophy due to malnutrition and atrophy resulting from immobilization of a body part (for example an arm or leg that has been immobilized in a cast).

atropine — a drug made from the *Atropa belladonna* plant. Atropine blocks many of the effects of acetylcholine (ACh) on the parasympathetic nerves. Consequently, it is used in the treatment of parkinsonism, in the prevention of motion sickness, and as a preanesthetic. It relaxes smooth muscles, dilates the pupils of the eyes, and reduces acid secretion in the gastrointestinal tract.

Atropine has several unpleasant side effects such as dryness in the mouth, sensitivity to light, etc.

audiogenic seizure — an attack or seizure similar to an epileptic attack but brought on by auditory stimulation. The sound is usually a very high pitch.

audiologist — a specialist professionally trained for testing, rehabilitation, and counseling of people with hearing disorders.

auditory canal — the outer part of the ear.
See ear.

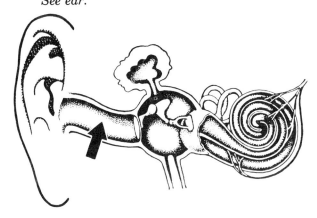

AUDITORY CANAL

Auenbrugger, Leopold Joseph — an Austrian physician (1722-1809) who invented the technique of tapping the surface of the body to determine the condition of organs beneath. The technique is called percussion and is an extremely important diagnostic tool.

See percussion.

aura — a sudden premonition warning the patient of an attack (usually an epileptic attack). Because it is subjective, it can not be measured or qualitatively described; however, many epileptics experience the phenomenon and use it to prepare for the attack.

See epilepsy.

aural — of or pertaining to the ear.

auricle — the part of the ear that projects out from the head.

Also, the upper chamber in each side of the heart (although strictly speaking, this is not correct).

auricular septum — the muscular wall dividing the left and right upper chambers of the heart which are called atria. The auricular septum is also referred to as the interauricular septum, or more properly, the interatrial septum.

See septum.

auriculoventricular bundle — *See atrioventricular bundle.*

auscultation — listening to the sounds within the body, especially of the heart and lungs, usually with a stethoscope, to help determine the physical condition of these organs.

Auscultation is an extremely important diagnostic tool.

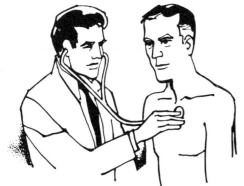

AUSCULATION

autism — a mental disorder which develops in childhood. The most striking symptom of the autistic child is his almost total withdrawal into himself. Ironically, autistic children often are very intelligent.

Until recently, there was little hope for curing autism. With patience and proper care and handling, more autistic children are being cured.

autoclave — a piece of equipment that sterilizes instruments by steam.

autodermic — a skin graft coming from the patient's own body. The patient is thus both donor and recipient.

autoimmunity — a condition in which the body has developed a sensitivity to some of its own tissues. The cause or causes of this reaction is not really understood.

autonomic nervous system — the relatively independent nervous system composed of the sympathetic and parasympathetic systems. The autonomic nervous system is often referred to as the involuntary nervous system or vegetative nervous system because it controls tissues not under voluntary control, such as the glands, the heart, the stomach, and the smooth muscles.

The sympathetic and parasympathetic systems have different effects on the same body organ. Frequently, they have opposite effects. For example, the effect of the sympathetic nerves on the intestines is to lower or reduce activity. The parasympathetic nerves will speed up or stimulate intestinal activity. On the other hand, the sympathetic nerves stimulate the heart, while parasympathetic nerves slow it down.

See sympathetic nerves, parasympathetic nerves.

A-V bundle — *See atrioventricular bundle.*

axilla — *See armpit.*

axillary artery — the artery of the armpit and shoulder.

axillary nerve — nerve involved in shoulder movement and general sensations in the shoulder area. The axillary nerve used to be called the circumflex nerve.

b

baby — a newborn child. A baby is usually from eighteen to twenty-one inches long and may weigh anywhere from two to three pounds to ten or more. Approximately seven pounds is the average size for babies in this country. Boys are apt to be a little heavier than girls. If a baby weighs less than five and a half pounds, he may need special care.

See premature baby.

baby blues — a feeling of depression and weepiness experienced by many new mothers. There are many reasons why a feeling of depression may occur.

Physical changes within the mother's body may trigger and deepen feelings of depression. Because the mind and the body are so delicately meshed, any profound physical readjustment is bound to be reflected in feelings and thoughts. The hormones secreted during pregnancy are no longer needed, and the supply of available energy may not match the increased demands of the day—and night.

To a lesser extent, fathers and older children in the family may have moments of depression, too.

Probably the best way to deal with ordinary baby blues is to be reassured that many mothers have them and that they are only temporary.

baby talk — the bridge between a child's words and adult language.

Children make up wonderfully expressive words, which become a part of the family vocabulary. An excited three year old, hearing a siren, shouts: "A sirengine." A breakfast cereal is christened "scrippies." As others in the family pick up these inventions, they help the child to fix meanings to words. Talking this kind of baby talk, in which the child's own words and simple sentence structures are copied by the adults, helps him to catch on to spoken language. He is baffled by long, elaborate sentences.

Children love to play with sounds long after they learn to speak, and three and four year olds giggle over nonsense such as "gaggle, goggle, zoom, zoom, zoom." A good beat to a string of nonsense is all that is required to keep a group of preschoolers amused. Along with their pleasure, they are perfecting difficult consonants and emphasize the last or middle syllables of words, which also improves their articulation of speech. These word games are good practice.

Neither of the above examples is to be confused with baby talk of the kind that keeps a child using immature sounds he long ago would have dropped had he not discovered that baby talk gets results from parents who think it is cute. Children who hear good speech tend to copy it. A child will usually outgrow baby talk when his parents do.

baby teeth — the first teeth, also called primary or milk teeth. The baby teeth are formed long before birth; the permanent teeth begin to form in the baby's jaw about the time he is born.

At about six months of age (earlier in some children, later in others), the first baby teeth appear, usually the lower front ones. These are followed at more or less regular intervals by the upper front teeth, the back teeth, and the cuspids (called eye or canine teeth).

There are twenty baby teeth and their presence in the mouth is essential until the permanent teeth are ready to take their place. The health and proper placement of the baby teeth influence the formation of the child's jaws and his appearance.

A child needs sound baby teeth for proper chewing of the variety of foods that promote his growth. Correct chewing is the first step in good digestion, without which the child's body cannot make full use of his food. This is vitally important because, in proportion to his weight, a child must eat three times the amount of food required by a grown person.

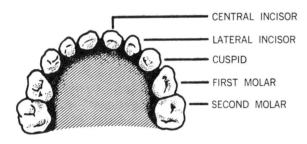
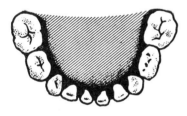

CENTRAL INCISOR
LATERAL INCISOR
CUSPID
FIRST MOLAR
SECOND MOLAR

BABY TEETH

The baby teeth need to be brushed. As early as possible, parents should teach the child the proper way to brush his teeth and gums, using a small brush and a small amount of pleasant-tasting toothpaste or tooth powder.

The primary teeth should not be neglected simply because they will be replaced later by permanent teeth. Those permanent teeth cannot come in straight and even if the baby teeth are prematurely lost.
See teeth.

bacillus — any bacterium shaped like a rod. Different bacilli (the plural of bacillus) are the cause of typhoid, tetanus, etc.
See bacteria.

bacitracin — an antibiotic usually used as an ointment for skin problems.
See antibiotic.

back — the rear portion of the body from the shoulders to the pelvis. The lower back is the area between the waist and the pelvis.

backache — an ache usually located in the lower back. Backaches generally fall into one of four categories: anatomical, mechanical, inflammatory, or reflex.

An anatomical backache is caused by a physical defect in the spinal column. The defect may be present at birth, or it may be the result of injury or certain types of diseases.

Backaches from mechanical problems are probably the most common. They are caused by poor posture, flat feet and fallen arches, etc.

An inflammatory backache is caused by an inflammation in the lower spinal cord — such as rheumatism.

A reflex backache may be caused by an inflammation or infection of the kidneys.

Almost all backaches can be aggravated by tension.

backbone — the spine.
See spinal column.

backflow — fluid moving in the opposite direction from the way it should be moving. A faulty or incompetent valve will allow blood to flow back in the wrong direction.

bacteria — a microscopic organism. Some bacteria

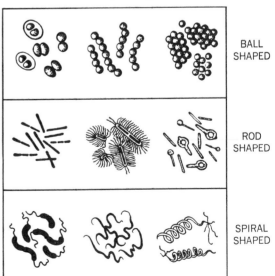

BALL SHAPED

ROD SHAPED

SPIRAL SHAPED

BACTERIA

are harmful to humans, others exist in harmony with humans, and still others play an important and necessary role within the human body.

Bacteria are shaped like rods (bacilli), spheres (cocci), or spirals (spirilla). They may occur as a congregation of single units, in clusters, or in chains.

bacterial endocarditis — an inflammation of the inner layer of the heart caused by bacteria. The lining of the heart valves is most frequently affected. Bacterial endocarditis is commonly a complication of an infectious disease, an operation, or an injury.

bactericidal — a term applied to any drug or agent that can destroy bacteria. Different bactericides destroy different bacteria.
See antibiotic.

bacteriostatic — a term applied to any drug or agent that inhibits the growth of bacteria. Different bacteriostats act against different bacteria.
See antibiotic.

bacterium — the singular of bacteria.
See bacteria.

bag of waters — the sac of fluid in which an embryo floats. The fluid keeps the fetus evenly warm and acts as a shock absorber to protect it from jolts and bumps.

Occasionally, a baby will be born with the bag of waters intact; however, the sudden gush of water from the vagina (indicating that the bag has broken) usually means that labor has begun. Whether it breaks early or later in labor makes very little difference to either the mother or the child and has nothing to do with the length of labor.

baking soda — *See sodium bicarbonate.*

BAL — abbreviation of British anti-lewisite.
See dimercaprol.

baldness — gradual loss of hair from the scalp. Baldness can be caused by disease, old age, or it can be an inherited condition.

There is very little that can be done to prevent natural baldness, and even less can be done to stop it once it has begun. It is, however, helpful to keep the flow of blood to the scalp unimpeded. Tight hats, caps, and wigs should be avoided.

An entire mythology has grown up about baldness. Such statements as "baldness is a sign of virility" are not true.

ballistocardiogram — a tracing of the movements of the body caused by the beating of the heart. The instrument that records these movements is called a ballistocardiograph.

ballistocardiograph — an apparatus for recording the movements of the body caused by the beating of the heart.

bandage — a piece of material used to hold a sterile dressing in place over a wound, to create pressure over a bleeding wound for control of hemorrhage, to secure a splint to an injured part of the body, or to provide support to an injured body part. It is important to realize the difference between a dressing, which is placed directly on a wound and therefore should be sterile, and a bandage, which is used to hold the dressing in place. A combined dressing and bandage in which a sterile gauze pad is fastened to an adhesive bandage is usually referred to as a dressing.

A bandage should never be applied directly over a wound; it should be used only to hold in place the dressing that covers a wound. A bandage should be applied firmly and fastened securely. However, it should not be applied so tightly that it stops circulation or so loosely that it allows the dressing to slip.

There are three general types of bandages: triangular bandages, roller bandages, and tailed or T-shaped bandages. From these three basic types many other shapes of bandages can be made by folding or lengthening.

bandaging — the application of a bandage to hold a sterile dressing in place over a wound.

Banti's syndrome — an anomoly of the spleen. It was once considered a separate disease, but today it is considered to be a complication resulting from some forms of hypertension.

barbital — a drug used to depress the central nervous system.

barbiturates — a class of drugs that produce a calming effect. They are made from barbituric acid. They are by far the largest group of drugs described as sedatives.

The first sleep-producing barbiturate was

synthesized in 1903. Today, there are over fifty commercial brands on the market.

The barbiturates vary in duration of action. They range from the very fast-acting thiopental, which can be used as an anesthetic, to moderately fast-acting pentobarbital and secobarbital, to the slow-acting phenobarbital.

Barbiturates, especially the short-acting ones, may lead to heavy abuse. Without careful medical supervision to avoid habituation, increasing doses are used to produce the desired effect, and physical dependence occurs. When sold on the street, they are called "goofballs," "sleepers," and "downers."

The principal response elicited by barbiturates is a depression of the central nervous system. They act upon the cerebral centers and interfere with the passage of impulses in the brain. They appear to affect the enzyme processes by which energy is acquired, stored in the protoplasm of the cells, and utilized. They depress brain function and in large doses depress the brain centers responsible for maintaining the rhythm of respiration.

Properly prescribed and taken as directed in small doses, they relieve tension and anxiety. In larger doses (three or four times as much) they produce drowsiness and sleep. They are also used medically for such psychosomatic conditions as high blood pressure, peptic ulcer, spastic colitis, and other psychophysiologic disorders.

ABUSE

Increasing use of barbiturates quickly produces tolerance, which means that more is required to produce the desired effect, thus leading to the strong desire to continue taking barbiturates in progressively larger amounts. Addiction to fifty or more sleeping pills a day has been reported. Those who take excessive amounts of barbiturates usually go into a coma. However, in persons used to taking large doses, instead of producing drowsiness or sleep, barbiturates may produce restlessness, excitement, and even delirium, resembling the excitation of the alcoholic. Persons intoxicated with barbiturates may appear to be inebriated and may be mistaken for "drunks." Their coordination is poor; their speech is slurred; and they become irritable, confused, and unsteady of gait. Ability to accomplish skilled, precise tasks is lost. Judgment, perception, and memory are impaired. In extreme cases disorientation, aggressive behavior, hallucinations, and paranoid delusions may develop.

Barbiturates are frequently used in conjunction with amphetamines, often to induce sleep after the amphetamine "jag" is over. Alternately, amphetamines may be taken to counteract the barbiturate "hangover." This results in a chemical attempt to regulate the sleep-waking rhythm, which often ends in failure.

Although the two types of drugs have opposite actions, some persons become dependent on both barbiturates and amphetamines because of their combined effect. Instead of completely neutralizing a "downer," an "upper" may not only take the edge off the jittery excitement but also may create a pleasant, mood-elevating effect, leading to habitual swallowing of large quantities of some combination of amphetamines and barbiturates.

While the majority of these drugs are legally used for medical purposes, an unknown but large quantity of barbiturates also enters illegal channels. Recent estimates indicate that of all the barbiturates manufactured in the United States more than half were diverted to illicit use. A good share of the "goofballs" being distributed today on the black market are capsules that were legally manufactured but found their way into illicit channels by theft, exportation and reimportation from a foreign country, hijacking, and indiscriminate sales to unauthorized persons.

Persons who are tense and anxious, or who have trouble with insomnia, may become overinvolved with sedatives and come to depend on them. Those who get in the habit of using these pills routinely may find themselves using increasingly large amounts. The largest group of persons using prescribed barbiturates and tranquilizers have been adults over twenty, principally those in the forty to sixty age group. However, today they are also being used more and more frequently by teenagers, who find them in the family medicine cabinet or obtain them from black-market sources.

Many cases of barbiturate or tranquilizer misuse begin in the physician's office. A doctor may fail to examine adequately the basis of complaints for his patient's symptoms, may overprescribe pills, or may permit multiple refills of the prescription without his supervision to assure they are being properly used.

Heroin addicts may take barbiturates to supplement or substitute for their preferred drug. Amphetamine users who become jittery may take them to ease their tension.

DANGERS

The barbiturates are highly dangerous when taken without medical supervision. Because they are commonly prescribed by doctors, many people mistakenly consider them safe to use freely and carelessly. They are not. Death may result from the use of barbiturates, either from overdose or sudden withdrawal.

A common mode of suicide with drugs is with sleeping pills. Some 3,000 barbiturate suicides occur each year. Accidental deaths from taking a larger number of pills than intended are not uncommon.

Death can also occur when a number of barbiturate capsules are swallowed by someone intoxicated with alcohol. These drugs act as synergists and are additive in their effects. Coroners have found a number of instances in which neither the barbiturate nor alcohol levels in the blood were sufficient to produce death, but the combination did.

A regular, heavy user who has built up tolerance to the drug and requires large amounts to obtain the desired effect suffers withdrawal symptoms when the drug is suddenly stopped. The severe withdrawal state resembles delirium tremens. The user is agitated, restless, and may have muscle cramps, nausea, and convulsions. In addition, he may see things that are not there and have delusional, confused thoughts.

It has been mentioned that less than lethal doses of alcohol and sleeping pills, taken together, may be fatal. This is also true of combinations of barbiturates with anesthetics, narcotics, or tranquilizers. These drugs act to potentiate, or intensify, each other's effects. They may depress vital functions such as breathing and heart action to the point where they cease. Past a certain point, even persons whose bodies have acquired tolerance to barbiturates risk death from an overdose.

TREATMENT FOR CHRONIC USE

The treatment of chronic barbiturate intoxication consists of the slow decrease of the drug under medical supervision. Sudden barbiturate withdrawal is a serious medical emergency and requires hospitalization. It is more dangerous than heroin withdrawal and can be deadly.

Certain kinds of barbiturate addiction are regarded by many medical authorities as more difficult to cure than narcotic addiction. Withdrawal requires careful medical and nursing supervision. After withdrawal, psychiatric help is frequently needed. Like other drug abusers, the chronic barbiturate abuser usually suffers from an inability to cope with the stress of living and finds facing reality difficult. Considerable social and psychological support, often most successfully provided through group therapy and relating to others who have "kicked the habit," is helpful.

Despite their longtime use, just how barbiturate drugs act on the body, brain, and nervous system is not fully understood. Much remains to be learned about the effects of massive doses. Basic studies are underway to determine the precise mechanism through which the drugs work and how tolerance develops. New analytic techniques are being applied to assess changes that occur in body organs and cells as a result of chronic heavy use.

barbituric acid — the acid from which barbiturates are derived.

barium — a toxic metallic element.

barium sulfate — an insoluble substance used as a contrast medium in X-rays. The barium sulfate is swallowed and X-rays are taken of its progress through the gastrointestinal tract.

Barnard, Dr. Christiaan Neethling — first surgeon to successfully transplant a human heart. The heart transplant was done on December 3, 1967 at Groote Schuur Hospital in Capetown, South Africa. The donor, a twenty-four-year-old woman, had died as a result of injuries from an automobile accident. The recipient, Louis Washkansky, was dying from progressive heart failure. In an operation that lasted less than five hours, Dr. Barnard (born in 1923) removed the damaged heart from his fifty-five-year-old patient and replaced it with the undamaged heart from the body of the young woman.

The patient was given drugs and radiation to suppress his body's natural rejection mechanism. He lived for eighteen days after the operation, but died from pneumonia.

See heart, heart transplant.

basal ganglia — part of the nervous system located in the brain. They play an important role in the transmission of impulses involved in voluntary muscular movement. When damaged, or diseased (as in Parkinson's disease), coordinated

muscular movement becomes difficult and movement often becomes involuntary.
See Parkinson's disease.

basal metabolic rate — the rate of basal metabolism expressed in a mathematical formula.

basal metabolism — the amount of energy needed to keep the body alive when it is at rest.
See metabolism.

base — *See alkali.*

Basedow's disease — a goiter (thyroid enlargement) condition which includes a rapid pulse and nervous symptoms. It is named for Carl A. von Basedow, a German doctor who described the condition. The technical name for Basedow's disease is exophthalmic goiter.
See goiter, thyroid.

battered-child syndrome — *See child abuse.*

bedbug — an insect found in temperate and tropical climates. Bedbugs are usually flat and red. They live in houses, particularly in furniture and beds, and feed on human blood.

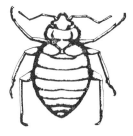

BEDBUG

bedsore — an ulceration of the skin and the tissues below it caused by continuous pressure which prevents the proper amount of blood carrying oxygen from circulating in the area.

The condition is called bedsores because of the tendency of bedridden patients to develop this problem.

The areas most likely to develop bedsores are the heels, shoulder blades, buttocks, and elbows.

bee sting — the painful reaction to the injection of a small amount of venom from a bee. Bee stings usually are not serious. However, a small proportion of the population is allergic to this venom, and their reaction to it can be very serious. While most people can tolerate the sting from several bees, people who have been attacked by a swarm of bees need a doctor's care immediately.

First aid for a bee sting should include removal of the stinger (when it is visible) and application of household ammonia to the sting.

behavior — generally, anything a person says or does. Behavior is the physical or outward manifestation of inner feelings.

belladonna — a drug derived from *Atropa belladonna,* the deadly nightshade. Belladonna is used in the treatment of Parkinson's disease, motion sickness, bronchial asthma, peptic ulcer, etc.

The classic side effects include dryness of the mouth and dilation of the pupils of the eyes.

Bell's palsy — a facial paralysis caused by injury or disease involving the facial nerve. Bell's palsy comes on very rapidly, leaving one side of the patient's face paralyzed. Just as there is no apparent cause, there is no really effective treatment. The paralysis can last from two weeks to two years; it is very infrequently permanent.

belly — *See abdomen.*

bemegride — a central nervous system stimulant which is used as a respiratory stimulant and as one of the antidotes for barbiturate poisoning.

bends — *See decompression sickness.*

benign — a term used to denote tissues or tumors that are not malignant, not recurrent, and are favorable for recovery.

benzalkonium — an antiseptic.

benzedrine — a stimulant referred to as a "benny" or "bennies" on the street. Benzedrine is an amphetamine.
See amphetamine.

benzothiadiazine — a drug used to increase the output of urine by the kidney.
See diuretics.

benzpyrene — a chemical of a type known as polycyclic hydrocarbon. It produces cancer in animals. It has been isolated from coal tar and is found in the smoky atmosphere of industrial cities and the exhaust of internal-combustion engines.

beriberi — a condition resulting from a dietary or nutritional deficiency of thiamine (one of the B vitamins). The symptoms include neuritis, paralysis, and anemia. The treatment is the same as the prevention — thiamine.

Beriberi is most common in areas where polished rice is a dietary staple, because polishing removes the thiamine from rice.

See vitamin B.

beta-naphthylamine — a chemical of a type known as aromatic amine. It is a cause of bladder cancer among workers in aniline dye plants.

biceps — strictly, any muscle that has two heads or branches. There is a bicep muscle in the thigh, but the bicep muscle of the arm is the one with which most people are familiar. The biceps of the arm is responsible for flexing the forearm and rotating the hand; the one in the thigh flexes the leg and extends the thigh.

Bichat, Marie Francois Xavier — French physician (1771-1802) who is credited with making histology and pathology sciences.

bicuspid valve — a valve of two cusps or triangular segments, located between the upper and lower chamber in the left side of the heart. It is usually called a mitral valve.

bifocals — eyeglasses that serve the dual purpose of correcting both near and far vision. This is accomplished by means of lenses with an insert in the lower half that is used for near vision. The remainder of the lens is used for distance vision.

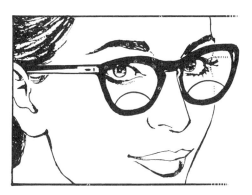

BIFOCAL GLASSES

bilateral — having or pertaining to two sides.

bile — the liquid secretion of the liver. It flows from the liver to the gallbladder and then into the intestine, where it acts as an aid to digestion by breaking down fats.

See gallbladder.

bilharzia — *See schistomiasis.*

binaural hearing-aid system — a hearing-aid system consisting of two complete hearing aids — microphone, amplifier, and receiver — one for each ear. For some people, the binaural system increases the directional sense and helps to separate wanted sounds from unwanted background noise.

See ear, hearing aid.

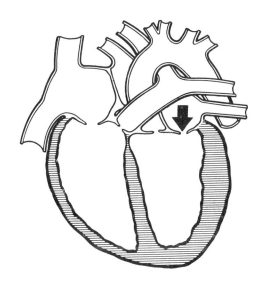

BICUSPID VALVE

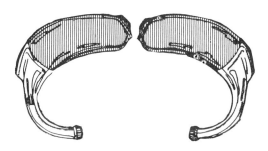

BINAURAL HEARING AID SYSTEM

biochemistry — the science of the chemistry of living organisms and of their vital processes.

biomedical — an adjective referring to both biology and medicine.

biopsy — a surgical procedure involving the removal and microscopic examination of tissue from the living body for purposes of diagnosis.

A small piece of suspect tissue is removed, placed in a preservative, cut in very thin slices, placed on a glass slide, stained with special dyes, and examined under the microscope. The biopsy may be performed quickly in the operating room so that the operation can be continued for removal of the tumor and surrounding tissues if the presence of a malignancy is established.

birth — the process of being born.
See labor.

birth canal — the canal a baby passes through during the birth process. The canal consists of the cervix, vagina, and vulva.

birth certificate — the legal record of a child's birth, date of birth, and citizenship.

birth defect — any defect that is already present when a child is born.

bites — *See snake bites, rabies, etc.*

blackhead — *See acne, comedo.*

blackout — a loss of consciousness, usually lasting only a short while, that is caused by an insufficient circulation of blood to the brain.

bladder — a sac that holds fluids. The gallbladder is discussed under its own entry. The urinary bladder is usually referred to as the bladder. It serves as the reservoir for urine.

The bladder receives urine from the kidneys through the ureter tubes (one from each kidney). Urine is stored in the bladder until the volume has stretched the bladder to an uncomfortable limit. At that point the body becomes aware of the need to urinate. Adults can, by an effort of will, refrain from urinating for a time even after the bladder has begun to send signals. However, even the strongest will cannot hold the bladder in check for long.

Either voluntarily or involuntarily, the circular muscle at the bottom of the bladder relaxes, allowing urine to pass from the bladder into the urethra and then out of the body.

The average person's bladder will hold up to a pint of urine, but the urge to urinate will be felt before that volume is reached.

The urge to urinate is caused by slight contractions of the wall of the bladder. Urination takes place when the circular muscle relaxes and the bladder contracts.

At times, it is necessary to empty the bladder artificially. This is done by inserting a catheter into the bladder.
See catheter, kidney, ureter, urethra.

bladder control — the ability to control the urge to urinate. From birth on, the bladder empties automatically. To empty it is the natural thing to do. To hold back is somewhat harder and takes training. Most babies are not ready to master such delicate timing until long past one year of age.

It is possible to lose control of the bladder through malfunction, old age, or disease. Extreme fright can also cause a momentary loss of control.

bland — a term used to describe something very mild, such as a bland diet.

blastocyte — a cell in an embryo. Blastocytes are nonspecific or primitive cells that later become more specific or differentiated.

bleeder — *See hemophilia.*

bleeding — blood escaping from the circulatory system.

The average adult body contains about five quarts of blood. One pint of blood can usually be lost without harmful effect — in fact, this is the amount usually given by blood donors. The loss of two pints of blood by an adult usually is serious, and the loss of three pints may be fatal.

The term bleeding is usually used to indicate bleeding from capillaries when blood trickles or oozes from a wound. The term hemorrhaging usually indicates bleeding from an artery or from a vein. The difference is one of degree — hemorrhaging is always serious, and if unchecked it is often fatal. Bleeding can result from a small cut or wound and will usually clot of its own accord.
See coagulation, hemorrhage.

blindness — loss of the ability to see. Blindness can be partial or total. Visual impairment may result from one or more of the following: disease, defective functioning of the various parts of the eye, defects in the shape of the eye, congenital defects, irritation, injury, and accidents.

Visual ability for distance vision is measured in terms of Snellen notations; i.e., the ability of the individual to read certain standard charts at standard test distances. Twenty feet is used for distance vision. Snellen notations are not fractions, although they are written similarly. The first figure, 20, is usually constant and indicates the distance at which the test was made. The second figure is based on the ability of the normal eye to read at various distances. A notation of 20/50 means that the eye being tested sees at twenty feet what the normal eye can see at fifty feet.

A person who is legally blind has a visual ability of 20/200 with correcting eyeglasses.

See color blindness, eyes.

blister — a collection of fluid immediately below the surface of the skin. Blisters can be caused by burns, freezing-cold temperatures, and by friction.

block — an obstruction or blockage. The term is also used to refer to an anesthesia that goes deep into the tissues but is restricted in area.

blood — the oxygen-carrying fluid that circulates throughout the body.

The normal adult of average weight has from ten to twelve pints of circulating blood. Pumped by the heart through miles of blood vessels, the blood carries oxygen, water, and food to all the cells of the body. It also serves the body as a temperature regulator, distributing heat produced by the working muscles.

The microscope shows that blood is made up of three types of cells — red cells, white cells, and platelets — all of which are suspended in a straw-colored liquid called plasma.

RED CELLS

There are about thirty trillion red cells in the bloodstream. Their main function is to carry oxygen from the lungs to all the cells in the body. On their return trip, the red cells pick up carbon dioxide and carry it to the lungs to be expelled. They repeat this cycle many times an hour (in a healthy person, with the body at rest, the heart contracts about seventy-two times a minute), traveling at high speed through the arteries and veins, some of which are smaller than the blood cells. Because of the rough life they lead, red blood cells live only about 120 days.

It is estimated that red cells are worn out and removed from circulation at the rate of ten billion an hour. In order to replace them, the bone marrow of the body must produce the same number of red cells in the same period of time. Iron is essential for red-cell building. It is supplied by the food we eat, especially meat, green-leaf vegetables, and whole-grain bread and cereals.

WHITE CELLS

White cells are among the important agents by which the body defends itself against disease. When the body is attacked by invading disease bacteria, the white cells go to work. One group destroys the bacteria by engulfing them. As many as twenty or more bacteria have been found inside a defending white cell. Another group forms a barrier in the body tissues to keep the infection from spreading.

There is only one white cell to every six hundred red cells, and they live a much shorter time — from eight to ten days.

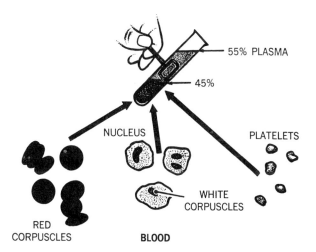

RED CORPUSCLES

NUCLEUS

55% PLASMA

45%

PLATELETS

WHITE CORPUSCLES

BLOOD

PLATELETS

Platelets are small, colorless bodies that enter the bloodstream from the bone marrow. They play an important part in the coagulation, or clotting, of blood, which is necessary to stop bleeding when injury to the body causes a blood vessel to break.

Platelets are smaller than red cells and fewer in number — about one to every ten or twenty red cells. They are believed to live only three to four days.

PLASMA

Plasma is the fluid part of the blood in which the red cells, white cells, and platelets are suspended. It is composed of ninty-two percent water and seven percent protein. The remaining one percent consists of fat, carbohydrates, and various mineral salts necessary for life. Plasma also contains essential hormones, vitamins, and enzymes in small amounts.

If the blood cells and clotting agents in plasma are allowed to combine and settle out, a clear fluid called serum remains.

ANTIBODY

When a foreign material enters the bloodstream, a substance called an antibody develops in the plasma. Any foreign matter that causes an antibody to develop is known as an antigen.

When the body is invaded by disease-producing organisms, two protective mechanisms are activated. One is the action of white cells, and the other is the development of antibodies. Antibodies protect the body from the foreign organisms by dissolving them or causing them to clump so that they cannot circulate freely through the bloodstream. Sometimes they simply inactivate the invaders so that white cells can destroy them. Antibodies develop against each type of disease-causing invader to which the body is exposed. They may remain in the blood long after the invader has been destroyed, and, for as long as they remain, the body is immune to that specific disease.

BLOOD GROUPS OR TYPES

In 1900 Dr. Karl Landsteiner of Vienna discovered that all human blood is not alike. The discovery was made in a simple experiment. Landsteiner took blood from a number of persons, separated the red cells from the plasma, and placed the cells and plasma of each person in separate test tubes. Then he took the plasma of one person and mixed it with the red cells of another. He continued to do this until he had mixed plasma from each person with red cells from each of the others.

Dr. Landsteiner found that the cells and plasma in some tubes remained mixed, just as they were when first combined. In other tubes, the cells separated from the plasma and settled to the bottom in a solid cluster or clump. By observing which plasma-cell combination clumped, he was able to divide his mixtures into four definite groups.

Dr. Landsteiner determined that the four blood groups were due to the presence of two substances in the red blood cells. He called these substances antigens A and B. The two specific antibodies to these substances, which he knew to be present in the plasma, he called a and b.

Various combinations of these substances and antibodies gave four possible blood groups:

1. Group A blood has antigen A in the red cells and antibody b in the plasma. This type of blood can be given to persons who have type A or type AB blood.

2. Group B blood has B in the red cells and antibody a in the plasma. Type B blood may be donated to people who have type B or type AB blood.

3. Group AB blood has both A and B in the red cells and neither antibody a nor b in the plasma. AB blood can only be given to people with type AB blood.

4. Group O blood has neither A nor B in the red cells and has both antibody a and b in the plasma. This blood is sometimes known as the "universal donor" for emergency purposes.

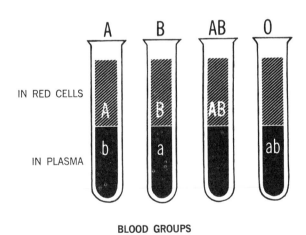

BLOOD GROUPS

It was many years before the significance of Dr. Landsteiner's discovery of differences was recognized. If the recipient of a blood transfusion belongs to a different blood group than the donor, an antigen-antibody reaction can take place. This can lead to agglutination (clumping) of the red cells, and the transfusion may be fatal. With

Dr. Landsteiner's discovery it became possible to match a donor's blood with the recipient's blood before a transfusion was given.

In the years since Dr. Landsteiner's discovery of blood groups, other differences in human blood have been discovered, including the Rh factor which Dr. Landsteiner and Dr. Wiener of New York discovered in 1940.

Blood differences such as blood groups and the Rh factor are inherited and never change.

See Rh factor.

blood chemistry — the chemical makeup of the blood. During a heart attack, the damaged heart muscle signals the degree of its distress by releasing enzymes into the bloodstream. The chemical measurement of these enzymes is most useful in determining recent heart injury. The presence of other elements indicates other factors.

blood count — a count of the number of cells (red, white, and/or platelet) in the blood used as an aid to diagnosis and as an indicator of general health. The count is made by withdrawing a small amount of blood and actually counting the cells within one cubic millimeter of the blood.

blood group — *See blood.*

bloodletting — a very old method for treating disease. It involved cutting the patient and allowing him to bleed. The idea was that the disease would leave the body with the escaping blood. It is used today in a very few cases of heart trouble to reduce the amount of blood and hence the amount of work the heart is required to do.

blood poisoning — *See septicemia.*

blood pressure — a measurement of the pressure of the blood in the arteries, usually by an instrument called a sphygmomanometer. Blood pressure is measured when the heart muscle is contracted — systolic blood pressure. Blood pressure is also measured when the heart muscle is relaxed between beats — diastolic blood pressure. Blood pressure is generally expressed by two numbers, as 120/80, the first number representing the systolic and the second the diastolic pressure.

Normal pressure varies for different people and at different times. Temperature can cause changes in blood pressure. In warm weather, the blood vessels close to the skin will dilate, tending to reduce blood pressure; in cold weather, these same blood vessels will constrict, raising the pressure. Other factors altering the blood pressure are emotions such as fear and physical conditions such as fatigue.

The brain is constantly monitoring the blood pressure. By means of the sympathetic nervous system, the brain constricts or dilates blood vessels to help keep the blood pressure as close to normal as possible.

HIGH BLOOD PRESSURE

High blood pressure, or hypertension, is a common disorder that shows up in the heart and blood vessels of the body. In itself, high blood pressure is not a disease, but it is a sign that something is wrong. If the blood pressure remains consistently high for a long period of time, however, it can result in serious damage to the heart, the kidneys, and other organs of the body.

What causes high blood pressure is still a medical mystery. For some unknown reason, the tiny branches of the arteries (arterioles) that carry blood to all the tissues of the body begin to tighten up. The passageway for blood becomes smaller, and the heart has to work harder to push the blood through to the tissues. After a time, the walls of the blood vessels toughen and lose their elasticity, and the heart muscle thickens because of the extra work load.

The heart, however, is a remarkably tough organ, and normal arteries are strong enough to withstand tremendous pressures. Hence, high blood pressure rarely means a sudden breakdown in either the heart or arteries. Rather, the chief risk is that if pressure continues to be high for a long period of time, the walls of the blood vessels will toughen. When the blood-vessel walls do toughen, blood pressure may remain high.

There seems to be some connection between high blood pressure and the tensions of modern living. People who work under constant strain or who worry too much over unsolved problems are often susceptible. Heredity is probably a factor. The condition occurs most often in persons between thirty and fifty.

Symptoms are not a reliable guide to the presence of high blood pressure. There are probably millions of people in the United States who have high blood pressure and don't know they have it. There may be no symptoms at all, or there may be symptoms such as headaches and dizziness. But these can also be symptoms of other conditions.

Science has not yet found any one reliable treatment for high blood pressure, but in recent years there have been very encouraging results from drugs, surgery, psychotherapy, and special diets. Which treatment is used depends on the particular patient, and only a doctor can advise the right prescription.

LOW BLOOD PRESSURE

Low blood pressure hardly ever causes trouble. The number of people in whom low blood pressure is a serious and dangerous condition is comparatively small. When it does occur, it is generally a symptom of some specific disease which can, in most cases, be treated successfully.

See hypertension.

blood tests — there are many different kinds of blood tests. Some of them are performed to determine the patient's blood group, others determine whether or not the patient has a particular infection. Other tests show what enzymes have been released into the blood. Blood tests are among the most important diagnostic aids a physician uses.

blood transfusion — a technique for replacing a patient's lost, diseased, or ineffective blood with fresh blood from a healthy donor. Before a blood transfusion, both the patient's blood and the donor's blood are tested to be sure that their blood-group types are compatible.

blood vessels — the vessels that carry blood throughout the body. There are three major blood-vessel types: arteries, capillaries, and veins.

Arteries carry oxygen and food away from the heart. The major artery, the aorta, branches off into smaller arteries. These branches divide and subdivide until they become very small and terminate in threadlike vessels known as capillaries. The smallest arteries are called arterioles.

In the capillaries the oxygen and food are exchanged for carbon dioxide and waste products. After the exchange, the blood returns to the heart by means of the third type of vessel — the veins. The smallest veins, called venules, receive blood from the capillaries and pass it on to larger veins, which then join until the very largest veins are formed, returning blood to the heart.

See artery, capillary, vein.

blotch — a spot, usually red or pink. There are any number of causes, including measles.

blue baby — a term applied to a baby born with a blue tinge to the skin, called cyanosis. The condition is caused by insufficient oxygen in the blood. This often indicates a heart defect but may have other causes, such as premature birth or impaired respiration.

See congenital heart defects.

BMR — abbreviation for basal metabolic rate.

See basal metabolism.

boil — a small abscess caused by infection that is usually located in a hair follicle. At first it appears as a hard red bump below the skin surface. As it grows, it becomes more pointed and develops a white head. This breaks open, allowing collected pus to escape. A few days after this happens, the hard core of the boil will come out. The remaining cavity will usually fill out with normal tissue.

bone — a highly specialized type of connective tissue that forms the rigid framework designed to bear body weight, provide fixed points for muscle action, and protect vital portions of the body.

Bone is composed of calcium, phosphorus, other mineral salts, and an inorganic substance called ossein. When a human bone is soaked in acid until all the inorganic mineral salts are washed out, all that remains is a flexible piece of tissue which can be bent and twisted without difficulty. Bone, therefore, depends on inorganic mineral salts such as calcium and phosphorus for its strength and hardness.

Bone structure consists of a hard outer shell and an inner spongy and porous center. The center is called a medullary canal and contains the marrow. There are two types of marrow — red and yellow. Yellow marrow is ordinary bone marrow in which fat cells predominate; red marrow is the manufacturing center of the red (and some of the white) blood cells of the body. When the body is actively engaged in growing, all bones produce red and white blood cells. However, when the body reaches adult size, only certain bones still produce these cells.

At the ends of the long bones is a smooth, glossy tissue which forms the joint surfaces. This tissue is called articular cartilage because these surfaces articulate with, fit into, or move in contact with similar surfaces of other bones.

The thin outer membrane around bone, called periosteum, is important in the nourishment of bone. Capillaries and blood vessels flow through the periosteum and send branches into the substance of the bone to supply it with blood. It is from the periosteum that new bone is formed. This area also has highly sensitive nerves which make it the pain center of the bone. In cases of fractures, the pain sensation arises from the periosteum and not from the bone itself.

Bone is both hard and elastic. Two-thirds of the bone is mineral matter (lime salts) to give it hardness; one-third is organic matter that contains protein to give it elasticity. A child's bones contain more organic matter than an adult's and are therefore more flexible and not so readily broken. As age increases, however, the proportion of mineral matter increases and bones become more brittle and more easily broken.

There are 206 distinct bones in the human adult body. In a child there are more, but in later life some of the bones fuse or become joined.

booster inoculations — shots given at intervals to maintain a level of immunity. Booster inoculations are usually given for diphtheria, whooping cough, tetanus, and polio.
See DPT, polio.

boric acid — a mild germicide used as an ointment for burns and minor skin infections, as a dusting powder, in solutions for mouthwash, and as an irrigating solution.
Despite its mildness, boric acid can be poisonous in large doses.

Bornholm disease — *See epidemic pleurodynia.*

bottle-feeding — the nourishment a child takes at the beginning of his life when he is not breast-fed.
Milk, other than breast milk, has to be specially prepared to make it suitable for feeding babies. Water and sugar, or another carbohydrate, are added. It is frequently heated to make it more digestible. This mixture is called a formula.

botulism — a very serious type of food poisoning. Botulism is caused by the toxin from the bacteria *Clostridium botulinum.* Botulism is usually the result of eating contaminated foods from cans. The bacteria that cause botulism are anaerobic. This means that they grow only in an oxygen-free atmosphere. Therefore, canned foods provide an ideal growing place for them.

The bacteria are usually killed by high temperatures during the cooking process. However, when they are not killed before being sealed in a can, they multiply within the can.

In recent years consumers have been cautioned against buying any can that is bulging outward. Symptoms of botulism include vomiting, stomach pain, impaired vision, etc.

bovine tuberculosis — a severely crippling bone and gland disease caused by dairy cows. Scofula, large masses of neck glands, and hunched backs resulting from infected vertebrae were symptomatic of the disease. Bovine tuberculosis can be transmitted by raw milk. The disease is very rare today because regular testing of cattle for tuberculosis and the removal of any infected animals from the rest of the herd is now required by law.

bowel — *See intestine.*

bowleg — a leg that curves outward, usually below the knee.

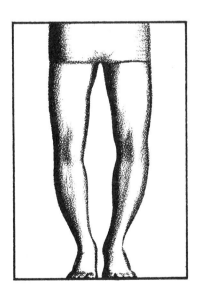

BOWLEG

brachial — of or pertaining to the arm.

bradycardia — an abnormally slow heart rate. Generally, anything below sixty beats per minute is considered bradycardia.

brain — the nerve tissue situated in the cranium. The brain is almost entirely enclosed in the skull, but it is connected with the spinal column. The brain has two major divisions: the cerebrum and the cerebellum.

The cerebrum occupies nearly all of the cranial cavity. It is divided into two hemispheres by a deep cleft. The outer surface is sometimes called "gray matter" because the nuclei of nerve cells make it appear gray in color. Beneath this layer are connective axons or nerve fibers that form the medulla or central portion of the brain. This is called "white matter" because the fat cells that protect it are white in color. The cortex or surface of the brain is thrown into folds called convolutions that are separated from each other by grooves or fissures.

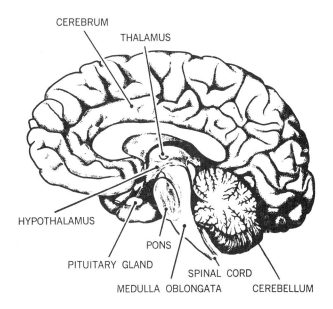

CEREBRUM
THALAMUS
HYPOTHALAMUS
PONS
PITUITARY GLAND
SPINAL CORD
MEDULLA OBLONGATA
CEREBELLUM

BRAIN

Certain areas of the cerebrum are localized for certain functions, including those concerned with sensation; thought, associative memory that allows the brain to store, recall, and make use of past experiences; and the initiation or management of those motions that are said to be "under the control of the will."

The cerebellum is situated beneath the rear or back portion of the cerebrum. It is chiefly concerned with bringing balance, harmony, and coordination to the motions initiated by the cerebrum.

Two smaller divisions of the brain, vital to life, are the pons and the medulla oblongata. The pons consists chiefly of a mass of fibers connecting the other three parts of the brain — the cerebrum, the cerebellum, and the medulla oblongata. It acts as a bridge between the members; its name is the Latin word for bridge.

The medulla oblongata is the lowest portion of the brain, the last division before the beginning of the spinal cord. In it are the centers for the control of heart action, breathing, circulation, and other vital processes such as the control of body temperature.

Inside the brain are small cavities, the ventricles, which contain cerebrospinal fluid. The outer surface of the brain is covered with three layers of membranes collectively called the meninges. The three layers of the meninges are the dura mater, pia mater, and arachnoid.

Cerebrospinal fluid is formed by a network of blood vessels in the central ventricles of the brain. It is a clear, watery solution similar to blood plasma. The total quantity in the cerebrospinal system ranges from 100 to 150 ml., and the amount produced daily may range up to several liters. This fluid is constantly being produced and reabsorbed. It circulates over the surface of the brain and spinal cord and serves as a protective cushion as well as a means of exchange of food and waste materials.

The central nervous system is much like a great telegraph system. The brain is its central office; the spinal cord and ganglia are substations; the nerve trunks are cables. The nerve fibers are like separate wires making connections in or between the central office and the substations, or going out to all parts of the body. Like the office of the telegraph system, the brain may send out orders in response to messages it receives. It also has the power to send out orders without first receiving messages.

See cerebellum, cerebrum, hypothalamus, medulla oblongata, pons, thalamus.

break — *See fracture.*

breast-feeding — feeding a newborn child with human milk from the mother's breast. It is probably the safest and most desirable way to nourish a child, because nobody has ever improved on the formula that the breast secretes to nourish the baby. However, breast-feeding should not be relied on exclusively for complete nutrition for much longer than the first four months of life.

Even breast-fed infants require supplementation with vitamin D and need additional iron early in life.

The decision to feed a baby by bottle or breast is a personal one for the mother and her family. However, the use of breast-feeding seems to run in cycles. At times it is very popular; at other times it is out of favor.

For a few days after a child's birth, the mother's breast secretes a yellowish liquid called colostrum. This is gradually replaced by the more typical whitish milk. Milk from the breast does not look like cow's milk. It is more watery-looking and bluish. But this does not mean it is not "rich" enough.

breasts — the mammary glands. Both males and females have breasts. The major difference is that the female breast develops to the point where it is capable of producing and secreting milk to feed a newborn child. The male breast is usually flat, with a slightly raised nipple. The normal female breast grows as it develops, until it is shaped like a comma. However, the size and shape depend on heredity and weight. The weight of the individual is a factor because of the amount of fat tissue found in the adult female breast.

BREAST CANCER

Cancer of the breast is extremely rare in children and occurs only occasionally in men. Most cases are found in women after the age of forty-five, when numerous changes taking place in the body in some way affect the breast. Among American women, breast cancer occurs more often than any other form of cancer. Over 65,000 new cases are diagnosed annually.

Surgery and radiation are both used for the treatment of breast cancer. In some cases only one of these methods is preferred. In others the doctor may use both.

Most women whose cancer is believed to be confined to the breast undergo an operation known as a mastectomy (removal of the breast). This operation is performed in a manner designed to prevent or arrest spread of the disease.

A precaution surgeons sometimes take following mastectomy is to apply radiation to the site of operation in order to destroy any cancer cells that surgery alone might not have been able to remove.

Radiotherapy (treatment by radiation) is used alone in very special cases. It is also sometimes used before surgery to reduce the size of breast tumors that are to be removed.

At the time of breast surgery, or later, the patient's ovaries may be removed. These organs are the principal source of female sex hormones affecting the growth of breast tissue. Also, synthetic hormones developed in the laboratory are often beneficial in treating breast cancer.

There are no known causes of breast cancer. Perhaps because this form of cancer has been so long recognized, notions that are really "old wives' tales" have often been accepted as facts. Many a patient, when examined, mentions a blow to the breast and believes that this is related to the subsequent development of a tumor. Scientists agree that a single injury, such as a blow, has never been proved to produce breast cancer. It is possible that such an injury simply attracted a patient's attention to her breast and she then felt a tumor that was already there but had not been noticed before.

There is some evidence that daughters or sisters of breast-cancer patients run a somewhat greater risk of developing the disease than women in whose families there is no history of this malignancy. Scientists do not yet know to what extent this is true and just what role family relationship may play. Statistical studies also suggest that the risk of developing breast cancer is lower for married women than for single women and lower still for married women who have borne children.

breast self-examination — a woman herself is often the first to discover a lump in her breast. Because most women see a doctor no more than once a year, many doctors believe that every woman should learn to examine her breasts regularly at the end of each menstrual period.

breathing — the process of bringing air into the lungs and removing carbon dioxide from the lungs.

Breathing is an act over which we exert little control. It occurs in the healthy adult from twelve to fifteen times a minute when the body is at rest, but the rate per minute may be increased by exercise, labor, and a number of other causes. The amount of air entering and leaving the lungs during each respiration varies, as does the rate of breathing, according to whether the person is at rest or engaged in work or exercise. At rest,

61

adults breathe twenty-five to thirty cubic inches of air per respiration, whereas during strenuous effort the amount may be increased by several times that breathed when at rest.

Breathing consists of two separate acts — inspiration (an enlargement of the chest cavity with a lowering of the pressure within the cavity), during which air is drawn into the lungs; and expiration (a lessening of the chest cavity and increasing of the pressure within the cavity), during which air is driven out of the lungs. In inspiration, which is chiefly a muscular act, the ribs are raised, and the arch of the diaphragm falls and becomes flattened, increasing the capacity of the chest cavity and tending to produce a vacuum, causing air to enter. In expiration, an act performed with slight muscular action, the ribs fall to their normal position, the arch of the diaphragm rises (lessening the capacity of the chest cavity), and air is forced out.

breech presentation — a baby born buttocks or feet first. Most babies are born head first. This is the easiest way, for a baby's head is the biggest part of its body and can be molded into a narrow, slightly elongated shape. When the baby is not in the head-first position, the birth can be more difficult for both mother and baby. However, a doctor is often able to turn the baby before he is born, so that the head will come first.

Bright, Richard — an English physician (1789-1858) who demonstrated the association of heart disease with kidney disease.

Bright's disease — any malfunction of the kidney in which there is also edema and the presence of protein is detected in the urine. Named after Richard Bright (1789-1858), an English physician.
See nephritis.

broad-spectrum antibiotic — any antibiotic that is effective against many different types of bacteria.

broken bones — *See fractures.*

bromide — any one of several drugs that produce a calming effect. Bromides are classified as sedatives or hypnotics.

For many years they were used in the treatment of epilepsy. Today, however, less-toxic drugs are used in most cases. However, bromides are still used in some difficult cases of epilepsy.

bronchi — the large bronchial tubes.

bronchial tubes — the large tubes (bronchi) that lead from the windpipe and carry the air that has been breathed in through the mouth and nose. These large tubes divide into smaller and smaller ones (bronchioles) until they are the size of small threads. Each one ends in a tiny air space. Here, the air comes into close contact with the thin-walled capillaries which carry blood through the lungs. The tiny air spaces and the lung capillaries make up a very important area. It is here that oxygen from the air enters the blood. In this same area, waste gas (carbon dioxide) is removed from the lungs and breathed out.

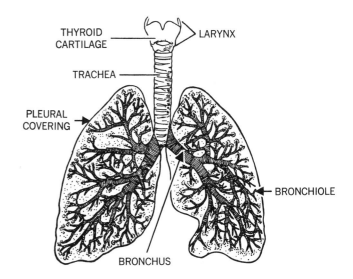

BRONCHIAL TUBES

The choked breathing of the asthma sufferer is caused by a narrowing of the small bronchial tubes during the asthma attack. This may be caused by swelling of the membrane that lines the tubes, by spasm of the tubes, or by mucus plugging the tubes.
See asthma, bronchitis.

bronchioles — the small branches of the bronchial tubes. Some are so small that they are the size of fine threads.

bronchitis — an inflammation of the bronchial tubes caused by a viral or bacterial infection.

Chronic bronchitis is a serious lung disease that impairs the ability to breathe. It causes irritation, inflammation, and eventual obstruction of the bronchial tubes leading to the lungs.

In chronic bronchitis, there is persistent inflammation of the smaller air tubes in the lungs (bronchioles). The onset of the disease may be slow, at first assumed to be "smoker's cough" ar a "winter cold." By the time the patient realizes something is wrong, the delicate lung tissue may be damaged.

The moist linings of the bronchial airways are protected by millions of tiny hair-like cilia, which sway along the surface of the linings. Mucous secretions bathe these linings. The cilia sweep foreign particles and excessive secretions upward through the windpipe and out of the lungs.

If the airway linings are constantly irritated by tobacco smoke and other air pollutants or are infected with viruses and bacteria, the cilia can become paralyzed or even be destroyed. The irritation can cause over-secretion of mucus, and the flow of air through the branches of the bronchial tubes can become obstructed.

Exactly why chronic bronchitis occurs is uncertain. There appears to be a susceptibility in certain people which makes them unable to withstand continued lung irritation. The link between cigarette-smoking and chronic bronchitis is very strong. When chronic cough and shortness of breath appear, cigarette-smoking compounds the irritation.

Long-term exposure to dusts, fumes, and similar lung irritants in polluted air, and repeated chest colds, influenza, allergies, or other respiratory illnesses irritate delicate lung tissue. The damaging spiral of chronic cough, excessive mucous secretions, and shortness of breath develops. It is also believed that chronic bronchitis may lead to emphysema.

See bronchial tubes.

bronchodilator — a drug or agent that helps the air passages of the lungs to expand, allowing freer breathing.

bronchopleuropneumonia — a case of pneumonia that is complicated by bronchitis and pleurisy at the same time.

bronchopneumonia — *See pneumonia.*

bronchorrhagia — hemorrhaging in the bronchial tubes.

bronchoscope — a lighted tube used to examine the bronchial tubes.

bronchus — *See bronchial tubes.*

brucellosis — a contagious disease of animals; it can be transmitted to humans. Fairly widespread throughout the world among cattle, hogs, goats, and sheep, the disease is caused by *Brucella* bacteria that live in some of these animals. Many farmers know brucellosis as Bang's disease, or contagious abortion. In humans, the disease was formerly called undulant fever because the fever that accompanies it undulates, or comes and goes in waves. Infected hogs are the cause of most of the brucellosis in the United States, although sheep and goats spread the disease more in other parts of the world.

Anyone can get the disease. Most cases, however, are among people who work on hog farms and in meat-packing or meat-processing plants. The infection rate in some areas is estimated to reach as high as twenty percent of the hog producers. A few cases occur among families who drink unpasteurized milk.

SYMPTOMS
Brucellosis in humans may begin in several ways. Some patients have a general feeling of tiredness and possibly a slight fever without being aware they have the disease. Others may have a sudden onset of chills, night sweats, pain in the joints, nervousness, and fever that comes and goes.

The disease may last only a few days, several weeks, or many years, depending on the severity of the case. Patients usually recover but are sometimes disabled. Recovery from the disease does not always mean that the patient will not get the disease again. In some cases, he may have a flare-up of his earlier symptoms — which is actually an allergic response to contact with the *Brucella* organism. Less than two percent of brucellosis patients die from the disease.

PREVENTION
Brucellosis is prevented in several related ways. Public health officials maintain rigid inspection programs in meat-processing plants to prevent the spread of the disease. They work to educate farmers, packinghouse and slaughterhouse workers, butchers, and milk-processing-plant workers about the dangers of handling infected materials. Veterinarians

periodically examine livestock herds to search for infected animals and segregate them from the herd. Infection among hogs generally requires slaughter of the entire herd.

To protect the human population against brucellosis-infected milk, all milk sold in many cities and towns must be pasteurized. When only raw milk is obtainable, it is wise to boil it before drinking it.

Because the bacteria that cause the disease are readily killed by normal cooking temperatures, humans cannot contract brucellosis by eating cooked meat products. Smoked ham, generally processed at high temperatures by modern meat-processing methods, cannot transmit the disease.

Bruce's septicemia — *See brucellosis.*

bruise — the most frequent injury suffered. Bruises are responsible for the discolorations that almost always accompany injuries to bones, joints, and muscles. Bruises (also called contusions) are caused by some blunt instrument or object striking the body or by the body coming in contact with a hard object, as in a fall or bump. Usually, the skin is not broken, but the soft tissues beneath the skin are injured. Small blood vessels are ruptured, causing blood to seep into the surrounding tissues. This produces swelling, at first red but later turning darker — to a blue or purple discoloration. Finally, perhaps several days later, the skin is yellowish or greenish in color. The bruised area is usually very tender. If a larger blood vessel is broken, much blood gathers under the skin, causing greater swelling and discoloration.

The symptoms of bruises are immediate pain from injury to the nerves; swelling; rapid discoloration; and, later, pain on pressure or movement. A bruise may be only the external evidence of a more serious injury to deep-lying structures.

The treatment should attempt to limit swelling and decrease pain. Apply cold applications, such as an ice bag or a towel wrung out in cold water. Elevate the injured part, and place it at complete rest. Make sure there is no other injury, such as a broken bone or dislocation. Severe bruises should have the care of a physician.

bruxism — grinding the teeth.

bubo — a swelling from infection that occurs in a lymph gland (especially in the groin area). Bubos are often a symptom of gonorrhea or syphilis.

bubonic plague — plague with bubos (swollen lymph nodes).
   See plague.

Buerger's disease — an inflammation of the blood vessels, frequently affecting the legs. The inflammation obstructs the flow of blood and can lead to gangrene.

Buerger's disease, also called thromboangiitis obliterans, seems to be a disease of young men.

bundle of His — a bundle of specialized muscle fibers running from a small mass of muscular fibers (atrioventricular node) between the upper chambers of the heart, down to the lower chambers. It is the only known direct muscular connection between the upper and lower heart chambers and serves to conduct impulses for the rhythmic heartbeat from the atrioventricular node to the heart muscle. It is named after Wilhelm His, a German anatomist, and is also called the auriculoventricular bundle, the atrioventricular bundle, or the A-V bundle.

bunion — a deformity or swelling of the joint of the big toe caused by unnatural pressure from shoes that do not fit properly. As a result of the pressure, the sac that covers the joint becomes swollen and forces the toe out of position. An extremely deformed joint may require minor surgery.

burn — an injury caused by dry heat, fire, heated objects, electricity, friction, hot solutions, steam and vapors, and chemicals such as strong acids or strong alkalis. Burns more commonly are the result of contact with dry heat, electricity, friction, and chemicals, whereas scalds more commonly are the result of contact with hot solutions, hot vapors, or steam. Electricity may cause burns either by current passing through the body or by electric flashes.

Dry skin offers about twenty times more resistance than moist skin to the passage of electric current; when the skin is dry, therefore, the local heating effects (burns) are greater, even though the total damage to the body is less than when the skin is wet.

It should be noted that burns and scalds are essentially the same type of heat injury. When the injury is caused by dry heat, it is called a burn; when caused by moist heat, it is called a scald. Treatment is the same in both cases.

CLASSIFICATION OF BURNS

Burns are classified in several ways: by the extent of the burned surface, by the depth of the burn, and by the cause of the burn. Of these, the extent of body surface burned is the most important factor in determining the seriousness of the burn and plays the greatest role in the patient's chances for survival.

1. Extent of burned surface

In calculating the extent of burned surface, the rule of nines is used. These figures aid in determining the correct treatment for the burned person. Shock can be expected in adults with burns of over fifteen percent or in small children with burns of over ten percent of body surface area. In adults, burns involving more than twenty percent endanger life, and thirty-percent burns are usually fatal if adequate medical treatment is not received.

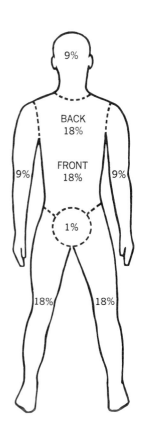

RULE OF NINE

2. Depth of injury

The depth of injury to the tissues is spoken of in degrees.

   a. First-degree burns are the mildest, producing redness, increased warmth, tenderness, and mild pain.

   b. Second-degree burns redden and blister the skin and are characterized by severe pain.

   c. Third-degree burns destroy the skin and may destroy muscle tissue and bone in severe cases. Severe pain may be absent because nerve endings have been destroyed. The color may vary from white and lifeless (scalds) to black (charred from gasoline explosions).

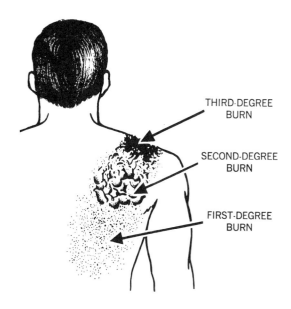

DEGREE OF BURNS

It is important to remember that the size of the burned area may be far more important than the depth of the burn. A first-degree or second-degree burn that covers a very large area of the body is almost always more serious than a small third-degree burn. A first-degree sunburn, for example, can cause death if a very large area of the body is burned.

3. Cause of burn

The cause of a burn is generally classified as thermal (heat) or chemical, or as resulting from sunburn, electric shock, or radiation. Whatever the cause of the burn, shock always results if the burns are extensive.

TREATMENT OF BURNS

First aid for all burns involves the following

main items: relieve pain, prevent or treat shock, and prevent infection.

In electric shock, the burn may have to be temporarily ignored while resuscitative measures are performed. Otherwise, the treatment is the same as for heat burns. Also, local treatment for chemical burns varies, depending on the agent that caused the burn.

As an emergency measure, ice water provides immediate relief from pain and also seems to lessen the damaging effects of burns.

Second- and third-degree burns are, in effect, open wounds and must be covered to reduce the possibility of infection. Every effort should be made to use a sterile covering. Ointments and other medicines should not be used on these burn wounds. Using these agents may make later treatment by a physician difficult or impossible.

bursa — a small sac of specialized tissue containing a viscous fluid. Bursae are located at various places in the body where friction would ordinarily occur between skin and bone, tendon or ligament and bone, or between muscles. Bursae may become inflamed (bursitis), and movements then elicit pain. There are three principal places where bursae are located. The subdeltoid bursa is situated in the shoulder between the deltoid muscle and the head of the humerus. The prepatellar bursa is found in the front of the kneecap. The olecranon bursa is located in the elbow between the bone and the skin.

bursitis — a condition in which a bursa becomes inflamed. Bursitis, which in some lines of work is an occupational hazard, can be quite painful. *See bursa.*

buttocks — the rounded portion of the lower back which joins the thighs. The buttocks are usually padded with fat to protect them from the pressure and weight they must withstand when the body is seated.

B vitamins — See vitamin B.

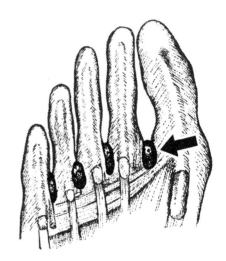

BURSAE

C

cacation — defecation.

cachexia — general physical decline and loss of weight, usually resulting from chronic disease.

cachinnation — a state characterized by excessive hysterical laughter.

cacomelia — deformity of a limb. Cacomelia is congenital.

cacotrophy — malnutrition.

cadaver — a dead body. They are used to help teach anatomy to medical students.

Caesalpinus, Andreas (1519-1603) — first to use the term "circulation" in connection with the movement of blood. However, he still believed in many of the classical theories taught by Galen.

caffeine — an odorless, bitter compound found in coffee and tea. It is used as a stimulant, a diuretic, and in the treatment of migraine headaches.

cal. — abbreviation for calorie.

calamine — a compound of zinc oxide and ferric oxide applied to the skin to soothe itching. Also used as an astringent.

calcaneus — the largest bone in the foot — also known as the heel bone.

calcification — a hardening of organic tissue caused by a deposit of calcium salts.
   See calcium.

calcitonin — a recently discovered hormone that seems to have the opposite effect of parathyroid hormone.

calcium — a yellow metal found in various compound forms in the body. One calcium compound forms the hard part of bones and teeth. Another is active in blood-clotting.

   Calcium is one of the elements the body can store. A deficiency of calcium weakens the bones and can lead to rickets. A surplus of calcium can lead to deposits of calcium in tissues other than bone.

   The best dietary source of calcium is milk; however, a well-balanced diet will supply the minimum requirements of calcium.

calculus — an abnormal, insoluble mass that can form in hollow body organs such as the gallbladder, bile ducts, kidneys, and bladder.
   See gallstones.

callosity — a thickening and hardening of the skin caused by friction, pressure, or other irritation.

callus — a callosity. The term is also used to refer to a substance formed around fragments of broken bone; it is eventually replaced by hard bone.

calomel — mercurous chloride. At one time calomel was a very widely used purgative; however, its purgative effects are now felt to be uncertain, and other drugs are safer. At present calomel has no valid use.

calorie — a unit of heat.

1. Large calorie (abbr. Cal.) — the amount of heat needed to raise the temperature of one kilogram of water one degree centigrade.

2. Small calorie (abbr. cal.) — the amount of heat needed to raise one gram of water one degree centigrade.

See diet, energy.

camphor — a compound extracted from the wood and bark of the camphor tree. It is used locally as a liniment to relieve itching and also as an analgesic. Camphor is an ingredient of paregoric and has been used for centuries by the Chinese for a variety of medical purposes.

camphor test — test for liver disease. When camphor is given orally, glycuronic acid will appear in the urine. Absence of this reaction indicates a disease of the liver.

canal — a narrow passage through which a substance moves or flows — such as the birth canal.

cancer — a malignant disease characterized by abnormal, uncontrolled cell growth.

Normal growth is a process that takes place when cells reproduce themselves by dividing in a regulated manner to build tissue in the growing individual, to replace worn-out cells in maintaining body structure and function, and to repair damaged tissue. If this damage is too great, or if it involves cells that are unable to divide, special connective-tissue cells complete the repair by forming scar tissue. Both in the development of an individual from a fertilized egg and in the process of healing, the remarkable feature is that the cells "know" when to stop dividing. The orderly nature of this growth distinguishes normal cells from cancer cells.

In abnormal growth, cells reproduce without constructive purpose, building up into masses of tissue called tumors, which compress, invade, and destroy adjacent normal tissues.

Tumors that do not invade or spread to adjacent tissues are called benign, because they usually do not endanger life.

Malignant tumors, such as cancer, always endanger life. They choke out normal tissue as they extend to adjacent tissue layers. They may also spread to other parts of the body. New growths thus related to the original tumor are called metastases. Cancerous cells can spread throughout the body via the blood and lymph systems.

Normally, the circulatory lymph systems are a part of the body's defense against infection, but, in the case of cancer, they serve as conduits for its spread.

TYPES

Malignant tumors are divided into two main classes: carcinomas, which develop in the lining and covering tissues of organs; and sarcomas, which develop in the connective and supportive tissues of the body. Bone cancers are sarcomas.

Sometimes cancer cells do not form tumors but instead affect the blood-forming tissues of the body and cause a form of cancer known as leukemia.

At the present time at least one hundred different types of cancer have been classified by their appearance under the microscope and by the site of the body in which they arise. Some of these grow very slowly and destroy neighboring tissue by limited spread. Others spread rapidly to distant sites.

Scientists know a great deal about some cancers and can prevent their occurrence. However, their knowledge regarding the cause of many cancers is still entirely lacking.

Cancer cells do not necessarily appear strikingly different from normal cells. The body's normal repair (regeneration) of damaged tissue may for a limited time look quite "wild" in appearance under the microscope. On the other hand, a tumor that could be fatal if located in a vital area, such as the brain, can seem benign or innocent in microscopic appearance. Again, although cancer tissues are generally characterized by a rapid growth rate, cell division and tissue growth in normal pregnancy may proceed at a greater pace. The most important difference is that the normal process stops when it has reached its end point, as in the healing of a cut or the completion of a pregnancy, whereas the cancerous process is uncontrolled.

CAUSES

Most investigators do not believe that exposure to any one agent, by itself, causes all cancers of a specific type. They point out that not everyone exposed to a cancer-causing agent (carcinogen) develops cancer. They think that multiple factors and one's degree of immunity may determine whether the exposed person will develop the disease.

However, there are some agents that frequently do produce cancer.

1. Industrial chemicals

Working in laboratories, chemists have manufactured several hundred pure chemicals that produce cancer in animals. The air in a limited area such as a mine or industrial plant is sometimes polluted by specific substances. If certain of these, such as dust, arsenic, coal tar, pitch, soot, carbon black, and asbestos, are inhaled or absorbed in enough concentration for a long time, they may result in cancer.

Chemical carcinogens include many types of compounds that act in different ways. Some produce cancers at the site of contact, perhaps by direct, specific injury to the cells. Others produce cancers at distant sites. Some are incomplete or weak in their action and need the action of other chemicals in order to induce tumors.

2. Environmental hazards (pollution)

Growing attention to environmental hazards in a pollution-conscious era has brought to light potential hazards in new combinations of chemicals and cruder products to which many people are exposed. These combinations include drugs, food additives, cosmetics, and insecticides, as well as smoke and residue of all kinds from industrial and consumer "air pollution."

The Food and Drug Administration of the United States Department of Health, Education and Welfare conducts and evaluates tests for carcinogenic activity of such compounds. Laws administered by the Food and Drug Administration prohibit the addition of any amount of known cancer-producing chemicals to food.

Mold and bacteria growing naturally on food products used by man may represent one source of environmental carcinogens. For example, recent research has shown that strains of a common mold that grow on wet peanuts and corn make compounds called aflatoxin. When fed to rats, these compounds produce cancer of the liver.

Hazards to which industrial groups are exposed also have some implications for the general population. For example, air pollution from industrial wastes and automobile exhausts represent a potentially important source of carcinogens. When the air contains impurities, our lungs ordinarily are rid of them by coughing or by more complicated processes within the lining of the bronchial tubes or lung tissue. However, excessive or continuous exposure to inhaled impurities brings about changes in the bronchial linings and the lungs; these changes may eventually result in disability and illnesses. If the impurities contain cancer-producing substances, prolonged exposure can lead to cancer.

3. Radiation

In the 1890's, German scientists felt that excessive exposure to sunlight was related to skin cancer. In 1928 English investigators produced skin cancer in experimental animals by exposing them to intense sunlight.

The cancer-producing effects of the ultraviolet rays of sunlight appear to be limited to the skin. It has been observed that the incidence of skin cancer is highest in the southern and western parts of the United States and lowest in the north and is related to the amount of sunshine in the area. Furthermore, skin cancer occurs more frequently among people who work outdoors, such as sailors and farmers, than among people who can guard themselves against excessive exposure to the sun.

Related to the cancer-causing effects of sunlight was the discovery of the cancer-producing effects of ionizing radiation from radium and X-rays. This discovery was actually made on human beings. Pioneer radiologists developed dryness, ulcers, and, eventually, cancer of the hands. In 1910, a French worker produced skin cancer in a rat following application of radium to the skin.

Ionizing radiation can cause several forms of cancer. Radiologists and others exposed to increased doses of radiation are more likely to develop leukemia than are people not so exposed. Information obtained in studies of the survivors of the atomic bombs on Hiroshima and Nagasaki leaves no doubt that a single radiation exposure at high dosage can produce leukemia in man.

Radium salts deposited in bone give rise to cancers of the bone. A tragic example of this was the death from bone cancer of factory women who used their lips to point the brushes they used in painting watch dials with radium.

Ironically, radiation is one of the techniques used by scientists to cure or retard cancer.

4. Viruses

Government scientists at the National Institutes of Health have succeeded in isolating from mouse leukemia tissue another agent that produced salinary-gland cancer in mice. After the agent had been grown in tissue culture, it produced many different types of tumors, not only in mice, but in several other rodents. This "polyoma" (or many-tumor) virus removed all previous doubts about virus research in cancer. The question of viruses as a cause of human cancer has assumed new significance.

Today, in various animal species, at least a dozen types of cancer have been shown to be caused by viruses. Considerable knowledge has been obtained of the structure and chemical composition of these viruses. Recent studies on the structure of animal cells are beginning to reveal what takes place when viruses invade cells.

Under the electron microscope, particles that resemble animal cancer viruses have been found in blood or tissue preparations from persons with various forms of cancer. But such evidence is insufficient. The mere presence of viruses does not prove they caused the disease. Such particles could be contaminants unrelated to the cancer process.

It is possible that some human cancers will be found to be caused by viruses and that such discoveries may lead to the development of protective vaccines. However, there is no scientific evidence that any type of human cancer is "catching"; that is, that it can be transmitted from a cancer patient to others by contact or direct means of infection.

5. Cigarette-smoking

Chemists have isolated and identified at least a dozen carcinogenic chemicals of the hydrocarbon type in the "tars" from tobacco smoke.

The membranes lining the lungs absorb cancer-producing chemicals from tobacco smoke. The protective mechanisms by which the lungs rid themselves of impurities are first paralyzed and then destroyed by tobacco smoke. Prolonged exposure of animals to tobacco smoke produces changes in cells that resemble early stages of cancer development.

While cigarette-smoking is a major cause of lung cancer, other uses of tobacco are associated with cancers of the oral cavity among cigar-smokers, and cancer of the lip among pipe-smokers.

In 1964, an expert committee appointed by the Surgeon General of the United States Public Health Service to assess the hazards of smoking concluded:

"Cigarette smoking is causally related to lung cancer in men, far outweighing all other factors. The data for women point in the same direction.

The risk of developing lung cancer is greater for pipe- and cigar-smokers than for nonsmokers, but much less than for cigarette smokers."

TREATMENT

There are three major ways to cure or arrest cancer: surgery, radiation, and chemotherapy. Frequently, a combination of two or three methods is used to help a patient.

1. Surgery

Surgical removal of internal cancers became possible after different forms of anesthesia were developed and the necessity for maintaining sterile procedures in operating was understood. Further improvements of surgical techniques and the introduction of blood transfusions and antibiotics have now made it possible for surgeons to operate on all areas of the human body.

A cancer is operable if it is fairly localized. However, once the original cancer has spread to other areas of the body, surgery loses its effectiveness. Therefore, in operating on cancer, a surgeon will attempt to remove every cancerous cell. This is based on the fact that all the descendants of a cell in which a malignant change has taken place continue to be malignant.

2. Radiation

Treatment by radiation makes use of various forms of ionizing radiation, including X-rays. It is often used after surgery to kill any remaining cancerous cells.

3. Chemotherapy

Chemotherapy is treatment by drugs. It is used when tumors cannot be destroyed by radiation doses in amounts that can be given safely to a patient, or when a tumor cannot be entirely removed surgically without destroying a vital organ. It is also used for patients whose cancer has spread to distant organs of the body or for those with a generalized form of the disease, such as leukemia. Chemical compounds that selectively hunt out and destroy cancer cells, or in some way provide the body with the ability to render such cells harmless seem to be the only solution to the problem of generalized forms of cancer.

Long remissions — periods when the patient is free of symptoms and the disease seems to have disappeared — are often obtained with the use of drugs.

EARLY WARNING SIGNS

The following are the early warning symptoms

of cancer:
1. Unusual bleeding or discharge.
2. A lump or thickening in the breast or elsewhere.
3. A sore that does not heal.
4. Change in bowel or bladder habits.
5. Hoarseness or cough.
6. Indigestion or difficulty in swallowing.
7. Change in a wart or mole.

If the symptom lasts longer than two weeks, a doctor should be consulted.

The statistics suggest that a greater percentage of patients are being cured every year. This is possible because of new and better techniques, and because with early detection, many forms of cancer respond well to treatment.

TESTS

There are several ways that a doctor can test for cancer.

The "Pap" smear is used in the detection of cancer of the uterine cervix. It is named for Dr. George N. Papanicolaou, who developed the technique. This test involves the microscopic examination of cells scraped from the cervix or collected in fluid from the vagina. The "Pap" test is given to all adult women.

The proctosigmoidoscope is used to detect cancer of the colon and rectum. The physician inserts a narrow, lighted tube through the rectum and passes it up the colon. This procedure can be performed in a doctor's office.

Doctors use two tests for breast cancer. A mammograph is basically an X-ray. A thermograph measures heat. If cancer is present, the breast will show a higher temperature in the cancerous area.

Every cancer diagnosis made by a physician is subject to confirmation by a biopsy. In this surgical procedure, a small piece of suspect tissue is removed, placed in a preservative, cut in very thin slices, placed on a glass slide, stained with special dyes, and examined with the microscope. The biopsy may be performed quickly in the operating room, so that the operation can be continued for removal of the tumor if the presence of cancer is established.

FREQUENCY

Cancer appears most frequently in men and women over thirty-five, but younger people and even babies are affected. Among children, leukemia is a major cause of death. Overall, cancer is the second leading cause of death in the United States.

RESEARCH

In the United States alone, billions of dollars and thousands of scientists are involved in cancer research.

A most encouraging and exciting area of research in the causation of cancer concerns viruses. The artificial boundaries between tumor viruses, animal viruses, and ordinary viruses that may infect and change human cells are now chapters out of the past. Scientists seems to be at the very threshold of the final step of showing a direct relationship between some human cancers and viruses. With the identification of a virus responsible for any form of human cancer, the way may be opened for the development of vaccines for the prevention of the cancer.

Research is also being conducted on hormones and their relationship to the development of cancer and on the development of new drugs to destroy a tumor.

Cancer research is proceeding along many lines. Some are concerned with cures, some with finding better tools for diagnosis.

Among most scientists, there is little doubt that research will eventually unlock the key to the puzzle of cancer.

cancrum oris — gangrene of the mouth.
See noma.

Candida — a yeast-like fungus found in the mouth and intestine. This fungus can cause an infection called thrush, characterized by white patches in the mouth. In the healthy body *Candida* live in harmony with other bacteria. When other bacteria are disturbed, as for example by antibiotics, *Candida* will multiply, causing infection.
See thrush.

canker — ulceration of the mouth or lips. This problem can range in severity from one or two occasional mild sores to weekly outbreaks of many painful blisters. Little is known about the cause, cure, or prevention of cankers.
See aphthous stomatitis, erythema multiforme, herpes simplex, pemphigus.

cannabis — the dried, flowering tops of the hemp plant. Also called marihuana and hashish.

cantharide — dried Spanish fly bug. Used externally, it is a strong irritant. Used internally in small doses, it stimulates the urinary organs, acting as a diuretic. However, in large doses canthardes are lethal. At one time it was used as an aphrodisiac because it irritated the whole urinary system. Unfortunately, this can lead to kidney failure and death.

canthus — the angle formed at either side of the eye where the upper and lowers eyelids meet.

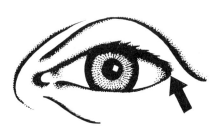

CANTHUS

capillary — the smallest blood-carrying vessel in the body. The capillaries serve as the crossing point between the small arteries (arterioles), which carry oxygenated blood from the heart, and the small veins (venules), which return blood to the heart.

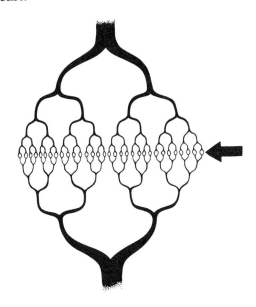

CAPILLARIES

The walls of capillaries are semipermeable, allowing the interchange of water, salts, glucose, etc., between the blood and tissue fluid.

Not all capillaries are used on each blood circuit. There are enough capillaries to handle the maximum flow of blood through a given part of the body. For example, many more capillaries are used during digestion than during sleep.

capsula — a sheath of fat, fibroid, cartilage, or membrane that covers or encloses a body organ. Sometimes called capsule.

capsule — the soluble container for a dose of medicine.
See capsula.

caput succedaneum — edema or an abnormal collection of fluid in and under the scalp of a newborn baby. The condition is a result of pressure during labor and usually lasts only a few days.

carbachol — a drug first synthesized by Kreitmair in 1932. It is similar to acetylcholine (ACh), but it is more selective and its effects are more prolonged. It is used primarily in the treatment of disorder of the gastrointestinal tract and the urinary bladder. It is also applied locally to constrict the pupil of the eye.

carbohydrates — compounds of carbon, hydrogen, and oxygen. They serve as sources of energy for the human body — to do external (physical) and internal work and to maintain body temperature.

The common sources of carbohydrates are cereals and products derived from them, such as bread and other baked goods, breakfast cereals, rice and noodles, and also most vegetables and fruits, sugar, jams and jellies, candy, soft drinks, and honey.

Carbohydrates are the most economical sources of body energy. This explains why they are the foundation and mainstay of most diets everywhere in the world.

When more carbohydrates are eaten than necessary, the excess is converted into fat and stored in the form of fatty tissues. Thus, eating more carbohydrates than are needed to supply the energy requirements for daily activities may lead to obesity.

Foods supply carbohydrates chiefly in three

forms — starches, sugars, and celluloses (fibrous materials). Starches and sugars are major sources of energy. Celluloses furnish bulk in the diet.

Glucose, commonly called blood sugar, is the form in which starches and sugars are mainly used by cells to furnish energy for body processes and to support activity and growth.

Carbohydrates spare proteins by supplying energy, thereby saving protein for tissue building and repair and for other special jobs. Carbohydrates also help the body use fats efficiently.

Different carbohydrates produce different effects in the body, depending on the heredity of the eater and the rest of his diet. The type of carbohydrate not only affects fat metabolism but may influence the progress of degenerative diseases, such as atherosclerosis, associated with cholesterol deposits.

carbolic acid — *See phenol.*

carbon dioxide — an odorless, colorless gas. Carbon dioxide is found in the air and is produced in the body tissues when cells burn fuel. It is carried in the blood to the lungs, where it is removed and exhaled.

The amount of carbon dioxide in the blood determines the rate of breathing. During a normal day, the rate of breathing changes several times. When the body is stationary, it uses a "normal" amount of energy; consequently, there will be a "normal" amount of carbon dioxide produced and a "normal rate" of respiration. When the body is in motion — running for example — the body requires more energy than "normal," and more carbon dioxide is produced. In order for the body to discharge the carbon dioxide and to take in more oxygen, the rate of respiration will increase. Conversely, when the body is asleep, little energy is used, and the rate of respiration is less than "normal."

carbon-dioxide poisoning — a result of an increase in the percentage of carbon dioxide in the body over six per cent. This causes the rate of respiration to increase to the point where it can strain the heart, slow reflexes, and cause unconsciousness and death. In a healthy body this is uncommon, because the body will compensate by increasing the rate of depth of breathing.

carbon monoxide — a colorless, odorless, tasteless gas, which is produced as a result of incomplete combustion of organic material, such as takes place in a car engine.

carbon-monoxide poisoning — when inhaled, carbon monoxide will combine with hemoglobin. Because hemoglobin has a greater affinity for carbon monoxide than for oxygen, the carbon monoxide will take the place of oxygen in hemoglobin. Thus, carbon-monoxide poisoning is a shortage of oxygen in the blood.

The symptoms of carbon-monoxide poisoning are a bright-red color of the fingernails and face, weakness, dizziness, headache, and nausea.

The most important treatment is pure oxygen or fresh air. It is also important to keep the patient warm and quiet.

carbuncle — an infection of the skin and subcutaneous tissue, usually caused by staphylococci bacteria. A carbuncle differs from a boil in that the infection goes deeper and covers a wider area. The diameter of a carbuncle can be two or three inches. The area is inflamed and painful for about a week. After that time, the center will begin to soften, and pus will be discharged from several drain sites within the carbuncle.

Surgery is often used to open and remove them.

Carbuncles occur most frequently on the back of the neck, the shoulders, and the back.

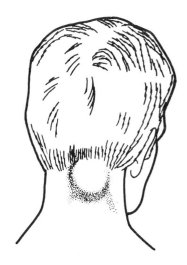

CARBUNCLE

carcinogen — any substance or agent that causes cancer.

carcinoma — one of two general types of cancer. Carcinoma is a cancer found in the lining or covering membranes of body organs.

See sarcoma.

cardiac — of or pertaining to the heart.

cardiac arrhythmia — irregular beating of the heart.

cardiac catheter — a diagnostic device for taking samples of blood, or pressure readings within the heart chambers, that might reveal defects in the heart. A cardiac catheter is a thin tube of woven plastic or other material to which blood will not adhere. It is inserted in a vein or artery, usually in the arm, and is threaded into the heart. It is guided by the physician, who watches its progress by means of X-rays falling on a fluorescent screen.

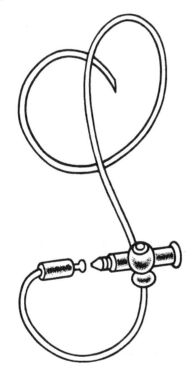

CARDIAC CATHETER

cardiac cycle — one total heart beat; i.e., one complete contraction and relaxation of the heart. In man, this normally takes about 0.85 seconds.

cardiac massage — a procedure instituted when the heart has stopped beating. There are two types of cardiac massage: open and closed. In open cardiac massage, the doctor actually massages the heart with his hands. In closed massage, rhythmic pressure is applied to the breastbone. This pressure squeezes the heart against the backbone and produces a pulse. The purpose of both types of cardiac massage is to keep blood and oxygen circulating.

cardiac opening — the opening between the esophagus and the upper part of the stomach.

cardiac output — the amount of blood pumped by the heart per minute.

cardiology — the branch of medicine that deals with the heart and its function.

cardiovascular — of or pertaining to the heart and the blood vessels.

cardiovascular disease — any disease that affects the heart and the blood vessels.

cardiovascular system — the heart and the blood vessels. The cardiovascular system is the circulatory system for transporting blood throughout the body.

caries — decay or death of bone (usually applied to dental decay). In serious cases of dental decay, it can include inflammation and abcesses. In mild form, caries can be a cavity.

carminative — a medicine for relieving flatulence.

carotene — a pigment (yellow or red in color) found in carrots, sweet potatoes, leafy vegetables, milk, and eggs. The body can convert it to vitamin A.

carotid artery — the main artery of the neck is called the common carotid artery. This artery splits into the interior and the exterior carotid arteries.

The interior carotid artery supplies blood to the middle ear, pituitary gland, and part of the brain.

The external carotid artery supplies blood to the neck, face, and skull.

Although the carotid arteries are not the sole source of supply for blood to the brain, injury to them can cause severe brain damage.

carotid gland — a small gland located between the internal and external carotid arteries. It reacts to

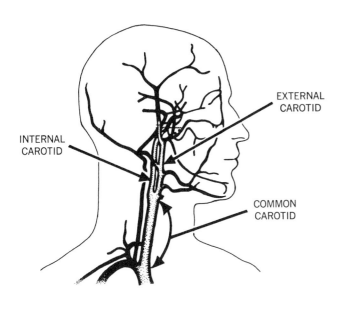

INTERNAL CAROTID

EXTERNAL CAROTID

COMMON CAROTID

CAROTID ARTERY

the levels of oxygen and carbon dioxide in the blood. When there is an imbalance, the carotid gland secretes a hormone that changes the rate of respiration.

carotid sinus — an enlarged portion of the internal carotid artery (but occasionally located at the end of the common carotid artery) which contains nerve endings that are stimulated by changes in blood pressure. If it is squeezed, blood pressure will drop, resulting in unconsciousness.

carpal tunnel — the passage in the wrist for the median nerve and the flexor tendons in the wrist. *See wrist.*

carpus — the place where the arm and hand join — the wrist. Made up of eight small bones.

carrier — a person who harbors in his body the infectious organisms of a disease without suffering any of the disease symptoms. Because the person carrying the disease feels normal, he moves around and comes in contact with many other people who are thus infected by the disease.

The classic example of a carrier is the infamous Typhoid Mary who infected thousands of people without herself suffering from typhoid.

A person can also be a carrier during the incubation period of many infectious diseases.

Females are carriers for sex-linked disorders such as color blindness and hemophilia.

car sickness — *See motion sickness.*

cartilage — a fibrous connective tissue commonly known as gristle. There are three types in the human body — hyaline, fibrocartilage, and elastic cartilage.

Hyaline cartilage forms most of the skeleton of an embryo. As the embryo grows, bone begins to replace the cartilage. When a child is born, some of the bones are still cartilage, which are gradually replaced by hard bone. In an adult, hyaline cartilage is the flexible semi-elastic tissue that covers the moving parts of joints such as the elbow.

Fibrocartilage is a fibrous tissue found between the vertebrae and also between the bones of the knee.

Elastic cartilage is more flexible than hyaline cartilage. It is found in the elastic tissue of the ear.

Cartilage differs from bone in that it has no blood vessels. If it is cut or torn, the damage must be repaired surgically.

cascara sagrada — a drug obtained from the dried bark of *Rhamnus purshiana,* a tree found in the western part of the United States. It is used as a purgative.

castor oil — obtained from the seeds of *Ricinus communis,* a bush found in the subtropics and used as a purgative. Castor oil combines with juices in the stomach to form ricinoleic acid, which stimulates the small intestine. It works so quickly that it is seldom used at bedtime. In recent years the use of castor oil has decreased. This decrease is due in part to its unpleasant taste.

Castor oil is also used on the skin as an emollient.

castrate — a nonmedical term used to indicate removal of the gonads in the male, or in female castration, removal of the ovaries. Castration leaves an individual incapable of sexual reproduction.

catabolism — any chemical process by which the body reduces complex substances into more simple ones. This happens frequently in digestion.

catalepsy — a condition in which there is a rigidity of the muscles that causes the patient to remain in a fixed position or posture. Catalepsy can be self-induced.

catalyst — a substance that produces a chemical reaction but which is not changed by that reaction. In the body, enzymes are catalysts.

cataplasm — a poultice, usually medicated.

cataract — an opaqueness in the lens of the eye. A cataract interferes with normal vision and is usually progressive. It is not a film growing over the lens, but a change in the lens itself. The cloudiness of the lens blocks the normal passage of light rays through the pupil to the retina.

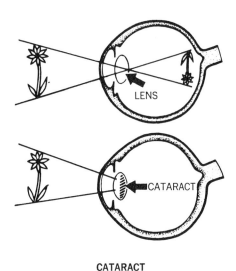

CATARACT

An early symptom of cataracts may be blurring of near and distant vision, but the symptoms depend on the location of the cataract. In many cases both eyes are affected, although not at the same rate.

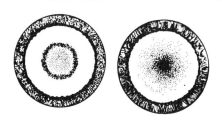

CATARACT

Among the known causes of cataracts are injury, general diseases such as diabetes, or neglected glaucoma of the eyes. Children may be born with cataracts from hereditary influences or because the mother had German measles during the first three months of pregnancy. Approximately two-thirds of all cataracts are found in people over fifty-five years of age, for which no cause has been proven.

Most cataracts can be cured by surgery. The surgeon removes the clouded lens entirely from the patient's eye. After the operation, the function of the eye lens is replaced by eyeglasses or by contact lens.

catarrh — the inflammation of a mucous membrane with a discharge of mucus, especially an inflammation of the mucous membranes of the head and throat.

Catarrh is no longer used very much as a scientific term. It has been replaced by more specific terms.

catatonia — a severe form of mental illness. Catatonia is listed under schizophrenia. The patient may be totally withdrawn, to the point where he is completely unaware of his surroundings. Another reaction is wild excitement, and in this case, the patient will often have to be tranquilized.

Perhaps the most striking aspect of catatonia is the catatonic trance or posture. A patient will assume a position and hold it despite all attempts to move him. The postures can sometimes be quite bizarre.

catgut — surgical "thread." It is obtained from sheep's intestines and made into aseptic cord. Depending on the way it is to be used, a surgeon will choose different thicknesses of catgut. One of the biggest advantages of using catgut in surgery is that the tissues will eventually dissolve it entirely.

catharsis — a cleansing or purging. In his method of treatment, Freud recommended a catharsis by means of stream of consciousness, thus purging the individual of his repressed thoughts.

cathartic — a medicine that causes or increases defecation. Cathartics work by stimulating motor activity in the intestines. They are stronger than

laxatives and are generally available only by prescription.
See laxative, purgative.

catheter — a thin tube that is inserted into the body to withdraw fluids. A catheter is frequently used to withdraw urine from the bladder.

catoptric test — a test for cataracts. It is made by observing reflections from the eye lens and cornea.

cat-scratch fever — a somewhat serious inflammation of the lymph nodes. It is caused by a virus and usually occurs after the patient has been bitten or scratched by a cat.

cauliflower ear — a deformity of the ear caused by injury and infection. As a result of the injury or infection, excessive scar tissue forms.

cautery — a hot iron, an electric current, etc., applied to kill tissue. Cauterization stops bleeding by sealing the damaged area. The technique was very popular until the end of the middle ages. Today, the principal behind cauterization is applied to the use of a laser beam in treating a detached retina.

c.c. —abbreviation for cubic centimeter, units of which are used in medicine dosage.

cell — the basic unit of plant and animal life, consisting of a small mass of protoplasm, a nucleus, and surrounded by a semipermeable membrane. A cell can build chemical compounds, break down compounds, and transform energy.

The cell as a unit was first discovered by a British scientist, Robert Hook, in 1665. With the aid of a very primitive microscope, he noticed that cork was arranged in more or less regular divisions. But as Hook used the term, a cell was the wall around a cell rather than the matter within the wall. It was several centuries later that the importance of his discovery and a fuller understanding of the anatomy of the cell were realized.

Although there are bacteria that consist of only one cell, higher animals and plants contain a multitude of cells. Higher animals that multiply by sexual reproduction begin with the union of male and female sex cells. In the case of the human, the resultant divisions of this union eventually develop into an adult body comprising billions of cells. Each of these cells is marked with the identity of that individual, yet the cells can be as different as those that make up the tissue of the brain, the liver, and the skin.

Although cells can be different shapes and sizes and can perform incredibly complex functions, they are so small that they can be seen only under a microscope.

Food and oxygen are absorbed through the semipermeable membrane of the cell, and waste products are expelled. When a cell is destroyed through injury, the remaining cells divide to bridge and repair the damage. With the major exception of the nervous system (including the brain), almost all cells in the body are capable of reproducing themselves.

The act of cell-reproduction or cell-division is called mitosis, and in an adult it results in two completely identical cells for every one cell that divides. An embryo starts with one cell and rapidly divides. In the beginning the cells are general or nonspecific, but as the embryo develops, the cells begin to become very specific — they become nerve cells, or muscle cells, etc.

See cell membrane, DNA, genetics, mitosis, molecules, nucleus.

cell membrane — the semipermeable wall surrounding an individual cell. It is composed of protein and fat molecules that carefully regulate admission to the cell.

cell theory — the doctrine that states that all plants and animals are composed of cells.

cellular pathology — the belief that the cell is the starting point of disease.

cellular tissue — loose connective tissue that has large interspaces and is found under the skin, peritoneum, etc.

cellulitis — an inflammation occurring in cellular tissue, especially in subcutaneous tissue. Cellulitis is often caused by streptococci and is then treated with penicillin.

celology — the study of hernias.
See hernia.

Celsus, Aurelius Cornelius — a Roman author (1st

77

century A.D.). He is best known medically for his description of the four classical symptoms of inflammation — pain, redness, swelling, and heat.

cement — a substance used by a dentist as an adhesive between a cavity and the filling.

cementum — the bony cover for the root of a tooth.

central nervous system — the part of the nervous system that includes the brain and the spinal cord. The central nervous system includes the twelve pairs of cranial nerves and the thirty-one pairs of spinal nerves.
See cranial nerves, nerves, spinal nerves.

centrifuge — a machine that rotates at high speeds and is used to separate substances according to their densities.

cephalalgia — headache.

cephaloridine — a drug used as an antibiotic, with many properties similar to penicillin.

cephalotractor — a forceps used by an obstetrician during delivery.

cerebellum — the portion of the brain concerned with coordinating the muscular activities of the body. In conjunction with the inner ear, it controls the sense of balance. The cerebellum is a

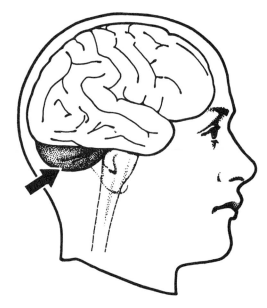

CEREBELLUM

part of the central nervous system. It is located under and in back of the cerebrum, so that it is situated in the lower rear quadrant of the brain. The outer portion of the cerebellum is covered with deep convolutions or folds and is gray in color.

cerebral palsy — a broad term used to describe a variety of chronic conditions in which brain damage, usually occurring at birth, impairs motor function and control.

SYMPTOMS
Symptoms may range from mild muscle incoordination to more severe physical handicaps. Impairments of motor function may involve upper or lower extremities, or both, and may affect one or both sides of the body.

Although the primary symptom in cerebral palsy is motor damage, there may or may not be other manifestations of brain damage. However, most cerebral-palsied individuals show destruction of brain tissue.

TYPES
The two most common types of the disorder are the spastic form and the athetoid type. The spastic form is characterized by tense, contracted muscle; the primary symptom of the athetoid type is involuntary and uncontrolled movements of arms and legs.

Among associated disabilities that may occur in cerebral palsy are intellectual impairment, convulsive seizures, speech defects, disorders of vision and hearing, and certain other brain-centered disorders, including specific learning difficulties and behavioral abnormalities.

EARLY DETECTION
Neurological or sensory signs of the child's abnormal development are sometimes detected at birth but in other instances do not become apparent until months or even several years later. Early detection and diagnosis of cerebral palsy in the infant or young child is crucially important in helping to prevent or lessen the extent of handicapping effects.

CAUSES
The different forms of cerebral palsy are rooted in multiple causes of injury or disease of brain tissue, many of which are essentially unknown or only suspected. Some of the causes of cerebral palsy occurring in the period before, during, and after birth have been identified or implicated:

1. Chronic or acute anoxia (oxygen deprivation) is one of the leading factors known to precede the condition of cerebral palsy and other serious neurological disorders of childhood.

2. Rubella (German measles) contracted by the expectant mother early in pregnancy can do serious damage to the developing nervous system of the fetus.

3. Obstetrical complications, such as breech birth and twin delivery, can figure in the cause of cerebral palsy.

4. Prematurity is strongly associated with cerebral palsy. The premature infant, particularly of low birth weight, is susceptible to asphyxia from respiratory distress. (Asphyxia implies not only a lack of oxygen but also excess carbon dioxide and other changes in blood and metabolic processes.)

5. Jaundice of the newborn may produce an illness called kernicterus, in which mild or severe damage of the central nervous system may occur. Most cases of kernicterus are caused by incompatibility of the red-blood-cell Rh factor between the developing fetus and the mother, or other blood-type conflict.

6. Toxemia of pregnancy, maternal diabetes, and other maternal illnesses are predisposing factors to cerebral palsy in the developing fetus.

7. Postnatal infection, such as encephalitis or meningitis, during infancy or early childhood may produce symptoms of cerebral palsy.

RESEARCH

Because of its diffuse causes, cerebral palsy takes in a wide research spectrum. Each of its origins must first be identified and controlled before the multitude of conditions known as "cerebral palsy" can be overcome. Simultaneously with discovering and conquering the conditions responsible for cerebral palsy, methods must be developed to train and treat those who now have the disorder to utilize their remaining motor skills.

Even if the causes of cerebral palsy were soon eliminated, many people in the country who already suffer the effects of destruction of important elements of the central nervous system would continue to need help in overcoming their handicaps. In order to understand and develop the best methods for retraining a damaged brain to compensate for lost function, scientists must acquire complete knowledge of the intricacies of the brain.

Research has contributed to forestalling measures against some causes of cerebral palsy. These include blood-compatibility tests in the prenatal period and exchange transfusion of the baby at birth, where necessary, to counteract the Rh factor and other blood-type incompatibility; emphasis on maintaining good maternal health during pregnancy; preventive measures — where these are now possible — against prematurity, and maximum protection of the prematurely newborn against disease or infection; alertness to the dangerous consequences to the fetus of rubella and other viral infections, and a stepped-up effort to vaccinate everyone against German measles.

Meanwhile, for the hundreds of thousands of children and adults who have cerebral palsy, various forms of therapy, depending on their individual type of the disorder, can help lessen handicaps.

REHABILITATIVE THERAPY

A combination of therapeutic measures is often prescribed, including physical and occupational therapy, drugs to reduce muscle spasms, orthopedic surgery, special braces, and other programs involving speech and hearing therapists and other specialists in physical medicine and rehabilitation. All such programs need to be geared to developing the individual's total capacities and remaining motor skills to the fullest extent possible.

RESEARCH OUTLOOK

Recovery from the effects of brain damage is still an enormous medical challenge. Nevertheless, scientists are striving to find ways to repair injury sustained to the central nervous system and thereby provide a possible cure for cerebral palsy and other serious disorders.

cerebral-vascular disease — a disease affecting the blood vessels of the brain. There are several things that can happen to these vessels. A blood vessel may rupture, or it may become blocked, causing blood flow to the brain to be reduced and even to stop. The common results of cerebral-vascular disease are headaches, difficulties of vision, dizziness, fainting spells, numbness of hand or face, weakness, paralysis, difficulty in speaking, poor memory, difficulty in thinking, personality changes, and mental disturbances. Any of the above symptoms may be caused by conditions other than cerebral-vascular disease, and not all of them are always present in any one patient with cerebral-vascular disease. The symptoms present depend on the severity of the disease, the areas of the brain that are affected, and other variable factors.

TYPES

1. Hemorrhage

The wall of an artery of the brain may break, permitting blood to escape and thus damage the surrounding brain tissue.

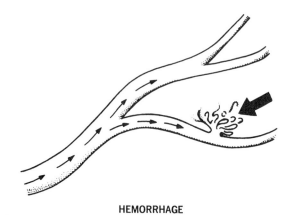

HEMORRHAGE

2. Thrombosis

A clot of blood may form in an artery of the brain and may stop the flow of blood to the part of the brain supplied by the clot-plugged artery.

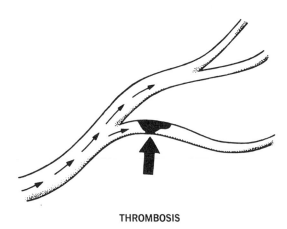

THROMBOSIS

3. Embolism

A clot from a diseased heart or, less commonly, from elsewhere in the body may be pumped to the brain and stop up one of the brain's arteries.

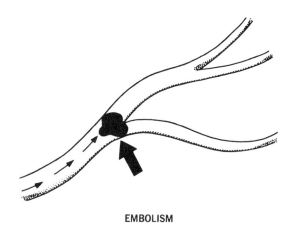

EMBOLISM

4. Compression

A tumor, swollen brain tissue, or a large clot from another vessel may press upon a vessel of the brain and stop its flow of blood.

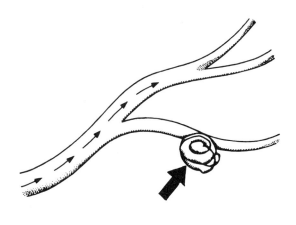

COMPRESSION

5. Spasm

An artery of the brain may constrict and thus reduce the flow of blood to an area of the brain. If the spasm is of short duration, permanent damage does not necessarily occur.

CAUSES

There are a number of causes for the different ways in which the circulation of blood to the brain may be disturbed. These include defects of the vessels, which may develop before birth; physical injury; infections of the blood vessels; general infections; blood diseases; heart disease; hardening of the arteries; and high blood pressure.

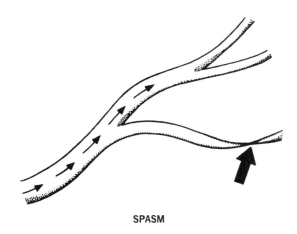

SPASM

cerebral-vascular system — the blood-vessel system of the brain.

cerebrospinal fever — an acute infectious form of meningitis, also referred to as epidemic cerebrospinal meningitis. In addition to inflammation of the membranes of the brain and spinal cord, there is usually an eruption of hemorrhage spots on the skin. It is caused by bacteria known as *Neisseria meningitidis* and is treated by antibiotics.
See meningitis.

cerebrospinal fluid — a colorless fluid composed primarily of glucose and salts. This fluid circulates through the central canal of the spinal cord, the four ventricles of the brain, and the subarachnoid space (space in the brain between the innermost and the intermediate layers of meninges).

It is manufactured in the small blood vessels of the ventricles and is absorbed or formed as needed to keep the pressure constant. When the pressure rises, too much fluid can accumulate in the brain.

An examination of the cerebrospinal fluid is often ordered to help diagnose meningitis as well as other diseases and conditions occurring in the brain.

cerebrum — the main portion of the brain. It occupies the entire top of the cranium and is divided into two cerebral hemispheres. The right hemisphere is responsible for the left side of the body; the left hemisphere is responsible for the right side. Each hemisphere is further divided into areas that serve as motor centers and sensory centers.

Part of the dura mater is situated in the cleft between the two hemispheres and is called the falx cerebri. One of the functions of the falx cerebri is to keep the hemispheres from pressing against each other when the head moves.

The surface of the cerebrum is covered with convolutions, or deep folds, and is gray in color. A fold is called a gyrus; the area between two folds is referred to as a sulcus. The whole of the surface area is known as the cortex and is approximately one-eighth of an inch thick. The cortex controls the higher mental processes such as memory and intelligence. Beneath the surface lies the medulla or central part of the cerebrum. This is white in color and contains groups of nerve cells, including the thalamus and the basal ganglia.

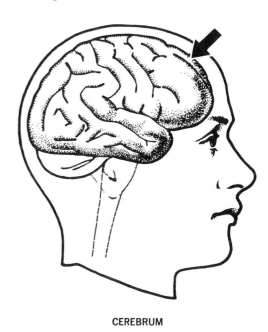

CEREBRUM

Different areas of the cerebrum are responsible for different functions. For example, the center for hearing is close to the ear, while the area concerned with vision is located at the back of the cerebrum.

cervical — of the neck, or pertaining to any cervix.

cervix — the constricted part of any body organ.
See cervix uteri.

cervix uteri — the narrow lower portion of the uterus. The cervix uteri connects with the vagina. During delivery, the cervix uteri expends greatly to allow the baby to pass from the womb to the vagina.

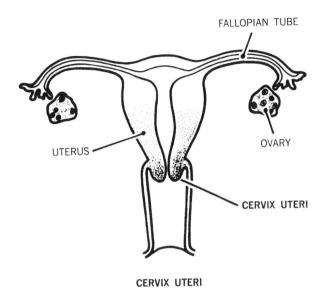

FALLOPIAN TUBE

UTERUS

OVARY

CERVIX UTERI

CERVIX UTERI

A "Pap" test for cancer consists of the examination of cells scraped from the cervix uteri.

cesarean section — an operation used as an alternative to normal delivery when a normal delivery would be difficult or dangerous for the mother. The operation is usually fairly simple and involves cutting through the walls of the abdomen and uterus to remove the baby.

Chagas' disease — a form of trypanosomiasis that affects people in South America, particularly Brazil. It is caused by the parasite *Trypanosoma cruzi* and is transmitted to humans by insects. Chagas' disease is frequently fatal.
See trypanosomiasis.

chancre — the first sore of the venereal disease syphilis. The chancre occurs at the site where the infection entered the body.
Often it is not painful and disappears without the patient's knowledge.
See syphilis.

chancroid — an infection of the genitals that is caused by *Haemophilus ducreyi*. The original sore is at the site of infection and can be quite painful. The infection can spread to the lymph nodes of the genital area. It is treated with sulphonamide drugs and sometimes with tetracycline.

change of life — *See menopause.*

chapped hands — a condition in which the hands are dry, cracked, and often split. This condition is usually the result of exposure to cold.

charcoal — a black carbon that results from the burning (or charring) of organic material. Activated charcoal is a fine black powder used internally to absorb gases and in emergencies to treat certain kinds of drug poisoning. The major drawback to activated charcoal is that it does not discriminate — it will absorb almost anything.

Chauliac, Guy de — a famous French surgeon (1300-1368). His book *Chirurgia Magna* was the standard work on surgery until the sixteenth century. He was one of the first men to operate for hernias and cataracts and was also one of the first to use narcotics on patients prior to surgery.

chaulmoogra oil — an oil obtained from the seeds of trees belonging to the order *Flacourtaceae*. For centuries it was one of the two drugs used to treat leprosy. It has been replaced by more effective drugs.

chelating agent — a drug used as a heavy metal antagonist. Heavy metals such as lead and mercury are toxic if taken internally. A chelating agent will combine with such a metal and the resulting compound will be less damaging to the body.

cheloid — *See keloid.*

chemical burn — a burn caused by acids, alkalies, or other chemicals. The chemical burn is not caused by heat but by direct chemical destruction of the body tissues. First-aid treatment for chemical burns should begin immediately by washing off the chemical that is causing the injury. The next steps depend on what particular chemical is involved.

chemotherapy — the treatment of disease by chemicals or drugs. The drugs act against the invading organisms without harming the body. Antibiotics and sulphonamides are two types of drugs used in chemotherapy. The importance of chemotherapy in the treatment of cancer has increased tremendously in the past few years.

chest — a nonmedical term indicating the area of the body contained within the ribs.
See thorax.

Cheyne-Stokes respiration — breathing that is characterized by changing depths of respiration. The patient will breathe very deeply and then gradually start to breathe shallowly. This occurs in a pattern and is accompanied by spells of apnea. It is often found when the nervous centers have been injured. It is named after the two physicians who described it — John Cheyne (1777-1836) and William Stokes (1804-1878).

chickenpox — one of the mildest of the childhood diseases. In adults the disease is more severe. It is an infectious disease and spreads so rapidly that most children have it before they are fifteen years old. It is very rare for a person to have chickenpox more than once.

The disease is spread from one person to another by secretions from the patient's mouth and nose and by fluid from the skin blisters. The incubation period for chickenpox is two to three weeks after exposure to the infectious secretions.

SYMPTOMS

In some cases, the child coming down with chickenpox has a slight fever, headache, and loss of appetite for a day or two before the rash develops; in other cases, the rash is the first symptom. Pink spots of various sizes appear first on the trunk, then on the face and, in severe cases, all over the body. The spots soon change to blisters which break and become crusted with scabs. The blisters do not all appear at the same time, but come in successive crops. Each crop of scabs takes three to four days to blister, break, and crust over. Eruptions that resemble small ulcers form on the lining of the mouth and throat.

TREATMENT

A physician should be consulted early when chickenpox is suspected, to make sure that the illness is not smallpox — the symptoms are somewhat alike. A diagnosis by a physician is particularly important for adults, because most of them have had chickenpox as children, and a second attack is unlikely.

Although a child with chickenpox is rarely seriously ill, he requires careful attention for a few days to keep him from scratching and infecting the eruptions.

The patient's clothes and bedding should be kept fresh and clean. His hands should be washed often and his fingernails kept short. Wearing mittens on the hands or paper tubes over the elbows will help to keep very young children from scratching. In applying soothing ointments or powders prescribed by a physician, any possible eruptions on the scalp or sex organs should not be overlooked.

Chickenpox does not usually leave scars unless a scab has been irritated. The disease will normally last a week, but the patient is contagious until all of the scabs have fallen off.

chigger — an insect also known as harvest mite and red bug. The bite of a chigger produces an irritated red swelling which is very itchy. They are usually found in tall grass and underbrush. Chiggers are different from jiggers and chigoes.

chigoe — the sand flea. A small insect found in warm climates such as the southern United States. The female of the species burrows into the skin (particularly into the feet and the legs) and causes itchiness and irritation.

chilblain — a swelling of portions of the skin on the fingers, toes, or ears due to cold weather. The affected areas itch and can be painful. The condition is caused by the lack of blood in the skin, which follows the constriction of blood vessels exposed to cold. The best treatment is also the best prevention — keep the areas warm.

child — the term used to denote human offspring from the time of infancy to puberty.

child abuse — the willful injury of a child by parents or guardians. The methods employed range from malnutrition and physical neglect to outright violence, sometimes leading to permanent crippling or death.

The physical symptoms include malnutrition, poor skin hygiene, bruises, abrasions, cuts, lacerations, burns, fractures, dislocations, and hemorrhages. Child abuse often manifests itself through irritability, repressed personality, etc.

Available information indicates that in about half of the cases the abuse is repeated. Therefore, scars, scab-covered areas, recurring injury, or fractures should be investigated for possible child abuse. The diagnosis of child abuse depends on physical examination, X-ray findings, and a high index of suspicion on the part of the physician.

The individual incident of abuse is related more to the parent's emotional state at the time than to any antisocial behavior by the child. The abuse of the child frequently is an explosive emotional reaction by an immature parent, triggered by an irrelevant cause. Other characteristics of the abusing parent are hostility, agression, dependency, insecurity, rigidity, depression, lack of warmth, and rejection of the child or children.

Accurate data on the amount of child abuse is limited. Only a small proportion of maltreated children are taken to a hospital or a physician, and many injuries are often explained away as being the result of falls or accidents. Some experts believe that the incidence of child abuse is increasing. Most cases occur in children under three years of age. The death rate is substantially higher in children under two years of age. In many cases, only one child in the family is the regular target for assault.

Child abuse occurs at all levels of society. There has been no correlation between the incidence of this problem and the amount of education, economic level, or social status. Because of their lack of resources, people at the lower end of the economic scale may be reported more frequently to legal authorities.

The overriding consideration in the treatment of child abuse is protection of the child. In cases where the abuse is obvious and the parents deny assaulting the child, immediate court action to remove the child from the home should be instituted. Otherwise, the incident may be repeated, with the child in danger of permanent crippling or death.

child development — each child develops at his own pace and may reach an activity level in advance of or later than the stated period. The order of events does not change with individual children; however, there can be a considerable difference in age at accomplishment within normal limits.

AGE	ACTIVITY
2 months	Coos and smiles
3 months	Holds head up
5 months	Rolls over, babbles
7 months	Sits up unaided
9-10 months	Crawls
10-11 months	Pulls self up
11 months	Walks with help; stands alone
12-13 months	Walks alone
18 months	Runs; has a ten-word vocabulary
24 months	Daytime control of bowel and bladder
36 months	Night control of bladder

childhood diseases — diseases that are commonly contracted by children. They are usually highly contagious — one of the prime reasons so many children have them. When contracted by an adult, they can be quite serious. Chickenpox, German measles, measles, and mumps are the most familiar childhood diseases.

chill — an attack of shivering caused by an involuntary contraction of muscles. The patient feels cold and loses color. A chill is one of the ways the body responds to infection.

Chinese medicine — *See acupuncture.*

chiropractic — a system of treatment based on the theory that disease and discomfort are the result of abnormal functioning of the nerves and nervous system. The theory states that manipulating various parts of the body (especially the spinal cord) relieves pressure on the ends of the nerves.

chloral hydrate — a drug discovered in 1832; it is used as an hypnotic. It works as a depressant to the central nervous system. For a while the use of chloral hydrate was replaced by the barbiturates, but recently it has been used more frequently. It has a strong odor and a bitter taste and should not be taken on an empty stomach. Chloral hydrate is one of the drugs prescribed for insomnia.

chloramphenicol — an antibiotic produced from cultures of *Streptomyces venezuelae*. This drug can also be produced synthetically. It is effective against typhus and other infections.

chlorine — a yellow-green poisonous gas. It is used in compounds as a disinfectant and antiseptic. However, the use of chlorine compounds for antiseptic purposes has decreased in favor of other less-irritating substances. Chlorine is also used to sterilize water. During World War I it was used in chemical warfare.

In undiluted forms, chlorine can be very harmful and even fatal if inhaled or taken internally. The lungs are particularly susceptible to damage from chlorine.

chloroform — a colorless liquid that was frequently used as an anesthetic. Its use is limited today because it can cause serious side effects.

It was first used as an anesthetic to be given during childbirth.

chloroquine — a compound drug used in the treatment of malaria. It was discovered by United States scientists during World War II when the problem of malaria was quite acute. It had been secretly researched by German scientists prior to that.

Chloroquine does not prevent malaria, but it is useful because it helps stop malarial attacks. It is also used in cases of cardiac arrhythmia, infection of the liver by ameba, and rheumatoid arthritis.

chlorosis — a condition that seems to be caused by iron deficiency. It occurs primarily in females during puberty and includes a yellow-greenish skin color.

chlorothlozide — a chemical compound that increases the output of urine. One of the diuretics sometimes used in the treatment of edema or waterlogged tissues.

chlorpromazine — one of the most widely used drugs. It is frequently used to control nausea and vomiting. It is also used as a tranquilizer for mental illness.

choking — an interruption of normal respiration caused by an obstruction or irritation somewhere in the respiratory system. The normal reaction to the obstruction or irritation is a cough or an attempted cough.

cholecystis — the gallbladder.

cholecystitis — a term used to denote an inflammation of the gallbladder.

cholera — a disease caused by the bacteria *Vibrio cholerae*. The disease attacks the intestines and causes severe diarrhea. The actual cause of death is loss of body fluid and electrolyte imbalance.

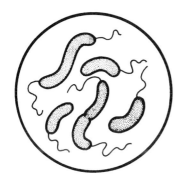

CHOLERA

The incubation period may be only a few hours or as long as seven days. The disease is usually transmitted through unsanitary conditions, and in underdeveloped countries cholera can become a fatal epidemic.

Treatment of cholera requires the replacement of lost fluids and the lost electrolytes.

People traveling to underdeveloped areas should receive a vaccination shortly before departing; any stay longer than six months will probably require a second vaccination.

cholestasis — a condition in which the flow of bile from the liver is stopped or suppressed. *See jaundice.*

cholesterol — a fat-like substance made in the body and found in every cell. It is a normal constituent of blood and tissues. In addition to the cholesterol made in the body, smaller amounts come from food. The cholesterol content of the diet is but one of many factors that influence the cholesterol level in blood.

Several studies have indicated that the incidence of coronary heart disease is greater among men with cholesterol levels above the average range. Thus, some physicians will prescribe treatment to decrease the amount of blood cholesterol if it is considered abnormally high.

Most medical scientists agree that the amount of cholesterol circulating in the blood can be increased or decreased by the amount and kind of fat in the diet.

Food fats and oils contain three kinds of fatty acids; saturated, mono-unsaturated, and poly-unsaturated. These fatty acids appear to affect blood cholesterol in different ways. Saturated fatty acids tend to raise the level of cholesterol in the blood; polyunsaturated fatty acids tend to lower it; and mono-unsaturated fatty acids seem to have no effect. Although a single food fat may contain varying amounts of all three kinds of fatty acids, it will usually be classified as predominantly one or another. For example, the solid animal fats are high in saturated fatty acids; most vegetable oils, as well as fish oils, are high in polyunsaturated fatty acids.

Liquid vegetable oils that have been made solid by hydrogenation have lost much of their polyunsaturated fatty-acid content. However, some recently developed margarines and solid cooking fats have been specially treated to retain these cholesterol-lowering fatty acids.

Cholesterol is found only in foods of animal origin. It is not present in fruits, vegetables, cereal grains, vegetable oils, or other foods coming from plants. Organ meats, such as brains, liver, kidney, and egg yolk contain the largest amount of cholesterol of any foods. Shellfish supply appreciable quantities. Other foods of animal origin contain smaller quantities.

When there is too much cholesterol in the body, the cholesterol will form deposits in the arteries and may form some types of gallstones.

choline — a substance that helps keep the liver free from deposits of fat. It is found in many forms of food, including meat and vegetables. Choline can be ingested or it can be synthesized by the body. There is some disagreement as to whether or not choline is a B vitamin.

chondro — a prefix meaning cartilage.

Chopart's amputation — an amputation of part of the foot.

chordae tendineae — fibrous chords that serve as guy ropes to hold the valves between the upper and lower chambers of the heart secure when forced closed by pressure of blood in the lower chambers. They stretch from the cusps of the valve to muscles called papillary muscles in the walls of the lower heart chambers.

chorea — a group of diseases characterized by involuntary jerky movements that occur constantly.
See Huntington's chorea.

choriocarcinoma — a cancer occurring in a part of the placenta sometimes retained in the uterus following pregnancy.

chorion — the outermost layer of the embryo. It acts as a protective cover and also provides nutrition.

chorionitis — an inflammation of the inner layer of skin.

chromatid — one of the pair of spirals of a chromosome.
See chromosome, mitosis.

chromosome — one of several small more or less rod-shaped bodies in the nucleus of a cell. The chromosomes contain the hereditary factors (genes) and are normally constant in number in each species. In man, there are forty-six chromosomes — twenty-two pairs and two sex chromosomes. In the case of a female, there are actually twenty-three pairs, because the sex chromosomes of the female are a pair of X's. The sex chromosomes of a male are an X and a Y.

The chromosomes are tightly coiled, double strands of molecules of deoxyribonucleic acid, or DNA for short. These strands carry the genetic orders that determine whether the cells develop into men, mice, or whales; whether the individual has blue or brown eyes; and whether he will or will not be susceptible to one or another disease. Additionally, they direct all the essential processes of the life of the cell.
See DNA, genes, genetics.

chronic — a term applied to any disease or condition that lasts a long time. A chronic disease or condition is not necessarily serious.

chronic bronchitis — *See bronchitis.*

chrysarobin — a drug obtained from the *Andira araroba* tree. In ointment form, it is sometimes used to treat psoriasis.

chrysoderma — a pigmentation of the skin resulting from deposits of gold. The pigmentation is permanent.

chrysotherapy — the treatment of a disease or condition with gold salts.

chyle — a milky fluid consisting partly of fat from foods. Chyle passes from the intestines into the veins, where it can be stored.

chylomicron — a minute particle of fat that is found in the blood during digestion.

chyme — the semiliquid, partially digested form in which food leaves the stomach and enters the small intestine.

cilia — microscopic waving hairs. The action of the cilia aids in trapping dust and foreign objects. The cilia also propel secretions.

ciliary muscle — the muscle that surrounds the eye lens and helps the eye to focus by changing the shape of the lens.

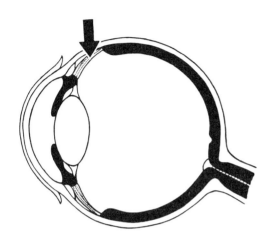

CILIARY MUSCLE

cinchona — a tree found in South America. Quinine, a drug used in the treatment of malaria, is extracted from the cinchona bark.

circle of Willis — a circular system of arteries that helps supply blood to the brain.

circulation — movement or flow within a defined area, such as the circulation of blood.

circulatory system — the system that consists of the heart, the arteries, the veins, and the capillaries. Through this system, blood is carried to and from all parts of the body.

The right side of the heart pumps blood to the lungs, where oxygen is added and carbon dioxide is discharged. The blood then returns to the left side of the heart. This oxygenated blood is then pumped from the heart into the major artery or aorta. From the aorta, the blood is dispersed to the rest of the body, through arteries to capillaries and then to veins, which return the deoxygenated blood to the right side of the heart.

As blood passes through the intestines, it picks up digested food to pass on to the rest of the body. The blood then goes to the liver, which takes some of the food and adds some important ingredients to the blood. Blood entering the kidneys is filtered of waste products.
See arteries, blood pressure, heart, veins.

circumcision — the removal by surgical means of the foreskin of the penis.

There is some evidence that the wives of men who have been circumcised are less likely to have cancer of the cervic than wives whose husbands are uncircumcised.

circumflex — a term used to denote a part of the body that winds around or bends around another part of the body.

cirrhosis of the liver — a disease of the liver in which the cells are destroyed and replaced by scar tissue, thus impairing function. It is the most common disease of the liver and is two of three times more common in men than in women. Age at onset is most often between forty-five and sixty-five.

While the specific cause in unknown, cirrhosis is associated with prolonged malnutrition. Most cases are related to excessive consumption of alcohol and lack of adequate nutrition; however, the disease also occurs among non-drinkers.

The onset of cirrhosis is gradual. The symptoms are often vague and ill-defined. Nausea, vomiting, weight loss, indigestion, flatulence, and abdominal pain represent the most common symptoms in the early phase of the disease. In advanced stages there is jaundice and swelling of the ankles, knees, and abdomen, as well as bleeding tendencies.

Therapy consists of bed rest, adequate diet, and abstinence from alcohol. All efforts are directed toward prevention of complications such as hemorrhage, intercurrent infection, and hepatic coma.

The number of people with cirrhosis of the liver could be reduced by activities directed toward the prevention of alcoholism and the promotion of good nutrition. Early detection and adequate medical care reduce the complications associated with the disease.
See liver.

citric acid — a mild acid found in citric fruits such as lemons and grapefruit. It plays an important role in metabolism.

clap — a slang term for gonorrhea.
See gonorrhea.

claudication — a term used to denote limping or lameness. Intermittent claudication is a condi-

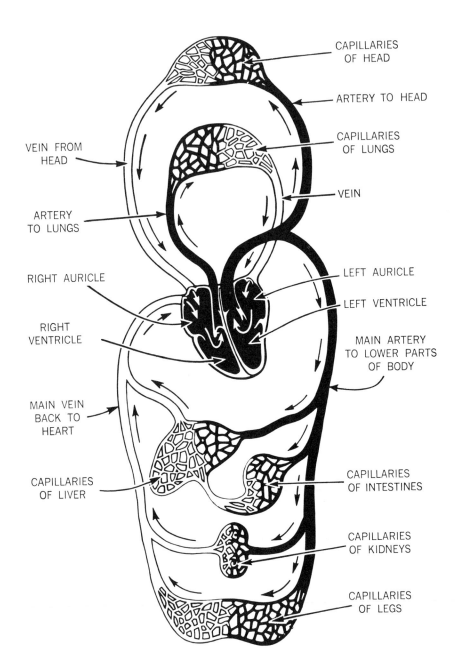

CAPILLARIES OF HEAD

ARTERY TO HEAD

CAPILLARIES OF LUNGS

VEIN FROM HEAD

VEIN

ARTERY TO LUNGS

RIGHT AURICLE

LEFT AURICLE

LEFT VENTRICLE

RIGHT VENTRICLE

MAIN ARTERY TO LOWER PARTS OF BODY

MAIN VEIN BACK TO HEART

CAPILLARIES OF LIVER

CAPILLARIES OF INTESTINES

CAPILLARIES OF KIDNEYS

CAPILLARIES OF LEGS

CIRCULATORY SYSTEM

tion of the limbs in which there is no pain when the limb is at rest, but increasing pain when the limb is in motion.

claustrophobia — the fear of being closed into a confined space. People who suffer from claustrophobia often cannot tolerate being in a room with the door closed.

clavicle — the collar bone. It is joined to the sternum (or breastbone) and the scapula (or shoulder blade) by strong ligaments. One of the purposes of the clavicle is to prevent the shoulders from drooping forward. Because of its position and its closeness to the skin, the clavicle is frequently broken.

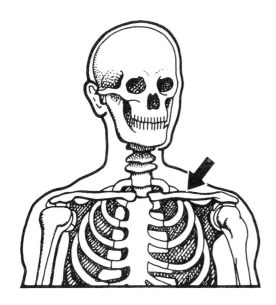

CLAVICLE

cleft — an opening that runs lengthwise.

cleft lip — *See harelip.*

cleft palate — a birth defect, the cause of which is unknown. As a child develops before birth, the parts that form the roof of the mouth meet and grow together. However, sometimes these parts fail to unite.

A cleft palate is usually more complicated than a harelip. It can affect such important functions as breathing, chewing, swallowing, and producing speech sounds. In some cases, the cleft palate may be operated on when the child is about

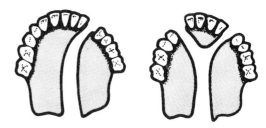

CLEFT PALATE

two years old. In other cases, the operation may be delayed until the fourth or fifth year, or it may seem better not to operate on the cleft at all.

When the operation is performed what is actually done depends on the speed and pattern of growth of the palate and jaw and the kind of cleft, as well as other factors.

There are several different kinds of clefts. Some are single openings, some are double, some are short, and some run the full length of the mouth from front to back. The cleft may or may not involve the gum ridge that contains the future teeth.

A child born with a cleft palate will differ from other children only in the way he talks, and perhaps in the appearance of his face. With the help of surgery and speech therapy, the child can develop normally.

climacteric — one of the points in a person's life when major change occurs in sexual activity. In the female, this is known as menopause, and during this period the female reproduction system shuts down; in the male it is the point at which sexual activity begins to decline.

clinical — having to do with a clinic or bedside. Knowledge or diagnosis gained clinically differs from knowledge gained experimentally or through tests.

clinotherapy — treatment of a patient's complaints by bed rest.

clithrophobia — claustrophia.

clitoris — a small, elongated protusion located where the folds of the vulva meet. The clitoris in the female corresponds with the penis in the male. It is very sensitive during sexual intercourse.

clomiphene — a drug used to increase fertility. It

works by stimulating the production of gonadotropin in the pituitary.
See hormones, pituitary.

Clostridium — a genus of bacteria that is anaerobic (lives without oxygen). One type causes botulism, another causes gas gangrene, and a third is the cause of tetanus in humans.

clot — a semisolid viscous lump, such as a clot of blood, which results from coagulation.

clubbed fingers — fingers with a short, broad tip and overhanging nail, somewhat resembling a drumstick.

clubfoot — *See talipes.*

coagulation — the process of forming a clot. Coagulation can be a blessing or a curse. When the body bleeds, blood-clotting is one of the ways the body stops the flow of blood from the wound. However, a clot that breaks loose can cause a coronary thrombosis.

In the normal healthy body, coagulation will occur about five minutes after bleeding starts.

If coagulation does not occur, as in the case of people who have hemophilia, the patient can bleed to death.
See blood, hemophilia.

coaguloviscosimeter — an instrument that measures the amount of time the blood takes to coagulate.

coarctation — narrowing or constricting.

coarctation of the aorta — *See congential heart defects.*

cobalt — a metal. Cobalt is found in Vitamin B^{12}. Doctors frequently use cobalt in their treatment of cancer patients.

cocaine — a drug derived from the coca bush, a plant that grows in the uplands of Bolivia, Peru, and Chile. It has been used for centuries by Andean Indians, who rely on its anti-fatigue and anti-hunger effects to sustain them through a life of toil and deprivation in the rarefied atmosphere.

In the Western world, cocaine was used as a local anesthetic; however, at present, effective synthetics have been developed, without the unfavorable side effects of cocaine.

Today, cocaine has reappeared on the United States drug scene. In large doses it produces violent stimulant, hallucinatory, and ecstatic effects. Overdoses are not rare and may cause death from cardiac or respiratory arrest. The favorite methods of taking cocaine are by "snorting" or sniffing and by injection.

The body does not develop a tolerance for cocaine, but marked psychic dependence results. Cocaine is highly addictive. As with amphetamines, severe depression occurs as the effects of the drug wear off, impelling the abuser to continue its use.

Chronic use results in nausea, digestive disorders, loss of weight, insomnia, skin abscesses, and occasional convulsions. Prolonged sniffing perforates the septum of the nose. Paranoid delusions, with auditory and visual hallucinations, occur. The mental disturbances often trigger compulsive, violent antisocial acts.

cocci — a type of bacteria that are spherical in shape. "Cocci" is used as a suffix for denoting specific bacteria. There are three major ways the cocci appear. When they occur in pairs, they are

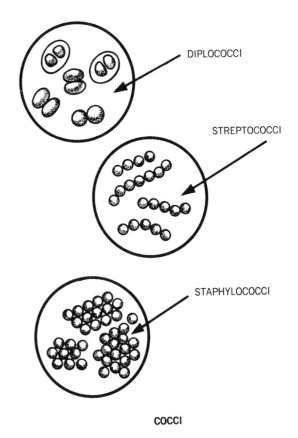

COCCI

called diplococci; when they occur in clusters, they are called staphylococci; and when they occur in chains, they are called streptococci.

Coccidioides — a genus of fungi that can cause infection in the lungs.

coccyx — the small bone located at the bottom of the backbone. It is normally formed by four (sometimes three or five) very small vertebrae joined together.

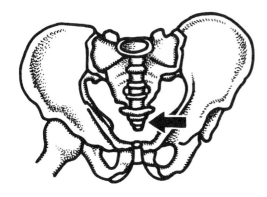

COCCYX

cochlea — the most important hearing organ. A spiral tube, similar to a snail shell, it is part of the structure of the inner ear.
See ear.

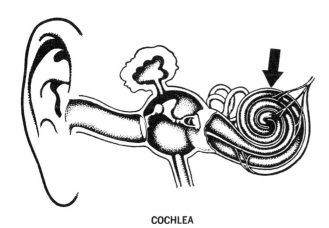

COCHLEA

codeine — a drug used as an analgesiac (to relieve pain) and frequently found in cough medicines. Codeine is effective in treating coughs because it acts as a depressant on the respiratory system. It is a derivative of opium and can be addictive.

coitus — sexual intercourse between a man and a woman.

coitus interruptus — a method of contraception in which the penis is withdrawn before the semen is ejaculated.

colchicine — a drug derived from the plant *Colchicum autumnale* (also known as autumn crocus or meadow saffron). It is one of the best drugs known for treating acute attacks of gout. Colchicine gives dramatic relief within hours.

cold — a low amount of heat. The effects of cold on the body vary with the exact temperature. For instance, when the temperature is 15°F., the body can feel cold, but if properly dressed, it will make the proper adjustments to withstand the cold. However, prolonged exposure when the temperature is −20° F. can be lethal.

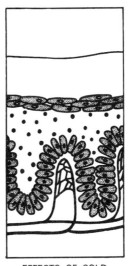 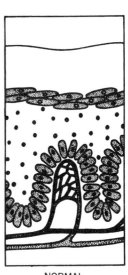

EFFECTS OF COLD ON CAPILLARY	NORMAL CAPILLARY

Capillaries constrict. Less blood flows to the part. Circulation is lessened. Pain is relieved (anesthetic effect).

EFFECTS OF COLD ON SKIN

When the body is chilled, the small arteries close to the skin contract. This helps to retain body temperature because it restricts the flow of blood to exposed areas. At the same time, the nerves seem to lose some of their ability to communicate — in effect, numbing exposed areas. Increased epinephrine is secreted, causing the heart to beat faster and finally generate more body heat.

The body's attempt to maintain body heat under cold conditions can be very tiring.
See common cold.

cold abscess — an abscess that develops slowly and shows little sign of inflammation. A cold abscess is generally tuberculous.

cold sore — *See herpes simplex.*

colic — a condition of severe abdominal pain in adults. It is caused by involuntary contractions in the abdominal region, which in turn are caused by an infection or a blockage.

However, the term colic is also used to refer to a condition in which a baby has hard crying periods soon after being fed. Babies with this condition may be called "colicky." Many babies have colic during the first three or four months. It is less frequent after that.

The cries of the colicky baby are unmistakably those of pain. The baby may draw his arms and legs up, his face gets red, and his abdomen may feel hard while he's having cramps that make him scream.

Many things can cause this discomfort, but many times not much can be done about the causes. Some, such as an immature digestive system, can only be cured by time. However, the condition should always be brought to a doctor's attention for investigation.

colitis — inflammation of the colon (the large intestine from the cecum to the rectum). The most frequent cause of colitis is food-poisoning. Symptoms include diarrhea and acute stomach pains. It is usually treated as acute diarrhea would be.

One form of colitis, ulcerative colitis, is particularly serious. In this type, the wall of the bowel is actually ulcerated. Treatment for ulcerative colitis includes antibiotics and, usually, complete bed rest.

collagen — a protein. It is the main part of all connective tissues. A collagen disease is one in which tissues containing collagen are involved. This would include rheumatic fever.

collateral — a secondary or alternative path for the flow of blood. These are used when more blood is needed in a particular part of the body, or when the primary route is blocked.

Colles, Abraham — an Irish surgeon (1773-1843) and professor of anatomy. His work in anatomy resulted in a description of the abdominal fascia, which is named after him. He wrote an important treatise on fractures, and in conjunction with the French physician Pierre Baumes, he propounded Colles' law.
See Colles' fracture, Colles' law.

Colles' fracture — a fracture of the lower end of the radius. The broken portion is displaced backward. It is treated by reducing the fracture and immobilizing the area by means of a cast.
See radius.

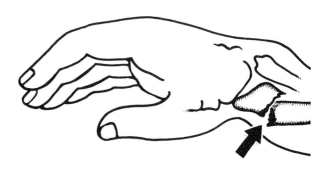

COLLES' FRACTURE

Colles' law — a law that states that a child with congenital syphilis will not infect its mother.

coloboma — a defect. Usually used to indicate a congenital defect of the eye.

colocynth — a drug made from the dried pulp of *Citrullus colocynthus*. It has been used as a purgative for centuries. However, it is not used much today because it is too irritating.

colon — the large intestine from the cecum to the rectum.
See intestine.

color blindness — a congenital and hereditary condition in which the eye is unable to distinguish between certain colors. The most frequent problem is inability to distinguish between red and green. Sometimes the difference between blue and yellow is affected. Very few people are entirely color blind. It is possible to be partially color blind and not know it.

One of the ways to detect color blindness was devised by a Japanese professor. This test consists of several different cards printed with dots of two different colors. The dots are arranged to show a number in the middle. A person who is color blind will be unable to perceive the number because its component dots (printed in one color) will not seem to differ from the background dots (printed in another color).

Color blindness is carried by women but primarily affects men. It is thus a sex-linked characteristic.

See genetics.

colostomy — a surgical procedure that reroutes the colon to bypass and avoid the rectum. A temporary or permanent opening also called a colostomy is made in the abdominal wall to permit elimination of solid body wastes. The wastes are then collected in a plastic bag worn by the patient. Bowel function is not impaired by this operation, and, after adjusting to some inconvenience, the patient can lead an otherwise normal, active life.

While this operation is performed for several reasons, it is most frequently used in cases of cancer of the colon or rectum.

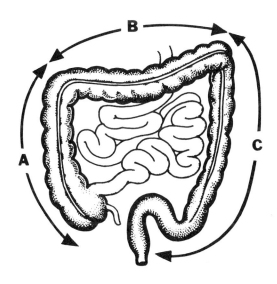

COLON

A ASCENDING COLON
B TRANSVERSE COLON
C DESCENDING COLON

coma — a condition in which the patient is unconscious and can not be aroused by any means. It may be caused by injury, disease, pressure, or some form of poisoning. In addition to being a serious condition, a coma is a symptom that something is very seriously wrong somewhere in the body.

The patient in a coma should be watched very carefully. Because part of the brain is not functioning properly, it is possible for the patient to suffocate from saliva inhaled into the lungs.

In some cases, a coma is the body's way of protecting the brain while it recuperates from injury, and the patient will come out of the coma when the brain has healed.

In other cases, the coma will become progressively deeper unless something is done to treat the disease or to lower the pressure on the brain. If nothing is done, it is possible for the coma to become so deep that the brain ceases to function altogether, and the patient dies.

comedo — a dried deposit of sebum in the pore of the skin. Also called a blackhead.

See acne.

commensal — a term used to denote an organism that lives on or within another organism without causing harm to the host. An example would be the bacteria that normally inhabit the human body without causing disease or infection.

commissurotomy — an operation to widen the opening in a heart valve that has become narrowed by scar tissue. The individual flaps of the valve are cut or spread apart along the natural line of their closure. This operation is often performed in cases of rheumatic heart disease.

See mitral valvulotomy.

common cold — a viral infection of the throat and nasal passages. It is the most common of all human illnesses.

The patient usually has a sore throat before the rest of the symptoms appear. This condition will generally improve once the other symptoms begin. Following the sore throat, the patient experiences one or more of the following: runny nose, congestion, sneezing, watering eyes, a slight rise in temperature, and an achy feeling.

Colds are not caused by one or even a few viruses. At least twenty viruses have already been identified as important causes.

There is no known cure for the common cold. In most people, the cold will run its course (which differs in length in different people from three to seven days or more), regardless of treatment. In the past, the treatments have included: feed a cold, starve a cold, fruit juice diets, and every advertised drug.

TREATMENT

Today, the recommended treatment is:

1. When possible, the patient should go to bed when he first feels a cold coming on. He will be more comfortable, less likely to develop complications, and will not spread the disease. He will be safer in bed if the illness turns out to be one of the diseases that mimic a common cold at the start.

2. The patient should be kept warm and protected from direct drafts and changing temperatures.

3. Drink plenty of liquids such as water, soups, milk, and fruit juices.

4. Eat moderately.

5. When blowing the nose, blow gently. Do not force infection into the sinuses and the canals that lead to the ears.

6. Cover sneezes and coughs with paper tissue and then dispose of them so that they need not be touched again and are not sitting out in the open air.

7. Aspirin is approved for use, but do not use other medicines without consulting a doctor. If the condition warrants it, a doctor can prescribe medicines to relieve some of the symptoms and to treat complications.

PREVENTION

Because colds are highly infectious, it is impossible to escape them entirely unless one can avoid all contact with other people.

People who brag about never giving up for a cold, will go about their business and recreation as usual, spreading colds as they go. Even the most considerate person is a source of infection at times, because a cold is contagious before symptoms warn of its presence. You catch a cold, not from an occasional few germs, but from taking more of them into your body than your defense forces can conquer. If you can keep out of range of massive doses of viruses that will be sneezed your way and keep your resistance high, you should have fewer colds. The following are sensible preventive measures:

1. Avoid people with colds whenever possible. Keep at a distance from them when they cough and sneeze or shake out a used handkerchief for another blow. These precautions would mean staying away from crowded amusement places during cold epidemics.

2. Wash your hands often, especially before eating and after touching a patient with a cold.

3. Don't use a drinking glass or towel that may have been soiled by a person with a cold.

4. Keep your general health as good as possible. Avoid chilling, wet feet, and fatigue. Eat well-balanced meals. Give your body every possible advantage when there are more than the usual number of colds around you.

SPREAD

The viruses that cause colds are present in great numbers in the throat and nasal secretions of the infected person. The disease is spread when these secretions leave the sick person's body and enter the mouths and noses of other people. There are many ways this can happen. The most frequent is through sneezing or coughing germ-laden spray into the air for nearby persons to inhale. (Pictures taken by high-speed photography show that a sneeze sprays nasal secretions a distance of about three feet.) Other ways of transmitting the disease are through kissing and through the common use of drinking glasses, towels, and other objects that have been freshly soiled by these secretions. Handkerchiefs that have been soiled by a person with a cold are believed to be storehouses of germs. From one to three days after the viruses get into the mouth or nose, cold symptoms appear. The most infectious stage of a cold is when a person is coming down with it and for the next day or two.

compensation — a change made by the body to compensate for some abnormality. For example, an adjustment of the size of the heart or the rate of heartbeat, made to counterbalance a defect in structure or function.

compound fracture — a fracture of the bone in which

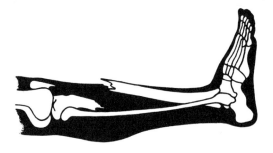

COMPOUND FRACTURE

the broken bone pierces the skin. This is much more dangerous than a simple fracture because of the possibility of infection and because it can be more difficult to reduce.

See fracture.

compression — squeezing or pressing together.

compression sickness — *See decompression sickness.*

conception — the fertilization of an ovum by a sperm forming a zygote or fertilized egg which develops into an embryo. In humans, conception usually occurs in the fallopian tube.

Because an ovum lives for only a few days, conception can only occur several days out of every month. By figuring the amount of time between menstrual periods and then finding the midpoint (when ovulation occurs), it is possible to approximate the times when conception can take place.

See contraception.

concussion — a violent physical shock to the brain. This can be caused by an injury to the head or to the neck.

A person suffering from a brain concussion will usually experience a period of unconsciousness. How long this lasts depends on how much damage has been done to the brain. Symptoms such as nausea, dizziness, restlessness, and some forms of amnesia are common.

condom — any covering used on the penis during sexual intercourse to prevent conception or avoid infection.

See contraception.

condyle — the rounded protuberance at the end of a bone.

congenital — a term applied to any condition, disease, or defect existing at birth. The term has nothing to do with the cause or source of the problem.

congenital heart defects — a defect existing at birth, resulting from the failure of an infant's heart or of a major blood vessel near the heart to develop normally during pregnancy. There are many types of inborn heart defects. Each may occur alone, or the heart may be crippled by a combination of several defects.

CAUSES

The exact reason why a few babies have defective hearts at birth is still unknown.

A small percentage of congenital heart abnormalities apparently may result from the mother having had German measles during the first three months of her pregnancy. This and other environmental or "outside" influences that could lead to imperfect development of the human embryo are under widespread study.

A twist of heredity may also be involved in producing an inborn heart defect. No conclusive answer to this has been found, however, and the role of genetic transmission is still a subject of extensive medical research. Scientists feel that an inborn defect is not caused, however, by "bad heredity" in either the mother's or the father's family. It is unusual for more than one child in a family to have this type of heart condition.

SYMPTOMS

The doctor who delivers a baby sometimes recognizes immediately that the newborn may have a heart defect. One signal is a blue tinge to the baby's skin — called cyanosis. "Blue babies" have heart defects that prevent enough blood from getting to their lungs to pick up oxygen. Most often the "blue baby" name is used for a defect known as tetralogy of Fallot, but other defects can also cause blueness. In mild cases, cyanosis may appear in the lips and fingertips when the child exerts himself.

Blueness, or any one of the other symptoms of an inborn defect, may be present in some instances, absent in others. Symptoms can also show up at varying ages. An inborn defect may prevent a child from growing and gaining weight normally. He may tire easily or feel weak. There may be spells of breathing difficulty, with the child having to stop often to catch his breath. The baby or youngster may squat frequently, as this posture helps him breathe more easily.

Any of these symptoms could also be an indication of some other problem, or they might mean nothing whatsoever. However, they should always be brought to the doctor's attention, since the earlier a defect is diagnosed, the better are the child's chances.

TYPES AND TREATMENT

The defects described below account for approximately three-fourths of all inborn heart abnormalities. Fortunately, surgical procedures are available today to completely or partially correct each of them. Whether or not an individual patient can benefit by one of these operations must of course be decided by his doctor.

1. Patent ductus arteriosus

Every newborn baby has a passageway — a "patent ductus" — between the two major blood vessels that adjoin his heart: the pulmonary artery and the aorta. This connection, useful during fetal life, normally closes before the baby is many weeks old. When it fails to do so, some of the blood that should be circulated through the body will instead shuttle uselessly back and forth between the heart and lungs. This means that the heart must work harder to pump sufficient blood through the body to nourish all tissues and organs. Before a child with patent ductus arteriosus reaches school age, normal circulation can usually be established with an operation to tie shut or cut the passageway that nature left open.

2. Septal defects

A septal defect is another inborn heart imperfection that results in an added burden on the heart in furnishing enough oxygen-laden blood throughout the body. This abnormality is an opening in the muscle wall, the septum, that separates the interior of the heart into a left and right side. The hole may be between the two upper heart chambers (atrial septal defect) or between the lower chambers (ventricular septal defect).

Unless it is small, either defect means interference with normal blood circulation. How much increase this places on the heart's work load depends on the size and location of the defect, but sometimes the heart cannot meet the demand that it work much harder.

With the aid of a heart-lung machine, open-heart surgery is now successful in sewing shut these septal openings, or in closing them with synthetic patches. Other openings are being improved with a surgical technique known as pulmonary banding. This technique helps ease the circulation work of the overtaxed heart until the patient reaches a size and age when the defect can be fully repaired.

3. Coarctation of the aorta

The aorta is the largest artery in the body, carrying the full load of blood away from the heart to begin its distribution to all areas of the body. When the aorta is narrowed, or coarcted, at birth,

the amount of blood it can transport may be seriously reduced.

When symptoms of such a harmful constriction of the vessel appear, surgery can usually be performed to remove the narrowed vessel segment. Surgeons then sew together the two ends of the natural aorta, or, if a long section has been cut out, they may replace this part of the aorta with an artificial vessel made from modern synthetic materials. A slight inborn coarctation of the aorta may cause no trouble and never require an operation.

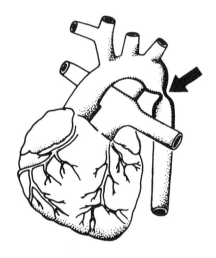

COARCTATION OF THE AORTA

4. Valvular stenosis

Some babies may be born with a narrowing, or stenosis, of one of the valves regulating blood flow inside the heart. Narrowing may occur in the valve itself (most commonly in the aortic and pulmonary heart valves) or in an area near a valve. Normal, smooth flow of blood is obstructed by the constriction. This necessitates an increase in the heart's pumping work to push blood through the crippled valve, or possibly an inadequate oxygenation of the blood. Stenosed valves are cut open in thousands of operations today, and many irreparably damaged valves are being totally replaced with man-made artificial valves developed in recent years.

5. Transposition of the great vessels

In this defect the two "great vessels" — the pulmonary artery that carries blood to the lungs to pick up oxygen, and the aorta transporting blood to the body — originate on the wrong sides of the heart, opposite their proper source. Almost without exception, the outlook for a newborn infant with this defect used to be extremely grave. Doctors now help some of them by surgically creating a second defect, an atrial septal opening, thus helping balance the circulation mix-up the baby had at birth.

Total correction of a transposition of the great vessels, possible in some cases today after the patient has reached a favorable size and condition, is one of the major surgical feats of recent years.

6. *Tetralogy of Fallot*

This name is given to a combination of four defects causing a blue baby: a ventricular septal opening; an "overriding aorta" that straddles both ventricles instead of originating solely in the left ventricle; a stenosed pulmonary valve; and an enlarged right ventricle. The main result is a short-circuit of the blood flow inside the heart so that not enough blood gets to the lungs to pick up oxygen. Oxygen-poor blood thus circulating in the body gives the skin a blue color and deprives the body tissues of as much oxygen as they need.

Several closed-heart operations have been in use for a number of years that relieve a blue baby's condition but do not correct the heart defects themselves. In these operations, surgeons provide a channel through which more blood can reach the lungs. Today it is possible, when the patient is of proper age and condition, to completely cure more and more cases of tetralogy of Fallot with open-heart operations in which the narrowed pulmonary valve is cut open and the septal defect sealed with a plastic patch.

In all, there are now known to be about thirty-five kinds of inborn heart defects. Today nearly twenty of these can be cured or improved by surgery. Some not already mentioned are tricuspid atresia, vascular ring, pulmonary vascular atresia, and total anomalous pulmonary venous drainage. Surgeons strive continually to correct more and more of these abnormalities and constantly seek new operations and improvement of those now in use.

congestion — an excess of blood in part of the body. The word is also used to indicate the stuffy feeling associated with the common cold.

congestive heart failure — a condition that is the eventual outcome of most forms of heart disease. It is the result of inefficiency of the heart muscle or incompetent valves in delivering blood to meet the demands of the body. The weakened heart cannot get enough blood to the tissues, and excess blood accumulates in certain organs.

It is the damaged heart that fails first. Any pump that becomes damaged will lose some of its effectiveness. The heart is, in reality, two pumps beating together. One side (the right side) pumps blood to the lungs, where it receives oxygen and returns to the other side (the left side) of the heart, which pumps blood to the rest of the body. Either pump can fail separately, or both may fail together. When the efficiency of the heart muscle decreases and is not able to keep up with the demands of the body, the patient begins to develop the symptoms. If the left side fails, fluid backs up in the lungs and he becomes short of breath. If the right side fails, fluid backs up in the abdomen and legs. If both fail, the patient may have shortness of breath caused by fluid in the lungs and edema due to fluid in the legs.

The exact mechanism that leads up to the condition is poorly understood. The kidney and certain hormones play an important part in bringing on the signs and symptoms of congestive heart failure.

In congestive heart failure the kidney has the unique ability of retaining all the sodium in salt and other substances delivered to it by the bloodstream. This means that all the sodium eaten is retained, whereas the normal kidney can usually excrete the same amount of sodium as the body takes in. Sodium retention in itself presents certain problems, but a more serious problem is the capacity of sodium to retain water. Thus, the sodium retention leads to water retention. The water retention leads to an increased volume of body fluid. The heart, already damaged and not functioning efficiently, is asked to pump harder. This is not possible, so it fails further, and fluid accumulates in tissues such as the legs, abdomen, and lungs. It is this fluid that creates the major problem of congestive heart failure and the one to which therapy is frequently directed.

The heart often tries to accommodate itself to this failure. It may beat faster (tachycardia), and this may be felt as palpitations. It may become larger (dilate), or it may develop thicker walls (hypertrophy). But when these mechanisms no longer serve to maintain the cardiac output, then congestive heart failure ensues.

SYMPTOMS

Congestive heart failure may be acute, but

usually it comes on gradually.

Onset is occasionally precipitated by a slight respiratory infection, overeating, excitement, or exertion on top of a heart condition. In attempting to compensate, the heart enlarges. Shortness of breath, increased by exertion or by assuming a reclining position; accumulation of fluid in the chest or abdomen; swelling of ankles; loss of appetite; nausea or vomiting; irritability; restlessness; and short attention span are characteristic of the disease.

TREATMENT

1. Digitalis

Digitalis is a drug used almost exclusively in congestive heart failure. Its main purpose is to increase the cardiac output by stimulating the heart muscle to contract more forcibly. As a result, there is an increase in cardiac efficiency. Often this is the only drug necessary to relieve the patient of his symptoms and to correct the problem.

2. Diet

A diet that restricts sodium is often recommended. Frequently the doctor will recommend cutting down on table salt, which is forty percent sodium. He may recommend the maximum amount of sodium that shoud be included in the diet. This amount is not the same for every patient and may even vary from time to time with the same patient, depending on the severity of his condition.

The recommendation for sodium restriction is based on the principle previously mentioned: in congestive heart failure, the kidney retains almost all the ingested sodium. By limiting the amount of sodium taken, it is possible to prevent an accumulation of sodium, and likewise water, in the body. Restricting water in itself serves no purpose.

3. Diuretics

These drugs are recommended because of their ability to promote excretion of water. Most of them work by removing sodium from the body, and with it they remove the water. Some may be given as injections for immediate effects, and some may be taken by mouth for less-rapid action or for convenience. Various preparations using the same principle may have different effects and, because of this, may be altered or changed by the physician. Like digitalis, they should be taken in the amount and with the frequency prescribed by the physician.

Diuretics do not take the place of digitalis or diet. They may be used in conjunction with them. Frequently they permit patients to follow a diet with less-severe restriction of sodium, but some degree of sodium control is almost always necessary.

4. Activity

Activity, either physical or emotional, contributes toward increased cardiac activity. Consequently, the physician must consider these factors as part of the patient's therapy. The amount of physical activity he recommends is determined by his appraisal of the condition and what his experience and knowledge have taught him to allow in the condition. It is best to maintain the prescribed degree of activity. Just as it is wrong to be overactive, it is also wrong to be inactive. In acute cases bed rest may be prescribed. This is done to permit the heart to rest and require that it pump only enough to maintain minimal body requirements. As the condition improves, more and more activity will be recommended. By taking the medicines and following the diet as prescribed, most patients can return to their normal activities. The patient should never do more than is prescribed, even though he feels well. Emotional stress forces the heart to work harder.

EARLY WARNING SIGNS
1. Sudden or gradual unexpected weight gain.
2. Shortness of breath on exertion.
3. Swelling of the ankles or abdomen.
4. Frequent urination at night.
5. Need to sleep in an upright position.
6. Unexplained, persistent cough.
7. Unexplained loss of appetite.

conjunctiva — the membrane lining of the eyelid and outer surface of the exposed portion of the eyeball. The membrane is very delicate.

conjunctivitis — an inflammation of the conjunctiva. The most familiar type is known as pinkeye. This type is highly contagious. The eye looks red or pink (hence the name), and there is usually a discharge.

connective tissue — the supporting tissue for the cellular layers of the body. This type of tissue, with its many varieties, is the most widespread tissue in the body. It surrounds cells, encases internal organs, sheathes muscles, wraps bones, encloses joints, composes the blood, and provides the supporting framework of the body. Structures of connective tissue differ widely. Delicate, tissue-paper-thin membranes; strong, tough cords; rigid bones; liquid blood - all are made of connective tissue.

constipation — a condition in which the bowels are opened infrequently or with difficulty.

The great problem in defining constipation lies in the fact that bowel-movement rhythm is an individual characteristic.

A movement every day, or twice a day, may be good bowel function for one person; for another, it may be one movement every three or four days. In fact, there are people in excellent health whose bowels move regularly only once in five or eight days.

Laxatives are not the cure-all for constipation. They frequently help in both temporary and habitual constipation — but a physician should be consulted first. People who diagnose their own ailments and constantly take laxatives will often increase rather than cure their troubles. It is actually possible to cause constipation by the cathartic habit. The habitual use of cathartics is responsible for a good deal of disease of the rectum.

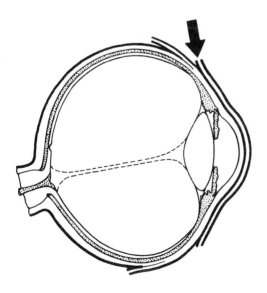

CONJUNCTIVA

As for taking a laxative to cure an acute pain in the abdomen — that is not only extremely dangerous — it can be fatal. A violent bowel action caused by a cathartic is often more than an inflamed appendix, ready to rupture, can stand. If the appendix does rupture, peritonitis, and frequently death, may follow. Laxatives should be avoided if there is acute pain, cramps, or soreness in the abdomen. These symptoms may be a warning of heart attack, kidney stone, gallbladder colic, or appendicitis.

People who have always had good bowel movements should see a doctor if constipation develops suddenly. It may be an early symptom of serious disease, possibly even cancer. A complete physical examination is highly important.

When bowel movements are difficult or painful, or when evacuation feels incomplete, the trouble may be more than simple constipation.

By starting treatment early, most constipation can be relieved without resort to drugs. It is not natural for the colon to be completely empty. Only a doctor should prescribe a purge or colonic irrigation.

Enemas are less upsetting to the system than cathartics for many people. However, they should be considered, like laxatives, as crutches — temporary aids to correct bad habits and to restore good bowel function.

To reestablish good bowel habits, doctors generally recommend making a habit of going to the bathroom at the same time every day. Right after breakfast is usually best — provided that enough time is allowed so that there is no feeling of being rushed or hurried. The important thing is to establish a regular habit and to relax. Be prompt and efficient in attending to this function, but do not hurry.

It is important to go to the toilet whenever the need is felt. Never ignore or put off that impulse. Constipation is often caused and aggravated by disregarding nature's signal that the bowel is ready to be emptied.

Children rarely need laxatives, and they should not be started on the cathartic habit. Overanxious mothers who give their favorite physic to their youngsters cause constipation more often than they cure it. A child will not become ill from a temporary lapse in the regularity of his bowel movement. Normal bowel activity usually reestablishes itself spontaneously in a day or two, especially if no anxiety is shown by the parents. A regular routine, with the child going to the toilet every morning at the same time, and a matter-of-fact attitude on the part of the parents, generally prevents or controls constipation.

constriction — narrowing.

constrictive pericarditis — a shrinking and thickening of the outer sac of the heart, which prevents the heart muscle from expanding and contracting normally.

consumption — a term applied to a disease associated with severe weight loss. This term is often used in referring to pulmonary tuberculosis (tuberculosis of the lungs).
  See tuberculosis.

contact lenses — a substitute for or an alternative to wearing eyeglasses. Contact lenses are usually round disks, concave in shape, to fit on the convex surface of the eyeball. The disk floats on the fluid of the eye and serves the same purpose as the lenses from a pair of eyeglasses — helping to adjust impaired vision.
  Some doctors feel that contact lenses are better than glasses, because they are worn closer to the eye. The disadvantage is that contact lenses can usually be worn only for a certain amount of time (particularly at first) before the eyes become somewhat irritated.

contagion — the communication of an infectious disease from a person who has or is carrying it to another person who does not have it.

contagious disease — a disease that can be passed on by people who have it or who are carriers for it.

contaminate — to soil or infect.

contraception — the prevention of the act of conception or of the impregnation of a fertilized ovum (zygote).
  See contraceptive methods.

contraceptive methods — methods to prevent contraception or impregnation. There are several methods.
  1. Spermicides are used to kill the sperm before they can fertilize the ovum.
  2. "The pill" contains hormones that lead the body to believe that it is pregnant. Because there is no ovulation during pregnancy, "the pill" pre-

vents conception by inhibiting ovulation.
  3. Rubber devices worn on the penis to prevent the sperm from entering the female body.
  4. I.U.D. (intrauterine devices) are coils, loops, or barbs that are implanted within the uterus. They do not prevent conception; rather they prevent the fertilized ovum from attaching itself to the womb.
  5. Coitus interruptus or interrupted coitus is the physical withdrawal of the penis before ejaculation.
  6. The rhythm method is based on the fact that conception can take place only during the few days during which the ovum lives. Thus, the rhythm method necessitates abstaining from sexual intercourse immediately before and after ovulation.
  See conception.

contractile protein — the protein substance within the heart muscle fibers responsible for heart contraction by shortening the muscle fibers.

contraction — shortening or tension.
  See labor.

contracture — a shortening or shrinking of tissues or scars. Contracture of tissues usually means there will be a loss of mobility in the affected area. Muscles in the affected area do not stretch well. Contracture can occur when a limb is immobilized over a period of time.

contraindication — a condition or factor that indicates that a particular treatment or drug is unsuitable for use in a specific case.

contrecoup — injury on one side as a result of a blow on the other side.

contusion — an injury below the skin (sometimes quite deep) caused by a blow that does not break the skin.
  See bruise.

convalescence — the period following an injury, illness, surgery, etc., during which the patient is recuperating.

convolutions — curved and winding inward folds, such as the surface of the cerebrum or the intestines.

convulsion — a violent, involuntary contraction or

series of contractions of muscles. A convulsion is the result of an irritation of an area of the brain.

Cooley's anemia — also called thalassemia and named for Thomas B. Cooley (1871-1945), an American pediatrician.
See thalassemia.

cord — a long, flexible, connective organ.
See spinal cord, vocal cord, etc.

corium — the layer of skin under the epidermis, also called the dermis. The corium contains connective tissue, blood vessels, and nerves.

corn — a thickening of the skin, usually caused by pressure or friction (as for example from shoes that do not fit correctly). The corn extends into the corium and can be very painful.

cornea — the part of the eye that covers the iris and pupil. It is circular in shape and is transparent. The transparency allows rays of light to pass through it. When the cornea loses this transparency, various forms of blindness occur. When the cornea is flawed in shape (i.e., not perfectly spherical), the result is a condition called astigmatism.

Cornea transplants are generally relatively simple and are usually very successful.
See astigmatism.

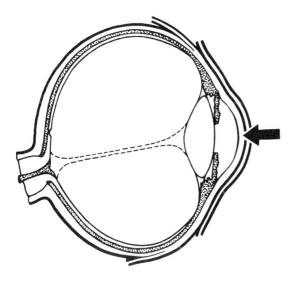

CORNEA

corona — a crown or halo. Under certain conditions, the eye will see a corona around a bright light.

coronary arteries — the two arteries that conduct blood to the heart muscle. They arise from the aorta and arch down over the top of the heart. When the flow of blood through these arteries is not sufficient for the needs of the heart muscle, a condition known as angina pectoris arises.
See angina pectoris.

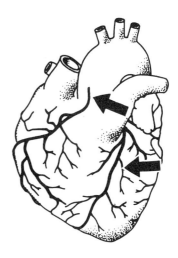

CORONARY ARTERIES

coronary atherosclerosis — an irregular thickening of the inner layer of the walls of the coronary arteries. The internal channel of these arteries becomes narrowed, and the blood supply to the heart muscle is reduced.
See atherosclerosis.

coronary heart disease — the common name for coronary atherosclerosis.
See coronary atherosclerosis.

coronary occlusion — any obstruction in a branch of one of the coronary arteries that hinders the flow of blood to some part of the heart muscle. This part of the heart muscle can then die because of lack of blood supply. It is sometimes called a coronary heart attack, or simply a heart attack.

coronary thrombosis — the formation of a clot in a branch of one of the arteries that conduct blood to the heart muscle. The clot hinders the blood flow to some part of the heart muscle. This part can then die because of lack of blood supply.

Coronary thrombosis is not necessarily fatal, and the chances for recovery increase with every extra day the patient lives after the attack.

Symptoms include sudden pain in the chest lasting for longer than half an hour and sometimes for days. Shortness of breath; cold, clammy skin; and a weak, irregular pulse are common.

The most important part of treatment for coronary thrombosis is complete bed rest. Additionally, oxygen and anticoagulants may be given.

Coronary thombosis is also called myocardial infarction.

coroner — the official responsible for determining the cause of death in unexplained deaths.

cor pulmonale — heart disease resulting from disease of the lungs or the blood vessels in the lungs. This is caused by resistance to the passage of blood through the lungs.

corpuscle — a small mass or body.

corpus luteum — a yellow substance secreted by the ovary after an ovum has been released. If the ovum is not fertilized, the corpus luteum is sloughed off during menstruation. When the ovum is fertilized, the corpus luteum increases and survives during the first few months of pregnancy.

The corpus luteum serves the function of secreting the hormone progesterone. The lining of the uterus is stimulated by the progesterone and grows a thick layer, ready to receive the fertilized ovum. If the ovum is not fertilized, the lining is sloughed off along with the corpus luteum.

corrigent — any substance that makes a drug milder in strength or taste. Used particularly when a drug is too strong.

corrosion — a slow, destructive process usually involving tissue. An eating-away.

cortex — the outer or external layer of a body organ, such as the cerebral cortex (the outer layer of the brain) or the renal cortex (the outer layer of the kidney).

corticosteroids — hormones secreted in the adrenal cortex. Corticosteroids can also be synthesized.

They play an important role in metabolism, electrolyte and water balance, and they influence the cardiovascular system as well as other systems and organs. The adrenocorticotropic hormone (ACTH) regulates the secretion of corticosteroids.

As synthesized hormones, corticosteroids are used in the treatment of acute bronchial asthma, rheumatoid arthritis, eye and skin diseases, and hyperallergic reactions. Corticosteroids are very helpful in reducing inflammations. They are also prescribed in cases of adrenal insufficiency.

Great care is given in administering corticosteroids. While one dose seems to have no adverse effect, treatment over an extended period must be very carefully regulated.

See adrenocorticotropic hormone.

corticotropin — a hormone that stimulates the adrenal cortex. Corticotropin can be synthesized.

cortisone — a hormone that regulates carbohydrates. It is manufactured in the adrenal cortex and can be synthesized. Cortisone is a corticosteroid hormone.

Corvisart, Jean Nicholas — French physician (1755-1821) who reintroduced the use of percussion in diagnosis. He was Napoleon's favorite physician and is probably best known for his treatise on cardiac diseases. He was the first man to call himself a "heart specialist."

Corynebacterium — a genus of bacterium. The bacterium causing diphtheria belongs to this genus. *Corynebacteria* are straight or slightly curved rods.

coryza — a condition in which there is discharge from the nasal mucous membranes — usually associated with the common cold and hay fever.

costa — a rib.

costae — the twenty-four bones (twelve on each side) that form the rib cage.

couching — a technique used in the treatment of cataracts. Instead of stripping the lens from the eye, the surgeon displaces or moves the cataract into a position where it cannot block light rays.

cough — a voluntary or involuntary expulsion of air and foreign materials from the lungs.

A cough is said to be productive when it brings

up foreign matter or mucus out of the lungs or respiratory system in general. There are many different types of coughs. For example, the barking cough, the hacking cough, and the cough resulting from the disease whooping cough all sound different.

The cough that will not go away is a sign that something is wrong with the breathing system. As such, it is one of the most important symptoms of chronic bronchitis, emphysema, and other serious illnesses.

cough medicine — a drug given to suppress coughing or to make it more productive.

A drug that suppresses coughing is called an antitussive. Antitussives work by suppressing the cough reflex center. Narcotics such as codeine are often used in cough medicines for this purpose, although there are some non-narcotic antitussives.

Cough medicines given to increase the productivity of coughing work by forcing the membranes to dilate and loosen the mucus.

coumarin — a class of chemical substances that delay clotting of the blood. An anticoagulant.

counterirritation — the application of an irritant to reduce or relieve another irritation.

Counterirritation can involve the use of drugs in the form of ointments or the use of heat. Counterirritants are usually applied to the skin and seem to work by producing an inflammation, thus increasing the flow of blood to the affected area.

Coutard's method — a method of X-ray treatment, using very slight doses over a long period of time. It is named for Henri Coutard, a French radiologist (18766-1950) who worked in the United States.

cowpox — See smallpox.

coxa — the hip or the hip joint.

cradle cap — an accumulation of a thick, greasy crust, usually on the scalp; but it may occur behind the ears, on the eyebrows or eyelashes, at the corners of the nose, on the cheeks, or even on the trunk. Cradle cap occurs in the first months of infancy.

cramp — a painful muscle contraction or spasm that is involuntary. A cramp can be caused by working in intense heat without replacing lost fluid and salts and by lack of an adequate flow of blood to a part of the body. Usually, when the cause is removed, the cramp will cease. For instance, when a cramp is caused by a narrowing of the blood vessels in the legs, the cramp will ease when the legs stop moving. With angina pectoris, a cramp of the heart muscle, when the flow of blood is returned to normal, the pain goes away. A painful cramp in an overworked muscle will loosen when the muscle is rested.

cranial nerves — twelve pairs of nerves directly connected to the brain. They are:

1. The olfactory nerves, which terminate in the mucous membrane of the nose, are responsible for the sense of smell.

2. The optic nerves terminate in the retina and transmit vision.

3. The oculomotor nerves are connected with the eye muscles and are responsible for their movement.

4. The trochlear nerves are connected to the superior oblique muscle of the eyeball, which rotates the eyeball down and out.

5. The trigeminal nerves divide into three branches.
   a. The ophthalmic branch goes to the forehead, nose, and eye.
   b. The maxillary branch goes to the eye and upper teeth.
   c. The mandibular branch goes to the ear, tongue, and lower teeth.

6. The abducens nerves are connected to the rectus muscles of the eyeball and control rotation of the eyeball up and inward and down and inward.

7. The facial nerves control movements and expressions of the face.

8. The auditory nerves terminate in the ear and control balance and hearing.

9. The glossopharyngeal nerves end in the tongue and throat and transmit sensations from there.

10. The vagus nerves branch into the lungs, liver, stomach, and bowels.

11. The accessory nerves are responsible for the neck muscles.

12. The hypoglossal nerves are responsible for controlling the movement of the tongue.

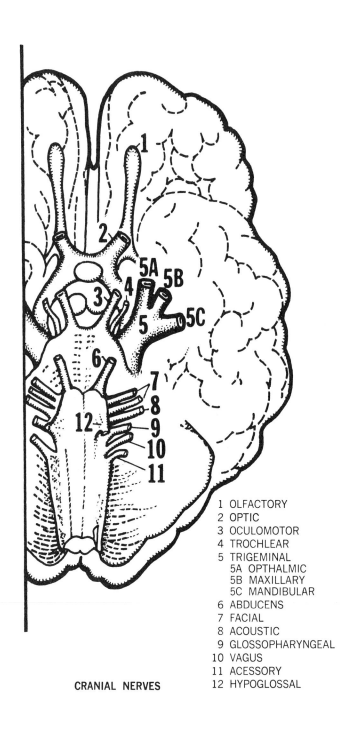

1 OLFACTORY
2 OPTIC
3 OCULOMOTOR
4 TROCHLEAR
5 TRIGEMINAL
   5A OPTHALMIC
   5B MAXILLARY
   5C MANDIBULAR
6 ABDUCENS
7 FACIAL
8 ACOUSTIC
9 GLOSSOPHARYNGEAL
10 VAGUS
11 ACESSORY
12 HYPOGLOSSAL

CRANIAL NERVES

cranium — the bones that make up the head. The skull.

creatine — a compound of nitrogen manufactured in the body. When creatine is in a phosphate form, it stores energy.

cretin — a person who has cretinism.

cretinism — a chronic congenital lack of thyroid function, which manifests itself in retarded growth — both mental and physical.

cricoid — shaped in a ring.

cricoid cartilage — cartilage that forms the lower and back sections of the larynx.

crisis — the turning point in a disease. That point where a definite change takes place. Either there is tremendous improvement in the condition, or the patient's condition seriously deteriorates.

Crohn's disease — regional ileitis.
See ileitis.

cross matching — a method used to be sure that the recipient and the donor involved in a blood transfusion are compatible blood types.

croup — a condition caused by an obstruction in the larynx. The restricted flow of air causes strained breathing and usually a barking cough. The obstruction can be the result of an allergic reaction, an infection, a growth, or a foreign body stuck in the passageway.

crude death rate — the ratio of total deaths to total population during a given period of time. Also called crude mortality rate.

crust — a solid outer layer that forms when a secreted body fluid dries out. In a sense a scab from a would is a crust.

crux — the juncture of the walls in the heart between the right and left sides and the upper and lower chambers.

cryalgesia — a pain caused by the application of a cold substance to the body.

cryanesthesia — the inability to feel or perceive anything cold.

cryptorchidism — failure of the testes to descend from the abdomen into the scrotum.

cryptoxanthin — a substance found in yellow corn; the body can convert it to vitamin A.

C.S.F. — abbreviation for cerebrospinal fluid.

cubitus — the elbow; also the forearm and hand.

Culex — a genus of mosquitoes that carry different diseases.

culicide — any substance that kills gnats and mosquitoes.

culture — the growth of bacteria or cell tissue on a specially prepared medium. Cultures are used to help identify bacteria and thus aid in diagnosis. The physician uses a cotton swab to remove a sample of bacteria from the infected area. The swab is then rubbed onto the culture medium and allowed to grow until it can be identified.

curare — the poison extracted from various species of *Strychnos* by South American tribes and used to poison arrowheads.
    Curare paralyzes muscles in all parts of the body. It works by blocking nerve impulses to the muscles, including the diaphragm. The effects are not long-lasting, and the victim can be saved by artificial respiration.
    Today, it is used as a drug to relax muscles. It is given, in conjunction with a general anesthesia, to relax muscles during surgery, particularly in operations involving the abdominal wall. This is important, because it allows the use of a much lower level of anesthesia.
    Curare is also used in the treatment of tetanus to relax muscle spasms, as well as for other diseases and conditions where there is muscle rigidity or spasms.

curet — an instrument used in the surgical removal of growths or other matter from the wall of a body organ or part.

curettage — the surgical removal of growths or other matter from the wall of a body organ or part. A curet is usually used to do this.

Curie, Marie — Polish chemist (1867-1934) who won

the 1911 Nobel Prize in physics for her discovery of radium.

curvature of the spine — a condition in which the spine is curved out of place.

Cushing, Harvey — Boston surgeon (1869-1939) who was one of the first doctors to specialize in brain surgery. With his techniques and skill, Cushing dramatically reduced mortality rates in brain surgery.

Cushing's law — the law that states that an increase in pressure in the brain produces an increase in blood pressure. Named for and propounded by Harvey Cushing.

cusp — a tapered protrusion, such as the tapered points on teeth.

cuspids — the canine or sharply pointed teeth.

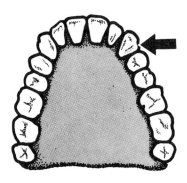

CUSPID

cut — a wound in which the skin is broken by a sharp cutting instrument or by material such as a knife, razor, piece of glass, or the edge of a piece of paper.
See incisions.

cutaneous — of or pertaining to the skin or the surface of the skin.

cuticle — the epidermis or outer layer of skin.

cutis — the outer layers of skin, including the epidermis and the dermis (or corium).

cyanide — one of the fastest-acting poisons known to man. Cyanide prevents the transfer of oxygen from the blood to the cells. It has a very distinctive odor, not unlike almonds. A fatal dose can cause symptoms within seconds and death within minutes. The symptoms include headache, cyanosis, and unconsciousness. If the patient is to be saved, immediate action must be taken. The two best antidotes are sodium nitrate and sodium thiosulfate.

cyanocobalamin — vitamin B_{12}. It is an essential requirement for normal growth and nutrition. Vitamin B_{12} is not a natural vitamin; it must be synthesized by living organisms. The body will store cyanocobalamin, and cooking does not destroy it. The best sources are organ foods, such as livers and kidneys.

Vitamin B_{12} is used in the treatment of pernicious anemia.

cyanosis — blueness of the skin caused by an insufficient supply of oxygen in the blood. Oxygen is carried in the blood by hemoglobin, which is bright red when saturated with oxygen. When hemoglobin is not carrying oxygen, it is purple and is called reduced hemoglobin. The blueness of the skin occurs when the amount of reduced hemoglobin exceeds five grams per one hundred cubic centimeters of blood.

cyclarthrodial — a term applied to any joint that can rotate.

cycle — any disease, condition, or phenomenon that reoccurs in a regular, predictable pattern.

cyclomethycaine — a chemical preparation used as a local or surface anesthesia.

cyclopropane — a gas used as a general anesthesia. It is highly inflammable and has a distinctive odor and taste.

cyst — a sac within the body. It can be a body organ or part or an abnormal growth. Cysts are usually filled with fluids or semiliquid matter.

cysticercus — a larval type of tapeworm.

cystic fibrosis — an inherited disease of children and adolescents that affects the exocrine, or externally secreting, glands of the body. These are glands that discharge their secretions onto the skin (sweat glands) or into organs that connect to the outside of the body (lungs, intestines, etc.), either directly or through special ducts or openings. In cystic fibrosis the mucus-producing glands do not yield their normal, clear, free-flowing fluid. Instead, they ooze an abnormal, thick, sticky mucus, which tends to clog up and block the ducts. This thick mucus accumulates in various parts of the body and interferes with other normal bodily functions, such as breathing and digestion.

The mucus-producing glands are not the only ones affected. Another basic abnormality is found in the glands that secrete sweat, saliva, and tears. In the cystic fibrosis victim the secretions of these glands usually contain an excessive amount of salt.

Cystic fibrosis is basically a childhood disease, for only in recent years has a victim had any chance of reaching adulthood. It is equally common among boys and girls.

People with cystic fibrosis were born with it. The disease is inherited from parents who carry the trait. Such a carrier can pass this trait to his children, but does not necessarily show any symptoms himself. It is not an infectious disease and cannot be caught from or given to others by contact.

When only one of the parents is a carrier, their children will not inherit the disease (although some of them may be carriers). However, if both parents are carriers, the chances are that their offspring will have cystic fibrosis. In families where one child is already afflicted, the chances soar to one-in-four that later offspring will also have the disease.

Children and adults who are symptom-free carriers of this disease also have an abnormality in their sweat secretion. This has led scientists to believe that many adults with lung and intestinal symptoms not attributed to cystic fibrosis may actually have the disease in a partial form.

Cystic fibrosis is now thought to be one of the most common health menaces of childhood, and it is one of the most serious. As a cause of death in children it kills more victims than do some of the better-known maladies, such as rheumatic fever, diabetes, and poliomyelitis.

Although recognized as a separate disease only within the last twenty-five years, cystic fibrosis is now being diagnosed with increasing frequency throughout the world. In the United States it is estimated that anywhere from two to twenty percent of the populace may be carriers. Approximately one of every one-thousand newborns is afflicted.

SYMPTOMS

The major symptoms, almost always apparent within the first few months of life, result from the sticky mucus secretions interfering with normal breathing, normal digestion, or both. About ten percent of cystic fibrosis patients are born with their intestinal tract obstructed by an accumulation of abnormal, thickened meconium (a mucus-like substance present to some degree in all newborns, but voided by a healthy child within a few days following birth). This abnormal condition in the cystic fibrosis victim proves fatal unless recognized promptly and corrected by surgery.

The pancreas is an important gland that furnishes digestion-triggering enzymes to the intestinal tract. In about eighty percent of cystic fibrosis cases, the ducts of this gland become clogged with a thickened secretion, and this seriously interferes with food digestion. Most of the food eaten then passes through the body undigested, providing no nutritive value, and produces bulky, fatty, foul-smelling stools. Abdominal pains are often present.

The child's appetite is usually excellent. He may actually be very hungry and double his food intake, but, since much of it is not digested, signs of malnutrition frequently appear.

Almost all patients develop chronic lung disease at some time during the course of their illness. Thick mucus deposits clog passages in the lung, causing it to stretch out of proportion. The air sacs of the lung eventually collapse, resulting in rapid, labored breathing. Mucus that lodges in the branches of the windpipe will cause obstructions and a chronic cough. As time goes by, bacterial infections set in, and the child is likely to have chronic bronchitis and a lingering cough. The patient is usually extremely susceptible to frequent, acute lung infections and can easily succumb to pneumonia. The obstructed, damaged lung tissues tend to impede blood circulation and, in some cases, result in death from chronic heart strain.

The constant, excessive loss of salt by sweating leads to heat exhaustion in the summer. This condition, at times, is severe enough to be fatal. Weakness and listlessness because of loss of salt are also fairly common symptoms.

A cystic fibrosis patient who has all the symptoms of the disease is an undernourished child with bulky, fatty, foul-smelling stools, who is especially subject to serious respiratory infections accompanied by fitful coughing and poor sleep. In severe cases additional symptoms such as clubbed fingers, bluish lips, and a barrel chest will appear.

In recent years it has become increasingly apparent that many cases of cystic fibrosis do not show all of the usual symptoms. A number of patients will show only partial symptoms, such as difficulty in breathing or abnormally high salt content in perspiration, tears, and saliva.

Partial and nondisabling signs of the illness, especially excessive salt secretion, are sometimes found among carriers, usually relatives of the afflicted children.

TESTS

The diagnosis of cystic fibrosis is usually based on four findings:

1. An abnormally high salt content in the patient's perspiration.

2. A lack of enzymes from the pancreas.

3. A chronic lung condition.

4. A suspicious history of cystic fibrosis symptoms, or the finding of abnormal, high-salt perspiration among members of the family.

The finding of an abnormally high-salt content in the sweat is the simplest and most reliable test and usually confirms the diagnosis when the usual disease symptoms are present. In about eighty percent of patients, the examination of material taken from the upper intestine will also show that pancreatic enzymes are either absent or deficient.

TREATMENT

The severity of the respiratory condition usually determines the fate of cystic fibrosis patients; consequently, treatment of this symptom is the most important part of therapy. This treatment is very often long and expensive. It frequently consists of the use of a variety of antibiotics to combat lung infections. At times these are administered by inhalation, using vaporizing equipment.

When there are not enough enzymes present for proper digestion, and food is not absorbed, the missing pancreatic enzymes are replaced by giving the patient commercially available pancreatic extracts to be taken with meals. Extra quantities of a well-balanced diet are also usually given to offset such a condition, although fats are moderately restricted to avoid the offensive stools caused by improper digestion and absorption of fats.

Extra salt is given to offset the excessive loss of salt in perspiration. This is particularly important during hot weather, since the loss of salt may have grave consequences if permitted to go unchecked.

Surgery is required for those infants born with their intestines obstructed by accumulations of abnormal, thick, tenacious meconium.

The outlook depends primarily on the severity of the lung disease and the extent to which the treatment with antibiotics proves successful. About ninety percent of deaths from cystic fibrosis are due to the long-term, progressive, lung disorder. Early detection of the disease and prompt treatment before the lung disorder has a chance to cause permanent damage is essential.

The death rate from cystic fibrosis is still very high. Nevertheless, the outlook has become increasingly favorable, and with newer treatments and earlier recognition, up to twenty percent of afflicted children now survive to adolescence or young adulthood.

cystine — one of the compounds in a protein molecule. It is occasionally found in the urine and kidney and can form crystals or stones in the bladder. Cystine is an amino acid.

cystitis — an inflammation of the urinary bladder. It can be caused by an allergic reaction, a bacterial infection somewhere else in the body, irritation from the presence of a foreign body in the urinary bladder, and irritation caused by crystal deposits.

cystoscope — a lighted tube used in the examination of the urinary bladder.

cytochrome — a group of compounds found in animal and human tissues; they play an important role in the movement of oxygen from the blood to the cells.

cytology — the study of cells, including their anatomy, physiology, pathology, and chemistry.

cytoplasm — the protoplasm of the cell exclusive of that of the nucleus.

d

daltonism — a form of color blindness in which a person has difficulty perceiving the difference between red and green.
See color blindness, genetics.

D and C — the abbreviation for dilation and curettage, a minor surgical procedure often performed after a miscarriage. The procedure involves scraping the womb to remove the remaining bits of placenta.

dandruff — a condition in which dry skin on the scalp peels off in small flakes. It can be caused by excessively dry skin or by minor infection. A greasy skin condition does not preclude dandruff.

dapsone — one of the sulfone class of drugs used in the treatment of leprosy.
See leprosy.

Darwin, Charles Robert — English naturalist (1809-1882) who set the world on its ear with his theory of evolution. Darwin maintained that man is descended from lower forms of life. Thus, in his view, man is closely related to apes. He also stated that evolution was a process of natural selection and survival of the fittest.

deafness — partial or total loss of hearing.

TYPES

When sound waves are not conducted properly to the inner ear, all sounds seem to be muffled, and the person's hearing loss is called conductive. The cause may be an obstruction in the auditory canal, such as an accumulation of wax, or a blockage caused by swelling and pus.

Occasionally, with children, doctors find a marble or a bean in the ear, and not rarely, with adults, a forgotten wad of cotton. (Only on direct orders from your doctor should you ever put cotton in the ear, and then only a large piece that cannot possibly get lost in the ear canal.)

Much more commonly the trouble in conductive hearing loss occurs in the middle ear, and again swelling and pus are one cause of hearing loss.

If sound waves do reach the inner ear but are not properly converted into a message that can be passed on to the brain, the loss is called sensorineural (sensory-neural) or neurosensory. Other terms are nerve deafness and perceptive deafness. A person with such a loss generally hears low-pitched tones better than high ones. The sounds are often distorted.

Many persons with poor hearing have a mixed loss: a combination of conductive and sensory-neural impairments.

Sometimes the trouble lies beyond the ear itself. The signals from the ear may not be reaching the brain because of trouble along the cochlear nerve, or the brain may not be properly interpreting the signals. Persons affected in such a way are said to have a central hearing loss. They may hear speech but have difficulty understanding it.

Nerve deafness or sensory-neural hearing loss can occur at any age, from the newborn to the elderly. If it is partial, a hearing aid may offer great assistance, especially to babies who should be learning language through listening to speech. A total hearing loss is rare, but in such cases hearing aids are useless. Sometimes, particularly in elderly persons, the hearing problem may involve "understanding" rather than volume of sound, and in this situation also hearing aids may not help.

For most kinds of nerve deafness, resulting from such causes as infections, noise, heredity, or a blow on the ear, prevention but not cure is possible.

Hearing loss from sensitivity to certain medicines or other irritants may be controlled by stopping their use. Active research both on the inner ear and on aging throughout the body may contribute directly to means of avoiding hearing loss due to nerve damage in the later years.

CAUSES

Some common childhood diseases (such as measles, German measles, scarlet fever, whooping cough, and mumps) can lead to impaired hearing of the sensory-neural type, as can other virus infections and meningitis.

The most common cause of childhood hearing loss, however, is inflammation of the middle ear, known as otitis media. When a child has a cold and complains that his ear bothers him, the chances are he has an earache from otitis media. In this case, the patient's eardrum may break from pressure of fluid collecting in the middle ear, causing a "running ear" and a partial hearing loss. When the eardrum is closed by nature or a plastic operation, the hearing may be restored to normal.

Otosclerosis is another cause of deafness, particularly during young adulthood. In this condition, new bone starts growing on parts of the bony capsule in which the organ of hearing lies. In ten percent of these cases, it anchors the stapes and prevents this tiny bone from properly transmitting sound waves to the inner ear.

When a mother has German measles during her pregnancy, the baby's hearing may be damaged or totally missing.

The term presbycusis is often used to describe a hearing impairment first noticed after sixty years of age. The higher tones frequently begin to fade during the thirties and continue to fade as the years go by, while the tones necessary to understand speech may show no great change for decades.

See ear, hearing, prelingual deafness.

decidua — the lining of the uterus; it is expelled during menstruation.

decompensation — the inability of the heart to maintain adequate circulation. This usually results in a waterlogging of tissues. A person whose heart is failing to maintain normal circulation is said to be "decompensated."

decompression — a gradual reduction in atmospheric pressure. Deep-sea divers must undergo decompression to avoid decompression sickness (the bends).
See decompression sickness.

decompression sickness — a condition caused by a rapid decrease in atmospheric pressure. Deep-sea divers must be very careful about surfacing too quickly.

The sickness is brought on by an excess of nitrogen in the blood and body tissues. Under high pressure, body liquids will absorb more nitrogen, oxygen, and carbon dioxide than at normal pressures. As the pressure drops, these gases emerge in the form of gas bubbles. The body quickly rids itself of the excess carbon dioxide and oxygen. However, the body requires a longer amount of time to rid itself of excess nitrogen. When the pressure is lowered gradually, there is no problem. When the pressure drops too quickly, the nitrogen bubbles impair circulation.

Symptoms of decompression sickness include ear pain, sinus pain, and pain in the joints, bones, etc. The term "bends" is frequently used to describe the condition because of the tendency of the arms to bend into a fixed position.

Decompression sickness can be avoided by allowing enough time for the body to adjust to the pressure change.

The usual treatment for decompression sickness is to place the patient in a high-pressure chamber and then gradually reduce the pressure within the chamber until the pressure inside is the same as the normal atmospheric pressure.

defibrillator — any agent or measure that stops irregular contractions of the heart muscle and restores a normal heartbeat. Electrical shocks are often used for this purpose.

deformity — a disfigurement or distortion of a body part.

dehydration — a serious loss of body fluid. Vomiting and diarrhea are two common causes of dehydration.

delirium — a condition in which the patient is confused and incoherent. Delirium often causes the patient to hallucinate. It is a symptom of brain damage or injury, high fever, etc.

delivery — the natural or artificial removal of a child from the mother's body.
See labor.

dementia — a broad term used to indicate mental deterioration.

dementia praecox — the old term for schizophrenia.
See schizophrenia.

demulcent — a substance that soothes. Demulcents are used in the treatment of poisoning by mouth to soothe the stomach and delay absorption of the poison.

dens — a tooth.

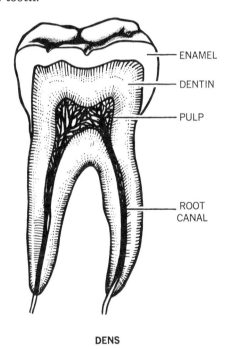

ENAMEL

DENTIN

PULP

ROOT CANAL

DENS

dental caries — tooth decay. It is the most prevalent disease in the United States, afflicting ninety-eight percent of the population. By the age of fifteen, the average American has had an average of eleven cavities.

A tremendous number of bacteria are present in the mouth at all times. Certain types of germs form adherent deposits on the tooth surfaces if a person does not clear food residues after eating, or if he allows products containing sugar to remain in the mouth for long periods of time. These deposits are known as plaque.

When highly soluble and fermentable foods, such as sugar or other refined carbohydrates, are metabolized by bacteria in this plaque, as well as in crevices in the mouth, acids are formed. These acids may then dissolve the enamel of the tooth and initiate its breakdown. Research findings indicate that acids form within five minutes after sweet foods are eaten. Harmful acid levels build up within fifteen minutes.

Cavities may form underneath the "invisible" sticky bacterial deposits (plaque). Caries can be prevented if the germs are removed thoroughly. It usually takes several days for a thick clump of the germs to form on a tooth surface. This happens in the sheltered areas between the teeth, near the gum line, and in the crevices or grooves on the surfaces of the teeth.

Once the cavity has started (i.e., the enamel is dissolved by acid), decay proceeds from the enamel into the dentin (the ivory-like substance forming the body of the tooth), and then into the pulp, which is made up of nerves and blood vessels. When the pulp is affected, the infection may be painful, and eventually an abscess may form at the tip of the root. Once a cavity has formed, the tooth cannot repair itself. Only professional treatment by dentists is effective.

Three conditions are necessary for tooth decay. One is a susceptible individual, which includes nearly every American. This susceptibility may be related in part to hardness and other qualities of the enamel and dentin, which may influence resistance to decay. Another condition is the presence of decay-producing bacteria found in plaques, which are allowed to remain on the teeth. Equally important is a caries-producing diet with large amounts of carbohydrates, particularly sugar, taken into the mouth frequently.

PREVENTION
There are several ways to help prevent dental caries. They include the use of fluoride, a good diet, removing the germs, and regular visits to a dentist.

1. Fluoride
Fluoridation of drinking water is one decay preventive that does not depend on the economic means or knowledge of the parents or on the availability of dentists. While not intended as a substitute for proper individual care

of the teeth, fluoridation of the water supply is the most-effective and least-expensive preventive dental-health measure available. Its major benefits, which may continue throughout life, are obtained by children who drink the fluoridated water from birth through the years their teeth are developing.

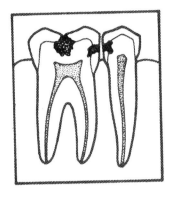
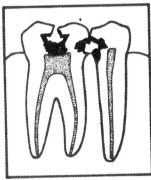

DENTAL CARIES

2. Removing the germs

Since decay occurs only under bacterial plaques, one protective measure is to remove such deposits before they grow to a size and thickness that favors the development of enough acid to damage the teeth.

Brushing the teeth immediately after eating helps remove food particles and bacteria before the bacteria can act upon any sugars present to form acids.

3. A good diet

A well-balanced, nutritious diet is important to general health, but in preventing tooth decay, what is left out of the diet is more important than what is included. The frequent eating of products containing sugars is one dietary pattern known to be associated with cavity formation. Reducing the frequent intake, especially between meals, of sweetened drinks, candies, syrups, jams and jellies, pastries, and other confections will help protect the teeth and will not harm nutrition.

Foods that require thorough chewing are called detergent foods, because they are forced over the teeth and gums, helping to clean them. Firm, crisp, raw vegetables or fruits may have this cleansing effect. However, they should not be considered as a substitute for brushing after eating.

4. Regular visits to a dentist

"See your dentist at least twice a year" is familiar advice. Nevertheless, half the children in the United States under fifteen years of age have never been to a dentist.

Decay may start as soon as the child's teeth appear, and it can increase rapidly. Most dentists advise bringing a child for his first visit shortly after all his primary teeth are in, at the age of two and a half or three. The child thus has a chance to get acquainted with the dentist on a friendly basis, probably before any extensive dental work is needed.

Regardless of the age, dental defects can be corrected more easily and with less discomfort and expense in the early stages. A visit to the dentist on a regular schedule, usually every six months, is therefore advisable. Beginning decay is hard to find, because the affected area is small and may be in a place that is difficult to see. To find such cavities, it is sometimes necessary for dentists to take X-rays of the teeth.

No matter how effectively one uses a toothbrush, it is important to have the teeth cleaned periodically by a dentist or a dental hygienist. This cleaning is called dental prophylaxis. Its purpose is to remove calculus and stains that cannot be removed by ordinary cleaning. This helps prevent injury to the gums and helps the dentist find beginning decay.

dentifrice — a substance used to clean the teeth. Toothpastes and powders are good mechanical aids in cleaning the teeth. With fluoride added, they provide some extra measure of decay prevention. A safe dentifrice will not always change the color of the teeth, either in one brushing or over a period of time. Tooth bleaches are not safe to use.

No toothpaste or powder will change the chemistry of the mouth for very long. None of them will cure bad breath, pyorrhea, or any other disease.

dentin — the substance under the enamel layer of the tooth. Dentin is softer than enamel and is the cover for the pulp chamber of the tooth. The dentin of the tooth, if exposed by decay or a crack in the enamel, is likely to be sensitive to hot or cold foods, to pressure, or to sudden shock. The closer the decay approaches to the pulp chamber, the more painful is the tooth.

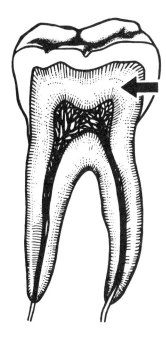

DENTIN

dentist — a licensed person whose specialty is the teeth.

deoxyribonucleic acid — *See DNA.*

depressant — any drug that decreases functional activity.

depression — a feeling of melancholy, hopelessness, and dejection. Everyone has feelings of depression, but a normal, healthy individual will bounce back from a mood of depression. The difference between normal depression and depression as a sign of mental illness is both the intensity of the depression and the length of time the depression lasts.
See manic-depressive psychosis.

dermatitis — any inflammation of the skin. The term is used to cover a wide range of skin disorders, but it is usually used to mean a skin disorder that is not caused by infection.

dermatologist — a physician whose specialty is the skin.

dermatosis — any disease of the skin and/or its appendages (hair follicles, sebaceous glands, sweat glands). These diseases are usually characterized by alterations in the normal structure, by irritation, and by inflammation.

Except in a few instances, they do not progress rapidly but manifest themselves gradually after continued exposure to the causative agent.

dermis — the true skin.
See skin.

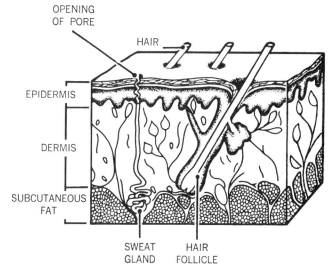

DERMIS

Descartes, René — French author (1596-1650) of the first physiology textbook that accepted the theory of the circulation of the blood as described by William Harvey in 1628.

desensitization — a series of injections given to a patient who has an allergy. The injections contain small traces of the substances to which the patient is allergic. The amount of these substances in the injection is gradually increased until the person develops an immunity.
See allergy, immunity.

desquamation — the shedding of skin.

deterioration — the process of losing ground, or of getting worse.

dexiocardia — *See dextrocardia.*

dextrocardia — one of two different types of congenital phenomena.

1. A condition in which the heart is slightly ro-

tated and lies almost entirely in the right (instead of the left) side of the chest.

2. A condition in which there is a complete transposition, the left chambers of the heart being on the right side, and the right chambers on the left side, so that the heart presents a mirror image of the normal heart.

dextrose — *See glucose.*

diabetes — a condition in which an excessive amount of urine is produced. There are several types of diabetes the most common type is diabetes mellitus.
See diabetes mellitus.

diabetes mellitus — a disorder of carbohydrate metabolism characterized by excessive sugar in the blood and urine and associated with a disturbance of the normal insulin mechanism.

Insulin, which is produced in the pancreas, helps convert food into usable energy. Normally, the sugars and starches in foods are changed by digestive juices into a sugar called glucose. This is absorbed by the blood and, with the help of insulin, is used to nourish the body.

In a person with diabetes, however, this bodily mechanism is defective. Either the body does not produce enough insulin or it does not make proper use of the insulin that is produced. As a result, unused sugar collects in the blood; some of it may overflow into the urine. Too much sugar in the blood is a sign of diabetes.

SYMPTOMS

In children, the onset of diabetes may be abrupt and may manifest itself as an acute illness. In older people, the disease is usually insidious and is discovered only on routine examination of blood or urine. If symptoms do occur, they are usually mild and do not cause the patient to seek medical care. The more common symptoms are frequent urination, increased thirst, itching, hunger, weakness, and weight loss.

The exact cause for diabetes is obscure. However, it is generally accepted that the disease is a result of insulin deficiency. Contributing factors in insulin deficiency are heredity, obesity, and disorders of hormone-producing glands other than the pancreas. Infections may be a common predisposing factor. Diabetes develops in people from all age groups. But those who are most likely to have it are overweight, over forty, or relatives of diabetics.

TESTS

Even when there are no symptoms, the physician can discover the presence of diabetes by testing small samples of the blood for sugar. Many physicians make these tests regularly for their patients, especailly for those over forty, who have relatives with diabetes, who are overweight, or who are the mothers of large babies. If these tests suggest the presence of diabetes, the doctor will make additional tests before his diagnosis.

In addition, an increasing number of communities are offering diabetes screening programs in which large numbers of people are tested. Those whose tests indicate the possibility of diabetes are referred to their own physicians for diagnosis and treatment. Estimates indicate that about twenty out of every one thousand persons in the United States have diabetes. Half of these people do not know that they have it.

CONTROL

Before the discovery of insulin in 1921, the person with diabetes had very little hope. Today, the disease can be controlled so successfully that the diabetic who is willing to take the necessary extra care of himself can expect to live a full, productive life.

Insulin frequently plays a major role in control. This insulin, taken from the pancreas of animals, is used to bring the body's supply up to normal. It must always be injected under the skin. Insulin cannot be taken by mouth, because the digestive juices destroy it.

Since 1957, chemical compounds in pill form have become available. These are not insulin tablets, but they can stimulate the body's own production of insulin in some diabetics.

Both insulin and oral drugs should be taken only as the doctor prescribes. Each individual patient's needs must be determined by a physician before treatment is begun.

Diet is important in diabetes. Some people, particularly the overweight, can control their diabetes by diet alone. A diabetic can eat most of the foods the rest of his family eats. Such foods include milk, meat, fish, eggs, cheese, breads and cereal products, vegetables, fruits, and fats. The doctor, however, must decide the amounts of each of these foods to be eaten each day and give the diabetic a meal plan. The amounts of food on the meal plan will be tailored to meet the patient's own needs. Considerable variety in the diet can be obtained by selecting different fruits, vegetables, meats, and breadstuffs. Lists of foods in the different groups have been prepared to help the patient make these exchanges.

Exercise in the form of work and play is also important for the person with diabetes. A normal amount of regular exercise increases the ability of the body to use food and lessens the amount of medication needed. But here again, the doctor must decide what is best for the patient.

Most people with diabetes are asked by their doctors to test their urine every day. This daily record enables the doctor to watch the condition. There are several ways to test urine for sugar at home.

COMPLICATIONS

Diabetes may have many serious complications. Special care must be taken of the feet, because poor circulation in the extremities, injury, or infection could result in amputation. Good oral hygiene is required, as well as close medical supervision of eyesight. A complication of poorly controlled or advancing diabetes is pain because of nerve involvement affecting the extremities.

The two most dangerous complications of diabetes are diabetic coma and insulin shock. Coma is the result of metabolic imbalance caused by an accumulation of toxic substances due to insufficient insulin or infection, whereas shock is the result of excessive insulin, producing a low blood sugar.

diagnosis — the process of finding and recognizing a disease. Physicians employ numerous techniques to help them diagnose diseases. Some of the techniques are very specialized, such as the tests for syphilis; others are very general, such as blood-pressure measurement.

A physician generally starts the process by taking the patient's medical history. He then moves on to some general tests to help him narrow down the possibilities. Finally, he will use specific tests to establish or confirm his diagnosis.

The ability to diagnose illnesses quickly is the hallmark of the good physician, but sometimes a patient's problem can be very difficult to diagnose. This is frequently the case when the patient has more than one problem. For example, a patient with a history of heart trouble presents special problems when he develops certain diseases that resemble heart trouble.

In diagnosing illnesses, a doctor uses his eyes (to observe skin tone), his ears (in auscultation), his hands (to feel the shape of body organs), and even his nose. Sometimes a doctor's instincts are as important as his senses.

Because of the elaborate equipment and trained personnel required, some diagnostic procedures are not done in a doctor's office, but in a hospital or clinic. These procedures are resorted to when examination in the physician's office cannot establish the diagnosis or when detailed information on the nature, location, degree, and physiological consequences of the disease is needed to determine treatment.

See auscultation, X-ray, etc.

dialysis — a method of separating substances in solution form. Dialysis is one of the methods physicians use in treating patients with kidney diseases or disorders. Dialysis is used to cleanse the blood of impurities and helps restore the normal chemical balance.

One type of dialysis, peritoneal dialysis, uses the lining of the patient's abdomen as a filter to remove waste products from the body. Another type of dialysis, hemodialysis, employs an artificial kidney machine for the same purpose.

diaphragm — the dome-shaped muscular wall

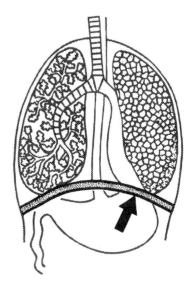

DIAPHRAGM

separating the thoracic region from the abdominal cavity. The action of the diaphragm, which is triggered by the brain, plays a major role in the breathing process.

The contraction of the diaphragm causes the chest to expand. This lowers the pressure in the lungs, causing air to enter the lungs. When the diaphragm relaxes, the chest returns to its original size and raises the pressure in the lungs. The higher pressure forces air out of the lungs.

diarrhea — loose, watery bowel movements. Diarrhea can be caused by many things, including infection in the bowel or elsewhere in the body. It is more of a symptom than a separate disease or condition. However, a prolonged spell of diarrhea can be serious, because it can lead to dehydration and acidosis. This is especially true in the case of small children.

Diarrhea that persists longer than a day or two should be treated by a physician.

diastole — the period of relaxation of the heart in each heartbeat. Auricular diastole is the period of relaxation of the atria or upper heart chambers. Ventricular diastole is the period of relaxation of the ventricles, or lower heart chambers.

diet — daily allowance or intake of food and drink.

From simple, one-celled plants to highly complex human beings, all living things need food. Food is necessary to support growth, to repair constantly wearing tissues, and to supply energy for physical activity. Unless the food consumed supplies all the elements required for normal life processes, the human body cannot operate at peak efficiency for very long. If an essential nutrient is missing from the diet over very long periods of time, deficiency diseases such as rickets, scurvy, or certain anemias may develop.

However, a diet that includes too much of any one element can also be damaging.

The food choice of civilized man is influenced by many factors, such as cultural background, habit, taste preference, susceptibility to advertising, family finances, economic situation, and many others.

The nutrients in food that are necessary for good health can be divided into certain groups: proteins, carbohydrates, fats, vitamins, minerals, and water. Most common foods consist of combinations of the above. Foods that are good

sources of one food element usually also contribute other essential elements as well, but no one food supplies all needed nutrients in sufficient amounts. For good nutrition all essential food elements must work together. Therefore, well-balanced nutrition calls for a well-chosen variety of foods.

In general, diets high in fat content, especially animal and dairy fats, tend to raise the level of cholesterol in the blood. Many doctors and scientists feel that dietary changes that reduce the total intake of fat and substitute polyunsaturated fats for animal and dairy fats can have a beneficial effect on people suffering from or who are prone to heart trouble. However, what changes in diet should be made are best decided on an individual basis by a physician.

See amino acids, carbohydrates, fats, nutrition, proteins, etc.

dietetics — the science and art dealing with the application of principles of nutrition to the feeding of individuals or groups under different economic or health conditions.

dietitian — one skilled in the scientific use of diet in health and disease.

differentiation — a process of growth in the embryo from very general cells to very specific cells. Cancer is often a reversal of this process. Thus, in cancer, a very specific cell type reverts to a very simple or nonspecific type.

digestion — the process of reducing or converting food into usable energy.

The process of digestion begins in the mouth, where the teeth perform mechanical digestion, and saliva begins chemical disgestion. The food then passes through the pharynx and esophagus into the stomach, where it undergoes further digestion. From the stomach, the partially digested food is passed on to the small intestine, which is the major digestion organ. The usable material is absorbed in the small intestine. The remaining mass is moved into the large intestine, where the water is absorbed.

digestive tract — the system responsible for the body's breakdown and use of food. It is composed of the mouth, pharynx, esophagus, stomach, small intestine, large intestine (including the colon and rectum), and accessory glands.

See esophagus, pharynx, etc.

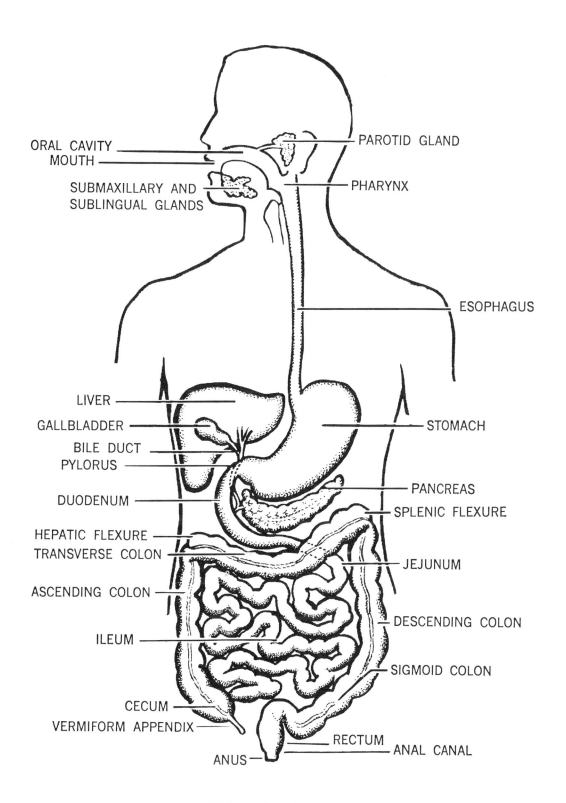

ORAL CAVITY

MOUTH

SUBMAXILLARY AND
SUBLINGUAL GLANDS

PAROTID GLAND

PHARYNX

ESOPHAGUS

LIVER

GALLBLADDER

BILE DUCT

PYLORUS

DUODENUM

HEPATIC FLEXURE

TRANSVERSE COLON

ASCENDING COLON

ILEUM

CECUM

VERMIFORM APPENDIX

ANUS

STOMACH

PANCREAS

SPLENIC FLEXURE

JEJUNUM

DESCENDING COLON

SIGMOID COLON

RECTUM   ANAL CANAL

DIGESTIVE TRACT

digitalis — a drug prepared from the leaves of the foxglove plant. It is used to strengthen the contraction of the heart muscle, slow the rate of contraction of the heart and to improve the efficiency of the heart.

dilation — a stretching or enlargement of a body part beyond the norm.

dilation and curettage — *See D and C.*

dimercaprol — a heavy metal antagonist. Drugs such as dimercaprol are used as antidotes to heavy metal poisoning. Dimercaprol is effective against metals such as mercury and arsenic. This drug is also known as British anti-lewisite or BAL because it was developed (primarily in Britain) as an antidote to lewisite (an arsenic derivative).

diphtheria — a very serious disease. Diphtheria was once one of the greatest scourges of childhood and dangerous to all age groups. Today, through immunization, this disease has almost been conquered in the United States.

In the 1880's and 1890's, about fifteen of every 10,000 people died of diphtheria each year, many of them in epidemics in large cities. In 1920 there were about 150,000 cases yearly, with about 15,000 deaths. Since that time the disease has declined gradually, although the germs are still present in many communities. They still infect about 1,000 people each year, causing fewer than one hundred deaths.

Formerly, two-thirds of the cases reported were in children under age ten, and two-thirds of those who died were under age five. This pattern still exists in some parts of the country, particularly in southern states, but in some northern and western states, a fairly large proportion of the cases occur among adults. Still most dangerous in the very young, diphtheria is now becoming almost equally fatal at the other extreme of life — in the very old.

SYMPTOMS

The first signs of diphtheria appear approximately two to five days after exposure. Ordinarily the disease develops in the throat, where a patch or patches of grayish membrane may form. Usually the throat is sore, and there is a slight fever. The membrane may interfere with swallowing or may extend to the windpipe and block the air passages, thus causing the patient to suffocate. Sometimes the lymph glands in the neck swell, adding to the difficulties in swallowing and breathing.

The germs produce and throw off a powerful poison called a toxin, which spreads throughout the body. In small amounts, toxin causes immunity to develop, but in large amounts it is particularly harmful to the heart, blood vessels, nerves, and kidneys and can injure them severely enough to cause death.

Serious complications often follow diphtheria if it is not treated, or if the treatment is inadequate or late. Diphtheria patients are particularly susceptible to bronchopneumonia; they may suffer paralysis lasting as long as three or four months; or their hearts, nerves, or kidneys may be permanently injured.

CAUSE

Diphtheria germs, in tiny droplets of moisture from the mouth, nose, or throat of someone infected, are usually spread by coughing, sneezing, or kissing. Infection can also be spread by drinking cups, eating utensils, handkerchiefs, towels, pencils, or anything that has touched the mouth of an infected person or been sprayed with discharges from his mouth, nose, or throat.

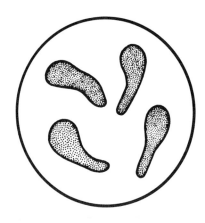

DIPHTHERIA BACILLI

An infected person can spread the disease after he seems entirely well. Half of the people who recover from diphtheria will continue to have the germ for more than two weeks; a fourth will be able to infect others for more than a month. Members of a patient's family may pass on the germ, whether or not they become ill. The disease can be spread by a carrier — an apparently healthy person who harbors the germs in his throat or nose.

Diphtheria germs grow easily in milk. Diphtheria cases or carriers can infect milk when it is being handled on farms, at dairies, or at distributing plants. Pasteurization kills the germs.

The disease is commonest in cold months, but an epidemic, once started, may continue regardless of the season.

PREVENTION

Some people, by repeated exposures to small numbers or mild forms of the germs, develop a resistance to diphtheria by building up an antidote or antitoxin. This antitoxin combines with the diphtheria toxin and renders it harmless. However, because diphtheria germs are scarcer now than they used to be, people have less chance of developing this natural immunity. Therefore, resistance through proper immunization is more important than ever.

Scientists can produce diphtheria toxin in the laboratory and then make it harmless by treating it with chemicals. When this treated toxin is injected under the skin of a person who has no immunity, his body is prompted to manufacture the disease-fighting antitoxin. Second and third injections will increase the protective effect. This active immunity usually is dependable for three to four years. Small booster doses are necessary at about three-year intervals to maintain a high degree of immunity throughout life. Actual infection with diphtheria germs acts like a booster dose of toxoid if the person has been properly immunized.

Most infants have "acquired immunity" at birth. This has been passed on to them by their mothers before they were born. However, this immunity disappears by the time the child is about six months old. After that, young children are highly susceptible to diphtheria unless they are immunized.

Immunization against diphtheria should begin at the age of two to three months. Diphtheria toxoid is usually given to infants in combination with tetanus toxoid and whooping cough vaccine. This requires three injections, one month apart, for best protection. Another injection is recommended three to twelve months after this primary series.

A child immunized as an infant should have a booster about every three years. It is particularly important that he have one before entering school. Once a child has completed an adequate primary series, he does not need to start over; one injection is enough. The primary series can be given at any time in childhood, but often, if a child is school age before beginning immunization, the whooping cough vaccine is omitted. When diphtheria and tetanus toxoids are given together, two injections are required, one month apart. Boosters should, of course, be given every three years thereafter. Older children and adults who have never been immunized should also be given injections of diphtheria toxoid. If they are sure they once had the complete series, they also need only one injection.

When exposure to diphtheria occurs, people who have been immunized previously should have a booster at once. People who have never been immunized can be given "passive immunity" by injections of antitoxin if they have come in close contact with a known case. This is an emergency measure, and it gives immunity for only two or three weeks. The first dose of toxoid should be given at the same time and should be followed by the other required doses so that more lasting immunity will develop.

diplopia — double vision. The vision is distorted, so that single objects are seen as two or double objects.

disc — *See disks.*

discharge — a liquid or semiliquid flow from a body opening. Every body opening can discharge a fluid. A discharge usually indicates an irritation or infection. Discharges should be taken as a warning.

discipline — a body of knowledge or field of study with distinctive rules and assumptions. Discipline is also the force (mental or physical) a parent or society applies to an individual to help him conform to an accepted pattern of behavior.

disease — the result of the invasion of the body by a foreign organism. Diseases have recognizable symptoms; in many cases they follow definite patterns.

disinfectant — a fluid used to kill bacteria and other microorganisms. Disinfectants are used only in cleaning inanimate objects; they are too strong to use on human or animal tissue. In fact, the basic difference between antiseptics and disinfectants is the strength—which in turn prohibits the use of the latter on living tissue.

disks — the pads (made of cartilage) that are located between each of the vertebrae. The disks protect and cushion the vertebrae and ultimately the brain from injury when the body is jarred.
See slipped disk.

dislocation — the forcible displacement of one or more bones from the normal joint. In some cases the bone slips back quickly into its normal position, but in other cases it becomes locked in the new position and remains dislocated until it is put back into place.

A dislocation is likely to bruise or tear the ligaments, blood vessels, tendons, and nerves near the joint. Frequently, the ligaments holding the bones in the proper position are stretched and sometimes torn loose. Dislocations result from force applied at or near the joints, from sudden muscular contractions, from twisting strains on joint ligaments, or from falls where the force of landing is transferred to a joint. The joints most frequently dislocated are those of the shoulder, hip, finger, and jaw.

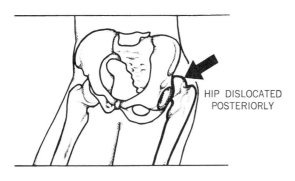

HIP DISLOCATED POSTERIORLY

DISLOCATION

SYMPTOMS
The parts forming the joint are held stiff and cannot be moved. The parts assume an unnatural shape and, when compared with the normal joint of the opposite side of the body, are misshapen. Dislocated extremities may be shorter or longer than normal. There is usually severe pain in the region of the joint, and the area is usually swollen.

TREATMENT
As a general rule, untrained personnel should not attempt to reduce a dislocation (that is, put a dislocated bone back in place) unless trained medical assistance cannot be obtained within three or four days. Unskilled attempts at reduction may cause great damage to nerves and blood vessels or may actually fracture the bone.

In first aid, no attempt should be made to reduce dislocations, except dislocations of the lower jaw, fingers, and toes.

displacement — a condition in which a body part has been moved out of its normal position.
See dislocation.

dissection — the separation and examination of body parts and tissues. Medical students dissect cadavers as part of their training in anatomy.

dissolve — to melt or liquify.

distal — remote or removed from. The opposite of proximal.

distention — an enlargement.

diuresis — an increased excretion of urine.

diuretic — a medicine that promotes the excretion of urine.

dizziness — a feeling of motion or loss of stability.

DNA — the abbreviation for deoxyribonucleic acid. DNA is one of the two nucleic acids found in all cells. (The other is RNA—ribonucleic acid.) Together, they exert primary control over life processes in all organisms.

The cell nucleus contains chromosomes — tightly coiled double strands of molecules of deoxyribonucleic acid. These strands carry the genetic orders that determine whether the cells develop into men, cows, or dogs; whether the individual will have blue or brown eyes; and whether he will or will not be susceptible to one or another disease. They also direct all the essential processes of the life of the cell.

dog bite — *See rabies.*

dominant trait — a trait that can be inherited from only one parent. A good example is eye color.

Brown eyes is a dominant trait. Therefore, if a child gets one brown gene he will have brown eyes. This is the opposite of blue eyes — a recessive trait. To have blue eyes, a child must receive a blue gene from both parents.

dope — a slang term applied to narcotic drugs when they are misused.

dorsal — of or pertaining to the back.

dosage — the amount or quantity of a medicinal aid that is administered at any one time.

The dose of medicine depends on the type of medicine, the patient's physical condition, and the particular illness the patient has.

Some medicines are too strong to be given in large doses: their good effects often have bad side effects in large doses. Some types of drugs are as effective in small doses as in large ones, because the body will absorb only a certain amount. When a patient is very weak or suffering from more than one complaint, the dosage may have to be somewhat limited because the patient cannot withstand the side effects. Depending on the type of illness, a physician may prescribe large or small doses of the same medicine. Some microorganisms are capable of surviving small doses; others will respond when a small dose of medicine is administered.

Whatever the prescribed dosage, it is important to follow the doctor's directions. Patients should never change the dosage they are taking unless ordered to do so by their physician.

double-blind — an experiment in which neither the patient nor the attending physician knows whether the patient is getting one or another drug.

douche — a cleansing technique. It involves sending a flow of water into a body cavity.

Down's syndrome — a form of mental retardation. Down's syndrome is also known as mongolism.

The brain and body damage of Down's syndrome probably is done before the eighth week of prenatal life. No remedy is presently available. The greatest hope is eventually to be able to prevent this disorder. Many children with Down's syndrome adjust well to life with their families and in their community.

Scientists have observed that most children with mongolism who lived with their families until five or six years of age walked and talked earlier than those who went directly to an institution at birth. Some with Down's syndrome who live to adulthood are earning money in protected situations or are happily assisting with work in the home.

One authority estimates that about one in every 700 live-born babies has mongolism. Such babies usually can be recognized at birth from a combination of signs, any of which occur in people of normal intelligence. Some of the signs include slanting eyes, flat nose, large tongue and protruding lower lip, and an unusual crease across the palm.

A chromosome study of the child with mongolism shows an abnormal number of chromosomes. Instead of the normal forty-six, there are forty-seven; or the count may be forty-six with extra material attached to one chromosome in a so-called translocation.

In instances where Down's syndrome is the result of translocation in the child's chromosomes, an abnormality of the mother's chromosomes is often present, or in a few cases the father has had a translocation of chromosomes. There is an increased risk that subsequent children of either of these parents might also be subject to Down's syndrome. Additionally, the risk rises sharply in mothers over forty.

For this reason, it is suggested that the parents of a child with Down's syndrome should have chromosome studies made in order to help predict the outlook for later pregnancies.

Children with Down's syndrome should have a medical examination at birth and at regular intervals thereafter, so that they may benefit from any research discoveries.

DPT and polio injection — a shot given to develop immunity to diphtheria, pertussis (whooping cough), tetanus (lockjaw), and polio (infantile paralysis). Some doctors give the DPT and polio shots separately.

A child may get whooping cough in spite of the shot, but it will be a much lighter or milder case. These shots produce a slight reaction in some children, but the reaction is a small price to pay for the protection they give. Slight fever, fussiness, tenderness, or swelling around the shot may occur, lasting for a few hours or a day or two. The shots do not cause colds or coughs. Any such symptoms are the result of an infection and have nothing to do with the injection.

Booster shots are needed to keep the immunity level high.

See diphtheria, pertussis, poliomyelitis, tetanus.

drainage — a rubber tube inserted in the body, which allows excess fluid or pus to escape instead of collecting. Drain tubes are often used after major operations.

dreams — flowing images that occur during sleep. The interpretation of dreams is a very controversial subject. Some authorities feel that it is vital in treating patients with mental disorders; others place much less importance on dreams.

One school of thought states that dreams are used to help ease sleep or to help the patient sleep. A simple example of this would be the person who dreams he is falling off a cliff. In reality he is falling or leaning off his bed. However, falling out of bed would disrupt sleep, and since the mind wants to stay asleep, it substitutes the dream for the reality. Another example would be that of a hungry person who dreams he is at a banquet. The dream takes the place of waking up (which would disturb sleep) and eating. This same school applies more disturbing and complicated dreams to a patient's mental problems.

dressing — a sterile pad, compress, sponge, or piece of material that is applied directly over a wound for the promotion of its proper healing. Since it is for use directly over an open wound, a dressing must be sterile; it must not only be clean in the ordinary sense of the word, but must be free of germs.

Dressings are used to cover the wound and protect it from bacteria, to control bleeding, to apply medication, to absorb excess moisture, and to conserve local heat. The material most commonly used in the making of dressings is gauze. Sponges and compresses are made of gauze or of cotton wrapped in gauze. Dressings may be generally classified as standard dressings for field and hospital use, commercially prepared and packaged dressings, and improvised dressings.

drinking — the swallowing of fluids.

See alcohol, alcoholism.

dropsy — an abnormal collection of excess water or fluid in body tissues or a body part.

See edema.

drowning — a form of asphyxiation or suffocation. The supply of air to the lungs is cut off completely by water. However, this does not mean immediate lack of oxygen, as there is a certain reserve supply in the air cells of the lungs, in the blood, and probably in the tissues that should maintain life for a short time. The amount of reserve oxygen varies; five minutes underwater sometimes produces death, and life usually is extinct after ten minutes' submersion.

It is important to start artificial respiration as soon as a drowning victim is removed from the water. Expulsion of air by artificial respiration tends to remove any water in the lungs, and care should be taken that the nose and mouth are low and unobstructed to prevent the water from reentering the air passages.

It is important to realize that it is possible to drown in a bathtub. It is not the depth of the water that is important; it is the ability to keep water out of the lungs that counts.

See artificial respiration.

drug — a substance used to diagnose, treat, or prevent illness.

Primitive man discovered by accident that some of the plants growing around him seemed useful to heal sores, relieve pain, or even cure diseases. These plants were the first drugs. Plants are still the source of some drugs, such as cascara, digitalis, quinine, and some narcotics.

Other important drugs, such as hormones and vaccines, are obtained from animals. But most of the modern drugs come from chemical combinations worked out by research scientists. Most people never see drugs in their simple form as chemicals; rather they see the end product: tablets, capsules, or liquids that contain the drug and other ingredients such as carrying agents.

Like primitive man, modern man uses drugs to get different results. Some drugs attack the organism that causes a disease and cure it by killing the organism. Other drugs relieve the symptoms of the disease (headache, pain, fever, or chills) and make the patient more comfortable.

Taking drugs is a complex business that can have serious consequences. A drug that kills a disease-producing organism may also cause other effects on the body. These are called side effects, because they are aside from the original effect intended for the drug. Sometimes these side effects seem trivial; for example, the drug may cause drowsiness. However, this can be dangerous when driving. A drug may be safe and effective for most people but may have a disturbing side effect on certain people. Physicians take these individual differences into account each time they write a prescription.

More than ninety percent of all prescriptions written today are for drugs that were not even on the market twenty-five years ago. In fact, many of the most important drugs that doctors prescribe today have been developed in the last fifteen years. Modern drugs are complex, specific, and potent. While powerful drugs can save lives that would have been lost a few decades ago, they can also harm or fail to help the ignorant or careless user.

USES

Drugs are used in many different ways, for a wide variety of purposes.

1. Drugs aid in the diagnosis of illness. For example, a patient may swallow a substance that will show up on X-rays to reveal a suspected growth in his intestines.

2. Drugs may give relief from symptoms of a disease; for example, reducing a high fever.

3. Drugs may treat a disease by combating its cause; for example, antibiotics that kill specific forms of bacteria.

4. Drugs prevent disease; for example, vaccination against smallpox.

5. Drugs affect the body's functions; for example, morphine depresses the central nervous system and alters the sensation of pain, and aspirin relieves moderate pain.

6. Drugs affect the function of parts of the body; for example, contraceptive drugs prevent ovulation and thus prevent pregnancy.

7. Drugs control disease conditions; for example, digitalis stimulates a weakened heart muscle, and insulin controls diabetes.

OVER-THE-COUNTER DRUGS

The nation's basic drug law (the Federal Food, Drug, and Cosmetic Act) divides drugs into two main classes: over-the-counter drugs and prescription drugs.

An over-the-counter drug is one that can be used safely without a doctor's supervision, if the directions on the label are followed. Examples of common over-the-counter drugs are aspirin, cough drops, antacids, and some antihistamines. The law permits the sale of these drugs "over-the-counter"; that is, without a doctor's prescription.

The law requires that these over-the-counter drug labels include the following information:

1. The name of the product.

2. The name and address of the manufacturer, packer, or distributor.

3. Adequate directions for safe use for each of the purposes for which the drug is intended to be used.

4. Any cautions and warnings needed to protect the user.

5. The established name of all active ingredients.

6. The quantity of some of the active ingredients and of certain other ingredients.

7. The name, quantity, and specific warning for any habit-forming drug contained in the products.

8. The net contents of the package.

PRESCRIPTION DRUGS

When a drug is one that should be used only under a physician's supervision, the law requires that it be sold only by prescription. Special tests or instructions may be needed. Also, drugs for serious diseases may require a prescription to ensure safe and effective use.

A prescription is as personal as a person's name. It is designed for one individual and is based on such factors as age, weight, general health, allergies, and other factors, as well as the specific illness.

It is a violation of the Federal law to sell a prescription drug without a prescription. A physician must write a prescription or phone it directly to the pharmacy. Otherwise a pharmacist is forbidden by law to fill it.

The following information will usually appear on a prescription drug label:

1. The patient's name.

2. The physician's name.

3. The pharmacy name, address, and telephone number.

4. The prescription number (given by the pharmacy).

5. How often and when to take the drug.

6. How much to take each time.

7. Any special instructions for use.

8. The name of the drug, if the physician tells the pharmacist to include it.

It is very important to follow the instructions

exactly. It is entirely possible that the patient will not get the desired effect by taking medicine after meals if the instructions were to take it before meals (some medicines are inactivated by food or by the digestive juices). If the doctor says to take a drug three times a day he does not mean three tablets once a day.

drug abuse — the deliberate act of taking a drug for other than its intended purpose, and in a manner that can result in damage to the person's health or his ability to function.

The misuse of drugs is not a new phenomenon. Different types of drug abuse have been present for years in the United States and other countries. The reasons that man has used drugs throughout history are mainly the same reasons for today's nonmedical drug use: to ease pain, to stop anxiety, to produce happiness, and to change experience and thought. Many of the reasons young people and adults use drugs are one and the same: for fun, to make social communication easier, to feel better, to relieve boredom and frustration, to escape from problems, and perhaps to protest.

Many people still seem to think of drugs as magic potions that have only the good effects they seek. However, almost every drug, even those not commonly thought of as drugs of abuse, is potentially dangerous at some dosage level for certain people under some circumstances. Some drugs can also be harmful when taken in dangerous combinations or by very sensitive people in small or ordinary amounts.

The drug problem is complex. There are few issues that arouse so many emotions as the abuse of drugs. In one respect, the problem is that we are a drug-oriented society, and people are using more drugs without understanding their actions.

The problem is also one of people and their feelings and beliefs about drugs. Just as no two people are exactly alike, no two drug users are the same. Many people tend to lump everyone who uses drugs into one category. However, not all drug abusers are at the same level of involvement, and distinctions must be made between the various types of users.

The experimenters have tried a drug, most likely marihuana, only a few times, often because of curiosity or peer-group pressure. This group does not plan to continue drug use, and their experience is usually not more than an occasional social exposure.

The moderate or social group uses drugs with some regularity; however, drugs have not become the most important factor in their lives.

The chronic users regularly take drugs, which have assumed a central role in their life-styles. This group consists of small proportion of all drug users, but they are the ones who are drug-dependent.

Drug dependence (physical or psychological) is a condition that results from chronic, periodic, or continuous use of various chemicals. There are many different kinds of drug dependence. They are differentiated by the type of drug used. Each type has specific problems associated with it.

Habituation is the psychological desire to repeat the use of a drug intermittently or continuously because of emotional needs. Many individuals come to use drugs habitually to escape from reality or just to feel better.

Addiction is the physical dependence upon a drug.

All drugs have many effects, and these vary among individuals, on different occasions in the same individual, with the amount of the drug, and the length of time the drug is used. Many factors not related to the chemical makeup of the drug cause varying effects. These include the expectations of the user, the circumstances or setting under which he takes the drug, and the meaning of drug use to the individual.

Even the same individual taking the same dose of a drug on subsequent occasions may have a completely different reaction. As the drug affects the individual, he becomes more susceptible to the moods of the people around him and the setting in which he takes the drug. These factors can markedly alter the drug's effects.

Some prescription drugs are so dangerous that they are included under a special law passed to control drug abuse. The Comprehensive Drug Abuse Prevention and Control Act of 1970 was the result of increasing national concern over the widespread abuse of four groups of drugs; narcotics, depressants, stimulants, and hallucinogens.

The law combines two methods to curb drug abuse:

1. All legal handlers of drugs designated as dangerous must keep records of their supplies and sales.

2. All suppliers of illegal drugs are subject to arrest and criminal prosecution.

drug addiction — physical dependence on a drug.

The definition includes the development of tolerance and withdrawal. As a person develops tolerance, he requires larger and larger amounts of the drug to achieve the same effect. Withdrawal occurs when the use of an addicting drug is stopped abruptly and is characterized by a wide range of distressing symptoms, such as diarrhea, vomiting, and cramps. Many drug users develop a compulsion to continue taking a drug to avoid the withdrawal symptoms.

Drug addiction results from a combination of two factors: the existence of a personality disorder and the availablity of addicting drugs.

Drugs other than narcotics can become addicting. They include barbiturates and certain tranquilizers. Stimulants in very large doses are addictive.

See amphetamine, heroin, etc.

duct — a tube or passageway for glandular fluid.

ductless gland — a gland without a duct. Fluid secreted from such glands enters the circulation directly from the gland.

ductus arteriosus — the passageway between the two major blood vessels that adjoin the heart: the aorta and the pulmonary artery. It serves the purpose of eliminating part of the blood flow to the lungs. This connection exists in the fetus until birth. Shortly after birth, the passageway closes. Failure to do so results in patent ductus arteriosus, a congenital birth defect.

See congenital heart defect.

ductus deferens — *See vas deferens.*

duodenal ulcer — *See peptic ulcer.*

duodenum — the first part of the small intestine. *See intestine.*

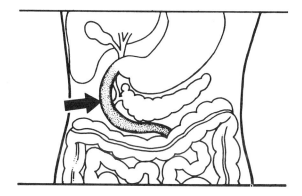

DUODENUM

dwarf — a person who is abnormally under average size. In some cases, this is caused by a lack of growth hormone.

dysentery — a general term used to describe disorders of the intestines produced by ameba, bacteria, or chemicals. The symptoms include frequent bowel movements (which are bloody and contain mucus) and pain in the abdominal region. *See amebic dysentery.*

dysmenorrhea — the pain before and during the menstrual period. Most women experience some discomfort with a menstrual period at one time or another. However, some women experience pain with every cycle. The pain can be caused by disorders (called secondary dysmenorrhea), or the cause may be unknown.

The pain is usually confined to the lower abdomen and lower back and is either a sharp, stabbing sensation or a prolonged feeling of intense pressure.

dyspepsia — a general term indicating any impairment of the digestive process or loss of the ability to digest food.

Dyspepsia can, however, be caused by nerves. When such is the case, the patient's own nerves are interfering with the eating and digesting process. Nervous dyspepsia can become a vicious cycle—the patient's nervous tension causes a lack of appetite; the lack of food in the stomach causes discomfort, which in turn decreases appetite. The cycle can best be broken by removing the cause of the nervous tension.

dysphagia — difficulty in swallowing. This is usually caused by an inflammation in or in the region of the esophagus.

dyspnea — difficult or labored breathing. Dyspnea usually refers to breathing problems that are abnormal under the existing circumstances. For instance, a person who has been resting should have no difficulty in breathing; if he does, that is properly classified as dyspnea. However, an athlete who comes off the playing field and has a little trouble catching his breath is not experiencing true dyspnea because he quickly resumes a normal breathing pattern.

ear — the organ of hearing. The ear consists of three different sections: the outer ear, the middle ear, and the inner ear.

THE OUTER EAR

The outer ear channels sound waves from the air inward through the external auditory canal. The external portion of the ear, called the auricle, is composed of cartilage covered by skin. The auricle projects from the side of the head and helps to funnel sound into the auditory canal. This canal terminates at a tightly stretched membrane, the eardrum.

THE MIDDLE EAR

Beyond the eardrum, in the middle ear chamber, are three tiny, linked bones called the malleus (hammer), incus (anvil), and stapes (stirrup). The outer bone, the malleus, is attached to the eardrum. The inner bone, the stapes, ends in a footplate that fits into the oval window, an opening in the wall of the bone housing the inner ear. The center bone, the incus, connects the malleus and the stapes so that when one moves, they all move.

THE INNER EAR

The inner ear is filled with fluid. The innermost portion terminates in a delicate spiral structure that is shaped something like a snail. It is called the cochlea. Inside the cochlea is an arrangement of thousands of tiny, specialized cells, each of which is equipped with many microscopic hairs. These hairs are immersed in the fluid that fills the cochlea.

HOW THE EAR FUNCTIONS

Sound waves enter the ear, travel through the auditory canal, and set up vibrations in the eardrum. The vibrations of the eardrum cause the bones in the middle ear to move back and forth like tiny levers. This lever action converts the large motions of the eardrum into the shorter, more forceful motions of the stapes.

The footplate at the inner end of the stapes moves in and out of the oval window at the same rate that the eardrum is vibrating. The movement of the footplate sets up motions in the fluid that fills the cochlea.

Thousands of sensory cells in one part of the cochlea are connected to fibers that make up the cochlear or acoustic nerve (nerve of hearing). Each sensory (receptor) cell has many microscopic hairs at one end. Movements of the fluid bend these tiny hairs. Movement of the hairs stimulates the hair cells to generate tiny electrical impulses that are carried along the fibers of the acoustic nerve to the brain. In the brain, the impulses are translated into the sensation of sound.

In short, the ear changes sound waves into electrical nerve signals to which the brain gives meaning.

SIZE

The smallness of the structures contributes to the difficulty of research on details of the hearing process. The three little bones of the middle ear, for example, could be held on the tip of a little finger. The whole middle ear is about as big as a string-bean seed (about three-sixteenths of an inch by three-eighths of an inch). The cochlea of the inner ear is even smaller than the middle ear.

However, the modern development of the elec-

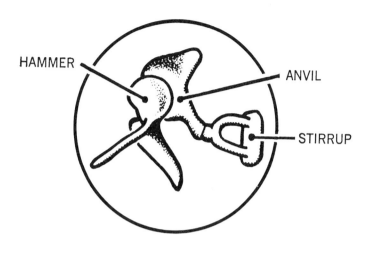

HAMMER

ANVIL

STIRRUP

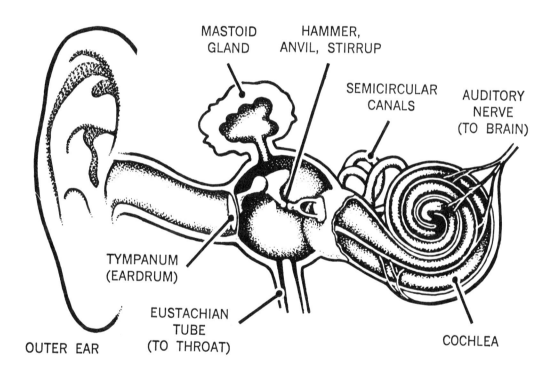

MASTOID
GLAND

HAMMER,
ANVIL, STIRRUP

SEMICIRCULAR
CANALS

AUDITORY
NERVE
(TO BRAIN)

TYMPANUM
(EARDRUM)

EUSTACHIAN
TUBE
(TO THROAT)

OUTER EAR

COCHLEA

EAR

tron microscope allows the research study of ear structures at practical magnifications up to 100,000 times. Furthermore, the ear surgeon can now use an operating microscope that enlarges his view of these tiny structures by as much as sixty times.

EAR INFECTIONS

Any infection of the respiratory tract can spread to the ear through the eustachian tube, which connects the back of the throat with the middle ear. Such common diseases of childhood as measles, German measles, scarlet fever, whooping cough, and mumps can lead to impaired hearing. So can other virus infections and meningitis.

See deafness.

eardrum — *See tympanic membrane.*

ECG — *See electrocardiogram.*

eclampsia — convulsions occurring during the latter stages of pregnancy. Eclampsia is a result of a type of blood poisoning called toxemia. This condition is more likely to develop in women who do not have good prenatal care or who do not follow their doctor's advice.

In moderately advanced cases of toxemia, doctors use certain drugs to lower the blood pressure and to ward off convulsions.

ecphyadectomy — appendectomy.

ecthyreosis — absence of or loss of function of the thyroid gland.

ectopic pregnancy — a pregnancy in which the fertilized ovum is not located in the proper place. Normally, the fertilized ovum attaches itself to the lining of the uterus. When this fails to happen, the mother usually has a miscarriage. However, an ectopic pregnancy can be dangerous. If, for example, the ovum lodges in the fallopian tube, it may continue to grow until it bursts the fallopian tube. The bleeding that follows can lead to death unless there is prompt surgical attention.

eczema — a red, thickened, rough patch on the skin. Eczema often begins on the cheeks or in the fold of the elbow or knees, but it may spread over a large portion of the body. It will itch, and scratching causes oozing, which forms crusts. While it is not contagious, the open sores may readily become infected. Eczema is one of the more common allergic reactions.

See allergy.

edema — swelling due to abnormally large amounts of fluid in the tissues of the body. Edema often follows heart problems.

When the heart fails, several mechanisms in the body are affected by its inability to pump blood normally. There is a backing up of blood in the veins; some of the fluid in the blood is forced into the body tissues; and the kidneys lose their ability to eliminate excess sodium in the urine. Excess sodium retained in the body holds water with it, causing accumulation of fluids (edema).

To reduce the edema or swelling, the physician may prescribe a drug (diuretic), a sodium-restricted diet, or a combination of the two. The diuretic will reduce the excess fluid quickly, which is often necessary in severe edema. The diet will cause a more gradual loss but is safer and more economical for long-term use.

While an excess accumulation of fluid and sodium in the body is undesirable, sodium is one of the basic mineral elements and is essential to normal health. It is found in the bloodstream and in the fluid that bathes the body tissues.

An average diet contains much more sodium than the body needs, but normally the excess is eliminated by the kidneys in the urine.

effort syndrome — a group of symptoms (quick fatigue, rapid heartbeat, sighing breaths, dizziness) that do not result from disease of organs or tissues and that are out of proportion to the amount of energy that is used.

effusion — the escape or leakage of body fluid into a body area in which it does not belong.

ego — an individual's conception of himself and the world around him. The ego is sometimes referred to as an individual's conscious mind.

ejaculum praecox — premature ejaculation in the male. This is usually a psychological problem rather than a medical problem.

EKG — *See electrocardiogram.*

elbow — the juncture and joint of the arm and the forearm. The elbow is the place where the bone of the arm (the humerus) meets the two bones of the forearm (the ulna and the radius).

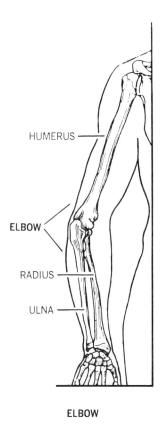

HUMERUS —

ELBOW

RADIUS —

ULNA

ELBOW

electric cardiac pacemaker — an electric device that can control the beating of the heart by a rhythmic discharge of electrical impulses.

electric shock — shock caused by electricity. Electricity causes shock by paralyzing the nerve centers that control breathing or by stopping the regular beat of the heart.

The symptoms of electric shock are sudden loss of consciousness, absence of respiration (which, if present, is slight and cannot be detected), weak pulse, and probable burns. Every second of delay in removing a person from contact with an electric current lessens the chance of resuscitating him. It is important to act quickly, but the rescuer must be careful not to come in contact with the current or a conductor.

In all cases, the wire or current must be removed from the patient or the patient from the wire promptly; if the patient is not breathing, artificial respiration should be started at once.

electrocardiogram — a graphic record of the electric currents produced by the heart. This graphic representation of the electrical activity of the heart is presented as a tracing produced on graph paper.

The electrocardiogram is one of the most important tools available to a doctor for the diagnosis of possible heart difficulty. It helps to provide information on the kind, extent, and location of injury sustained by the heart as a result of heart attacks.

An electrocardiogram is often referred to as an EKG or an ECG.

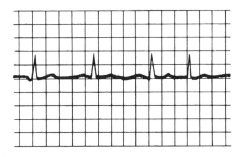

EKG GRAPH
(ELECTROCARDIOGRAM)

electrocardiograph — an instrument that records electric currents produced by the heart.
See electrocardiogram.

electroconvulsive therapy — a method of treating certain types of mental illnesses. Electroconvulsive therapy (ECT) involves passing an electric current or shock through the patient's brain. Though it seems to work, doctors are not sure how or why it works.

Electroconvulsive therapy is more commonly known as shock treatment or shock therapy.

electroencephalogram — a graphic record of the tiny electric currents given off by the brain (that is, by the approximately one-third of the brain whose electrical activity can be picked up from outside).

Electrodes, tiny flat disks, are pasted on the scalp. Each disk picks up an electric current from a different part of the brain. A fine wire carries each brain current to a device that looks like a large radio receiver, where the tiny current is amplified or increased. Each amplified current

129

moves a pen that is held against a moving band of paper. The record is a series of long, wavy lines—one for each section of the brain where "broadcasts" are being picked up. Each wave indicates an increase in the voltage. The higher the waves and the faster they come, the greater the electrical activity of the brain's nerve cells.

An electroencephalogram is often referred to as an EEG.

electrolyte — any substance that, in solution, is capable of conducting electricity by means of its atoms or groups of atoms, and in the process is broken down into positively and negatively charged particles.

The most important electrolytes in the body are sodium and potassium. When there is too little sodium and/or potassium in the body, the chemical balance of the entire body is upset. The loss of electrolytes (called electrolyte imbalance) is often caused by severe diarrhea. Electrolyte imbalance can be extremely dangerous if it is not speedily corrected.

electron microscope — an optical instrument using a beam of electrons directed through an object to produce an enlarged image (up to 100,000 × magnification) on a fluorescent screen or photographic plate.

elephantiasis — a disease caused by a type of worm called filaria. The disease results from the blockage of lymph channels. The skin and subcutaneous tissues thicken, enlarge, and sometimes are ulcerated. Elephantiasis is usually most severe in the legs and external genital areas, where gross swellings occur.

embolism — the blocking of a blood vessel by a blood

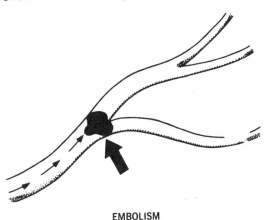

EMBOLISM

clot, air bubble, or other substance carried in the bloodstream. The clot or air bubble causes no serious problem until it reaches a blood vessel it is too big to pass through. At that point, it stops up the blood vessel. If the blood vessel is not a major vessel and is not located in a vital area, the damage can be minimal. If, however, an embolism lodges in one of the brain's arteries, in the lungs, or in any of the major arteries, death can occur very quickly.

embolus — a blood clot (or other substance such as air, fat, or tumor) inside a blood vessel, where it becomes an obstruction to circulation. An embolus causes an embolism.
See embolism, thrombus.

embryo — a term used to describe an unborn child from one week after conception through the second month. Before that time (that is, for the first week after conception), the recently fertilized ovum is referred to as a zygote. After the second month, the unborn child is called a fetus.

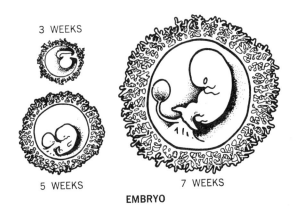

3 WEEKS

5 WEEKS

7 WEEKS

EMBRYO

About two weeks after conception an embryo is barely large enough to be seen with the naked eye. The place where a head and brain will later develop is growing very fast, however, and there are little indentations where the eyes will be.

At the end of four weeks the embryo is still only about a quarter of an inch long. This is a particularly important time because the internal organs—heart, liver, digestive system, brain, and lungs—are beginning to form. The heart begins to beat, although it is still inaudible.

At five weeks the embryo is the shape of a tiny quarter moon. The backbone has started to form. The head is growing much faster than the rest of the body and will continue to do so until after birth. Tiny limb-buds appear as the beginnings of the arms and legs.

At six weeks the embryo is almost half an inch long. The four limb-buds have grown into arms and legs.

By the seventh week ears and eyelids are forming, and the internal organs are moving into place. The embryo is now floating in a sac of fluid, which is sometimes called the "bag of waters." The fluid keeps the embryo evenly warm and also acts as a shock absorber to protect against jolts and bumps.

The embryo gets all the oxygen it needs, as well as blood and nutrition, from the mother through the umbilical cord.

After the eighth week the embryo is called a fetus.

See fetus, zygote.

embryology — the study of the development of embryos. Embryology is important to the study of evolution. During the early part of embryonic development, the embryos of man, rabbits, and pigs are very similar. According to the theory of evolution, this is because all three are descended from a common ancestor.

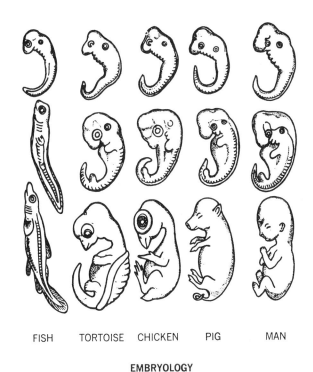

FISH   TORTOISE   CHICKEN   PIG   MAN

EMBRYOLOGY

emetic — a substance that causes vomiting. Emetics work in one of two ways. The first type promotes vomiting by irritating the stomach; the second promotes vomiting by way of a reflex in the brain. Among the first type are salt, warm water with soapsuds, etc. These are commonly used as antidotes to ingested poisons. Drugs such as morphine belong in the second group.

emphysema — a lung disease in which there is an impairment of the bellows action of the lungs.

In healthy breathing, the lungs efficiently extract waste gas (carbon dioxide) from the blood as it circulates through blood vessels in the lungs. Acting like an elastic bellows, the lungs exchange carbon dioxide with the atmosphere for fresh oxygen. The air must be distributed throughout myriads of small air spaces in this bellows system by a branching tree-like arrangement of tubes called bronchial tubes.

The tubes end as tiny bronchioles that feed elastic, bulb-shaped air sacs called alveoli. These are distributed throughout the lung tissue, giving it a sponge-like appearance. Healthy bronchioles and alveoli have elastic properties that allow them to expand or contract as one breathes, thus achieving the bellows effect. Covering all passageways from the nose to the tiny bulbous alveoli is a mucous blanket—thin, but present throughout.

Beneath the blanket and normally separating it from direct contact with the surface of the tubes are millions of microscopic hairs or cilia, constantly in motion in a watery layer. Known as the mucociliary mechanism, its responsibility is to protect the delicate tissues of the passages and, by its constant motion, propel foreign matter (such as dust, pollen, or other material) toward the throat, where it can be removed by clearing the throat.

Although there is much research yet to be done on emphysema, on the basis of current knowledge it seems that when emphysema sets in, this mechanism breaks down as noxious materials — bacteria and viruses — go to work on the cells that line the tubes. The cilia are destroyed; inflammatory cells invade; ulceration may occur; and the normal physical properties and architecture of the bronchioles and lung tissue are unfavorably altered. In addition, the walls of the alveoli are destroyed and broken down. This produces large, inefficient air spaces. As a result, resistance to airflow increases, and breathing is progressively more difficult. Late in the disease added expiratory effort can actually result in decreased airflow. Finally, there is a buildup of the toxic gaseous waste product, carbon dioxide. Meanwhile, the heart works harder to pump oxygen-poor blood to needy body tissues. In time, without diagnosis, adequate treatment and medical management, death may result from suffocation and an overworked heart.

SYMPTOMS

Generally speaking, emphysema does not strike its victims suddenly. It creeps up on them. Many patients are unaware of anything seriously wrong until much of their lung function is impaired. Initially, severe and repeated respiratory infections, followed by long periods of feeling "not quite up to par" are apt to occur, particularly in the winter. There is much coughing, accompanied by increasing amounts of phlegm, especially on arising in the morning. Each year the discomfort hangs on for a longer period. Finally, decreasing lung-breathing capacity, frequency of coughing spells, and shortness of breath send the sufferer to his doctor. At this point it is often too late to do more than slow down the harmful effects.

Other symptoms include wheezing, general weakness and a tendency to tire easily, dizziness, and a feeling of tightness in the chest.

If the patient's history and clinical examination suggest emphysema, the diagnosis can be confirmed readily by tests for pulmonary function. Preliminary tests can be carried out in the physician's office. More extensive procedures, including tests for blood gases, gaseous exchange capacity, and spare lung volume, are sometimes necessary to assess the degree of lung impairment. These require more complex equipment and laboratory skills, usually available only in a well-equipped hospital or clinic.

TREATMENT

The belief that all emphysema patients will inevitably grow worse and die from the disease is a common fallacy. Emphysema is a disease state of broad spectrum — that is, it ranges from mild, perhaps unnoted forms, to severe stages. It may be experienced in very mild form, and if treated with proper care in the earlier stages, it often can be arrested.

Treatment, for the most part, is directed toward relieving inflammation in the bronchial area. With this in mind, it becomes of great importance to remove all bronchial irritants from the air taken in. Any type of dust or air pollution may serve as an irritant. A chief offender for those who smoke, is, of course, tobacco smoke. Rarely is it too late to secure benefits by giving up this habit.

Infection, part of the bronchitis-emphysema problem, can be combated with antibiotics. Physicians may advise influenza vaccine as a precautionary measure if an epidemic is anticipated, because severe bronchitis and pneumonia may be associated with influenza virus infections.

Bronchodilators, drugs that produce dilation of the bronchi and reduce airway resistance, are often useful. Various hand instruments, or nebulizers, are available.

Sometimes the patient with emphysema may have episodes of acute pulmonary impairment. During these episodes, the doctor employs various specific measures. A special machine (called an intermittent positive-pressure breathing apparatus) may be used to maintain adequate breathing for the patient. Drugs that stimulate the brain to send impulses via the nerves to the breathing muscles are sometimes helpful. In addition, special nursing care may be required. Surgery in pulmonary emphysema may be helpful if large, balloon-shaped "blebs" are removed where they compress adjacent normal lung tissue.

Attempts at replacement of an entire lung, severely damaged by this disease, with a donor lung or artificial device are still on the frontier of research. There is much current research in this direction, but much more investigation will be required before such replacements become a reality.

Physicians sometimes recommend a change of climate on a trial basis. In making such a recommendation, the physician usually suggests desirable ranges in temperature, humidity, precipitation, and altitude.

REHABILITATION

The essential ingredients of rehabilitation are postural drainage—placing the body so that gravity helps drain the lungs—and breathing exercises. Breathing exercises emphasize use of the diaphragm and abdominal muscles instead of the chest muscles and allow the patient to make the best use of his limited breathing capacity. Both drainage and exercises, as prescribed by the attending physician, are important parts of long-term management of emphysema.

OUTLOOK

The expected outlook today for an individual patient varies greatly. His outlook depends on age, degree of lung damage, and cooperation with his physician in an effective disease-management and rehabilitation program. The older the patient and the greater his respiratory difficulty, the shorter is his life expectancy. For example, in one study of patients under fifty who had mild breathing difficulties when first seen, seventy percent were either improved or no worse five years later. Among patients over sixty with similar symptoms, twenty percent were improved or the same after five years. Among severely ill patients in the same age groups, the death rate was forty percent among those under fifty and sixty percent among those over sixty.

Life expectancy is also reduced by circulatory complications combined with emphysema. Especially serious are such added problems as right-heart overwork owing to high blood pressure in the pulmonary blood vessels and an abnormal increase in the number of red blood cells.

In most cases, the patient who stops smoking improves his life expectancy.

empyema — *See pleurisy.*

enamel — the outer covering of the part of a tooth that projects beyond the gums. Enamel is the hardest of all body tissues.

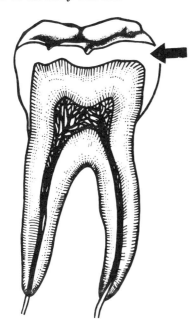

ENAMEL

encephalitis — an inflammation of the brain, usually caused by a virus.
See poliomyelitis, rabies.

endarterium — the innermost layer of an artery. It is also called intima.

endemic — a term used to describe a disease that is constantly present in or native to a particular region or locality.

endocarditis — an inflammation of the inner layer of the heart (endocardium) that is usually associated with acute rheumatic fever or some infectious agent.
See rheumatic fever.

endocardium — a thin, smooth membrane forming the inner surface of the heart.

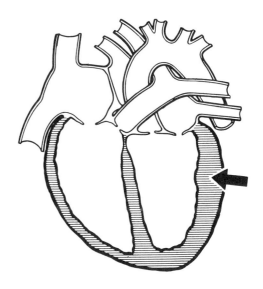

ENDOCARDIUM

endocrine glands — glands that are ductless; that is, their secretions enter the blood or the lymph system directly. There are seven endocrine glands: pituitary, thyroid, adrenal, parathyroid, ovaries, testes, and special cells in the pancreas.

The secretions of the endocrine glands are called hormones. The hormones of each gland enter the blood or lymph systems in one area but can affect many different parts of the body.

The pituitary gland regulates most of the endocrine glands.
See different glands, hormones.

endothelium — the thin lining of the blood vessels.

enema — the injection of water or a liquid substance into the rectum. Enemas are given to clean out the rectum and lower bowel, to supply nutrition, and to get medicines into the body.

Entamoeba — a microscopic ameba. One type, *Entamoeba histolytica,* causes amebiasis and the more severe amebic dysentery.
See amebiasis.

enteritis — an inflammation of the intestines, particularly of the small intestines.

enzyme — a complex organic substance that is capable of speeding up specific biochemical transformations or processes in the body, as in digestion. Enzymes are universally present in living organisms. They assist and regulate the many chemical reactions that go on constantly in the body. Several hundred enzymes have been identified, and many have been isolated and crystallized.

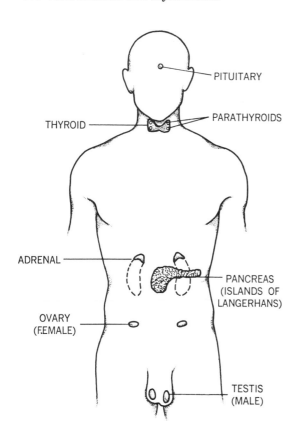

ENDOCRINE GLANDS

epicardium — the outer layer of the heart wall. It is also called the visceral pericardium.

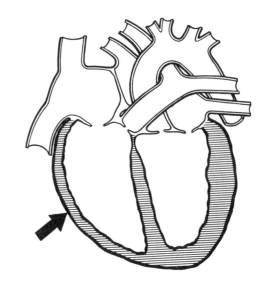

EPICARDIUM

epidemic — a disease that attacks a broad segment of a local community at about the same time and that spreads very rapidly.

epidemic pleurodynia — an epidemic disease caused by a virus. The disease causes pain in the region of the chest or abdomen, as well as fever. One of the typical symptoms of epidemic pleurodynia is a relapse occurring two to three days after the original attack. Epidemic pleurodynia is also referred to as Bornholm's disease.

epidermis — the outer layer of skin.
See skin.

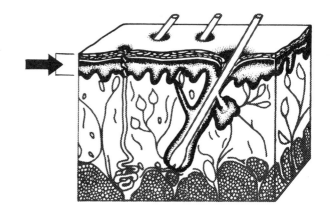

EPIDERMIS

134

epiglottis — the flap of cartilage that acts as a lid for the larynx. The epiglottis covers the opening of the larynx when food is being swallowed. This action keeps food from entering the larynx and consequently the trachea and the lungs. The epiglottis closes automatically during swallowing.

The movement of the epiglottis is what prevents breathing and swallowing from occurring at the same time.

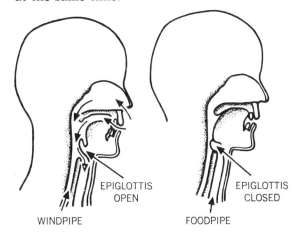

EPIGLOTTIS
OPEN

EPIGLOTTIS
CLOSED

WINDPIPE

FOODPIPE

EPIGLOTTIS (FOODPIPE)

epilepsy — a symptom of some disorder in the brain. The name of this condition comes from the Greek word for seizure. The brain has many millions of nerve cells, called neurons. that work together to control or guide the actions of the body. To do their work, the nerve cells build up a supply of electricity through the action of the chemicals they contain. Each cell has its own storage battery, which it discharges at the proper moment and then recharges instantaneously.

However, cells can become overactive and fire off irregularly. This disturbance can suddenly spread to neighboring areas or jump to distant ones or even overwhelm the brain. When it spreads, a seizure results. The great majority of the neurons soon begin working in harmony again, and the seizure is over.

Epilepsy is a condition in which seizures occur. A seizure itself is the sign of an abnormal release of energy within the brain.

DIAGNOSIS

An EEG or electroencephalogram is a record of the tiny electric currents given off by the brain (that is, by the approximately one-third of the brain whose electrical activity can be picked up from outside).

Each current moves a pen that is held against a moving band of paper. The record is a series of long, wavy lines—one for each section of the brain where currents are being picked up. Each wave indicates an increase in the voltage. The higher the waves and the faster they come, the greater the electrical activity of the brain's nerve cells.

When a baby is about three months old, the EEG shows from three to six waves per second. The adult pattern is about ten waves per second, at least until the sixties; it may begin to slow down after that.

Odd though it may seem, brain waves give no clue to a person's intelligence, thoughts, or mental health. However, they do provide strong clues as to whether or not a person has epilepsy. An EEG recorded during a seizure is likely to show unusually high bursts of energy coming either unusually fast or unusually slow. The pattern is likely to vary according to the type of seizure. Even between seizures, the EEG of most persons with epilepsy will show irregularity.

TYPES

There are three major types of epilepsy: grand mal, petit mal, and focal seizures.

1. Grand mal

This is the most prevalent and dramatic type. There may be a warning (aura) that consists of false perception of the sense of smell (e.g., geraniums) or hearing (e.g., bells), followed by a vocal cry, loss of consciousness, falling, and convulsions. There may be injury in the fall or if the person hits something hard as he thrashes around. The tongue may be bitten, and loss of control of bladder and bowel may occur. Typically, after the seizure, sleep, confusion, headache, or stomach upset may occur for a period of time.

In spite of its fearsome aspects, this type of epilepsy is generally the easiest to bring under control. The medical term, grand mal, is French for great sickness or major attack.

2. Petit mal

This type is especially prevalent in childhood. It is rare in persons over twenty years of age. The seizures are very brief periods of loss of consciousness and may recur fifty to one hundred times a day. Many children blink their eyes during an attack; others nod their heads or jerk their arms.

Brain-wave records indicate that, in this type of epilepsy, the disordered release of energy covers the entire brain, as in attacks of grand mal.

On the basis of brain-wave patterns, some neurologists consider two other types of seizures to be varieties of petit mal. In one of these, all the muscles suddenly go limp and the person falls to the ground. He then usually picks himself up and goes about whatever he had been doing. In the other type, the muscles of the arms or trunk suddenly begin to move jerkily, and then stop in a little while. Other authorities class these as minor motor seizures. In this class they also place infantile spasms or quivering spells.

3. Focal seizures

Some types of epilepsy are called *focal* because the abnormal electrical discharges can be traced to one small area, or focus, in the brain, or to a number of such areas.

In one of these types, called "Jacksonian," the overactive neurons are located in the part of the brain governing movements of the muscles. A seizure generally starts in the toes of one foot or the fingers of one hand or in one corner of the mouth. Suddenly the affected part trembles violently or just feels numb. As more and more neurons become affected, the trembling or numbness marches upward. It may stop at any time or, in a few seconds or a few minutes, cross to the other side of the body. Then the person loses consciousness and has an attack like that in grand mal.

A far more common type of focal seizure is the one generally known as psychomotor epilepsy, because the abnormally discharging cells act on the mental process as well as on muscles. There is a sudden alteration of mood and behavior, sometimes aggressive, followed by total amnesia during the attack.

When the EEG shows electrical discharges in one or both of the brain's temporal lobes, the area lying above each ear, this type is called temporal lobe epilepsy. It appears in a great variety of forms, most of which have one thing in common: a period of irrational or odd behavior that generally lasts only a few moments, but may continue longer, and is not remembered.

CAUSES

Epilepsy may result from many different causes: brain injury resulting from lack of oxygen, central nervous system infections or physical impact, chemical abnormalities, congenital malformations of the central nervous system, genetic abnormalities, or some other anatomical defect of the brain, such as tumors. In many instances, it is not possible to identify a specific cause. Seizures are often precipitated by drugs, emotional strain, or alcohol.

Many doctors are beginning to look upon epilepsy as a symptom rather than a disease. Abnormally discharging neurons can cause the symptom, and a lesion causes the abnormally discharging neurons. In ordinary language a lesion is an injury, but in medical terminology it is any variation from normal.

It may be a congenital malformation — something with which a person is born. It may be a scar that formed within the brain after a bullet wound or other injury. It may be damage to brain tissue from a childhood infection. One example of an infection is meningitis, an inflammation of the membranes covering the brain. Another example is encephalitis, an inflammation of the brain that may, but rarely does, follow measles, mumps, whooping cough, and other diseases.

Neurosurgeons occasionally find tumors and abscesses. Sometimes, too, they find evidence of damage that must have happened during an exceptionally difficult birth, although the seizures began a long time later.

All such lesions may irritate nearby nerve cells.

A probable cause can now be assigned in perhaps fifty percent of all cases of epilepsy, and this proportion is expected to rise as research continues. But there remains a puzzle: what causes epilepsy in one person is by no means sure to cause it in another person.

TREATMENT FOR EPILEPSY

About one hundred years ago, an English doctor discovered almost by accident that sedatives called bromides would do some good in epilepsy (although they tended to make patients dull). They were the first real anti-seizure medicines. Next, about fifty years ago a German doctor, again almost accidentally, found that another sedative, phenobarbital, worked better, although it caused drowsiness in some cases.

Approximately twenty-five years ago, a young American doctor asked: "Why not make a medicine to order?" He told drug companies what he had in mind: something chemically related to phenobarbital but without its sedative effect.

During the next few years an associate painstakingly tested scores of compounds. One stood out. It raised the seizure threshold of cats four times. This means that when cats were given this compound they would withstand an electrical shock, without getting convulsions, four times stronger than that which produced convulsions in untreated cats. And the new medicine rarely had bad side effects.

Since the discovery of diphenylhydantoin sodium—or Dilantin, as the medicine is generally known in this country—about twenty-five other drugs have proved effective and safe under medical supervision. Each new one has enabled doctors to control seizures in some patients who were helped only a little or not at all by the older medicines.

Even when the seizures themselves have been fully controlled, the brain waves generally show irregularities (except in the case of petit mal seizures that have been brought under control). Perhaps the drugs work not on the abnormally discharging neurons themselves but on the other neurons: they keep the electrical disturbance from spreading.

Once in a while an operation is recommended for temporal lobe epilepsy—but only when three circumstances hold true: the seizures originate wholly or in large part from an area in one of the temporal lobes that can be safely removed; the seizures are frequent and incapacitating; a long trial shows they cannot be controlled by present drugs. (Some less-common types of focal seizures may be operated upon, too.)

The EEG tells in a general way the location of the abnormally discharging neurons. Surgeons are guided also by records of electrical activity made directly from the surface of the brain and by other techniques.

During the course of such operations, a team of neurosurgeons using electrodes with tips only five microns across—about two ten-thousandths of an inch—has recorded the electrical activity of individual neurons. Each of those in the affected area appears to be firing off at a high rate but in its own fashion — without regard to what is going on around it.

TREATMENT FOR A MAJOR SEIZURE

In some cases where medication has not been very effective, a seizure apparently can be traced to a time of great nervous tension, a sudden noise, or a bright, flickering light. Generally, however, no clear precipitating cause can be found. When a seizure does occur, there are certain steps that should be taken.

1. Keep calm. Nothing can be done to stop the attack once it has started. The person is not going to die; he does not need a doctor (unless—and this does not happen often—he seems to pass from one seizure to another without regaining consciousness). His condition is not "catching." Ordinarily, the attack will be over in a few minutes.

2. Try to get the patient in a position where he will not hurt himself by knocking against something, but do not interfere with his movements.

3. If you can do it without using force, slip something like a folded handkerchief or a piece of rubber (nothing hard) between his teeth to keep him from biting his tongue or cheek.

4. Loosen tight clothing, particularly around the neck.

5. Once the convulsive movements stop, you may turn the person on his side to assist his tongue to fall forward and excess saliva to drain out of his mouth. As he recovers, let him rest if he wants to. Treat him matter-of-factly.

These points apply to grand mal seizures. Petit mal seizures require no special steps. Ordinarily, the best way to handle a psychomotor seizure is to let the person continue his activity without restraint.

epinephrine — a hormone secreted by the adrenal medulla of the adrenal glands; it can also be prepared synthetically. Epinephrine constricts the small blood vessels, increases the rate and strength of the heartbeat, and raises the blood pressure. It is called a vasoconstrictor or vasopressor substance.

The adrenal medulla secretes epinephrine in moments of stress to allow the body to meet added demands. For example, large amounts of epinephrine are secreted when a person is frightened, allowing the person extra energy to run or to fight. For this reason, epinephrine is known as the "flight or fight" hormone.

As a synthesized drug, it is used to help relieve respiratory problems, to give relief from acute allergic reactions, and in some cases it is given to restore normal heart rhythm.

The effects of epinephrine, natural or synthesized, do not last very long because the body absorbs or reabsorbs it very quickly.

See adrenal glands.

episiotomy — a surgical cut or incision in the vaginal opening. It is made to enlarge the area during delivery. This is done when the doctor feels that the tissues might tear as the baby comes out of the vaginal opening. This surgical cut heals better than a tear would. It is closed with a few stitches after the baby is born. The stitches are made of catgut and do not need to be removed. Most episiotomies heal soon and cause comparatively little discomfort.

epithelium — the covering layer of body surfaces—both internal and external.

erepsin — enzymes that act in the process of digestion, specifically in the digestion of protein.

erythema — a general term used to indicate redness of the skin or an inflammation of the skin.

erythema multiforme — one of the more severe forms of oral ulcerations. Because the skin and the mucous lining of the mouth are similar in structure, the same kind of sores will develop both on the skin and in the mouth. Erythema multiforme is common in children and young adults. It appears most frequently in the winter and spring months.

SYMPTOMS
Erythema multiforme may develop suddenly, causing a general sick feeling, sore throat, and arthritic or rheumatic pains. The patient may have a slight fever or a temperature of 104 to 105 degrees.

Sores develop first in the mouth, on the cheek, palate and tongue, and on the lips. The gums are not often involved. The affected areas show an intense reddening with the appearance of the sores, which are blisters of varying size. Later these blisters break, leaving an ulcerated, irregular surface, coated by a yellowish membrane. Sores on the lips become bloody and encrusted.

Similar blisters appear on the skin on almost any part of the body, frequently on the genital membranes. These blisters are bright reddish-purple at first, fading to deep purple as the disease progresses.

The patient may be acutely ill for three or four days. Because his mouth is very painful, he has great difficulty eating and drinking.

Several attacks of blisters may follow one another.

In a more rare form of the disease, the characteristic sores are called "bullae." These are very large blisters. When they break in the mouth, the whole area becomes very red, as if the patient had been burned.

In very severe cases, blisters may form in the eyes, perhaps causing blindness.

CAUSE
The precise cause of this disease is a mystery. Viral or bacterial infection and vitamin deficiency have been suggested. However, there is reason to believe that it is an allergic reaction. When a person is allergic to pollen, dust, etc., his whole system is affected, but for some reason just one part of the body reacts as a kind of "shock organ." Thus, the nose is the shock organ in the person suffering from hay fever. In the case of erythema multiforme, the mouth and skin are the shock organs, repeatedly reacting to some outside stimulus.

TREATMENT
No specific treatment is available for erythema multiforme. However, the disease usually runs its course in ten to twenty days. Mild mouthwashes, penicillin, sulfa drugs, and vitamin B complex have been used to reduce pain and make the patient more comfortable.

erythroblastosis — a condition brought about by an incompatability of Rh factors. The condition can cause severe anemia and a failing heart. The condition affects the newborn child but not the mother.
See Rh factor.

erythrocyte — red blood cell.
See blood.

erythromycin — an antibiotic drug with many of the same properties as penicillin. It is often used in diseases caused by bacteria that have developed a resistance to penicillin.

esophagus — a muscular tube about ten inches long that acts as the passageway between the pharynx and the stomach. By means of waves of muscular contractions called peristalsis, food is pushed along this tube to the stomach. When peristalsis is reversed, vomiting occurs.

essential hypertension — an elevated blood pressure not caused by kidney or other evident disease. Sometimes called primary hypertension, it is

commonly known as high blood pressure.
See blood pressure.

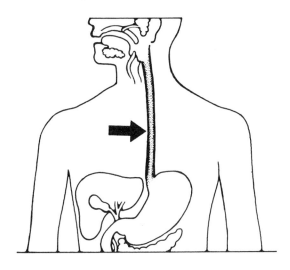

ESOPHAGUS

estrogens — female sex hormones. Estrogens have special importance at puberty, because they are responsible for the development of secondary sex characteristics—such as the growth of the breast. Estrogens also stimulate the growth of the lining of the uterus.

Any hormone that affects the monthly cycle of changes taking place in the female genital tract is considered to be an estrogen.

ether — a colorless liquid with a strong odor that is used as an anesthetic. Ether, discovered before 1795, was first demonstrated on a human in 1846.

Although ether is still one of the most potent anesthetics known, its use has declined because of some of its side effects. Ether is very irritating to the respiratory system and frequently leads to vomiting.

etiology — the sum total of knowledge about the causes of a disease.

eustachian tube — the tube that connects the pharynx with the middle ear. The function of the eustachian tube is to equalize the pressure in the middle ear with the atmospheric pressure.

examination — the physical investigation of a patient by a physician. A physician uses many different tools and techniques during an examination. The purpose of an examination is to deter-mine the health of the patient. If the patient is ill, the examination becomes a diagnostic tool.

excretion — elimination of waste materials.
See excretory systems.

excretory systems — the several different systems that eliminate waste products that enter or are formed within the body.

The residue of food taken into the digestive system, mainly indigestible materials, together with secretions from various glands emptying into the intestines, is gathered in the lower portion of the large intestines—the rectum—and eliminated as feces.

Excess water carrying dissolved salts either in excess in the system or formed as waste products is secreted by the kidneys, collected in the bladder, and expelled as urine.

Carbon dioxide and certain volatile products carried by the blood are exchanged in the lungs for oxygen and pass from the body in exhaled air.

The skin contains many small organs known as sweat glands. They range in number from 400 to 2,800 per square inch, according to position, over the body surface. These glands play an important part in eliminating body heat, excess fluid, and dissolved waste products from the body.

Life and health depend on the body throwing off waste products; interference with or lessening of normal functioning of any of the excretory systems results in illness and may even cause death.

exocrine glands — glands that have ducts and that deliver their secretions to a specific location.

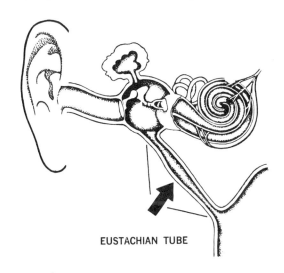

EUSTACHIAN TUBE

expectorant — a term applied to any drug that promotes productive coughing—that is, which helps the patient to cough up mucus or whatever is causing the trouble. Expectorants work by loosening the mucus so that it will move when the patient coughs; they do not cause the patient to cough.

extracorporeal circulation — the circulation of the blood outside the body as by a mechanical pump-oxygenator. This is often done while surgery is being performed inside the heart.

extrasystole — a contraction of the heart that occurs prematurely and interrupts the normal rhythm. *See blood pressure.*

extremites — the arms and legs. The arms are the upper extremities; the legs are the lower extremities.

Each upper extremity consists of thirty-two bones. The collarbone (a long bone, the inner end of which is fastened to the breastbone and the outer end to the shoulder blade at the shoulder joint) lies just in front of and above the first rib. The shoulder blade (a flat, triangular bone) lies at the upper and outer part of the back of the chest and forms part of the shoulder joint. The arm bone extends from the shoulder to the elbow and the two bones of the forearm extend from the elbow to the wrist. There are eight bones of the wrist that form the heel of the hand, five bones in the palm of the hand, and fourteen bones of the fingers (two in the thumb and three in each finger).

Each side of the lower extremities consists of thirty bones. The thighbone, the longest and strongest bone in the body, extends from the hip joint to the knee; its upper end is rounded to fit into the socket in the pelvis and the lower end broadens out to help form the knee joint. The kneecap, a flat, triangular bone, is in front of the knee joint. Two bones in the leg extend from the knee joint to the ankle. There are seven bones of the ankle or back part of the foot, five long bones of the front part of the foot, and fourteen bones of the toes.

The majority of fractures and dislocations occur to the bones of the extremities.

eye — the organ of sight, a specialized organ for the reception of light. It is assisted in its function by accessory structures such as the ocular muscles,

eyelids, conjunctiva, and lacrimal apparatus.

The eye is a hollow ball or globe that contains various structures that perform specific functions. The bulb of the eye, or eyeball, is composed of three layers of tissue:

1. The sclera is the protective outer layer—the white part of the eye. In the front of the eye, the sclera is transparent and known as the cornea. The exposed part of the eye is covered with a mucous membrane—the conjunctiva—which is a continuation of the inner lining of the eyelids.

2. The choroid is the middle, vascular layer of the eyeball. The iris, containing radiating and circular muscles, which reflexly make the pupil larger or smaller, is the colored portion of the choroid just behind the cornea. The opening in the iris is called the pupil.

3. The retina is the inner coat of the eye. It contains the light receptors (rods and cones). The site of the exit of the optic nerve, which lacks rods and cones, is called the "blind spot."

The portion of the optic globe in front of the lens is divided into an anterior chamber and a posterior chamber, separated by the iris. These chambers contain a watery solution called aqueous humor. The cavity of the optic globe behind the lens is filled with a jelly-like substance called the vitreous body, which helps maintain the shape of the eyeball.

The crystalline lens, enclosed in its capsule, is situated immediately behind the iris and in front of the vitreous body. It is held in place and its thickness regulated by the ciliary structures, a component part of which are the ciliary muscles.

A ray of light enters the eye through the cornea. It then passes through the aqueous humor, the pupil, the crystalline lens, and the vitreous humor, until it comes to the retina, where it is absorbed. As the ray of light moves through the eye on the way to the retina, it is bent or refracted so that a clear image or impression focuses on the retina. The important part of the refraction process takes place in the crystalline lens.

The eyelids provide mechanical protection for the eyeball, and by frequent closing, or blinking, distribute the secretions of the lacrimal glands over the surface of the globe. The conjunctiva, although delicate in appearance, rapidly regenerates when injured and provides protection for the transparent cornea. The muscles controlling the movement of the eyeball provide for focusing of both eyes on one spot at the same time, whether

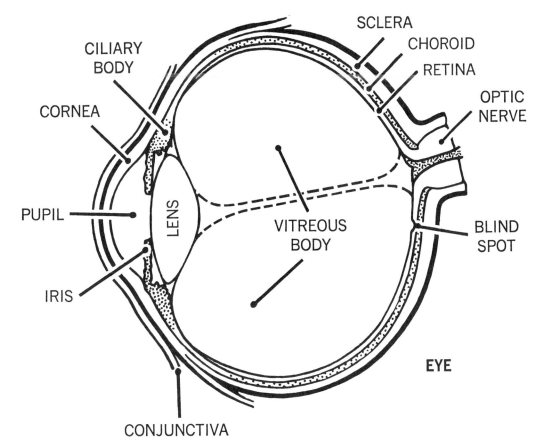

EYE

- CILIARY BODY
- SCLERA
- CHOROID
- RETINA
- CORNEA
- OPTIC NERVE
- PUPIL
- LENS
- VITREOUS BODY
- BLIND SPOT
- IRIS
- CONJUNCTIVA

distant or close. If it were not for the fine adjustment provided by these muscles, each eye would focus on a different spot, resulting in a dual or blurred image beng perceived by the brain.

The ability to see objects clearly at different distances is accomplished by reflex or automatic changing of the thickness of the lens and of the diameter of the pupil to bring an object into focus. This process of change is called accommodation.

The eye is like a camera: the pupil in front allows entrance of light, the lens behind the opening focuses the rays of light; and the retina in the back of the eyeball receives the image. The nerve endings for the sense of sight are tiny rods and cones standing on end, side by side, in the retina. They are so sensitive and so close together that points on the retinal image can be seen as separate points when they are less than four ten-thousandths of an inch (0.01 millimeters) apart. By a complex chemical reaction, these small organs act like the film in a camera, recording the picture for the brain. The optic nerve conveys the impulses from the retina to the visual area of the brain, where the visual image is consciously perceived.

eye drops — liquids instilled in the eyes. There are several different types of eye drops, and they are used for different purposes.

The eye drops an ophthalmologist puts (instills) into the eye to enlarge or dilate the pupil are medically a mydriatic. These drops relax the muscle that controls the lens shape and allow the doctor to distinguish farsightedness, etc. In this way, use of drops reveals faulty eyesight not detected under normal conditions.

The opposite effect on the iris is caused by miotics, which make the pupil tiny.

Several kinds of eye drops are prescribed by ophthalmologists as one of the treatments of glaucoma. Such drops may lower the damaging high internal eye pressure of glaucoma and must be prescribed individually for each patient.

Still other eye drops are used to anesthetize the eye briefly to make the tonometer test for glaucoma painless.

Antiseptic drops are prescribed for infections and, at times, to lessen the danger of a well eye becoming infected from a sick eye.

Plain tap water should be used to flood the eye as first aid treatment if anything splashes into the eye. Anything stronger should be prescribed by a doctor.

eyeground — the inside of the back part of the eye seen by looking through the pupil. Examining the eyeground is one means of assessing changes in the blood vessels. The eyeground is also called the fundus of the eye.

eyestrain — fatigue of the eyes, which frequently follows straining the eyes or the eye muscles.

f

F. — abbreviation for Fahrenheit, one of the systems for measuring temperature. In medicine, Fahrenheit is the preferred system.

Fabricius ab Aquapendente, Hieronymus — an Italian anatomist (1560-1634) and a teacher of William Harvey at Padua. He studied the valves of the veins. Harvey is reported to have credited the work of Fabricius with leading to his own concept of the circulation of the blood.

fainting — a temporary loss of consciousness caused by an inadequate supply of blood to the brain. Fainting is a mild form of physical shock. It may be caused by an injury, the sight of blood, exhaustion, weakness, lack of air, and emotional shocks such as fright. Some persons faint much more readily than others.

The patient feels weak and becomes dizzy, black spots appear before his eyes, his face becomes pale and his lips blue, and his forehead is covered with perspiration. He then sinks back in his seat or falls to the ground unconscious. The pulse is rapid and weak, and the breathing is shallow. The above symptoms usually occur in a few seconds.

Fainting is one of the more frequent occurrences that require first aid. A patient lying down seldom faints; therefore, in first aid it is always best to have the patient in the lying position. An injured person being examined in a sitting or standing position may faint suddenly and fall, either aggravating his original injuries or causing additional ones. Where early symptoms of fainting are noted, unconsciousness may be prevented by lowering the patient's head immediately. If a person is sitting, bend the body at the waist and bring the head down between the knees. Better still, if space is available, lay the person down with the head low.

fallopian tubes — two very small tubes curving away from the two upper corners of the uterus. They lead into the abdominal cavity, one to the right and one to the left. At the outer end, each spreads out in an umbrella-like formation close to a small almond-sized organ called an ovary. Conception actually takes place in a fallopian tube when a male sex cell (spermatozoa) fertilizes an ovum on its way down the tube to the uterus.

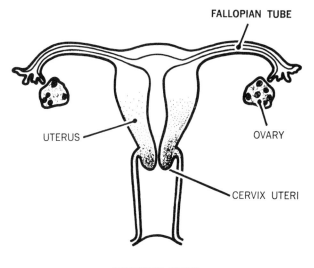

FALLOPIAN TUBE

UTERUS

OVARY

CERVIX UTERI

FALLOPIAN TUBES

Fallot, Etienne Louis Arthur — French physician (1850-1911) who gave an important description of a congenital heart defect known as tetralogy of Fallot.

See congenital heart defect, tetralogy of Fallot.

false labor — early contractions over a period of several hours or even days during pregnancy. The contractions are chiefly in the abdomen. They do not change much in intensity, but they come and go quite irregularly.

See labor.

farsightedness — difficulty in close vision. Distant vision is usually good, but the lens adjusts poorly for near objects.

See hyperopia.

fat — a concentrated source of energy. Weight for weight, fats give more than twice as much energy, or calories, as either carbohydrates or protein. Primarily, fats supply energy, but they also carry the fat-soluble vitamins A, D, E, and K and help the body use them.

Fats also make up part of the structure of cells. They form a protective cushion around vital organs. Additionally, fats spare protein for its special jobs in the body.

Certain fats supply an essential fatty acid called linoleic acid. This acid is found in valuable amounts in many oils that come from plants — particularly corn, cottonseed, safflower, sesame, soybean, and wheat germ. These are referred to as polyunsaturated fats or oils. Margarines, salad dressings, mayonnaise, and cooking oils are usually made from one or more of these oils. Nuts contain less linoleic acid than most vegetable oils; among the nuts, walnuts rate quite high. Poultry and fish oils have more linoleic acid than other animal fats, which rank fairly low as sources.

In planning daily meals, it is important to keep the total amount of fat at a moderate level and to include some foods that contain polyunsaturated fats.

In recent years studies have indicated that the incidence of coronary heart disease is greater among men with cholesterol levels above the average range. Most medical scientists agree that the amount of cholesterol circulating in the blood can be increased or decreased by the amount and kind of fat in the diet.

TYPES

Food fats and oils contain three kinds of fatty acids: saturated, mono-unsaturated, and polyunsaturated. These fatty acids appear to affect blood cholesterol in different ways. Saturated fatty acids tend to raise the level of cholesterol in the blood; polyunsaturated fatty acids tend to lower it; and mono-unsaturated fatty acids seem to have no effect. Although a single food fat may contain varying amounts of all three kinds of fatty acids, it will usually be classified as predominantly one or another. For example, the solid animal fats are high in saturated fatty acids; most vegetable oils, as well as fish oils, are high in polunsaturated fatty acids.

Liquid vegetable oils that have been made solid by hydrogentation have lost much of their polyunsaturated fatty-acid content. However, some recently developed margarines and solid cooking fats have been specially treated to retain these cholesterol-lowering fatty acids.

fatigue — a feeling of exhaustion that follows excessive exercise or prolonged periods without rest.

fauces — the area between the mouth and the pharynx.

febrile — a term used to indicate a patient suffering from a raised temperature.

feces — solid excrement.

femoral artery — the main blood vessel supplying blood to the leg.

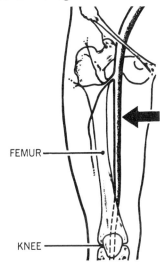

FEMUR

KNEE

FEMORAL ARTERY

femur — the thighbone. It is the longest and strongest bone in the body. The femur extends from the hip joint to the knee. Its upper end is rounded to fit into the socket in the pelvis, and the lower end broadens out to help form the knee joint.

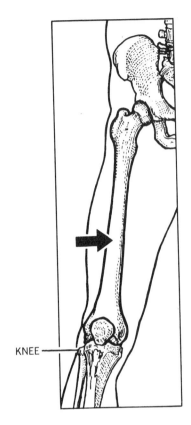

KNEE

FEMUR

fenestration — an operation to open a new window between the middle ear and the inner ear. Fenestration was performed for a condition called otosclerosis, but today an operation called a stapedectomy is more commonly used.

See otosclerosis, stapedectomy.

fertilization — the union of a spermatozoa (male sex cell) and an ovum (female sex cell).

Male sex cells enter the upper vagina in millions. These cells are much smaller than the ova and move by lashing their long, slender tails. Within ten to twenty minutes they swim through the cervix, into the uterus itself, and up through the fallopian tubes. If there is an ovum in either of the two tubes, a spermatozoa will usually succeed in entering and combining with it. This is fertilization.

The fertilized egg passes through the tube into the uterus in three to five days. At the end of about six days it sinks into a spot in the wall of the uterus. Now the fertilized egg is considered to be an embryo.

See embryo, fetus.

fetus — a term used to describe an unborn child from after the eighth week to birth.

In the third month of pregnancy, the fetus is about two and a half inches long and weighs about an ounce. The baby's fingers and toes are usually well formed by the fourth month, and tiny nails begin to show. His back is still curved like a bow, but his head is straightening up. A little hair, usually dark, is starting to grow on his scalp, and his teeth are forming deep in his gums. In both sexes, the external sex organs have now appeared. At sixteen weeks the fetus is four to five inches long and weighs about four ounces.

Sometime during the fifth month the doctor may hear the first, faint fetal heartbeat through his stethoscope. The fetus stretches his arms and legs, causing light fluttering movements. At twenty weeks the baby is about eight inches long and ten and a half ounces in weight.

By the sixth month the baby's movements are real thumps. Sometimes he lies on one side, sometimes with his head down, sometimes with it up. This movement continues until the fetus is about seven months, when he usually takes one position and keeps it until birth. Sometimes the pregnant mother may not feel him move at all. Babies have periods of waking and sleeping before they are born, just as they do afterward.

During the last two or three months of uterine life, a baby grows "tall" very fast, gets his body fat, and rounds himself out. From the sixth month on until shortly before birth, he is covered with downy fuzz. A soft, creamy substance called vernix begins to form on his body at about the seventh month.

During the eighth and ninth months he becomes more and more like the typical full-term child. The cartilages of his nose and ears develop. His nails, still paper-thin, grow beyond the tips of his fingers and toes. The bones of his skull become harder and are becoming more closely knit. The hair on his head grows longer. His eyes, like the eyes of all newborn babies, are slate-blue.

The fetus is now prepared to exist independent of the mother's body.

See embryo.

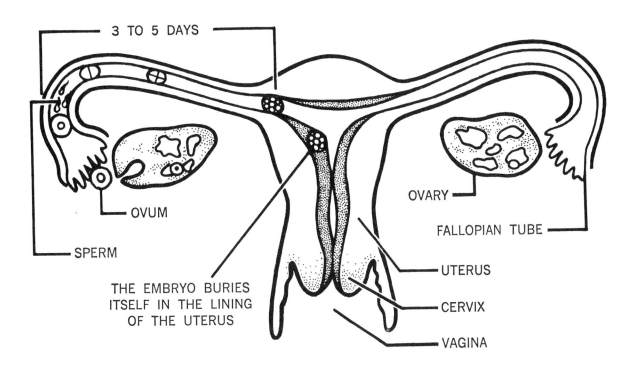

3 TO 5 DAYS

OVUM

SPERM

THE EMBRYO BURIES
ITSELF IN THE LINING
OF THE UTERUS

OVARY

FALLOPIAN TUBE

UTERUS

CERVIX

VAGINA

FERTILIZATION

fever — a raised body temperature, also called pyrexia.
See temperature, thermometer.

fever blister — *See herpes simplex.*

fever thermometer — *See thermometer.*

fibrillation — uncoordinated contractions of the heart muscle occurring when the individual muscle fibers take up independent irregular contractions. When fibrillation occurs, it is often necessary to use a defibrillator, such as electric shock, to stop the uncoordinated contractions and restore the normal heartbeat.

fibrin — an elastic protein that forms the essential portion of a blood clot.

fibrinogen — a soluble protein in the blood which, by the action of certain enzymes, is converted into the insoluble protein of a blood cot.

fibrinolysin — an enzyme that can cause coagulated blood to return to a liquid state.

fibrinolytic — an agent having the ability to dissolve a blood clot.

fibroids — benign growths of connective tissue. These are frequently found in the uterus.

fibrositis— the commonest rheumatic condition that does not affect the joints directly. The symptoms include pain, stiffness, or soreness of fibrous tissue, especially in the muscle coverings or sheaths. Attacks may follow an injury, repeated muscular strain, prolonged mental tension, or depression.
Fibrositis within the muscles is sometimes

called myositis. Lumbago is fibrositis in the lumbar region and low back.

The condition may disappear spontaneously or respond well to treatment, but some cases persist for years. However, chronic sufferers are rarely crippled. Fibrositis is not a destructive, progressive disease.

fibrous tissue — two types of connective tissue, both composed of fibrous cells. White fibrous tissue is dense and helps form tendons and ligaments. Yellow fibrous tissue is not as dense as white fibrous tissue. It is more elastic and can be found in arterial walls.

fibula — one of the two bones between the knee and the foot. The fibula is smaller than the other bone (the tibia).

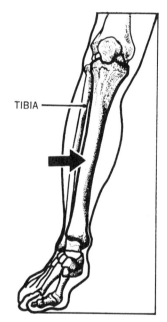

TIBIA

FIBULA

filament — a thread or a thread-like substance.

filtrate — the fluid that passes through a filter.

fingers — the five digits on each hand.

fingernails — *See nails.*

first aid — the emergency care of a person who is injured or ill. The aim of first aid is to prevent death or further injury, to relieve pain, and to counteract shock until medical aid can be obtained.

First aid is never taught to replace the physician or surgeon but only to protect the patient until medical or surgical aid can be obtained. One of the first things first-aid students learn is to send for medical aid in all cases of serious injury and even in minor injuries to be sure that the patient sees a physician as soon as possible.

First aid, rendered correctly, in many instances can restore natural breathing, usually check loss of blood, prevent or moderate shock, protect wounds and burns from infection, immobilize fractures and dislocations, lessen pain, and conserve the patient's strength; when medical aid can be obtained, the patient's chance of recovery is greatly enhanced.

The principal objects of first aid are:

1. Prevention of further injury.

2. Checking conditions known to be endangering life.

3. Protecting injuries from infections and complications.

4. Making the patient as comfortable as possible to conserve his strength.

5. Transporting the patient to medical assistance, where required, in such a manner as not to complicate the injury or subject him to any more discomfort than is absolutely necessary.

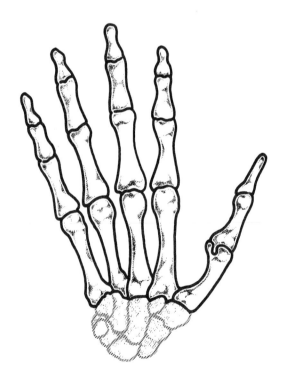

FINGERS

The imperative need for first aid in many injuries where medical aid is not immediately available makes it vital that everyone be able to give proper assistance until a doctor arrives or the injured person can be taken to a doctor.

fistula — an unnatural opening or passageway between two body organs or between a body organ and the skin. A fistula may result from infection or may be performed as a surgical procedure.

fits — *See seizures.*

flatulence — an excess of air or gas in the stomach or intestines. This causes a very uncomfortable feeling. Although flatulence can be caused by diseases and by fermentation in the intestines, it is usually the result of swallowing air. The patient feels that he can relieve the discomfort by burping, but actually all he does is swallow more air. This is a very typical cycle seen in nervous patients.

fleas — small, wingless insects that feed on the blood of animals and humans. Most species prefer one type of animal but will attack others, including man, if their normal host is not available. Most fleas—those that live on humans, dogs, and cats, for example—are important chiefly as pests that cause annoying bites. But one type, the oriental rat flea, is of particular health concern, because it is the chief transmitter of urban plague and murine typhus. These are diseases of humans as well as rodents. Because of vigorous campaigns to eliminate rats and insecticide dusting programs to control the fleas, plague very rarely occurs here, and murine typhus has been reduced to a few cases a year. Continuing watchfulness is necessary, however, since plague still exists in small, wild mammals in the western part of the United States, and murine typhus is a common disease of domestic rats in the southeastern states. Control of rat fleas is a technical operation usually done by health departments or other experts.

Fleming, Sir Alexander — Scottish bacteriologist (1881-1955) who discovered penicillin. Fleming was working on bacteria grown on a medium in a closed dish. He noticed that a mold on the medium was inhibiting the growth of the bacteria. On closer examination he discovered that the mold was actually killing the bacteria.

For his discovery, Fleming (along with Florey and Chain, who furthered his work) was awarded the Nobel Prize in medicine in 1945.

flex — bend.

fluorescent antibody test — a rapid and sensitive test for certain disease organisms and substances. Its value in the field of heart disease is that it speeds the recognition of harmful streptococci in a throat smear, so that immediate treatment might avert an attack of rheumatic fever. The test consists of "tagging" with a fluorescent dye the antibodies, i.e., substances in blood serum that have been built up against certain bacteria. This dyed antibody is then mixed with a smear taken from the throat of the patient. If streptococci are present in the smear, the glowing antibodies will attach to them, and they can be clearly seen in the microscope.

fluoride — a mineral that is important for sound tooth development and for the prevention of tooth decay. Two out of every three cavities can be prevented by drinking water containing the right amount of flouride.

Fluoride occurs naturally in many water supplies. It was noticed that this natural flouride water could prevent tooth decay, and this observation sparked investigation of the possibility of adding fluoride to water supplies not naturally endowed. Extensive studies begun by the United States Public Health Service in 1938, and confirmed by other research, led to the demonstration that when one part fluoride was added per million parts of their drinking water, children had, on the average, about sixty percent fewer decayed teeth than children living where the water did not have such a desirable fluoride content. These studies demonstrated conclusively that fluoridation is effective and safe.

Fluoridation of the drinking water is one decay preventive that does not depend on the economic means or knowledge of the parents or on the availability of dentists. Where not intended as a substitute for proper individual care of one's teeth, fluoridation of the water supply is the most-effective and least-expensive preventive dental-health measure available. Its major benefits, which may continue throughout life, are obtained by children who drink the flouridated water from birth through the years their teeth are developing.

Approximately one part of fluoride per million parts of water is the correct amount. Less than this does not provide protection against decay.

fluorine — *See fluoride.*

fluoroscope — an instrument for observing structures deep inside the body. X-rays are passed through the body onto a fluorescent screen, where the shadow of deep-lying organs can be seen.

fluoroscopy — the examination of a structure deep in the body by means of observing the fluorescence on a screen, caused by X-rays transmitted through the body.

fly — the housefly. This fly is a danger to the health of man and animals, principally because it carries and spreads disease germs that may be in the materials it breeds in, feeds on, or walks on.

This fly feeds and breeds most extensively in manure, garbage, and fermenting crop wastes. If disease germs are in these materials, or in others that they frequent, the flies get them on their hairy legs and feet and in their digestive tracts. If the flies have access to man's food, they contaminate it by walking over it and by leaving their excreta on it.

By contaminating food and water and by coming in direct contact with the hands and mouth, the flies spread typhoid, dysentery, and diarrhea. They have a part in spreading cholera, yaws, trachoma, and many other diseases. They can also transmit the eggs of various parasitic worms.

focal seizures — some types of epilepsy in which abnormal electrical discharges can be traced to one small area, or focus, in the brain, or to a number of such areas.

In one of these types, called "Jacksonian," the overactive neurons are located in the part of the brain governing movements of the muscles. A seizure generally starts in the toes of one foot or the fingers of one hand or in one corner of the mouth. Suddenly, the affected part trembles violently or just feels numb. As more and more neurons become affected, the trembling or numbness marches upward. It may stop at any time or, in a few seconds or a few minutes, cross to the other side of the body. Then the person loses consciousness and has an attack like that in grand mal.

In some persons who are not controlled well by medication, a seizure apparently can be traced to a time of great nervous tension, a sudden noise, or a bright, flickering light. However, no clear precipitating cause can usually be found.
See epilepsy.

follicle — a small sac or gland that either secretes or excretes.

fontanels — the soft, membrane-covered places between the bones on the head of a newborn baby. Portions of the skull have not hardened into bone. The incomplete areas allow for some squeezing during birth, and later for growth as the baby's brain becomes larger. A tough, elastic membrane covers the soft spots. One of these, located on the top of the skull, is large enough to be noticeable.

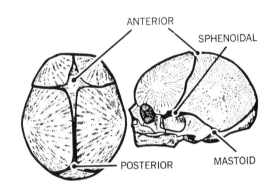

FONTANELS

food — the body's source of energy. Food is necessary to support growth, to repair constantly wearing tissues, and to supply energy for physical activity. Unless the food consumed supplies all the elements required for normal life processes, the human body cannot operate at peak efficiency for very long. If an essential nutrient is missing from the diet over very long periods of time, "deficiency diseases" such as rickets, scurvy, or certain anemias may develop.

The food choice of civilized man is influenced by many factors, such as cultural background, habit, taste preference, susceptibility to advertising, family finances, economic situation, and many others.

Supplying enough energy to support the many functions of the body at work and play is one of the chief jobs of food. This energy comes from the fats, carbohydrates, and proteins contained in foods.

Of the three, fat is the most concentrated source. It furnishes more than twice as much energy for a given weight as protein or carbohydrate does.

Food energy is measured in calories. All foods furnish calories, some much less in a given serving than others. Foods that contain appreciable amounts of water are relatively low in calories, because water, which has no caloric value, dilutes the energy-yielding nutrients in these foods. Many fresh fruits and vegetables are in this category. Calories climb, however, when sugar, fat (such as butter or margarine), or a fat-containing food like salad dressing or cream is added to them.

In cooking, fats add flavor and variety to many foods. Fats also make foods — and meals — satisfying, because fats digest slowly and delay a feeling of hunger.

Foods rich in fat, starch, or sugar—and beverages high in alcohol—are high in calories. When foods that furnish more energy or calories than are needed are eaten, the excess energy is stored in the body as fat. Continued overeating can lead to an unwanted gain in weight. If too little food is eaten to meet energy demands, the body's stored fat serves as an energy source. Weight loss results when there is a shortage of energy from food day after day. Body weight stays about the same when the energy from food matches the energy needs of the body.

See food elements, nutrition.

food allergies — allergies caused by sensitivity to one or more foods. The symptoms, which can appear shortly after the food is eaten, affect the skin, the digestive tract, or the respiratory system.

See allergy.

food elements — the different types of nutrients. The nutrients in food that are necessary for good health can be divided into certain groups — proteins, carbohydrates, fats, vitamins, minerals, and water. Most common foods consist of combinations of the above; foods that are good sources of one food element usually also contribute other essential elements. However, no one food supplies all needed nutrients in sufficient amounts. For good nutrition all essential food elements must work together. Therefore, well-balanced nutrition calls for a well-chosen variety of foods.

foot — the end of the leg. There are seven bones of the ankle or back part of the foot, five long bones of the front part of the foot, and fourteen bones of the toes.

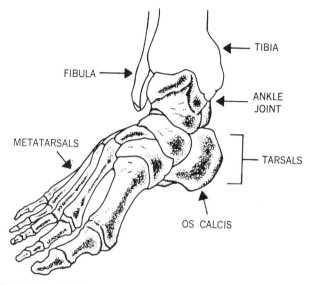

FOOT

foramen — a natural body opening or passageway.

foramen ovale — an oval hole between the left and right upper chanbers of the heart that normally closes shortly after birth. Its failure to close is one of the congenital defects of the heart, called a patent foramen ovale.

See congenital heart defects.

forearm — the part of the arm between the elbow and the wrist. The two bones of the forearm are the ulna and the radius.

formula — milk that is specially prepared so that it is suitable for feeding babies.

fracture — a break in a bone. There are two main kinds of fractures. A simple fracture is one in which the injury is entirely internal—that is, the bone is broken but there is no break in the skin. In simple fractures there is no considerable displacement of the ends of the broken bone.

A compound fracture is one in which there is an open wound in the soft tissues and the skin. Sometimes the open wound is made when a sharp end of the broken bone pushes out through the tissues and skin; sometimes it is made by an object piercing the skin and tissues and breaking the bone.

Compound fractures are more serious than simple fractures. They usually involve extensive damage to the tissues, and they are quite likely to become infected.

SYMPTOMS

It is not always easy to recognize a fracture. All fractures, whether simple or compound, are likely to cause severe pain and shock, but the other symptoms may vary considerably. A broken bone sometimes causes the injured part to be deformed or to assume an unnatural position; however, this is not always the case. Pain and moderate-to-severe swelling may be localized at the point of fracture, and there may be a kind of wobbly movement if the bone is broken all the way through. In fractures of the extremities, the limbs are usually shortened.

It may be difficult or impossible for the patient to move the injured part; if he is able to move it, he may feel a kind of grating sensation as the ends of the broken bone rub against each other. However, if a bone is cracked rather than broken through, the patient may be able to move the injured part without much difficulty. A compound fracture is easy to recognize if an end of the broken bone protrudes through the flesh. If the bone does not protrude, however, it is possible to see the external wound but fail to recognize the broken bone.

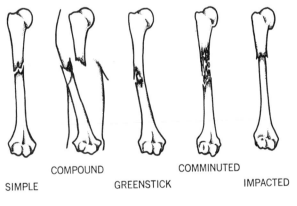

COMPOUND COMMINUTED
SIMPLE GREENSTICK IMPACTED

FRACTURE

Other types of fractures are: greenstick, comminuted, and impacted. With a greenstick fracture, the bone shaft is bent and cracked, but it is not broken through completely. In a commi-

nuted fracture, the bone is crushed, splintered, or broken into a number of fragments. The overlying skin may be either closed or open with this type of fracture. An impacted fracture occurs when one fragment of bone is forcibly driven into another piece of bone and remains more or less fixed in that position.

TREATMENT

Broken bones, especially the long bones of the arms and legs, often have sharp, sawtooth edges; even slight movement may cause the sharp edges to cut into blood vessels, nerves, or muscles, and perhaps through the skin. Therefore, by careless or improper handling, a simple fracture can be converted into a compound fracture; or, by damage to surrounding blood vessels or nerves, the injury can be made much more serious. A person handling a fracture should always bear that in mind. Damage from careless handling of a simple fracture may greatly increase pain and shock, cause complications that will prolong the period of disability, and endanger life through hemorrhage or pierced blood vessels.

First-aid care for fractures includes the following:

1. If there is any possibility that a fracture has been sustained, treat the injury as a fracture.

2. Get medical aid at the first possible opportunity. All fractures require medical treatment.

3. Do not move the patient until the injured part has been splinted, unless you must move him in order to save his life or prevent further injury.

4. Treat for shock.

5. Do not attempt to locate a fracture by grating the ends of the bone together.

6. Do not attempt to set a broken bone.

7. When a long bone in the arm or leg is fractured, the limb must be carefully straightened so that splints can be applied. Never attempt to straighten the limb by applying traction with any improvised windlass or other device. Pulling gently with your hands in the long axis of the limb is permissible and may be all that is necessary to get the limb back into position. If protruding bone ends are covered with dirt or other foreign matter which can be easily wiped off, they should be very gently cleaned with sterile cloth before the limb is straightened.

8. Apply splints.

9. If the fracture is compound, the wound and any bleeding must be attended to before dealing with the fracture.

10. Never attempt to force the end of the bone back into the wound.

freckle — a brown or dark pigmented spot on the skin. Freckles can be caused or increased by exposure to sunlight.

freezing injuries — *See frostbite.*

Freud, Sigmund — Viennese physician (1856-1939), considered by many people as the father of modern psychiatry. Freud was the first to describe the three levels of the mind—the ego, the id, and the libido. He was also responsible for developing psychoanalysis—treatment by free association.

Though some psychiatrists reject parts of his work, there is still a school of psychology based on his theories.

Friedman's test — a test for pregnancy that involves injecting the woman's urine into a rabbit.

frigidity — the inability to have or lack of desire for sexual intercourse. The term is usually applied to the female. Frigidity may be caused by a physical problem, but more often it results from an emotional problem.

frontal — of or pertaining to the forehead.

frostbite — the damage done to skin and tissues caused by exposure to severe cold. The nose, cheeks, ears, toes, and fingers are the parts most frequently frostbitten.

Frostbite is more likely to occur when a high wind is blowing, because the wind takes heat from the body rapidly.

At first the symptoms are burning, stinging, and then numbness. However, the victim may not be aware of frostbite of the cheeks, ears, or nose until someone tells him, or of frostbite of hands or feet until he removes his gloves or shoes.

Ice crystals in the skin cause a gray or white waxy color, but the skin will move over bony ridges. When the part is completely frozen, there are ice crystals in the entire thickness of the extremity, indicated by a pale, yellow, waxy color. The skin will not move over bony ridges. When the frozen part is thawed, it becomes red and swollen, and large blisters develop.

Frostbite may also be caused by contact with certain chemicals that have a rapid freezing action, such as liquid oxygen, carbon dioxide, and Freon. Although injuries caused by contact with these substances are often referred to as chemical "burns," the body tissue is actually frozen rather than burned. Cold injuries caused by contact with chemicals tend to be superficial and, as a rule, not very serious, unless the chemical comes in contact with the eyes. If the eye tissues are frozen, permanent impairment of vision may result.

TREATMENT

Do not rub the frostbitten part. Do not expose the part to high temperatures immediately. Until the patient can be brought indoors, the frozen part should be covered with woolen cloth or clothing, and the patient himself should be made warm with extra clothing or blankets. As soon as possible, the patient should be brought into a warm room.

The frozen part should be handled with great care in order to avoid injury to it. If it is still cold and numb, it should be rewarmed as rapidly as possible by immersing it momentarily in lukewarm, but not hot, water or by gently wrapping it in warm blankets. Hot-water bottles or heat lamps should not be applied, nor should the frostbitten part be placed near a hot stove. Excessive heat may increase the damage.

Warming should not continue beyond the time when thawing is complete. After warming, the affected area should be carefully dried. If possible, the frostbitten area should be slightly elevated. Blisters should not be disturbed.

All frostbites of the second and third degree should have medical care as promptly as possible.

fructose — a simple sugar that resembles glucose.

fundus of the eye — the inside of the back part of the eye, seen by looking through the pupil. Examining the fundus of the eye is used as a means of assessing changes in the blood vessels. The fundus of the eye is also called the eyeground.

fusion — an artificial union or joint performed surgically.

g

galactosemia — an inherited disorder caused by a missing enzyme. This enzyme is necessary for the digestion of milk or lactose to convert galactose into the useful glucose of the blood. This rare disorder, if untreated, may cause vomiting, diarrhea, and jaundice in the newborn, cataracts as early as three weeks, severe retardation, and probably early death.

A strict diet for the baby without milk, lactose, or glucose often makes normal health and mentality possible. However, for best results, tests should be performed to locate either mothers or fathers who are carriers, so that the galactose-free diet can be started in pregnancy and continued in the infant after birth.

Galen (Claudius Galenus) — renowned Greek physician (ca. 130-200 A.D.), whose theory that life and health depended on the balance of four "humors" in the body dominated medical practice for 1500 years. His concept of the ebb and flow of the blood that transported the humors to various parts of the body was not refuted until William Harvey's discovery of the circulation of the blood in 1628.

Much of his importance in the field of medicine is the result of his work in anatomy. Though he could not study the anatomy of humans (that was forbidden in his time), he did do extensive studies of other animals.

gallbladder — a little sac or pouch underneath the liver, in the upper right part of the abdomen. The gallbladder, as part of the digestive system, is used as a temporary storehouse for the bile. Its

duct, the cystic duct, joins the hepatic duct from the liver to form the common bile duct, which enters the duodenum.

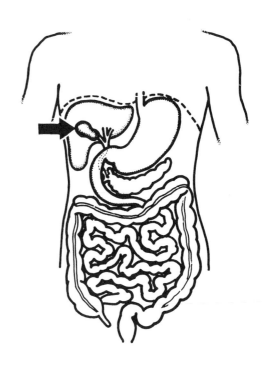

GALL BLADDER

gallop rhythm — an extra, clearly heard heart sound that, when the heart rate is fast, resembles a horse's gallop. It may or may not be significant.

gallstones — lumps of solid material that sometimes form in the gallbladder or in the ducts leading to or from it. These stones are composed of a fat-like substance, bile pigment, and lime salts.

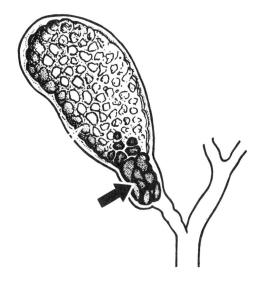

GALLSTONES

Gallstones occur more frequently in persons over forty years of age than in younger individuals and are more common in women than in men. It is generally believed that gallstones form as a result of infection, stagnation of the bile, or changes in the chemical composition of the bile. Overeating and poor eating habits contribute to the formation of gallstones.

Gallstones may occur singly or in the hundreds. They may be fairly large or so small as to be invisible to the naked eye. A single gallstone is usually rounded or egg-shaped. If there are several gallstones together, their sides are often flattened by pressure against their neighbors, so that the stones assume many-sided shapes.

SYMPTOMS

The stones may lie quietly in the bile ducts or in the gallbladder and cause little or no trouble. In fact, their owner may be unaware that he is harboring a miniature stone quarry. On the other hand, he may have a sense of fullness and pressure in the pit of his stomach after eating. He may notice a stitch in the side, a feeling of faintness, nausea, or chilliness. He may have attacks of indigestion.

If a large stone starts to move, its possessor will know that something is radically wrong. The movement of the stone may cause an attack of severe pain. One may suddenly feel a stabbing pain in the upper right portion of the abdomen. The pain may spread out—it may be felt on both sides, in the back, throughout the abdomen, where it shifts from side to side, and it may be felt in the right shoulder. This pain is often so intense that the sufferer may be in agony. He becomes wet with perspiration; he may vomit. Often he has a chill with a high fever. The upper right quarter of his abdomen may become very tender to pressure. An attack of this kind may be over in a few minutes or it may last a week.

If a gallstone is so located as to cause obstruction to the flow of bile into the intestine, the person may become yellow (jaundiced). An individual may have only one attack, or he may have several attacks at irregular intervals. Gallstones are rarely fatal, but such complications as rupture or perforation of the gallbladder, or acute obstruction of the intestines with stones, may have fatal results.

TREATMENT

If the patient has an attack of gallbladder colic such as the one described, a physician should be called immediately.

Until the physician comes, the patient should be made as comfortable as possible. He should be put to bed and his clothing loosened or removed. The physician may recommend that, while waiting for him, heat in some form be applied to the gallbladder region. A hot-water bottle can be used for this purpose, or towels wrung out of hot water can be applied to the painful area. The hot applications should be changed frequently in order to ensure their hotness, but great care should be taken that neither towels nor hot-water bottles are so hot that they burn. Heat should not be applied unless a physician orders it.

In some cases, a change of diet and proper exercise may be the only treatment necessary; in others, an operation may be required. An attack of gallbladder colic is a warning to the patient to change his living habits. He should not overeat or overindulge in rich foods such as pies, cakes, or fried foods. The physician may advise him to cut down on eggs and fats in his daily diet. Plenty of water and outdoor exercise are recommended. As the person with gallbladder disease is likely to be over forty years of age, the exercise he takes should not be too strenuous. Walking, gardening, and golf are especially suitable.

gamete — a female or male reproductive or sex cell; i.e., an ovum or a sperm.

gamma globulin — a type of protein in the blood that aids the body in resisting diseases. Gamma globulin forms the antibodies that help to fight specific diseases.

An intramuscular injection of gamma globulin containing the proper antibodies gives passive or temporary immunity to measles and infectious hepatitis. In the case of measles, gamma globulin will lighten the effects of the disease even if it is given too late to prevent it.

ganglion — a mass of nerve cells that serves as a center of nervous influence.

ganglionic blocking agent — a drug that blocks the transmission of a nerve impulse at the nerve centers (ganglia). Some of these drugs, such as hexamethonium and mecamylamine hydrochloride, may be used in the treatment of high blood pressure.

gangrene — the rotting or decay of body tissue. Gangrene is caused by a loss of blood flow followed by bacterial infection.

Gas gangrene is a more serious form of gangrene, in which the bacteria move from damaged tissue to healthy tissue. In this form of gangrene the bacteria produce a noxious gas as well as poisons.

Gangrene, including gas gangrene, always requires immediate medical attention—usually surgical—to remove the destroyed tissue and prevent further tissue decomposition. Because the bacteria that cause gas gangrene are anaerobic (i.e., they can live only in an oxygen-free atmosphere), the patient is often placed in a high-oxygen atmosphere.

gargoylism — a form of dwarfism with heavy facial features, damaged vision, and mental retardation. Gargoylism appears in infants who apparently inherit an abnormal carbohydrate or fat metabolism. No treatment has been successful as yet. Gargoylism is also known as Hurler's disease.

gas gangrene — *See gangrene.*

gasoline intoxication — inhalation of gasoline fumes. This causes a kind of intoxication similar to that produced by alcohol. The first stage of gasoline intoxication produces a false sense of well-being and security. The patient's movements become unsteady and uncoordinated, and his ability to think is impaired. Injury other than poisoning must be guarded against at this point—the patient is very likely to fall, or he may want to light a cigarette, not realizing that he is a highly inflammable object.

Later stages of gasoline intoxication result in unconsciousness and a serious depression of breathing, which may be followed by death from asphyxiation.

Treatment should include removing the patient to a well-ventilated place, giving oxygen or an oxygen-carbon dioxide mixture, and giving artificial respiration if the patient has stopped breathing.

Gasoline vapor is heavier than air and tends to flow downward. It is highly explosive and flammable when mixed with air.

gas poisoning — poisoning by noxious or toxic gases. Toxic gases cause asphyxia, or cessation of breathing. Although the occurrence of these gases and their physiological effects on the human system vary greatly, many lives have been saved by prompt and efficient use of artificial respiration.

These gases include carbon dioxide, sulfur dioxide, oxides of nitrogen, ammonia, hydrogen sulfide, carbon monoxide, hydrogen cyanide gas, and cyanogen compounds.

The first steps in treating poisoning by noxious or toxic gases are: remove the patient to fresh air as quickly as possible; apply artificial respiration if the patient has stopped breathing.

Inhalations of oxygen, when administered immediately, will greatly reduce the severity of the poisoning, as well as decrease the possibility of serious aftereffects.

See artificial respiration, carbon-monoxide poisoning.

gastrectomy — the surgical removal of all or a portion of the stomach.

gastric ulcer — *See peptic ulcer.*

gastritis — a general term used to indicate an inflammation of the stomach.

gastroenteritis — a term used to indicate an inflammation of the stomach and the intestines.

Gaucher's disease — a family disease, particularly found in Jewish families. The onset of Gaucher's disease occurs in infancy and consists of listlessness, bronze spots in the skin, retardation, and eventual paralysis. No specific treatment is yet available. The disease is also known as familial splenic anemia.

gene — the biologic unit of heredity that is located in the chromosomes.
   See genetics.

general anesthesia — *See anesthesia, anesthetics.*

genetics — the study of heredity. The hereditary factors (genes) are contained in the chromosomes. In man, there are forty-six chromosomes—twenty-two pairs and two sex chromosomes. In the case of a female, there are actually twenty-three pairs, because the sex chromosomes of the female are a pair of X's. The sex chromosomes of a male are an X and a Y. A child receives twenty-three chromosomes from each parent.

The chromosomes are tightly coiled, double strands of molecules of DNA (deoxyribonucleic acid). These strands carry the genetic orders that make each person different.

DOMINANT AND RECESSIVE CHARACTERISTICS
Because an individual's genetic makeup is based on the genetic makeup of his parents, he inherits certain traits and characteristics. Sometimes, however, two brown-eyed parents will produce a child with blue eyes. This can only happen when both parents have contributed a blue-eye gene, because blue eyes are a recessive characteristic. Recessive characteristics are characteristics that appear only when the individual receives the recessive gene from both parents. A person with one blue- and one brown-eye gene will always have brown eyes, because brown eyes are a dominant characteristic. Dominant characteristics always take precedence over recessive characteristics and consequently require that only one of the two genes be present in order for the characteristic to appear.

Dominant characteristics include brown eyes,

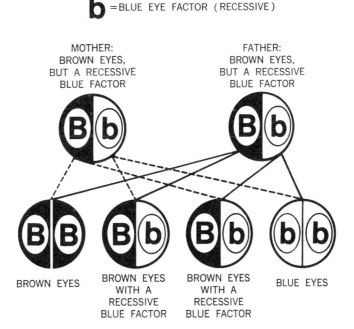

B = BROWN EYE FACTOR (DOMINANT)

b = BLUE EYE FACTOR (RECESSIVE)

MOTHER:
BROWN EYES,
BUT A RECESSIVE
BLUE FACTOR

FATHER:
BROWN EYES,
BUT A RECESSIVE
BLUE FACTOR

BROWN EYES

BROWN EYES
WITH A
RECESSIVE
BLUE FACTOR

BROWN EYES
WITH A
RECESSIVE
BLUE FACTOR

BLUE EYES

**DOMINANT & RECESSIVE CHARACTERISTICS
(EYE COLOR)**

curly hair, dark skin, and normal intellect. Recessive characteristics include blue eyes, straight hair, light skin, and feeble-mindedness.

SEX-LINKED CHARACTERISTICS

The sex of a child is determined by the sex gene. Even though both sexes have two sex genes, they only transmit one each to a child. A fertilized ovum thus has two sex genes—one from each parent. A female has two X sex genes; therefore, she can only transmit an X gene. However, a male has both an X sex gene and a Y sex gene. He

can transmit either the X gene or the Y gene. If the father transmits an X gene, the child will have two X genes (one from the mother and one from the father) and will be a female. If the male transmits a Y gene, the child will have an X gene (from the mother) and a Y gene (from the father) and will be a male.

In addition to determining the sex of the child, the sex genes determine certain other characteristics. These are called sex-linked characteristics because they are linked to or carried on the X sex gene. Only the X gene carries the characteristic; the Y gene plays no role in determining the presence or absence of these characteristics. It is a neutral factor.

A good example of these sex-linked characteristics is color blindness. With very few exceptions, color blindness occurs only in males. Like the other sex-linked characteristics, color blindness is recessive—but only in females. This is because a female can inherit a color-blindness-carrying X gene from one parent and a normal X gene (which will dominate it) from the other parent. The male who inherits a color-blindness-carrying X gene from his mother receives only a neutral Y gene (which has no effect) from his father.

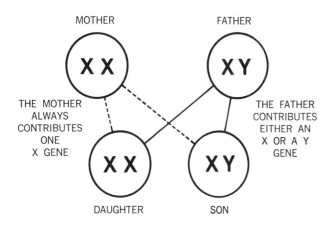

SEX DETERMINATION

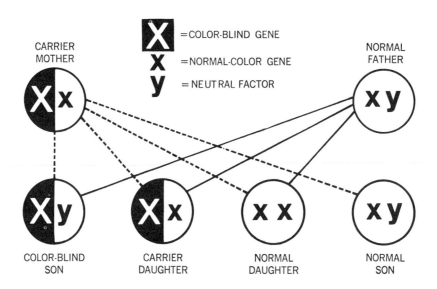

SEX-LINKED CHARACTERISTICS
(COLOR BLINDNESS)

A male who is color-blind passes on the characteristic to any female children he has. They inherit his X gene, which is the carrier gene. However, his female children are not color-blind, because the normal X gene from the mother will dominate the X carrier gene from the father. Instead they become carriers. Any male children these females have will have an even chance of being color-blind. They have an even chance of inheriting her X carrier gene or her normal X gene. Depending on which of these two genes they inherit, they will or will not be color-blind.

A male child whose father is color-blind is neither color-blind nor a carrier. He inherits the neutral Y from his father. The only way he can be color-blind is if his mother (from whom he inherits an X) is a carrier.

Other examples of sex-linked characteristics are hemophilia, some forms of nearsightedness, and some types of baldness.
See hemophilia.

genital organs — the sex organs; the organs of reproduction.

genitourinary system — the genital and urinary system.

geriatrics — the study of and the care of the aging.
See aging.

germ — a microscopic disease-causing organism.

German measles — one of the diseases usually contracted in childhood. German measles is a mild disease that is usually accompanied by a mild fever, sore throat, and cold symptoms. The patient breaks out in a rose-colored rash. Enlarged glands at the back of the neck and behind the ears are common. The incubation period is from two to three weeks (usually about eighteen days). The patient is contagious until the rash fades, which is usually about five days. German measles is not a serious disease, and complications are rare. Treatment is usually limited to bed rest if the fever is high.

If German measles is contracted in the early months of pregnancy, it may harm the unborn baby. Complications of this sort include deafness, cataracts, and mental retardation.

A vaccine has been developed to prevent German measles.

German measles is also known as rubella.

germicides — *See antiseptics, disinfectants.*

gestation — pregnancy. In humans this lasts approximately 266 days from conception to delivery.

gingivitis — inflammation of the gums.

gland — a body organ that excretes or secretes; also a body organ that traps germs. There are three types of glands. Exocrine glands, such as the sweat glands and the liver, are glands with ducts leading into localized areas, where the secretion or excretion is released. Endocrine glands, such as the thyroid and adrenal glands, are ductless glands, which release their secretions directly into the blood and which affect the entire body. The third type of gland is the lymph gland. These glands are part of the body's defense against disease.
See endocrine gland, exocrine gland, lymph gland.

glandular fever — *See infectious mononucleosis.*

glaucoma — a disease in which increased eye pressure crushes the nerves of sight. Prolonged high eye pressure can kill many nerve fibers in the eyes. Once destroyed, these nerve fibers are never usualbe again. The increased eye pressure, called increased intraocular pressure, strangles the optic (eye) nerve and the blood vessels that nourish it. A block in normal eye drainage is the usual cause of such increased pressure.

An estimated million Americans over thirty-five years of age have glaucoma without knowing it. Every year about four thousand more people in the United States go blind from glaucoma, which could have been controlled by early discovery and faithful treatment.

Glaucoma ranks second only to cataract as a cause of blindness in the United States and accounts for fourteen or fifteen percent of the blind. About one blind person in seven is needlessly blind from glaucoma.

SYMPTOMS
A person can read a wall chart with 20/20 central vision and still be blind around the edges of his eye field. He can have glaucoma for months or years before he notices any change. By the time glaucoma causes difficulties noticeable to the individual, vision loss has begun.

In acute glaucoma, the eyeballs turn stony-hard without warning. This causes one of the most agonizing pains known to man.

No one symptom that is noticeable indicates the presence of glaucoma. However, several are a warning for an immediate tonometer test. These include vague and changeable headache or eye aches, perhaps after seeing movies or TV in the dark; any fuzzy or blurred vision that comes and goes; watering or discharge of the eye; poor vision in dim light; any change in eye color; seeing rainbow halos around lights; and any loss of side vision (which will grow worse and cannot be restored).

Another warning for a checkup with a tonometer is family history of glaucoma. Relatives of those with glaucoma have this eye ailment five or six times as often as persons without glaucoma in the family.

Glaucoma is not cataract, is not contagious, is not cancer, and not caused by high blood pressure. However, among people over thirty-five, those with high blood pressure, heart ailments, or diabetes have glaucoma more than others. Glaucoma occasionally affects children and younger adults.

Glaucoma is more truly a symptom than a disease. The basic symptom is the increased eye pressure, which crushes the eye nerve. Some investigators believe glaucoma could be a general body disease of which the eye symptoms are the only ones yet discovered. Research may eventually tell whether this is true.

TESTS

One exception to the necessity for measuring eye pressure with a tonometer is recognized. A person having the excruciating pain of acute glaucoma does not need a tonometer reading. The immediate need for surgery to relieve such a stony-hard eye is obvious.

With this exception, all other persons must have a reading with a tonometer to determine their eye pressure (intraocular pressure or IOP or intraocular tension). The old method of pressing lightly on the closed eyelids revealed a difference in pressure if only one eye had glaucoma, or hardness in both eyeballs in advanced glaucoma. This finger-pressure test does not detect early glaucoma and could be compared to estimating fever by laying your hands on the sick person instead of using a thermometer.

In 1881, a Norwegian physician, Hjalmar Schiotz, invented an eye tonometer to measure eye pressure. Today the Schiotz tonometer is the most widely used instrument for early detection of glaucoma.

When a physician performs this painless, five-minute test, he first drops a local anesthetic in each of the eyes. The patient then sits in a chair, with his head tipped back, or he lies down. The physician carefully places the tonometer on each of the eyeballs in turn, because the pressure often differs in right and left eyes.

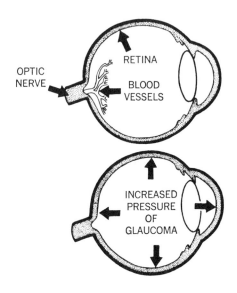

GLAUCOMA

A movable weight weighing less than one-fifth of an ounce (or about the weight of two dimes) indents the eyeball slightly. A little pointer moves along a scale to give the physician the reading of the eye pressure. The pressure is recorded as millimeters of mercury, and this record over the months and years becomes the guide to treatment to prevent blindness.

In doubtful cases of glaucoma, the eye doctor has the patient drink a quart of water in a short time, then remeasures the pressure to see whether the eyes can handle extra liquids without dangerous increase in eye pressure.

Another device for measuring pressure, the applanation tonometer, has certain advantages. The painless applanation-tonometer test also requires a drop of local anesthetic and a few minutes' time. In extremely nearsighted persons and other special cases, applanation tonometry may be more reliable than Schiotz tonometry.

Another test for glaucoma is tonography. An electric tonometer connected with a recording device is placed on the eye for perhaps four minutes. Instead of the single reading with a tonometer, a continuous reading is made that helps to measure the ease of outflow of the liquid (aqueous humor) that is causing the increased eye pressure. This outflow record assists in diagnosis of doubtful cases of glaucoma and helps the eye specialist watch cases under treatment. Information on a decrease in ease of outflow could warn of the need for glaucoma surgery to save eyesight.

TREATMENT

There are two basic methods of treating glaucoma. The first is surgery. For acute glaucoma this must be performed promptly, at least within a day or two, to prevent blindness from strangled eye nerves. The other treatment is for chronic glaucoma and involves the use of special eye drops several times a day, perhaps combined with a medicine taken by mouth.

Careless treatment of chronic glaucoma may necessitate an operation. Even people who are always faithful with their medical care of chronic glaucoma may need glaucoma surgery.

The doctor plans and directs the treatment, which usually includes one or more of these common goals:

1. Unblock with special eye drops the drainage system of the eye which dams back the outflow of eye fluid.

2. Decrease with medicine by mouth or eye drops the inflow of fluid into the eye.

3. If the drainage system cannot be unblocked, consider a new drainage outlet with surgery.

The task of controlling glaucoma usually requires several trips to the ophthalmologist, until the eye pressure comes down and stays down; then regular checkups with a tonometer and medical advice for the rest of the patient's life.

globulin — a class of proteins found in the human body.
   See gamma globulin.

glossa — the tongue.

glossitis — an inflammation of the tongue.

glottis — the part of the larynx that consists of the vocal cords.

glucose — a simple sugar. The process of digestion converts sugars and starches to glucose.

goiter — a disfiguring swelling of the thyroid gland at the front of the neck. It is usually caused by lack of iodine in the diet, but in some areas of the world goiter also may be caused by certain agents in the food. The number of cases in the United States and in many other countries has been greatly reduced in recent years by adding iodine to table salt.

In mountainous areas, or in places where the soil was brought by the last glacier, the plants and water are sometimes short of iodine. People who live in the Rocky Mountain states, the Great Lakes Basin, the upper Mississippi Valley, or any other section where there is little natural iodine are particularly liable to develop goiter unless they add iodine to their diet. The amount of iodine the body needs is small—ordinary rations of iodized salts are usually ample—but that small amount is vitally important.

Many centuries ago the Greeks burned sea sponges—which have a high iodine content—and fed the ashes to goiter victims. Not until 1914, however, was the exact relationship between iodine and goiter discovered. In that year, the nature of the internal secretion formed by the thyroid, known as thyroxin, was determined by chemical analysis. This substance, vitally necessary for normal growth and development, as well as for regulating the speed of most bodily processes, was found to contain sixty-five percent iodine.

CAUSES

When the body does not get enough iodine, the thyroid gland cannot produce thyroxin, and it enlarges in an apparent effort to make up the deficiency. When small, it is often seen most easily by swallowing with the chin raised. As this enlargement continues, swelling of the neck becomes noticeable, and the goiter may grow large enough to interfere with breathing or swallowing. In spite of its importance as a preventive measure, iodine usually will not make a goiter disappear once it has formed.

Though lack of iodine is usually the cause, sometimes improper functioning of the thyroid gland or certain inflammations may result in a goiter.

TREATMENT

If goiters are treated in early years, it is often possible to make them shrink or even disappear through the use of certain thyroid-containing medicines. In older people, particularly those who have had goiters for many years, medicines are not very effective, and removal by surgery may be the wisest course.

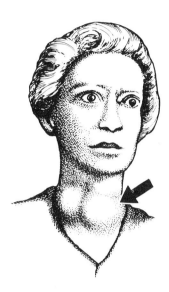

GOITER

Whenever an enlargement in the neck appears, no matter how small it may be, it should be examined by a doctor. Untreated goiters can be dangerous. Also, it is often difficult to distinguish a goiter from cancer of the thyroid. A physician can find out whether an enlargement in the neck is really a goiter, can usually determine its cause, and can decide what should be done about it.

gold — a heavy metal that is used as a drug to treat certain diseases and conditions. Gold salts have been used in the treatment of rheumatoid arthritis. The use of gold salts has provided remissions for many people suffering from this disease.

In the past, gold salts were used in the treatment of both tuberculosis and syphilis. However, new drugs have replaced gold salts for these diseases.

One of the problems associated with the use of gold as a drug is the relatively high incidence of unpleasant side effects.

gonad — a sex-cell-producing organ—an ovary or a testis.

gonadotropic — any substance that acts as a stimulant to the gonads. Certain hormones from the anterior pituitary have this effect.

gonococcus — the bacterium that causes gonorrhea.

gonorrhea — a venereal disease that may cause sterility, arthritis, blindness, and even death. Gonorrhea is a serious communicable disease. It is estimated that there are at least a million unreported cases of gonorrhea a year.

The incubation period is usually three to five days after exposure to an infected person.

SYMPTOMS

Because of severe pain, a man who is infected with gonorrhea will usually seek medical attention. The symptoms in the male are a painful, burning sensation during urination and a discharge or "tear drop" of pus from the sex organ.

The signs of gonorrhea in a woman are more difficult to detect. Women who have been infected rarely have a burning sensation during urination, and any pus discharge often goes unnoticed. Many times gonorrhea is not discovered in the woman until it has caused serious body damage. A woman with gonorrhea does not feel sick, and there is no sign of the disease until it spreads up through the uterus and into the fallopian tubes.

Because of this, a woman infected with gonorrhea can continue to have sexual intercourse and pass on the disease without realizing that she is doing so.

Gonorrhea from a mother can get into a baby's eyes, either while he is being born or afterward, causing blindness. The reason drops are put into the baby's eyes when he is born is to protect him against this possibility even when the mother is not known to have gonorrhea.

DIAGNOSIS

It is never easy to tell if a woman has gonorrhea. There is no blood test for gonorrhea, and even the laboratory test is not easy to do and takes several days.

Sometimes the germ may show at once in the "drop" from a man, because the pus is thick with germs. But in a woman, the germs may be few and far between, and so they must be grown and studied in a laboratory to decide whether they are the germs of gonorrhea.

The doctor takes a small smear of the pus from the sex parts with a cotton swab and puts it on a special dish. This dish is kept in the laboratory for a few days until the germs grow thickly enough to be found. They are then stained and examined under a microscope. At this point the doctor is able to make a definite determination of gonorrhea. Sometimes, this test is not necessary for men, because the germs grow so thickly in the man's organ that they may often be easily found and examined at once.

TREATMENT

The treatment for gonorrhea is usually by antibiotics. Because a case of gonorrhea in a woman can progress to the point of serious uterine and tubal involvement without her knowledge, surgery is sometimes necessary in the case of a woman.

MISCONCEPTIONS

There are a number of misconceptions about gonorrhea.

It is not possible to catch this disease from contact with a toilet seat, doorknob, shaking hands, etc. Gonorrhea is transmitted through sexual intercourse. It is possible to have gonorrhea any number of times. There is no immunity. Gonorrhea is not caused by straining or lifting heavy objects.

SYNONYMS

There are several slang terms for gonorrhea. Clap, strain, morning dose, a dose, and the whites are all used.

gout — an arthritic disease that usually affects the joints of the feet, especially the big toe. The disease causes inflammation and thickening of the linings of these joints. A susceptibility to it is inherited, and nearly all cases occur in men. The inherited factor is a disorder of metabolism, or body chemistry.

In diagnosing gout, a chemical test is used to detect a major effect of the altered metabolism — excessive uric acid in the blood.

Gout is sometimes referred to as the rich-man's disease, because it can be caused by excessive eating or drinking. However, gout may also follow minor injury, heavy exercise, or surgical operations. Often, attacks occur with no apparent provocation.

These attacks last days or weeks, during which the patient suffers acute joint inflammation. Between attacks he is free from symptoms. Many years after the onset, chronic arthritis may set in.

Acute gouty arthritis usually responds to colchicine given by mouth or by vein. Other drugs that physicians may prescribe are phenylbutazone and corticotropin (ACTH). In cases of chronic gout, several drugs, including probenecid and sulfinpyrazone, successfully reduce the excessive amount of uric acid in the blood and tissue. Also, these drugs can diminish the frequency of recurrent acute attacks of painful gouty arthritis, although they have no effect in reducing the inflammation and pain of these attacks. A special diet, rest in bed, and other measures may also be prescribed.

graft — a piece of skin or other body tissue that is transplanted from one area of the patient's body to another. This differs from a transplant, in which tissue from one person or patient is implanted in the body of another person or patient.

Grafts are used to replace lost tissue in cases of serious burns. The surgeon removes a tiny, paper-thin sliver of skin from a normal, healthy area and places it on the prepared burned area. Many grafts are made until there is enough grafted skin on the damaged area to begin to grow together.

The areas most frequently used to remove skin for a graft are the legs and the back of the neck.

The grafted area takes the place of the scar that would normally form. The advantage of the skin graft (aside from the cosmetic value) is that a grafted area will be more flexible than a scarred area.

grand mal — a type of epilepsy in which the patient has violent seizures.

See epilepsy.

graviditis — pregnancy.

gray matter — a slang term used to indicate the brain. The term is applicable because most of the brain belongs to the nervous system, and most nerve tissues are gray in color.

groin — the area of the body where the lowest part of the abdomen meets the thigh.

growth — the process of growing or increasing in size.

1. Human growth is greater during the last few months of prenatal life than at any other time.

During the first six months after birth a baby continues to grow rapidly — usually at the rate of two pounds per month. Between six months and a year the rate of growth is about one pound a month. The rate of growth slows to approximately one half pound per month during the second year of life.

Normal growth continues into the teen years, with the many individual differences becoming increasingly important. For example, a child may reach full height at thirteen or may keep growing until nineteen or twenty. Some children seem to grow gradually; others seem to experience growth in spurts.

While it is true that growing is going on in the body until death, it is not properly termed growth, because it is not an increase in size. Rather, it takes the form of replacing worn or damaged tissue.

2. A growth is one of the terms applied to extraneous or abnormal tissue growing in the body. A growth can be benign or it can be malignant. Benign growths do not threaten life. Malignant growths always threaten life if they are not removed. Growths are also called tumors.

See cancer.

gullet — the passageway from the mouth to the stomach. This area includes both the pharynx and the esophagus.

See esophagus, pharynx.

gum diseases — *See gingivitis, periodontal disease, pyorrhea.*

gums — the tissues and membrane surrounding the teeth.

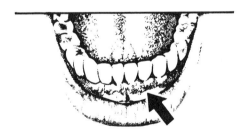

GUMS

gun-barrel vision — vision in which the field is narrow, as if the patient were looking through a tube.

The visual field is the total area perceived when the eyes are focused straight ahead. This comprises both the small area on which the eyes are focused for sharp impression (central vision) and the large area that is seen "out of the corner of the eye" (indirect or peripheral vision). In gun-barrel vision, the eye loses the ability to see "out of the corner of the eye"; that is, the eye loses the peripheral vision.

Gun-barrel vision is also called shaft vision or tunnel vision.

gustation — the sense of taste.

gynecologist — a physician whose specialty is gynecology.

gynecology — the medical specialty that treats the female reproductive tract. The field of gynecology does not include pregnancy. The medical specialty that treats pregnancy is obstetrics, but many physicians are both gynecologists and obstetricians.

gynecomastia — a condition in which there is excessive growth of the male mammary glands. This results in male breasts. The condition is usually caused by an imbalance of hormones, occurring most frequently during puberty. Normally the condition does not last very long.

gyrus — one of the convolutions of the cerebral cortex of the brain.

See cerebral cortex, convolution.

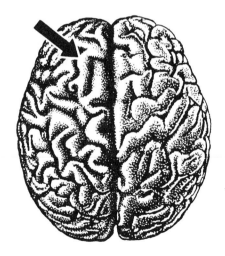

GYRUS

h

habituation — the psychological desire to repeat the use of a drug intermittently or continuously because of emotional reasons. Escape from tension, dulling of reality, and euphoria are some of the reasons drugs are used habitually.

See addiction.

hair — a thread-like substance that grows from the dermis layer of the skin. Each individual hair has a root. The shaft through which the hair grows is lubricated by secretions from the sebaceous glands, which are also located in the dermis.

Body hair has no nerves and is not supplied with blood vessels. However, the hair roots have both nerves and blood supply. This is the reason hair can be cut without pain, while pulling the hair does produce pain.

Hair color and quality (curly or straight) are inherited characteristics. Dark hair and curly hair are dominant characteristics. Light hair and straight hair are recessive characteristics.

hallucination — a change of sensation, thinking, or mental delusion that is not caused by any physical phenomenon.

hallucinogens — drugs capable of provoking changes of sensation, thinking, self-awareness and emotion. Alterations of time and space perception, illusions, hallucinations, and delusions may be either minimal or overwhelming, depending on the dose. The results of hallucinogens (also called psychedelics and psychotomimetics) are very variable—a "high" or a "bad trip" may occur in the same person on different occasions.

LSD is the most potent and best-studied hallucinogen. Besides LSD, a large number of synthetic and natural hallucinogens are known. Mescaline from the peyote cactus, psilocybin from the Mexican mushroom, morning-glory seeds, DMT, MDA, and dozens of others are known and abused.

Many drugs will cause a delirium, accompanied by hallucinations and delusions, when taken by people who are hypersensitive to them. Extraordinarily large amounts of certain drugs may also produce hallucinations. However, the mind-altering drugs are much more likely to induce hallucinations because of their direct action on the brain cells.

See LSD.

hamstring muscles — the collection of muscles at the back of either thigh.

hand — the part of the body consisting of the wrist, the palm, and the fingers. There are eight bones of the wrist that form the heel of the hand, five bones in the palm of the hand, and fourteen bones of the fingers (two in the thumb and three in each finger).

hangover — the body's reaction to an excess of alcohol. The associated symptoms of nausea, gastritis, anxiety, and headache vary by individual case, but a universal characteristic of all hangovers is fatigue. There is no scientific evidence to support the curative claims of coffee, raw eggs, chili peppers, steak sauce, vitamins, the "hair of the dog," or drugs. Doctors usually prescribe aspirin, rest, and solid food.

The best way to avoid a hangover is to drink carefully. That is, drinking slowly, with food in the stomach. It is also important to drink under relaxed social circumstances and to pay attention to the body's response to the alcohol so that intoxication is avoided.

See alcohol, alcoholism.

Hansen's disease — *See leprosy.*

harelip — a cleft lip. A harelip can sometimes influence the shape of the nose and cause its appearance to be different. Today this does not need to be a permanent factor. Plastic surgeons have developed remarkable skill in making the lip and nose look natural. The operation is performed soon after birth, and usually there is no further serious problem.

See cleft palate.

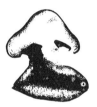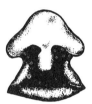

HARELIP

Harvey, William — the English physician (1578-1657) who discovered the circulation of the blood and described his theory in 1628 in his classic work *De Motu Cordis.*

Harvey's discovery is one of the milestones in medical history because it was such a radical departure from accepted knowledge.

hashish — *See marihuana.*

hay fever — an inflammation of the eyes and nasal passages caused by sensitivity (allergy) to some particular pollen, dust, or other substance. The symptoms are tickling, stuffiness, and a watery discharge in the nose; sneezing; and redness and itching of the eyes.

Hay fever is more than just an annoyance—it can be a serious matter. It can affect general health through loss of sleep and appetite. It can lead to infections of the sinuses, throat, and bronchial tubes and is sometimes accompanied by asthma.

TYPES

Perennial hay fever is a type of hay fever that may occur at any time of the year. It is caused by sensitivity to house dust, animal hair, feathers, certain foods, or other substances.

Seasonal hay fever is the most common type. It is due to certain pollens in the air and occurs only at the time of year when the plant that causes it is in bloom. Spring hay fever is caused by tree pollens. In the eastern states it begins in late March or early April and lasts through May. Summer hay fever, caused by pollens of grasses such as timothy and redtop, lasts from the end of May until the middle of July. Fall hay fever, usually caused by ragweed pollen, is the most widespread. It lasts from about mid-August until the first frost.

DIAGNOSIS

People who have hay fever may be sensitive to more than one thing. A doctor may be able to determine, by allergy tests, which substances are responsible. Often a patient may have to take a number of tests in order to be sure that all the causes have been found.

TREATMENT

There are several ways in which a physician may be able to help someone who has hay fever.

A series of hypodermic injections, or shots, will often reduce the sensitivity and prevent further attacks for some time. The injections must usually be given each year, a few days apart, during the months before the hay-fever season. Sometimes they can be given during an attack. A long series is time-consuming and rather expensive, but taking less than the complete series is a waste of time and money.

Removal of pollens from the air, particularly in the bedroom, may help. The physician may also recommend an air filter, an air-conditioning unit, or an electric pollen remover. Physicians occasionally suggest a filter mask or a small filter worn in the nose.

A change of location may be advisable in stubborn cases. Sometimes physicians recommend that patients go away during the hay-fever season. As a last resort, patients may be advised to consider moving permanently to another part of the country. However, a move of this type should be made in consultation with a physician, since it is possible to escape one kind of pollen only to encounter another to which the patient is also sensitive.

Medicines of various kinds may be useful in relieving hay fever. They may be given as drops in the eyes or nose, as sprays, or as pills or capsules. These drugs must be prescribed by a physician for each individual patient.

See allergy.

head — a nonmedical term used to indicate the part of the body above the neck, including the face, brain, ears, etc.

headache — a pain that lasts several minutes or hours; it may cover the whole head, one side of it, or sometimes the front or the back of the head. The pain may be steady or throbbing, barely noticeable, or completely prostrating. To add to the confusion about a definition, some people call any dizzy, tense, or queer feeling in the head a headache.

The medical term for headache — cephalalgia — does not explain anything more because it comes from three Greek words meaning "a condition of head pain."

Doctors feel that headache is not a disease by itself but rather a symptom. A symptom is a change in the body condition that points to something wrong. Doctors distinguish between symptoms that only the patient can feel (such as headache) and signs that anyone can observe.

Headache is important because it can be the symptom—perhaps the first warning—of a serious condition that probably could be controlled if detected early. Only a doctor is professionally trained to find out what the headache symptom indicates. If one removes the warning, day after day, with a pain-killer, it is possible to pass the point of easy control. The professional name for covering up a symptom is "masking," as when aspirin drops a mask between a headache and its cause.

Some of the headaches that are alarm signals for a prompt and thorough medical checkup are:

1. Sudden, severe headache "out of the blue."

2. Headache associated with fever.

3. Headache associated with convulsions.

4. Headache accompanied by confusion or lessening of consciousness.

5. Headache following a blow on the head.

6. Headache associated with local pain in the eye, ear, or elsewhere.

7. Headache beginning in the older person, previously free of headache.

8. Recurring headache in children.

9. Headache at any age that interferes with normal living.

10. Daily or frequent headache.

CAUSES

Only in the twentieth century have investigators studied the pathways and the processes that cause headache. Oddly enough, the brain tissue does not feel pain on direct stimulation, nor does the bone of the skull. Other structures of the head are extremely sensitive to pain, including the scalp, blood vessels, and certain of the brain coverings.

This is one way of classifying the mechanism of head pain:

1. Swelling (dilation) of the arteries in the head. Just as the ankle hurts when it is swollen, so the pain-sensitive blood vessels hurt (ache) when they swell inside or outside of the head. Headaches of migraine, fever, carbon-monoxide poisoning and other toxic states, hangovers, and hunger are some that relate to pain in the cranial arteries.

2. Pulling (traction) on pain-sensitive structures within the head. A brain tumor, abscess, or hemorrhage does not cause pain because of direct pressure on brain tissue but because it pulls on the arteries or other pain-sensitive structures.

3. Inflammation or irritation of pain-sensitive structures. Like an infected finger, an inflamed brain artery produces pain; an inflamed brain covering is accompanied by severe headache.

4. Prolonged contraction of neck muscles. Holding the head stiffly with tense neck muscles may be an instinctive reaction to events that cause anger or worry, or simply a poor posture habit. This produces one of the commonest of headaches—the muscle-contraction (tension) headache. Because a head already aching from swollen arteries or inflammation probably will be held stiffly, muscle-contraction headache often complicates and confuses the diagnosis of headaches from other sources.

5. Spreading pain. Pain may spread into a general headache from local pain in the eye, ear, nose, sinuses, or infected teeth.

These physical sources of headache may be duplicated by research experiment. When no physical mechanism to explain headache can be discovered, the source may be considered:

6. Psychogenic. An emotional conflict or anxiety is "converted" ("conversion reaction") into a body symptom: a "real" not an "imaginary" headache.

TYPES

Headache may be classified as acute or chronic. The acute headache occurs suddenly and occasionally and is an unpleasant part of many illnesses.

Chronic headaches recur more or less frequently, and doctors classify them in various ways, such as:

1. Migraine and other headaches caused by blood-vessel (vascular) changes. Headaches associated with blood-vessel (vascular) changes include the painful migraine or "sick" headache and its variations, such as cluster headache, which is also called histamine headache.

Research has proven that a temporary narrowing (vasoconstriction) of the blood vessels in the head marks the early, painless stage of migraine. Perhaps eight to ten percent of migraine patients experience a warning of the impending headache, such as jagged streaks of light or other "fireworks" of vision, numbness, tingling, and perhaps nausea. Some feel weak, tired, or overexcited.

This warning "aura" allows the individual to lie down in a dark, quiet room, or to take immediately the medicine his doctor has prescribed. These means may ward off the threatening head pain.

The second and painful stage begins in minutes or hours with a severe, throbbing, one-sided or two-sided headache and distended, throbbing arteries sensitized by certain chemical substances. Distension of arteries by the sun or a hot bath does not cause pain unless sensitization of the arteries also occurs. Medicine to contract dilated arteries may end a migraine attack.

A third stage, the steady headache, may follow. This is either part of the original migraine attack or a complicating muscle-contraction (tension) headache resulting from muscles held stiffly in the neck.

2. The muscle-contraction (tension) headache. Undoubtedly the commonest of chronic headaches is the muscle-contraction headache that comes from stiffly set muscles in the neck. A popular name is "tension headache."

The trigger that causes the person to hold these muscles stiffly is some kind of conflict or stress. It could be an emotional conflict when a person or event is hated or viewed with anxiety. Or, the trigger could be physical—a cold draft from an air conditioner, eye-muscle fatigue, straining to hear because of partial deafness, or pain anywhere in the body. Muscle-contraction headache can complicate other types of headache.

Muscle-contraction headache comes without warning symptoms or signs. It usually affects both sides of the head, or the back of the head and neck, or the forehead, face, or jaw muscles, or a band around the head. The pain is steady or pressing or "tight" rather than throbbing.

This type of headache may occur occasionally or frequently. Such a headache at times disappears quickly and at other times lasts for days or weeks. The pain can be mild or may be more severe than some "dangerous" headaches.

3. Headaches associated with various structural changes. A small but important group of recurring headaches are associated with a variety of structural changes. These include headaches caused by high blood pressure, virus infection, tumors, brain abscesses, defects and malformations of blood vessels, and certain diseases of the neck and spine.

Headache in persons with high blood pressure takes many forms, such as muscle-contraction or migraine headache, and can accompany sudden rises of blood pressure. A distinct type of hypertensive headache occurs in the morning on awakening and eases as the day goes on.

Certain headaches involving structural changes may resemble migraine, adding to the doctor's problem of diagnosis.

4. Other headaches involving special problems. Post-traumatic headaches follow an injury, commonly a fall or an auto accident. Structures on the outside or inside of the head may be damaged. Every person who has been knocked unconscious should have a medical examination. Medical guidance should be continued as long as headache continues after an accident involving the head.

The weekend headache can result from an extra rush to finish work on Friday, followed by too much letdown, almost to inertia.

Recreation, which should add joy to life, is full of hidden hazards of headache from an overexciting social life. Personality conflicts, smoke, bad ventilation, lack of sleep, and too much alcohol are invitations to headache.

Boredom headache is the opposite side of this coin. Activities that provide a moderate change or a moderate quantity of complete change prevent boredom headache.

The coffee-hunger headache (caffeine-withdrawal headache) afflicts heavy drinkers of coffee if they miss a usual cup. Relief comes from drinking coffee or eating a caffeine tablet. However, such individuals would be wise to taper off their coffee-drinking until they are no longer dependent on it. Coffee is a readily available emergency treatment for some headaches, if the individual is not such a heavy coffee drinker that its effect is dulled.

Hangover headache involves physical factors,

such as the swelling of blood vessels, a tolerance to alcohol that varies greatly in different persons, and an apparent sensitivity to some chemical by-products of some drinks. A bundle of psychological factors includes changed schedules, lack of sleep, exciting company, and futile regrets.

A headache from an allergy may be moderate and accompanied with swollen, runny nose, sneezing, and two-sided pain. It may be confused with a sinus-infection headache or certain forms of migraine.

TREATMENT
The broad kinds of treatment for headache are symptomatic, to relieve the immediate pain, and prophylactic, to prevent future headaches by treating the underlying causes and mechanisms. Muscle-contraction headaches may be treated with muscle relaxants and tranquilizers. Headaches accompanying infections may require antibiotics. The headache of high blood pressure (hypertension) is treated with medicines to reduce the blood pressure. When headache accompanies nasal disorders, a decongestant for the nose may bring relief. The headache of allergy often responds to antihistamines. All these chemical agents require a physician to make the diagnosis, prescribe the medication, and follow up its effects.

healing — the process by which a body part or tissue returns to a normal condition following an injury or a disease.
See clotting, inflammation.

hearing — *See ear.*

hearing aid — a unit containing tiny components working together as a system to amplify sound. It

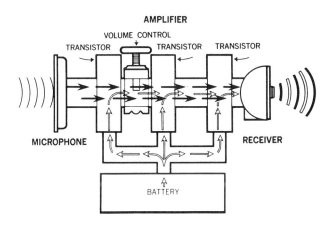

HEARING AID

is similar to a hi-fi set, but miniaturized and specially designed to be lightweight, inconspicuous, and highly efficient in bringing sound directly to the ear.

The system consists of a tiny microphone that picks up sound waves from the air and converts them into electrical signals, an amplifier that increases the strength of the electrical signals, a battery that provides electrical energy to operate the hearing aid, and a tiny loudspeaker called a receiver that converts the amplified signals back into sound waves and directs them into the ear through a specially fitted ear mold.

hearing impairments — hearing losses. There are two main types of hearing loss—conductive deafness and perceptive or nerve deafness. Conductive deafness exists when sound waves are blocked before they reach the inner ear. Perceptive or nerve deafness, which is much more serious, results when there is a defect in the inner ear or when there is damage to the nerve that carries the impulses to the brain, or injury to the brain itself.
See ear, otosclerosis, presbycusis.

heart — a hollow, muscular organ, somewhat larger in size than a closed fist. The heart is located in the lower left section of the chest cavity just behind the breastbone.

FUNCTION
By its pump action, the heart keeps the blood under pressure and in constant circulation throughout the body. In a healthy person, with the body at rest, the heart contracts about seventy-two times a minute. This varies with age, weight, sex, amount of exercise, and body temperature. Every day the heart beats approximately 100,800 times, propelling the total volume of blood through the body 1,440 times. The effect of the contractions can be noted by the pulse. This is most easily found on the thumb side of the inner surface of the wrist.

Each contraction of the heart is followed by limited relaxation. Cardiac muscle never completely relaxes but always maintains a degree of tone. Contraction of the heart is systole and is the period of work. Relaxation of the heart with limited dilation is called diastole and is the period of rest. A complete cardiac cycle is the time from the onset of one contraction or heartbeat to the onset of the next.

The heart is actually two separate pumps. The

right side receives unoxygenated blood into the atrium from the various regions of the body. Then the right ventricle pumps it into the lungs. There it receives a fresh supply of oxygen and releases carbon dioxide. This phase is called pulmonary circulation. The left side of the heart receives the oxygenated blood into the atrium. The left ventricle then pumps it into all regions of the body through the arteries. This phase is the systemic circulation. In a diseased or damaged heart, either pump can fail separately, or both may fail together.

STRUCTURE

The heart is divided into four main parts or chambers. The two upper chambers receive blood. The right upper chamber (called the right atrium) receives unoxygenated blood from the body. The left upper chamber (called the left atrium) receives oxygenated blood from the lungs.

The lower chambers, called ventricles, pump blood out of the heart. The left ventricle pumps oxygenated blood through the arteries to the body. The right ventricle pumps unoxygenated blood to the lungs through an artery known as the pulmonary artery. The pulmonary artery is the only artery in the body that carries unoxygenated blood.

Four veins, called pulmonary veins, return the oxygenated blood from the lungs (two veins from each lung) into the left atrium.

There are four valves in the heart that regulate the flow of blood into and out of the heart and the flow of blood within the four chambers of the heart. The pulmonary valve is formed by three cup-shaped membranes at the junction of the pulmonary artery and the right ventricle. When the right ventricle contracts, the pulmonary valve opens, and the blood is forced into the pulmonary artery leading to the lungs. When the chamber relaxes, the valve is closed and prevents a backflow of the blood.

The aortic valve is situated at the junction of the aorta (actually the aortic arch) and the left ventricle of the heart. Formed by three cup-shaped membranes (called semilunar valves), it allows the blood to flow from the heart into the aorta and prevents any backflow.

The mitral valve, sometimes referred to as the bicuspid valve, is composed of two cusps or triangular segments. It is located between the upper and lower chambers on the left side of the heart.

This valve controls the flow of blood between the two left chambers.

The tricuspid valve consists of three cusps or triangular segments and is located between the upper and lower chambers on the right side of the heart. Its position and function correspond to the bicuspid or mitral valve on the left side of the heart.

Two major veins return unoxygenated blood from the body to the heart. The superior vena cava conducts blood from the upper part of the body (head, neck, and thorax) to the right atrium of the heart. The inferior vena cava returns blood from the lower part of the body to the right upper chamber of the heart.

The upper chambers of the heart are divided by a muscular wall called the atrial septum or the interatrial septum. The lower chambers of the heart are divided by a muscular wall (thinner at the top) known as the ventricular septum or the interventricular septum.

The walls of the heart are formed by three layers of membrane. The endocardium, a thin, smooth membrane, forms the inner surface of the heart. The middle layer, the myocardium, is the thickest of the three layers of the heart. The myocardium is the muscular wall of the heart. The outer layer of the heart wall, the epicardium, is also called the visceral pericardium.

Finally, the heart and the roots of the great blood vessels are surrounded by the pericardium, a thin membrane sac.

heart attack — a serious decrease in the flow of blood to the heart muscle. Serious trouble occurs when hardening of the coronary arteries (the arteries supplying blood to the heart muscle) has progressed far enough to cause a heart attack. Such an attack can occur primarily in to ways.

Blood fighting its way through a narrowed and roughened coronary artery may form a clot that seals off the channel, halting further blood flow through that vessel and all of its "downstream" branches. With its source of life cut off, that segment of heart muscle normally fed by the blocked artery will die. Doctors call a heart attack occurring in this way a coronary thrombosis. A coronary thrombosis, the most common form of heart attack, can happen during sleep as well as during normal daily activity or in the midst of a stressful or exciting situation.

In the second type of heart attack, the fatty deposits themselves plug the vessel, without the

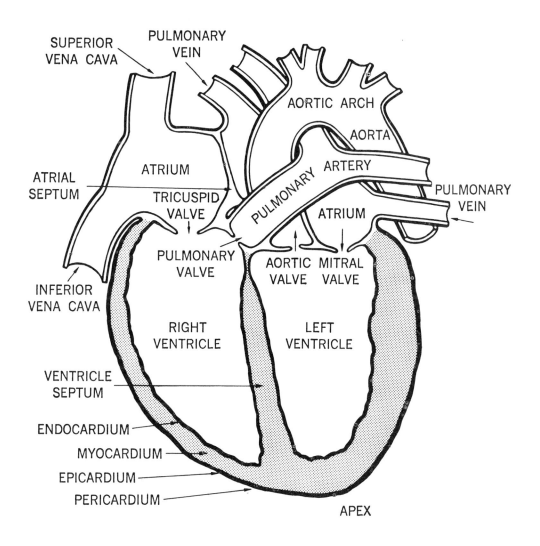

SUPERIOR VENA CAVA

PULMONARY VEIN

AORTIC ARCH

AORTA

ATRIUM

PULMONARY ARTERY

ATRIAL SEPTUM

TRICUSPID VALVE

PULMONARY

ATRIUM

PULMONARY VEIN

INFERIOR VENA CAVA

PULMONARY VALVE

AORTIC VALVE

MITRAL VALVE

RIGHT VENTRICLE

LEFT VENTRICLE

VENTRICLE SEPTUM

ENDOCARDIUM

MYOCARDIUM

EPICARDIUM

PERICARDIUM

APEX

RIGHT SIDE OF HEART

LEFT SIDE OF HEART

HEART

help of a clot. The deposits simply become so greatly enlarged that they merge and shut off the flow of blood.

An attack occurring in either way may be so mild that the victim doesn't notice it (although this is most uncommon), or it can be so severe that it causes sudden death. How serious it is depends on the size of the blocked vessel and the extent of the heart-muscle area damaged by blood starvation. This damaged or killed region of heart muscle is called a myocardial infarct.

The excruciating pain of a heart attack may last for several days. Other sysmptoms are usually an intense shortness of breath and heavy perspiration. Occasionally, the person suffering a heart attack also loses consciousness.

During the period of recovery a scar will form where the heart muscle has been damaged. In order to recover from a heart attack, it is imperative that the patient has plenty of rest, coupled with a physician's treatment. The patient should keep in mind that the repair job going on in his heart is like the knitting of a broken bone. It takes time. When recovery is complete, a rule of moderation in all things is required—no overworking, no overeating, no extremes of any kind—but most people can resume a normal daily routine.

If the heart-attack victim is willing to give himself proper care and follow his physician's advice, his chances are very good for many more years of enjoyable living.

heart block — interference with the conduction of the electrical impulses of the heart. This can be either partial or complete. A heart block can result in a lack of coordination of the rhythms of the upper and lower heart chambers.

heartburn — a form of indigestion in which there is a pain in the chest near the heart. Heartburn has nothing at all to do with the heart.

heart defects — *See congenital heart defects.*

heart-lung machine — a machine through which the bloodstream is diverted for pumping and oxygenation while the heart is opened for surgery.

heart transplant — an operation that replaces a severely diseased or malfunctioning heart with a healthy heart. The replacement heart comes from a donor who has died from causes that do not involve the heart, such as an automobile accident.

The operation makes use of a heart-lung machine from the time the patient's diseased heart is removed until the donor heart has been attached to his body. This machine keeps the blood circulating throughout the body and keeps the blood oxygenated.

Suprisingly, the operation is a fairly simple one. The heart is a complicated organ, but it is only attached to the rest of the body in a few places. Thus, when the new heart is in place, the surgeon need only attach the donor arteries and veins to the corresponding vessels in the recipient.

The major problem that has been encountered in heart transplants has been the attempt on the part of the recipient's body to reject the donor heart. Despite the fact that an effort is made to match the donor and the recipient, the new heart is perceived by the recipient's body as foreign matter. Consequently, the defense mechanisms of the body are alerted to repel the "invading" tissue. This rejection mechanism must be suppressed by drugs. The drugs (and other treatment, such as radiation) suppress the rejection mechanism but also weaken the entire defense mechanism. This leaves the recipient vulnerable to almost any bacterial or viral infection. To protect the patient until the new heart has been "accepted" by his body, he must be kept in isolation to avoid disease-causing microorganisms.

At present, research scientists are working on two possible solutions to this problem. The first is an artificial heart that would be accepted naturally by the recipient and thus avoid the problem. The second possibility involves the careful balancing of drugs so that the body's rejection mechanism is suppressed enough to accept the new heart but not so much that the recipient is left vulnerable to every possible infection.

Heart transplants are a fairly recent innovation. The first was performed by Christiaan Barnard on December 3, 1967 in Capetown, South Africa.

See Barnard, Christiaan; heart.

heat cramps — painful spasms of muscles, especially those of the abdomen and limbs, after prolonged exposure to high temperatures while engaged in strenuous labor. The spasmodic cramps may be simply a slight cramp in the abdomen or muscles of an extremity or so severe as to cause convulsions. Attacks may be brief or may last twelve to twenty-four hours; after being relieved, the spasms may be renewed by exposure to a cold draft or exertion.

Nature attempts to relieve a person working in high temperatures by sweating and evaporation of the sweat. Profuse sweating not only removes moisture from the body but a considerable amount of the salt content of the body fluids as well. Loss of the body's salt content from the body fluids excites irritation of the muscles, causing the spasmodic cramps.

Heat cramps can be prevented by drinking adequate amounts of water to replace the fluid lost in perspiration and at the same time replacing the salt also lost by taking salt tablets.

The treatment for mild heat cramps is increased salt intake, warm baths, and rest. If the cramps are severe and persistent, medical care is necessary.

heat exhaustion — collapse from the effects of heat—from the sun or any other source. It occurs more frequently when the humidity is high.

The patient is seldom unconscious but may complain of feeling very weak. His face is pale and anxious-looking and covered with cold perspiration. Frequently he vomits. He may complain of feeling chilly. His pulse is rapid and weak, and his breathing is shallow, with little chest expansion.

The treatment for heat exhaustion is the same as that for physical shock, but the patient should also be given salt.

Heat exhaustion is also called heat prostration.

heat prostration — *See heat exhaustion.*

heatstroke — a reaction to excessive heat.

Heatstroke (sometimes called sunstroke) is a very serious condition that results from a failure of the heat-regulating mechanism of the body. The body becomes overheated, the temperature rises to between 105° and 110° F., but there is no sweating and therefore no cooling of the body. The patient's skin is hot, dry, and red. Sometimes the patient may have preliminary symptoms such as headache, nausea, dizziness, or weakness; but very often the first signs are sudden collapse and loss of consciousness. Breathing is likely to be deep and rapid. The pulse is strong and fast. Convulsions may occur. Heatstroke may cause death or permanent disability; at best,

recovery is likely to be slow and complicated by relapses.

TREATMENT

The longer the patient remains overheated, the more likely he is to die. Therefore, all first-aid measures are aimed at lowering the patient's body temperature. The following steps should be taken:

1. Remove the patient to the coolest possible place.

2. Take off the patient's clothing.

3. Place him so that he is lying on his back, with his head and shoulders slightly raised.

4. Cool the patient. Sponge or spray his body with cold water and then fan him so that the water will evaporate rapidly.

5. If the patient regains consciousness, give him cool (but not cold) water to drink.

6. Get medical assistance.

hematology — the study of the blood.

hemiplegia — paralysis of one side of the body caused by damage to the opposite side of the brain. The paralyzed arm and leg are opposite to the side of the brain damage because the nerves cross in the brain, and one side of the brain controls the opposite side of the body. Such paralysis is sometimes caused by a blood clot or hemorrhage in a blood vessel in the brain.
See stroke.

hemodynamics — the study of the flow of blood and the forces involved.

hemoglobin — the oxygen-carrying red-colored substance of the red blood cells. Hemoglobin carries oxygen to the body tissues. If the amount of hemoglobin is below normal, not enough oxygen will get to the tissues.

When hemoglobin has absorbed oxygen in the lungs, it is bright red and is called oxyhemoglobin. After it has released the oxygen load in the tissues, it is purple in color and is called reduced hemoglobin.

hemolytic disease of the newborn — a condition caused by the destruction of the red cells in a baby; it occurs in some cases where a mother with Rh-negative blood has an Rh-positive baby.

The first signs are severe anemia and a failing heart. If the baby survives these disorders, a destructive form of jaundice, called kernicterus, may occur within forty-eight hours of birth. This afflicts an estimated two thousand newborn babies every year in the United States. About half of these babies die; the other half usually live with permanent brain damage.

See Rh factor.

hemophilia — a disease characterized by an inability of the blood to coagulate or clot. Thus, a hemophiliac (a person with this disease) can bleed to a serious degree, even to death. A relatively minor cut or abrasion, or such common events as a tooth extraction or tonsillectomy, may cause such bleeding. The rupture of a relatively small blood vessel inside the body can cause serious internal bleeding.

Hemophilia, or bleeder's disease, is the commonest of a rather rare, incurable group of hereditary blood disorders occuring almost exclusively in males but transmitted through women. Females themselves generally show no signs of difficulty.

HISTORY

Known since ancient times, the disease is scarcely recognizable even today in primitive societies, because afflicted male infants die young. In ancient Egypt a woman was not permitted to bear any more children if the first-born son bled to death from a minor wound.

Historically, Queen Victoria was perhaps the most famous carrier of hemophilia. She had nine children. One son, Prince Leopold, was a bleeder and two daughters, Alice and Beatrice, were known carriers. Victoria Eugenie, one afflicted granddaughter, introduced the disease into the royal family in Spain, while another, Alexandra, carried it to Russia's Romanoffs. At least eleven descendants of the Queen are known to have been afflicted. This is the reason that hemophilia is sometimes referred to as the royal disease. It is not, as many people believe, the penalty for inbreeding among Europe's royal families.

Because modern medicine has done so much for young children and infants, more hemophiliacs are reaching adulthood, marrying, and having children. This is only natural, but the laws of genetics are relentless. Daughters will be carriers with the ability to pass it on to the grandchildren. Some of the hemophiliac's daughter's sons may have the disease and some may not. Some of the granddaughters may be carriers, yet the disease can lie dormant for many generations. Generally, none of the sons of a hemophiliac will inherit or transmit the disease, although exceptions have been recorded.

No one can predict exactly how many children will be afflicted in the future, but from a statistical view, because the defect is a sex-linked recessive trait, each carrier will average one bleeder child to three nonbleeders. Although this results in a dilution of the inherited defect down through generations, it is also believed to account for the sudden appearance of a hemophiliac where it would seem that there is no previous family history of the disease.

DIAGNOSIS

Diagnosis can usually be made early in life as a result of prolonged bleeding of the umbilicus at birth or by episodes of severe or uncontrolled bleeding shortly afterward.

Normal blood contains some eight or more constituents that work together to form a blood clot and close small wounds within four to six minutes. In hemophiliacs, however, this can take several hours or days. Even then there is no guarantee that a clot, once formed, will not be dissolved or reopen, because the blood of a hemophiliac is deficient in one of at least three antihemophilic factors essential to normal clotting.

Thus, the disease is not one but three or more closely allied disorders of blood coagulation. Severe bleeding from a minor injury should always provide reason for suspicion and should be promptly reported to a physician. Diagnosis is relatively simple, especially if a family history of the defect is known.

TREATMENT

Loss of blood through an open cut or wound is rarely as serious or painful as damage resulting from internal hemorrhage. This can put pressure on a nerve and cause great pain or even paralysis. The area can swell to such an extent that the blood supply to a limb is cut off and gangrene results. Hidden bleeding in the head, chest, or abdominal cavity is often extremely difficult to diagnose and can prove rapidly fatal. Blood in the urine may also be a sign of trouble. In all such instances the help of a physician should be sought early.

Many adults are capable of self-treatment under a physician's guidance, using special blood-clot-stimulating materials (obtainable on prescription) that can be applied directly to small wounds.

Mothers of hemophilic children quickly learn that cold and pressure can work wonders with small wounds and that heat only accentuates hemorhaging. The only effective treatment for uncontrolled hemophilic bleeding at present is by transfusion of fresh or recently quick-frozen whole blood or plasma.

Scientists have found that there is enough of the required clot-forming substances in the plasma content of fresh whole blood to supply what is needed in the patient's system to control bleeding temporarily. Such blood or plasma cannot be stored or "banked" unless "freeze-dried" and kept under vacuum, because the necessary clotting ingredients are unstable.

In recent years many researchers have sought to concentrate or synthesize the active anti-hemophilic factor, much as insulin is produced and used daily for the treatment of diabetes. But the problems involved in hemophilia are very different and thus far have proved insurmountable.

Lacking an ability to choose their parents, grandparents, or earlier ancestors, hemophiliacs must strive to avoid those situations and activities that might lead to physical injuries. However, parents, relatives, and friends should seek (following their doctor's advice) ways to avoid raising psychological barriers in children that may arise from their being considered "different" and being overprotected.

A serious danger to be guarded against is the inclination to overlook an infant's propensity to flex his legs and hold them in a bent position in response to pain from blood collecting in the knees after injury. Failure to give such a situation prompt attention and treatment can mark the start of a crippling deformity sometimes more severe than the results of polio or arthritis.

Depending on the extent of his disease, the individual hemophiliac should take the disability into account in his daily life, abstaining from sports that involve bodily contact with others and paying prompt attention to all injuries that break the skin or cause swelling. When surgical operations or other emergencies arise, there may be a need for appropriate transfusions. Under these conditions, he can expect to live a useful and relatively normal life.

Once identified, every hemophiliac should wear an identity disc and carry a card spelling out his problem, his blood group, what to do in an emergency, and the name and telephone number of his physician.

See genetics.

hemorrhage — severe loss of blood from a blood vessel. In external hemorrhage, blood escapes from the body. In internal hemorrhage, blood passes into tissues surrounding the ruptured blood vessel.

Blood is circulated throughout the body by means of three different kinds of blood vessels: arteries, veins, and capillaries. Arteries are large vessels that carry the blood away from the heart; veins are large vessels that carry the blood back to the heart; and capillaries form a connecting network of smaller vessels between the arteries and the veins.

Hemorrhage (escape of blood) occurs whenever there is a break in the wall of one or more blood vessels. In most small cuts, only capillaries are injured. Deeper wounds result in injury to veins or arteries. Bleeding that is severe enough to endanger life seldom occurs except when arteries or veins are cut.

The average adult body contains about five quarts of blood. One pint of blood can usually be lost without harmful effect. In fact, this is the amount usually given by blood donors. However, the loss of two pints (one quart) will usually cause shock, and shock becomes greater and greater as the amount of blood loss increases. If half the blood in the body is lost, death almost always results.

Capillary blood is usually brick-red in color. If capillaries are cut, the blood oozes out slowly. Blood from the veins is dark red. If a vein is cut, the blood escapes in a steady, even flow. If an artery near the surface is cut, the blood will gush out in spurts that are synchronized with the heartbeats; but if the cut artery is deeply buried, the bleeding will appear to be a steady stream. Arterial blood is usually bright red in color.

In actual practice, it might be difficult to decide whether bleeding was venous or arterial, but the distinction is not usually important. A person can bleed to death quickly from a cut artery; prolonged bleeding from any large cut can, of course, have the same effect. The important thing to know is that all bleeding must be controlled as quickly as possible.

TREATMENT

The best way to stop serious bleeding is to apply pressure. In practically all cases, bleeding can be stopped if pressure is applied directly to the wound. If direct pressure does not stop the heavy bleeding, pressure should be applied at the appropriate pressure point. In those rare cases where bleeding is so severe that it cannot be controlled by either of these methods, pressure can be applied by means of a tight, constricting band called a tourniquet.

See pressure point, tourniquet.

hemorrhoids — enlarged, dilated veins inside or just outside the rectum. Hemorrhoids are also called piles. They are somewhat like varicose veins in the legs. The veins in the rectum are not buried deep in the flesh but lie close to the surface, where they can easily be pressed on and irritated. Any pressure that slows up the flow of blood through them or that irritates can cause piles.

CAUSES

A frequent cause is constipation that results in hard, dry stools accompanied by straining. During pregnancy, the enlarged womb sometimes presses on the nearby veins. A tumor can do the same thing. These are local causes of hemorrhoids. Sometimes the interference with the flow of blood is at some point distant from the rectum.

The veins in the rectum carry blood from the rectal area back to the heart. Part of this blood returns by way of the liver. The trouble may be in the liver or even in the heart itself. When the flow of blood through these veins is greatly interfered with, the delicately covered veins in the rectum can bulge and result in hemorrhoids.

It is never safe to take for granted that hemorrhoids are caused by nothing more serious than constipation. They may be nature's warning that liver disease, heart trouble, or a tumor is developing and needs medical attention.

Although hemorrhoids in themselves seldom endanger life, the condition that causes them can be serious and should be corrected. Another good reason for seeing a doctor promptly is the possibility that the trouble may be something other than hemorrhoids. There are a number of conditions that cause discomfort in or near the anus. Some are very easily corrected; others are serious. For instance, rectal symptoms sometimes attributed to hemorrhoids may actually be caused by cancer; therefore a thorough examination by a physician is necessary. Con-

trary to an old belief, however, hemorrhoids do not turn into cancer.

SYMPTOMS

Symptoms of hemorrhoids differ among individuals. There can be aching discomfort, extreme pain, itching, or bleeding. Sometimes the enlarged vein inside the rectum pushes out and can be felt.

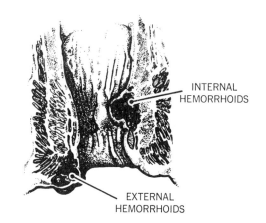

INTERNAL HEMORRHOIDS

EXTERNAL HEMORRHOIDS

HEMORRHOIDS

TREATMENT

Continued bleeding from hemorrhoids often causes anemia. If a blood clot forms in them, piles become extremely painful. If untreated, they can become inflamed, infected, and can rupture and cause a hemorrhage. Medical care for hemorrhoids not only gives relief but is necessary for safety.

Many cases of hemorrhoids can be relieved by methods other than surgery. Some require an operation. The operation is usually not a serious one.

hemp — *See marihauna.*

hepar — *See liver.*

heparin — a chemical substance that tends to prevent blood from clotting. It is sometimes used in cases of an existing clot in an artery or vein to prevent enlargement of the clot or the formation of new clots. Heparin is classified as an anticoagulant.

hepatitis — a swelling and soreness of the liver. Two types caused by viruses—infectious and serum hepatitis—are frequently found in the United States.

One is called "infectious" because a person with the disease can infect others by contact. This type is also spread by contaminated water and food, including raw clams and oysters harvested from polluted waters.

"Serum" hepatitis was first recognized in people who had been given medicines or vaccines that contained human serum. A person may develop serum hepatitis after receiving a transfusion of infected blood or its derivatives or after having contaminated needles, syringes, or other skin-puncturing instruments (including tattoo needles) used on him.

INFECTIOUS HEPATITIS

Infectious hepatitis is one of the more-common communicable diseases, especially in children. It may be compared to mumps in frequency and seriousness and in the fact that it is spread from one person to another. The closer the contact, the greater the chance that any susceptible individual will develop the disease. The risk of infection is small among children who have only classroom contacts; to adults who are exposed to the disease at work, the risk is even smaller.

Anyone who has not had infectious hepatitis may get the disease, but people who have once had hepatitis are usually immune to a second attack. Infectious hepatitis normally lasts only a week or two in children and is fairly mild. However, the disease is more severe in adults, frequently lasting four to six weeks. It is seldom fatal (the death rate rarely exceeds one half of one percent), but the deaths that do occur are usually among persons over thirty years of age. Autumn and winter are the times when epidemics are most frequent, but cases occur throughout the year.

SYMPTOMS

Symptoms of infectious hepatitis may appear any time from two to six weeks after the patient has been exposed to the disease. Loss of appetite, fatigue, a feeling of weariness, nausea (with or without vomiting), pain or a feeling of heaviness in the abdomen, and headache are common symptoms. Fever is a common early symptom but usually subsides after a few days. The liver becomes enlarged and is tender. Symptoms in children may be not at all typical or almost nonexistent.

A yellow tinge, usually first noticeable in the white part of the eyes, but also giving a yellow cast to the skin, is the most charcteristic feature of the disease. However, many persons with infectious hepatitis do not have this symptom. In mild cases and in children there is often no jaundice (yellow coloring of the skin and eyes). Moreover, since jaundice also occurs in other diseases, its presence does not always mean that the patient has infectious hepatitis.

It is extremely important to consult a doctor, even though the symptoms may be mild and may resemble those of other less-serious diseases. A physician should be seen at the first sign of illness, and his instructions should be followed carefully throughout convalescence—which is often long—to prevent a relapse.

TREATMENT

The treatment for infectious hepatitis usually recommended by physicians is rest in bed and an adequate diet. It may take a long time to recover fully from this disease. Recovery is especially slow in adults. Sometimes the convalescent period lasts several months, and in a few patients chronic liver trouble may develop.

REDUCING THE RISK

There is no vaccine available to immunize against infectious hepatitis. There are several ways, however, to reduce the risk of contracting the disease. Proper community sanitation and personal hygiene are important in this regard.

Once a person has been exposed to infectious hepatitis, gamma globulin provides temporary protection. Gamma globulin is the disease-fighting part of human blood. It contains antibodies that hold the infection in check while the body builds up its resistance of disease. Thus, an injection of gamma globulin given to a person who has been exposed to the disease will prevent or lessen the severity of infectious hepatitis. Gamma globulin is made from human blood, much of which may have been donated. Physicians use it as protection against infectious hepatitis only when exposure is sufficient to make infection very likely.

SERUM HEPATITIS

Serum hepatitis is caused by a virus that circulates in the blood of some persons for many years. Because it cannot be detected by tests and may not cause symptoms, infected persons can unwittingly transmit the virus by serving as blood donors.

The symptoms of serum hepatitis are similar to infectious hepatitis, but this disease is not transmitted in the same way. People get serum hepatitis from blood and plasma that contains a virus. It may be transmitted through transfusions of blood or serum. It may also be transmitted by medical instruments, tattooing needles, or any other skin-puncturing instrument that has come in contact with blood or serum and has not been properly sterilized.

The incubation period for serum hepatitis is quite long. It may take from two to six months for a person who has been infected to show any symptoms. The symptoms are similar to those of infectious hepatitis but come on more slowly and are often more severe and longer-lasting. However, mild cases also occur.

Gamma-globulin injections are not known to prevent serum hepatitis. People who have had either infectious or serum hepatitis should not donate blood to Red Cross or other blood-donor programs. Occasionally, when blood is to be fractionated, persons with a past history of hepatitis can donate, but they should be sure to tell the people at the donor center that they have had hepatitis. Even though it may have been years since a person had serum hepatitis, he may still be able to transmit the virus if his blood is used for transfusions.

Proper sterilization of all instruments that are used for penetrating the skin is the other and important method of preventing serum hepatitis.

An attack of serum hepatitis probably provides immunity, but a person who has had infectious hepatitis is not immune to serum hepatitis, nor is a person who has had serum hepatitis immune to infectious hepatitis.

See liver.

heredity — the sum total of inherited characteristics, qualities, and tendencies.

See genetics.

hernia — a protrusion of a portion of an internal organ, usually the bowel, through the muscular wall of the abdomen. Most hernias occur in or just above the groin, although they may occur at other places over the abdomen. Hernias are caused by muscular strains from lifting or pushing, violent coughing, sudden jars in jumping, and similar acts.

The symptoms of a hernia (also called a rupture) are a sharp, stinging pain and the feeling of something giving way at the site of the rupture. On examination, swelling is found—ranging in size from that of a marble to that of a doubled-up fist or even larger. The swelling is usually tender. Nausea and vomiting often occur.

A truss, or supporting belt, is sometimes used to keep the internal organs from protruding through the hernia. A more-active form of treatment involves the surgical repair of the weakened muscle wall.

heroin — morphine chemically altered to make it three to six times stronger. Heroin is an addictive narcotic (a drug that relieves pain and induces sleep). It accounts for ninety percent of the narcotic addition problem in the United States. Heroin is not used in medicine, and all heroin in the United States is smuggled into the country.

ADDICTION

When the user of heroin becomes "hooked" (addicted) his body requires repeated and larger doses of the drug. Once the habit starts, larger and larger doses are required to get the same effects. This happens because the body develops a tolerance for the drug.

A second sign of heroin addiction is withdrawal sickness. When the addict stops using the drug, he may sweat, shake, have chills, develop diarrhea and nausea, and suffer sharp abdominal and leg cramps. Modern treatment helps the addict through these withdrawal symptoms. Science now has new evidence that the body's physical addiction may last much longer than previously believed.

Typically, the first emotional reaction to heroin is reduction of tension, easing of fears, and relief from worry. Feeling "high" may be followed by a period of inactivity bordering on stupor.

Heroin is usually sold heavily "cut," or adulterated with milk-sugar, quinine, or other materials. Typically it is mixed into a liquid solution and injected into a vein ("mainlining"), although it can also be injected just under the skin ("skin popping") or sniffed through the nose. The latter methods of use are more common among "joy poppers" than among confirmed addicts. However, addiction is possible no matter which method is used. Taken in any way, the drug appears to dull the edges of reality. Addicts will relate that heroin "makes my troubles roll off my mind," and "it makes me more sure of myself." As the addict becomes more and more used to the drug, he requires increasingly larger doses to achieve a "high." Eventually, he doesn't even obtain a "high." Instead, he is forced to continue using heroin to avoid the withdrawal sickness. In other words, he uses heroin to feel normal.

The drug depresses certain areas of the brain and may reduce hunger, thirst, and the sex drive. Because addicts do not usually feel hungry, and because they spend their money for heroin, they can become malnourished and physically depleted. Pneumonia, tuberculosis, and venereal disease occur more frequently in addicts than in the rest of the population. The injection of contaminated material and the use of unsterile syringes and needles cause hepatitis and blood infections that may settle in the brain or heart valves or may spread throughout the body.

Withdrawal symptoms appear in the addicted person within twelve or sixteen hours after the drug has been last taken, and they become progressively worse. After two or three days they begin to subside, and within a week the addict is free from withdrawal symptoms.

The addict will admit that, once "hooked," obtaining a continued supply becomes the main goal of his life. His concentration on getting money and drugs frequently prevents the addict from continuing either his education or his job. His health is often bad. He may be sick one day from the effects of withdrawal and sick the next day from an overdose. Statistics indicate that his life-span may be shortened by fifteen to twenty years.

Medical authorities say that the addict is a sick person. He needs treatment for his personality problems, physical addiction, and withdrawal sickness. Then, he needs considerable help to keep him from going back to drug use after his withdrawal.

A number of rehabilitation approaches to the problem of addiction are being tested, including ex-addict self-help groups and narcotic substitutes. Rehabilitation means to rebuild — physical, mental, emotional, social, and vocational reconstruction. With many addicts, every aspect of existence needs rehabilitation.

One promising experimental effort to help addicts is through maintenance on methadone, a narcotic commonly used to treat withdrawal from heroin. When taken regularly, methadone eliminates the craving for heroin as well as its euphoric effects. In some neighborhoods, addicts are maintained on methadone by daily doses administered at a local community clinic. Close supervision is most important, including urine analysis to make sure the addict is following directions about taking no drug but methadone. Counseling, job retraining, and the building of a new way of life must be combined with methadone-maintenance treatment.

herpes simplex — a disease that causes recurrent sores on the lips. Because these sores frequently develop when the patient has a cold, or a fever of other origin, the disease has become known as fever blisters or cold sores.

The cause of herpes simplex is a virus or possibly several different viruses. Almost half the population suffers from fever blisters. In fact, the infection is considered by some to be second only to the common cold in prevalence.

PRIMARY HERPES
The herpes-simplex virus, which is highly contagious, enters the body early in life. The disease makes its first appearance in very young children, one to three years of age, although primary cases have occurred in older people.

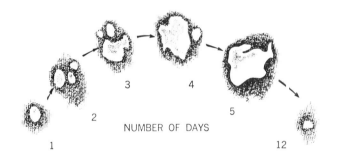

COURSE OF DEVELOPMENT OF THE PRIMARY HERPES SIMPLEX ULCER OVER A 12-DAY PERIOD

HERPES SIMPLEX (PRIMARY)

The primary infection may cause only one or two sores to develop. These frequently go unnoticed. In other cases, the child will have a slight fever, pain in the mouth, increased salivation, bad breath, and a general feeling of illness. The inside of his mouth becomes swollen and the gums inflamed. Many lesions, or sores, appear simultaneously on the lips, inside the cheeks, and on the tongue and gums. These sores are yellow and irregularly shaped. Later in the course of the disease, a red ring of inflammation forms around them.

This first attack of herpes simplex is the only time the sores occur over a widespread area within the mouth.

There is no specific treatment for primary herpes. Healing begins naturally within three days, and the illness is usually over in seven to fourteen days. Supportive measures can be taken to make the child more comfortable, relieve his pain, and prevent secondary infection.

RECURRENT LABIAL HERPES
Following this initial childhood infection, the virus of herpes simplex lies dormant, to reappear later in life as the familiar, recurring fever blister or cold sore. In this second stage of the disease, the characteristic sore usually appears on the outside of the patient's lip, at the point where the red part of the lip meets the adjoining skin. Thus the medical name—recurrent labial (lip) herpes. It is a peculiarity of the disease that in each succeeding attack the sore always develops at the same place. Recurrent fever blisters usually do not occur inside the mouth.

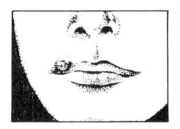

HERPES SIMPLEX (RECURRENT)

A burning sensation, itching, or feeling of fullness is usually noted about twenty-four hours before the sore actually appears. The lip becomes swollen and red. The sore of herpes is small and covered with a yellow scab.

Fever blisters erupt when the patient's general resistance is lowered or when he has a cold or fever. The attack may come when he has suffered some emotional or physical stress. Exposure to sunlight or a dry, cracked lip are also predisposing factors in these recurrent attacks. Some women have noted that fever blisters occur in connection with menstruation.

Recurrent attacks of fever blisters may occur as infrequently as once a year or as often as weekly or even daily. Just why the infection should behave in this way is not yet fully under-

stood. There is some scientific evidence, however, that more than one virus may be involved and that each succeeding outbreak of sores is actually caused by a different virus.

As in the case of primary herpes, secondary labial herpes sores heal by themselves in seven to ten days, leaving no scar. There is no specific treatment, although a new antiviral drug, now under study, shows promise as a means of hastening the healing process.

herpes zoster — an acute inflammation of nerve cells, producing pain and then a rash. For several days the pain may pull, nag, or burn in or under the skin, with no apparent explanation. Such pain on the abdomen has been mistaken for appendicitis or a gallbladder attack; on the chest, for heart disease or pleurisy; on the face, for neuralgia. Occasionally, besides suffering local pain, patients feel generally ill, with fever and headache; sometimes the local pain is so slight that it is overlooked at first.

Physicians call shingles herpes zoster or occasionally zona. From the ancient Greek and Latin words for "girdle" come the names "shingles," "zoster," and "zona." "Herpes" comes from a word for "creeping" and describes the spreading or creeping of the rash. Herpes zoster (shingles) should not be confused with herpes simplex, which is the common cold sore or fever blister.

The diagnosis becomes clear with the appearance of the rash of small watery blisters, closely grouped on reddened skin. The blisters usually are limited to one side of the body and follow along the course of the nerve that the virus of shingles has attacked. Later crops of blisters may continue to appear. Shingles occasionally occurs without a rash, zoster sine herpes, which makes diagnosis difficult.

Shingles affects both sexes and all races. It is usually an illness of adults but has been reported in children of all ages, even the newborn.

TREATMENT
Although the average person will recover from shingles without treatment, early care by a physician may provide immediate relief and prevent or lessen complications. The doctor may prescribe various pain relievers. A variety of powders or liquid dressings can be prescribed for use directly on the skin eruption. Presently known antibiotics appear to prevent secondary infections but do not lighten the course of shingles.

In shingles of the eye, an ophthalmologist (eye specialist with an M.D. degree) should be consulted at once to help prevent loss of vision.

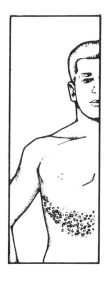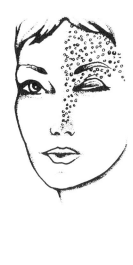

HERPES ZOSTER

In some encouraging published reports on treatment, gamma globulin started in the first two days of the shingles rash appeared to lighten the rash, control the immediate pain, reduce the course of the disease, and prevent lingering pain (postherpetic neuralgia). Because some other reports were discouraging, more research on gamma globulin is needed to clarify its possible treatment value in the early stages of shingles.

COMPLICATIONS

Probably the most common complication in adults, particularly older persons, is postherpetic neuralgia. The pain can last for weeks, months, or indefinitely in the area where the rash occurred. Fortunately, the pain may disappear spontaneously with time.

In certain cases where the pain persists, many medical and some surgical treatments have been tried, but none has proved entirely successful. Patients are advised to continue with a physician in whom they have confidence, for supervision as long as needed.

If a rash appears on the forehead, nose, or eyelid during the acute stage, shingles may affect the eye itself (ophthalmic zoster). An ophthalmologist will start immediate treatment that can often prevent scarring of the cornea and thus prevent loss of vision. If the ear is affected when shingles occurs on the face, a doctor may suggest an ear specialist (otologist or otolaryngologist). Medical treatment helps a patient avoid temporary or lasting loss of hearing.

Scarring of the skin may occur, particularly if the skin blisters develop a further (secondary) infection. Extreme fatigue may plague the person who is recovering from shingles.

hexamethonium chloride — a drug that lowers blood pressure and increases blood flow by interfering with the transmission of nerve impulses that constrict the blood vessels. One of the ganglionic blocking agents, it is one of the drugs used in the treatment of high blood pressure.

hiccups — involuntary contractions of the diaphragm (the muscular wall between the chest and the abdominal cavity). Hiccups may be caused by gastric upset, nervous upset, irritation of the diaphragm (usually from diseases), and chronic disease.

Hiccups can often be stopped by increasing the amount of carbon dioxide in the system. This can be accomplished by rapidly drinking a glass of water or by breathing into a paper bag. When the underlying cause is more serious, stronger measures may have to be taken.

high blood pressure — *See blood pressure, hypertension.*

hip — the joint between the pelvis and the thighbone. *See joints.*

Hippocrates of Cos — famous Greek physician (late 5th century B.C.) who is still thought of as the father of medicine. Hippocrates set down a standard of medical ethics that is still the basis of medical practice. He was careful in keeping records of his cases and in observing symptoms. *See Hippocratic oath.*

Hippocratic oath — the code of medical ethics set by Hippocrates which is still the standard followed by physicians.

"I swear by Apollo the physician, by Aesculapius, Hygeia, and Panacea, and I take to witness all the gods, all the goddesses, to keep according to my ability and my judgement the following Oath:

"To consider dear to me as my parents him who taught me this art; to live in common with him and if necessary to share my goods with him; to look upon his children as my own brothers, to teach them this art if they so desire without fee or written promise; to impart to my sons and the sons of the master who taught me and the disciples who have enrolled themselves and have agreed to the rules of the profession, but to these alone, the precepts and the instruction. I will prescribe regimen for the good of my patients according to my ability and my judgement and never do harm to anyone. To please no one will I prescribe a deadly drug, nor give advice which may cause his death. Nor will I give a woman a pessary to procure abortion. But I will preserve the purity of my life and my art. I will not cut for stone, even for patients in whom the disease is manifest; I will leave this operation to be performed by practitioners (specialists in this art). In every house where I come I will enter only for the good of my patients, keeping myself far from all intentional ill-doing and all seduction, and especially from the pleasures of love with women or with men, be they free or slaves. All that may come to my knowledge in the exercise of my profession or outside of my profession or in daily commerce with men, which ought not to be spread abroad, I will keep secret and will never reveal. If I keep this oath faithfully, may I enjoy my life and practice my art, respected by all men and in all times; but if I swerve from it or violate it, may the reverse by my lot."

His, Wilhelm — German anatomist (1831-1904) who discovered the muscle fibers running from the upper to the lower chambers of the heart. These fibers are known as the bundle of His.

    See bundle of His.

histamine — a protein substance found in the body. Histamine is released by the tissues when they are injured or damaged. This substance dilates the capillaries.

    See allergy, antihistamine.

histology — the study of the anatomy of the cells and minute structures of the tissues and organs.

hives — itching, raised welts on the skin that resemble mosquito bites. They normally appear and disappear suddenly. Hives are usually an allergic reaction.

    See allergy.

Hodgkin's disease — one of several malignant disorders of the lymphatic and other tissues that play a part in the individual's ability to fight infection. The disease was first described in 1832 by an English physician, Thomas Hodgkin (1798-1866). Though persons of any age may develop this rather rare type of cancer, young adults, aged twenty to forty, are most often affected.

SYMPTOMS

The most common first symptom is a painless, swollen lymph gland, usually in the neck. Normally, these glands are no larger than beans. They manufacture lymphocytes, a variety of white blood cells that fight the spread of infection and are found in greatest number in the side of the neck, the armpit, the groin, the midchest, and the abdominal cavity.

Because these lymph glands swell in the presence of infection as well as in Hodgkin's disease, severe reactions of the lymph nodes to such diseases as rheumatoid arthritis or mononucleosis often mimic Hodgkin's disease. Biopsy (the microscopic examination of a swollen node removed by surgery) offers the only method of diagnosis. In examining a thin slice of the affected node, pathologists look for distinctive abnormal cells known as the Reed-Sternberg cells. The presence of these cells is an indication of Hodgkin's disease.

Other symptoms of Hodgkin's disease are pain in the abdomen, back, or legs; fatigue; persistent sore throat; fever; loss of weight; and itching. As the disease progresses, blood changes may take place, and anemia (a reduction in the number of red blood cells) develops. The body is less able to combat infections, and damage to vital organs occurs.

Any lymph gland that remains significantly enlarged for three weeks or longer without the presence of infection should be brought to the attention of a physician.

TREATMENT

X-ray is the treatment of choice for early Hodgkin's disease that is confined to one area of the body. In fact, evidence is strong that X-ray is curative in many such cases. Recent studies have shown that thirty to forty percent of patients with early localized Hodgkin's disease, treated by X-ray, are alive and well as long as fifteen years after treatment.

For the later, more-widespread phase of the disease, physicians use X-ray or nitrogen mustard and related drugs. Recently, different types of drugs, such as vinblastine and vincristine, obtained from the periwinkle plant, and others, are also proving useful. In addition, the use of combinations of these agents offers a new approach, which appears promising at this point. Treatment with X-ray or drugs reduces the size of tumors and relieves symptoms.

The cause of Hodgkin's disease, like that of most cancers, is unknown. Research is directed toward discovering its cause and improving methods of treatment. Some scientists believe that if drugs or vaccines are eventually found that can cure or prevent any cancer, their initial success will be against such malignancies as Hodgkin's disease, But, even today, as a result of modern therapy, patients with Hodgkin's disease may lead normal, productive lives for a number of years; and it is possible that in some individuals the disease may be completely eradicated.

See cancer.

Holger-Nielson method — one form of artificial respiration. The patient is placed on his stomach with his elbows bent and his hands placed under his head. To force air into the lungs, the patient's elbows are lifted. To expel air from the lungs, pressure is exerted on the patient's back.

See artificial respiration.

homeopathy — a method of treating diseases that involves giving the patient a minute dose of a drug that normally causes symptoms similar to his own. The theory behind homeopathy and the methods used were developed by Samuel Hahnemann (1755-1843).

hookworm disease — a disease caused by microscopic worms. Hookworms thrive in areas where winters are mild and the soil is moist and sandy. Typically, they are found in soil surrounding unsanitary outhouses. The most common way of getting hookworm disease is by walking barefoot on infected soil or by handling such dirt.

It is impossible to feel the microscopic worms entering the body through the skin. After they have entered the body, the patient may itch where they have pierced the skin and bored through, or he may notice an itchy sore. These sores are most likely to appear between or under the toes or on the hands around the fingers. This is often called ground or toe itch, but it is generally a sign of hookworm disease.

Once the hookworms are in the body, they are carried by the blood to the heart and then to the lungs. There they bore through the membranes and get into the bronchial tubes and are coughed up into the throat. Even if some are expectorated, others are swallowed. Those that are swallowed go down through the stomach to the intestines, where they stay.

True. to its name, the hookworm has hooks—sharp teeth or cutting plates in its mouth. It is with these that it clamps onto the intestines and sucks blood to nourish itself. Thus housed and fed, hookworms grow to adults that lay thousands of eggs daily. These pass out of the body in the waste and get onto the ground, where they soon hatch into small worms, and the circle starts all over again.

Hookworm disease makes a person listless and weak, even in mild cases. As a result, many people are called lazy, when actually they are victims of hookworm disease.

People suffering from it grow pale and frequently complain of indigestion. Their skin may be pasty-yellow, their gums and lips almost colorless. Their legs, abdomen, and face may become swollen. They often develop abnormal appetites for things such as paper, chalk, thread, clay, and dirt.

Hookworm disease is no respecter of age. It attacks both old and young. When one person in a family has hookworm disease, the chances are that other members have it too, since they are all exposed to the same insanitary environment. It spreads rapidly in schools and communities where toilet facilities are inadequate or lacking entirely. It is apt to be found in small rural towns that do not have sanitary sewage systems.

There are only two requirements for eradicating hookworm disease.

1. Replacement of unsanitary outhouses.
2. Treatment of infected persons.

hooping cough — *See whooping cough.*

hormones — complex chemicals produced by the endocrine glands of the body; when secreted into body fluids, they have a specific effect on other organs. In many instances, they produce effects in remote regions of the body.

See endocrine glands.

humerus — the long bone of the upper arm. It extends from the shoulder to the elbow.

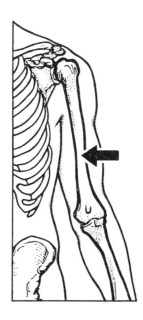

HUMERUS

Huntington's chorea — a rather rare inherited disease. The disease usually begins to manifest itself during middle age (forty to sixty), although it occasionally develops much earlier or later.

The symptoms include personality changes as well as jerky, twitching movements. The personality disorders can cover a very wide range: paranoia, obstinacy, moodiness, and euphoria.

As the disease progresses, both physical and mental processes become seriously impaired. There is no known prevention for Huntington's chorea. Once the symptoms have begun, there is no known effective treatment. Frequently the patient becomes unmanageable and has to placed in a mental hospital or a nursing home.

People whose parents or grandparents have had Huntington's chorea are usually advised not to have children in order to avoid passing on the disease to successive generations.

Hurler's disease — *See gargoylism.*

hydralazine hydrochloride — a drug that lowers blood pressure. An antihypertensive agent.

hydrocephalus — a condition that results from an abnormal collection of fluid within the cavities of the brain. In one type, the normal outlet channels

for this fluid are blocked. As a result, the fluid collects, enlarging the head and also pressing on the delicate brain tissue. Unless the pressure is relieved before permanent damage is done, mental retardation will result. Pressure may often be relieved through a shunt operation in which a tube is inserted to drain the excess liquid to other parts of the body where it can do no damage.

hydrogen peroxide — a strong antiseptic.

hydrophobia — *See rabies.*

hymen — the membrane that partially covers the opening of the vagina.

hyper — a prefix meaning too much or too high.

hypercholesteremia — an excess of a fatty substance called cholesterol in the blood.
See cholesterol

hypermetropia — *See hyperopia.*

hyperopia — farsightedness. A condition in which far vision is very good but near or close vision is poor because the focus of light rays is behind the retina. This is due to an abnormally short front-to-back diameter of the eye.

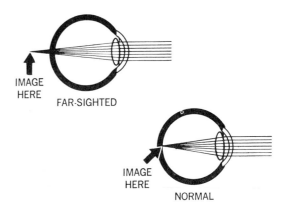

HYPEROPIA

hyperplasia — an abnormal increase of the number of normal cells. Hyperplasia is frequently the result of a hormone imbalance.

hypertension — a term used to describe blood pressure that is higher than the limits considered desirable. Generally speaking, hypertension is either primary or secondary.

Primary hypertension, the most common kind of high blood pressure, apparently is not related to any other disease and its cause is not known. Secondary hypertension is high blood pressure caused by an underlying disease.

In the early stages, an abnormal increase in blood pressure produces no permanent damage. If it is allowed to continue over a period of time, disease changes can usually be found in the small blood vessels. These may lead in time to damage of the larger vessels and the heart.

Treatment, which varies with causes and individual cases, may include surgery, drugs, weight reduction or other dietary restriction, or a combination of these.

Dietary treatment usually involves controlling calories to establish and maintain a desirable weight. Excess weight can be an added burden to an already overworked heart. Furthermore, the weight loss may be accompanied by a reduction in blood pressure.

Sodium restriction may also be prescribed in some cases of hypertension. However, dietary modification, like any other medical treatment, should not be self-prescribed and should be carried out under a physician's supervision.

See blood pressure.

hyperthyroidism — a condition in which the thyroid gland is overly active. This may eventually result in a speeded-up rate of heartbeat.
See thyroid.

hypertrophy — the enlargement of a tissue or organ owing to an increase in the size of its constituent cells. This may be caused by a deman for increased work.

hypnotic — any drug that induces sleep.

hypo — a prefix meaning too little or too low.

hypodermic — a term used to indicate the tissues under the skin. A hypodermic needle is used to inject medicines, blood, or nutritional fluids into the body.
See injection.

hypoglycemia — a condition in which the level of blood sugar is abnormally low or abnormally reduced. Hypoglycemia may be caused by many different factors. In the case of a diabetic, hypoglycemia is insulin shock resulting from an overdose of insulin or from an insufficient food intake. Other causes include infection, liver conditions, tumors, muscular exertion or overexertion, and pregnancy.

The symptoms begin with general weakness, sweating, hunger, dizziness, and trembling. If the attack continues, other symtoms appear. These may include emotional problems, slurred speech, convulsions, coma, and possibly even death. The treatment for an attack is usually limited to immediate intake of sugar to restore the blood-sugar level. However, the treatment of the condition requires careful dietary control.

hypotension — blood pressure that is below the normal range. This condition is commonly referred to as low blood pressure. The term is usually used to describe an acute fall in blood pressure such as occurs in shock.
See blood pressure.

hypothalamus — the part of the brain that exerts control over activity of the abdominal organs, water balance, temperature, etc. Damage to the hypothalamus can cause abnormal gain in weight, among other things.

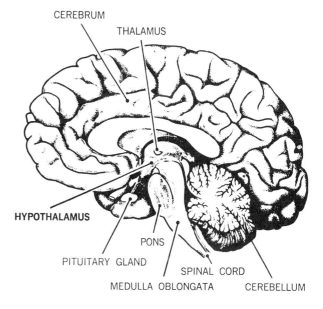

CEREBRUM
THALAMUS
HYPOTHALAMUS
PONS
PITUITARY GLAND
SPINAL CORD
MEDULLA OBLONGATA
CEREBELLUM

HYPOTHALAMUS

hypothermia — the deliberate lowering of the body temperature in order to slow the metabolic processes during surgery. In this cooled state, body tissues require less oxygen. Hypothermia is also referred to as hypothermy.

hypothyroidism — a condition in which the thyroid gland is underactive, resulting in the slowing down of many of the body processes, including the heart rate.
See thyroid.

hypoxia — a condition in which there is less than the normal content of oxygen in the organs and tissues of the body. At very high altitudes a healthy person suffers from hypoxia because of insufficient oxygen in the air that is breathed.

hysterectomy — the surgical removal of the uterus. Sometimes the ovaries and fallopian tubes are removed at the same time. This operation is usually performed when a woman has a history of fibroids.

i

iatrogenic — a term that literally means "caused by the doctor." A patient's belief that he has a disease or condition that is based solely on the physician's actions, manner, or other clues belongs in this category. An iatrogenic illness is based on the power of suggestion.

The term is also used to indicate any condition that follows or results from the treatment given a patient by a physician.

icthyosis — a skin condition in which the skin is dry, scaly, and rough.

ictus — *See stroke.*

ileitus — inflammation of the ileum.

ileum — the lower portion of the small intestine. *See intestine.*

iliac artery — a large artery that conducts blood to the pelvis and the legs.

immersion foot — a condition caused by exposure to cold water (50° F. and below) for twelve hours or more or to water of approximately 70° F. for several days. Inability to move about freely is also a contributing factor. These injuries are characterized by tingling and numbness, swelling of the legs and feet, bluish discoloration of the skin, and by blisters and pain.

The best treatment is to expose the affected areas to warm, dry air.

immunity — the body's ability to resist or overcome infection, whether it occurs naturally or is artificially induced.

Some of the greatest triumphs of medicine are closely associated with research on immunity, which has enabled physicians to protect people against a wide variety of bacterial and viral diseases.

It was long known that individuals recovering from diseases such as smallpox were nearly always safe from catching the disease again: they were immune. In the late 1700's Jenner observed that people infected by a mild disease, cowpox, were protected against a related disease, deadly smallpox. He put this knowledge to practical use by vaccinating a boy with pus from the hand of a dairymaid ill with cowpox. Eight weeks later Jenner inoculated the boy with smallpox, and no disease appeared.

In the nineteenth century Pasteur showed that killed or weakened forms of several types of bacteria and viruses, when injected into the body, could also produce protective reactions against subsequent exposure to disease-causing agents.

Research over the years has shown that an individual's ability to resist infection by bacteria or viruses is not expressed as an all-or-none reaction. Partial immunity to a specific agent is manifested by the development of mild disease or by infections that produce no recognizable symptoms. Such immunity, induced by deliberate exposure to many attenuated (weak) strains of agents, provides future protection against more-virulent strains.

TYPES

When an individual's own body provides im-

185

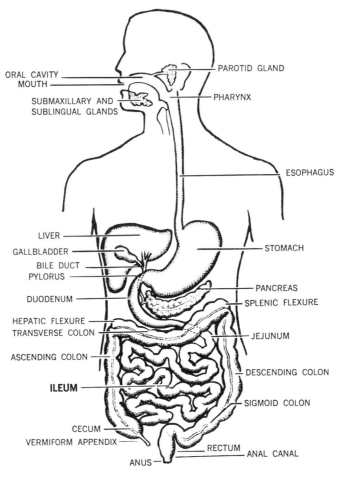

ILEUM

munity automatically, he is said to have a natural immunity to a specific disease. Some people can be exposed to an epidemic of diphtheria and not become infected. Others seem to have a natural immunity to measles. The difference between these individuals and people who do become infected is that in one case the body's own defensive system is protecting the individual, and in the other case the defensive system does not seem to have the proper defense.

There are two types of active acquired immunity. In one type, the person produces the antibodies (defensive agents) to defend the body. This often occurs after a person has had a particular disease—such as measles. In this type of immunity, one attack of the disease confers immunity against subsequent attacks. Another type of active acquired immunity is artificially induced. This is done by injecting the individual with weakened or dead bacteria or viruses. This

method is known as vaccination or immunization. The amount of bacteria or viruses is enough to force the body to develop antibodies against the injected substance but not strong enough to actually give the individual the disease. In this way the body is prepared to defend itself against the stronger form of the same disease.

Passive acquired immunity is obtained by injecting foreign antibodies into an individual. These antibodies usually come from an animal that has been vaccinated. This form of immunity is important in cases where an individual has already been exposed to a disease and needs immediate protection. Passive acquired immunity may be used against diseases such as tetanus and diphtheria.

immunization — the process of artificially conferring immunity to a specific disease. This usually involves injecting weak or dead organisms into the individual so that his body will develop antibodies to protect it against stronger forms of the same organisms. On occasion immunization involves injecting an animal's antibodies to help defend the individual.

See immunity.

impacted teeth — teeth that cannot grow properly because of the angle at which they are growing. The term is usually used in reference to the wisdom teeth. Impacted teeth must usually be extracted. However, because of their position, they cannot be pulled as easily as a normal tooth. The removal of impacted teeth is often a minor surgical procedure performed by a dentist or an oral surgeon.

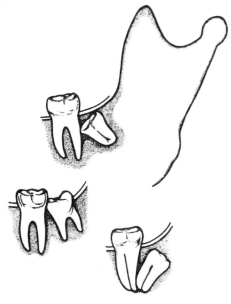

IMPACTED TEETH

impetigo — a very contagious skin infection. The disease usually starts on the face, with an itchy blister that oozes pus and then crusts over. The open sores look like a collection of blisters.

Impetigo spreads easily from one person to another and from one part of the body to other parts. The open sores contain germs that transfer the infection.

implantation — the attachment of the fertilized egg into the lining of the uterus. This happens between six and seven days after fertilization.

impotency — a lack of ability to perform sexual intercourse. The term is usually applied to a male.

Impotency can be caused by any number of physical problems, or is may be the result of a psychological problem.

incidence — the number of new cases of a disease developing in a given population during a specific period of time, such as a year.

incision — a wound made by a sharp cutting instrument such as a knife, razor, broken glass, etc. Incisions, commonly called cuts, tend to bleed freely, because the blood vessels are cut straight across. There is relatively little damage to the surrounding tissues. Of all classes of wounds, incisions are least likely to become infected, because the free flow of blood washes out many of the microorganisms (germs) that cause infection.

The term incision is also used to indicate a surgical stroke that cuts open part of the body.

incisor — *See teeth.*

incompetent valve — any valve that does not close completely and consequently allows blood to leak or flow back in the wrong direction. An incompetent valve is also called a valvular insufficiency.

incontinence — the lack of ability to control the bladder and/or the rectum. Incontinence is usually caused by a disease of or by injury to the nervous system. However, it may be caused by a problem within the affected organ.

incubation period — the usual amount of time that elapses between exposure to a disease and onset of the first symptoms. During the early incubation period of a contagious disease the patient is not usually contagious; however, toward the end of the incubation period he may be highly contagious.

The incubation period of a disease varies considerably. Bacterial diseases such as diphtheria usually have shorter incubation periods than do diseases, such as chickenpox, that are caused by viruses. The two major exceptions to this are the common cold and influenza.

The childhood diseases have fairly well-defined incubation periods. The incubation period for German measles may be two to three weeks but is usually eighteen days. Mumps may take eleven to twenty-six days but generally appears eighteen days after exposure. Between two and three weeks may elapse before chickenpox symptoms appear, but normally they arrive between thirteen and seventeen days after exposure. The incubation period for measles may be one or two weeks, but in most cases symptoms appear on the tenth or eleventh day.

incubator — a piece of equipment that is used to protect premature babies. An incubator provides a controlled environment in which the temperature and the humidity can be carefully controlled. The closed environment also helps to prevent the premature baby from being exposed to germs.

incus — *See anvil, ear.*

indigestion — a somewhat vague term used to indicate a wide variety of uncomfortable stomach symptoms. Flatulence, nausea, heartburn, and other similar symptoms are often classified as indigestion.

Indigestion may be a symptom of a serious disorder, or it may simply be caused by overeating. Indigestion frequently results from eating when emotionally upset or when rushed. At these times much of the blood leaves the digestive tract, as a result of strong emotion or for use by the muscles. Without a sufficient supply of blood, the digestive organs cannot perform properly. The result may be indigestion.

See dyspepsia.

infantile paralysis — *See poliomyelitis.*

infarct — an area of tissue that is damaged or dies as

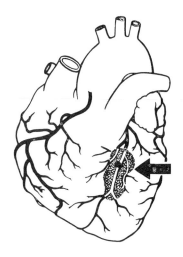

INFARCT

a result of not receiving a sufficient blood supply. The term is frequently used in the phrase "myocardial infarct," referring to an area of the heart muscle damaged or killed by an insufficient flow of blood through the coronary arteries that normally supply it.

infection — the invasion of the body by harmful microorganisms.

Any break in the skin or other body membrane (such as the mucous membrane that lines the nasal passages) is dangerous, because it allows microorganisms (germs) to enter the wound. Although infection may occur in any wound, it is a particular danger in wounds that do not bleed freely, wounds in which torn tissue or skin falls back into place and so prevents the entrance of air, and wounds that involve crushing of the tissues. Incisions, in which there is a free flow of blood and relatively little crushing of the tissues, are least likely to become infected.

Infections are dangerous in any part of the body but particularly so in the area around the nose and mouth. From this area infections spread very easily into the bloodstream, causing septicemia (blood poisoning), and into the brain, causing abscesses and infections there. Boils, carbuncles, and infected hair follicles just inside the nostril are perhaps the most common infections that occur in this area.

The general symptoms of infection include heat, redness, swelling, and pain around the wound or site of the infection. Pus is often (although not always) visible. If the infection is severe, there may be an increase of body temperature and swelling of the glands in the neck, armpit, or groin.

Infections are usually treated with antibiotics.

infectious hepatitis — *See hepatitis.*

infectious mononucleosis — an infectious disease. The major characteristic of infectious mononucleosis is constant fatigue. In addition, possible symptoms include fever (although this may be only a low, persistent fever), headache, sore throat, swollen glands, jaundice, and upset stomach.

One of the major problems with mononucleosis is the difficulty involved in proper diagnosis. Because the symptoms are fairly general, special tests must be made to diagnose infectious mononucleosis. The problem is further complicated because not all patients have the symptoms.

The incubation period for infectious mononucleosis is between five and fifteen days. Patients are contagious for two to four weeks, but, since the method of transmission is not clear, the amount of time a patient is contagious is sometimes difficult to gauge.

Infectious mononucleosis generally lasts anywhere from one to three weeks, but cases lasting two or three months are not uncommon. Occasionally, complications involving the liver develop. These complications can resemble hepatitis.

The treatment is almost always limited to bed rest and increased fluid unless complications develop. An attack of infectious mononucleosis usually confers lifetime immunity, but it is possible for a patient who has not been resting sufficiently to suffer a relapse.

inflammation — one of the body's natural defensive reactions. The classic symptoms of inflammation are redness, heat, pain, and swelling. Sometimes a loss of function in the inflamed area is also experienced.

When a part of the body is attacked by foreign organisms, the injured cells in the area release a substance called histamine. The histamine forces the blood vessels in the area to expand, thus increasing the flow of blood and fluid. This increase causes the redness, heat, and swelling. The additional fluid and swelling increase the pressure in the area and cause the pain associated with inflammation.

influenza — an infectious disease caused by a virus. There are several known main types of influenza virus. Each type has various strains, and each is somewhat different from the others. Sometimes new strains develop. These are very likely to cause epidemics, because people have had no experiences with them to help build up some degree of natural immunity against them. Because existing vaccines are ineffective against new virus strains, a special vaccine has to be developed, usually on short notice, to protect the susceptible population.

Single cases of influenza appear occasionally, but the disease usually occurs in epidemic form. People catch it from each other easily and develop symptoms quickly. During the first few days of an epidemic a large number of people in a community may come down with the disease. Cases build up rapidly, and the epidemic is usually over within a month. Epidemics may appear in a number of places in one country or throughout the world at the same time or closely following one another.

SYMPTOMS

Influenza attacks suddenly. The symtoms can be some or all of the following: fever, chills, headache, sore throat, cough, and soreness and aches in the back and limbs. Although the fever usually lasts only one to five days, the patient is often as exhausted or weakened as if he had gone through a long illness.

CAUSE

The viruses that cause influenza are so small that they can be seen only with powerful electron microscopes. The disease is acquired when these viruses get into the noses and mouths of people. When a person has influenza, or is just coming down with it, the fluids in his mouth and nose contain the viruses. They are most commonly passed to others through sneezing and coughing.

PRECAUTIONS

During an epidemic, when many people are becoming sick with influenza, the community air becomes laden with viruses. It is almost impossible to avoid getting in the path of a few coughs and sneezes. However, there are a few sensible precautions to take at such times. Practicing good health habits such as getting plenty of rest and eating regular, well-balanced meals will help keep up resistance to infection.

The only practical preventives known to medical science are the influenza vaccines. Vaccines that combine protection against the common strains are available.

Influenza is especially dangerous to people over sixty-five years of age, pregnant women, and persons of all ages who have chronic diseases such as those involving the heart, lungs, and kidneys and those that upset the body's normal chemical processes. Most of the deaths that follow epidemic waves of influenza occur in these people. People in these categories should discuss the advisability of the vaccines with their physicians.

TREATMENT

No known medicine will cure influenza. Sulfa, penicillin, and other antibiotics have no effect upon it, although they are used to combat some of the complications that may follow. Getting well without developing dangerous complications depends on giving the body every known advantage while it fights the influenza infection.

The best way to help the body is to get plenty of rest (in fact, bed rest is often recommended) and to stay warm.

injection — the introduction of a fluid (usually a medicine) into the body by means of a needle. The fluid can be injected into the muscles (intramuscular), into the subcutaneous tissue (hypodermic or subcutaneous), into a vein (intravenous), etc.

inner ear — *See ear.*

innominate artery — one of the largest branches of the aorta. It rises from the arch of the aorta and divides to form the right common carotid artery and the right subclavian artery.

inoculate — the deliberate introduction of a mild form of a disease into the body in order to develop antibodies against the disease.
See immunity, vaccination.

insect bites and stings — the injection of a toxic substance into the body by an insect.

Many insects bite or sting, but few are poisonous in the sense that their bite or sting can cause serious symptoms of itself. However, there are insects that do transmit diseases; these insects act as hosts to an organism or virus of diseases. For example, certain types of mosquitoes transmit malaria, yellow fever, and other diseases; certain types of ticks transmit spotted or Rocky Mountain fever; and certain types of biting flies transmit tularemia or rabbit fever.

Occasionally, stinging or biting insects have been feeding on or in contact with poisonous substances, and at the time of the sting or bite such substances may be injected into or come in contact with the wound thus made, causing a poisoned or infected wound.

The stings of bees, wasps, yellow jackets, and hornets and the bites of mosquitoes, ticks, fleas, and bedbugs usually cause only local irritation and pain in the region stung or bitten. Moderate swelling and redness may occur, and some itching, burning, and pain may be present.

Treatment usually consists of removing the stinger if it is left in the wound. Then a weak ammonia solution should be applied.

The effects of stings and bites of spiders, centipedes, tarantulas, and scorpions in some instances are much more severe than those of insects mentioned previously. They may cause alarming symptoms but, except for bites of tarantulas and black-widow spiders, seldom prove fatal.

The black widow is a moderately large, glossy, black spider with very fine hairs over the body, giving it a silky appearance. On the underside of the abdomen is a characteristic red or crimson marking in the form of an hourglass. Only the female is poisonous; the male, which is much smaller, is harmless.

The symptoms of the more poisonous insects' stings or bites are one or two small, pinpoint punctures of the skin, local swelling, and redness, with a smarting, burning pain. The swelling, redness, and pain increase rapidly; prostration, sweating, nausea, and pain in the back, shoulders, chest, and limbs develop within a few hours. In most instances the constitutional symptoms are mild and subside within six to twelve hours, but occasionally they are severe and end in collapse.

Treatment for these bites and stings may require medical attention.

insomnia — the inability to sleep. Insomnia may be caused by external sources such as noise, an unfamiliar bed, excessive heat or cold, etc. Pain can also cause insomnia. Surprisingly, being too tired (either mentally or physically) can also interfere with getting to sleep.

Overstimulation from coffee and tea keep some people awake. One of the most common causes of insomnia is emotional upset.

Physicians try to cure the cause of insomnia rather than try to cure the insomnia itself.

insufficiency — incompetency. In the term valvular insufficiency, it means an improper closing of the valves, which admits a backflow of blood in the wrong direction. In the term myocardial insufficiency, it means the inability of the heart muscle to do a normal pumping job.

insulin — a hormone formed in the islets of Langerhans of the pancreas. Insulin helps convert sugar into energy that can be used or stored. When there is a lack of insulin or the body is not using insulin properly, unused sugar collects in the blood. This condition is called diabetes.

Before the discovery of insulin in 1921, people with diabetes had very little hope. However, today a diabetic is given insulin taken from the pancreas of animals in order to bring the body's supply up to normal.

See diabetes, diabetes mellitus.

interatrial septum — the muscular wall that divides the left and right upper chambers of the heart, which are called atria. The interatrial septum is also called the auricular septum, interauricular septum, or the atrial septum.

See heart.

internal bleeding — bleeding within the body.

See hemorrhage.

intertrigo — an acute skin irritation and inflammation. Intertrigo is caused by two skin surfaces rubbing together. The friction is complicated by moisture or perspiration. Consequently, more cases occur in the summer than during cooler times of the year. This condition is found most frequently in people who are very overweight.

interventricular septum — the muscular wall, thinner at the top, that divides the left and right lower chambers of the heart, which are called ventricles. The interventricular septum is also known as the ventricular septum.

See heart.

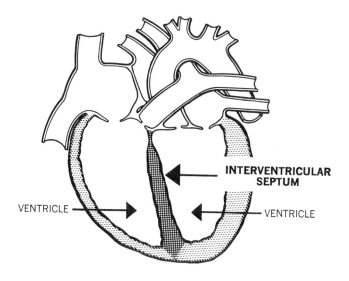

INTERVENTRICULAR SEPTUM

intestine — the bowels. The part of the alimentary tract from the pyloric opening of the stomach to the anus.

The intestines are composed of two major parts: the small intestines and the large intestines. The names "small" and "large" refer to the diameter of the tubes. In a living body, the small intestine is only five or six feet long. However, after death, the contraction relaxes, and it becomes apparent that the small intestine is actually about twenty-two feet long. In contrast, the large intestine is only five feet long.

The intestines finish the digestive process begun in the stomach and prepare the waste products for excretion from the body.

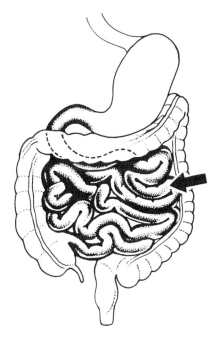

INTESTINE

SMALL INTESTINE

The small intestine begins as a short curve called the duodenum. This section of the small intestine receives the partially digested semiliquid food (called chyme) from the stomach. In the duodenum (which is about ten inches long) additional digestive juices are added to the chyme, as well as secretions from the pancreas and bile from the liver (or from the gallbladder, where bile is stored).

The next nine feet of the small intestine are known as the jejunum. This is followed by approximately twelve feet of small intestine known as the ileum. Most sugars, amino acids, and fats are absorbed as well as digested in the small intestine. Part of this digestion-absorption process is carried on by the villi—small finger-like projections that occur throughout the small intestine.

LARGE INTESTINE

The large intestine has three major sections: the ascending colon, the transverse colon, and the descending colon. These three sections designate the three geographic positions of the doorway-shaped large intestine. The large intestine receives the fluids and waste products from the small intestine. During the passage this material makes through the large intestine, the water is absorbed, and the material is prepared for excretion through the rectum.

The transfer between the small and large intestine takes place at the cecum, the first part of the large intestine. The cecum, at its lowest end, is actually a blind pouch. Attached to this "dead end" is the appendix.

The material moves up the ascending colon, across the transverse colon, and down the descending colon to the rectum.

The material, now called feces, is excreted through the anus, or rectal opening. The passage through the full length of the colon takes about twelve hours. During this passage, the bacteria in the large intestine ferment some of the remaining food. This decomposition process is responsible for the formation of the gases that give excretions an odor.

intima — the innermost layer of a blood vessel.

intussusception — a condition in which a segment of the intestine will fold in on itself, cutting off the passageway. Intussusception occurs more frequently in babies than in adults or in older children.

The baby will scream in pain and pull up his legs. When the pain goes away, though, he seems well or possibly pale and listless. Pain may return, next time with vomiting. The bowel movement, when it occurs, may be dark with blood. The condition requires immediate medical attention.

in vitro — a term used to indicate a phenomenon studied outside a living body under laboratory conditions. In vitro literally means "in glass," hence in a laboratory vessel.
See in vivo.

in vivo — a term used to indicate a phenomenon studied in a living body or in a living organism.
See in vitro.

iodine — a naturally occurring mineral that is necessary for the proper functioning of the thyroid gland. People who live away from the seacoast in areas where the soil is low in iodine sometimes fail to get an adequate supply of this mineral. Getting too little iodine can cause, goiter, a swelling of the thyroid gland.

Iodized salt and seafoods are reliable sources of iodine. Regular use of iodized salt is the most practical way to assure enough iodine in the diet.

ionizing radiation — radiation that tears molecules apart, leaving their fragments electrically charged. This type of radiation may cause both physical and genetic damage to the human body. Despite the possible dangers, ionizing radiation is being explored as a possible treatment for certain kinds of cancer.

ipecac — a drug used as an emetic (causing vomiting). It works by irritating the gastrointestinal tract. Ipecac has been used for centuries, originally in the treatment of diarrhea.

Ipecac is used in syrup form to induce vomiting following poisoning.

iris — the circular, pigmented membrane behind the cornea, which surrounds the pupil. The iris is responsible for controlling the size of the pupil. The iris is also the part of the eye that has color (brown, blue, or green).
See eye.

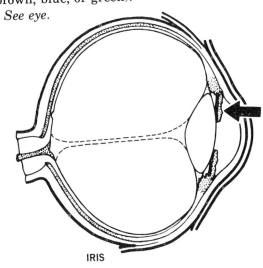

IRIS

iron — a metallic element that is needed by the body in relatively small but vital amounts. Iron combines with protein to make hemoglobin, the red substance of blood that carries oxygen from the lungs to body cells and removes carbon dioxide from the cells. Iron also helps the cells obtain energy from food.

Because of the normal monthly blood loss (menstruation), women need twice the amount of iron that men do.

Only a few foods contain much iron. Liver is a particularly good source. Lean meats, heart, kidney, shellfish, dry beans, dry peas, dark-green vegetables, dried fruit, egg yolk, and molasses also count as good sources. Whole-grain and enriched bread and cereals contain smaller amounts of iron, but when eaten frequently they become important sources.

irritants — substances that do not directly destroy the body tissues but cause inflammation in the area of contact. Some examples are zinc sulfate, iodine, and phosphorus.

When swallowed, irritants cause faintness, nausea, vomiting, and diarrhea. The vomited matter and stools frequently contain blood. There is also pain in the abdomen.

ischemia — a local, usually temporary, deficiency of blood in some part of the body. Ischemia is often caused by a constriction or an obstruction in the blood vessel supplying that part of the body.

islets of Langerhans — groups of specialized cells scattered throughout the pancreas. These special cells produce insulin.
See insulin, pancreas.

isotope — a term applied to one of two elements, chemically identical, but differing in some other characteristic, such as radioactivity. Radioactive isotopes are often used in medicine to help trace the course of substances in the body.

itch — *See scabies.*

j

Jacksonian seizure — a type of focal seizure caused by some types of epilepsy. It is the result of overactive nerve cells in the part of the brain that controls the movement of muscles. The seizure usually begins in the fingers or toes of one hand or foot, or sometimes in the corner of the mouth. The affected part trembles violently or perhaps becomes numb. As more nerve cells become affected, the trembling or numbness spreads. It may stop as suddenly as it began, or it may spread to the other side of the body. When the seizure spreads, the patient loses consciousness and has an attack similar to grand mal (another type of epilepsy).

See epilepsy.

jaundice — a yellow tinge, usually first noticeable in the white part of the eyes, but also giving a yellow cast to the skin.

Jaundice is the result of an excess of bile (which has a dark-yellow color) in the blood. There are several possible reasons for the excess of bile. Sometimes the blood is affected by disease (such as some types of anemia) and cannot absorb the increased bile. Occasionally the bile ducts themselves are blocked. Another type of jaundice occurs in newborn babies within a few days after birth. The yellow color shows that the baby's body is discarding the extra supply of red blood cells that were needed before the baby was breathing air. The red blood cells release a yellow pigment when they die off, and this colors the tissues for a time.

jaw — the two principal bones that form the mouth.

The bone of the upper jaw is the maxilla. The bone of the lower jaw is the mandibula.

jejunum — the part of the small intestine between the duodenum and the ileum.

See intestine.

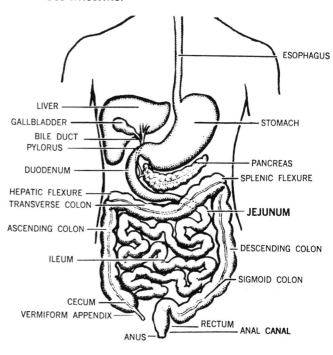

JEJUNUM

Jenner, Edward — English physician (1749-1823) who was the first to observe the process of immunity and to put the principle behind it into practice.

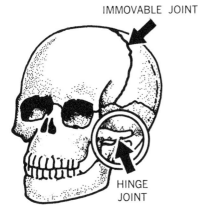

IMMOVABLE JOINT

HINGE JOINT

SKULL

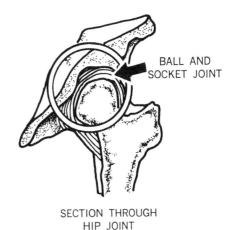

BALL AND SOCKET JOINT

SECTION THROUGH HIP JOINT

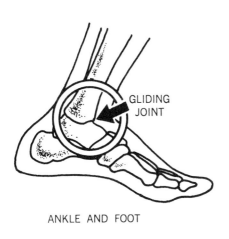

GLIDING JOINT

ANKLE AND FOOT

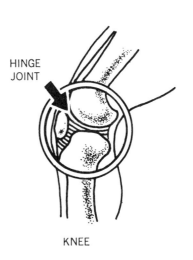

HINGE JOINT

KNEE

JOINTS

Jenner noticed that people who recovered from smallpox never got that disease again. He also noticed that people who had cowpox (a mild form of smallpox) never contracted smallpox. He tested his observations by vaccinating a boy with cowpox and then deliberately exposing the boy to smallpox. When no smallpox appeared, his theory was confirmed.
See immunity.

jerk — a reflex action, a sudden involuntary muscular movement.

joint — the place where two or more bones or cartilage come together. There are several types of joints, but there are two major classifications: immovable joints, such as the bones in the head; and movable joints, such as the elbow.

MOVABLE JOINTS
Movable joints are protected against friction by cartilage and by special fluids. The fluid is contained in small pockets or bursae. If the cartilage or bursae are injured or diseased, movement in the joint is limited and very painful. There are

195

four types of movable joints in the human body.

1. The ball-and-socket joint includes a rounded end of bone that fits into a pocket, or socket, of another bone. The joints between the thighbone and the hip and between the upper arm and the shoulder are ball-and-socket joints.

2. A hinge joint unites two bones in an arrangement similar to a door hinge, allowing movement chiefly within an up-and-down or back-and-forth area. Examples of hinge joints are the elbow and the knee.

3. A pivotal joint, such as in the lower arm, is one in which one bone rolls or rotates over another bone.

4. A gliding joint permits two bones to slide or glide over each other. The ankle and wrist are two examples of gliding joints.

jugular veins — veins that return blood from the head and neck to the heart.

k

kala-azar — an infectious disease transmitted by the sandfly, which bites man and transfers the microbes. Symptoms include fever, anemia, and spleen and liver involvement. Cases of kala-azar are usually limited to West Africa, India, Brazil, and similar locales.

kanamycin — a broad-spectrum antibiotic. Kanamycin occasionally produces a hearing loss.
See antibiotics.

keratin — the protein that is the principal component of nails, hair, and epidermis.

keratitis — inflammation of the cornea.
See cornea.

kernicterus — a condition of severe mental retardation that results from a blood incompatability involving the Rh blood factor.

Sometimes the blood of a pregnant woman will start to build up immunity against any conflicting blood type of her unborn child. A couple who have a potential blood conflict can have from one to five normal children before the increasing blood-sensitivity of the mother threatens to cause kernicterus in her child.

This disorder used to be responsible for an estimated one percent of the severely retarded in institutions; yet it can usually be prevented by treatment. Through repeated blood transfusions for the baby before or at birth, the exchange transfusions can wash out the hostile sensitized blood before brain damage occurs.

Rh-negative mothers may become sensitized to Rh-positive blood from having an Rh-positive baby, an Rh-positive miscarriage, or an accidental Rh-positive blood transfusion.
See Rh factor.

kidneys — two small but vital organs of the human body. A little larger than a man's fist and roughly bean-shaped, the kidneys lie in the small of the back on each side of the spine. They remove waste products from the blood and regulate the amount of water and the delicate balance of chemical substances in the body. These intricate functions are absolutely essential to human life. The kidneys also assist in regulating the production of red blood cells, which carry vital oxygen from the lungs to all parts of the body, and in maintaining normal blood pressure. The life of every human being depends as much on his kidneys as on his lungs or his heart.

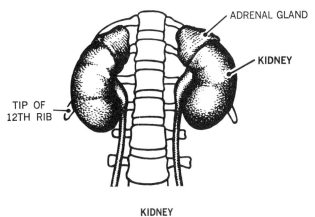

KIDNEY

While an individual normally has two kidneys, one of every one thousand persons is born with only one. Many others have had one of their kid-

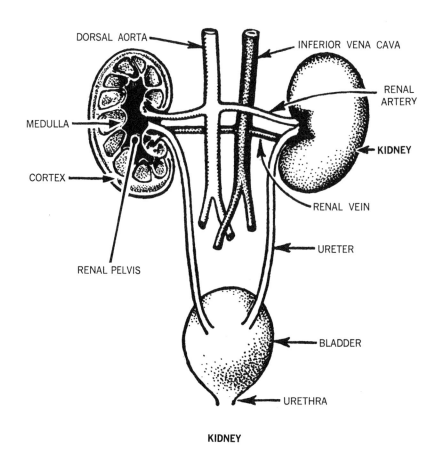

KIDNEY

neys removed for medical reasons or for donation to other kidney patients. People with a single kidney (which usually grows large and does the work of two) have no difficulty or restrictions as long as the kidney remains healthy.

About nineteen gallons of blood pass through the kidneys every hour. On the average, a person's entire blood supply is filtered through the kidneys twenty to twenty-five times per day. Within the outermost layers (the cortex) of the kidney the blood passes through an intricate network of arteries. These arteries grow progressively smaller, ending in microscopic units called nephrons.

A single kidney contains almost a million nephrons, each of them part of a filtering system that removes fluid containing waste products brought from all parts of the body by the blood. This is the first step in the complex function of the kidneys.

This waste-carrying fluid, called filtrate, is still rich in minerals and protein. Passing from the nephrons into an arrangement of coiled tubes, most of the filtrate and its essential min-

erals and proteins are absorbed back into the blood. This process takes place in the medulla.

The liquid remaining after these two steps have been completed is called urine. Urine collects in a pouch called the pelvis in the center of the kidney. From each kidney a tube called a ureter carries the urine to the bladder, where it is stored until it is discharged through another tube, the urethra. The entire system is called the urinary tract.

The kidneys are hard-working organs. The average man forms more than 180 quarts of filtrate every day. During passage through the coiled tubes, all but one and a half quarts are absorbed back into the blood.

DISEASES

Many diseases of different types attack the kidneys. Depending on its type, a particular kidney disease may begin by damaging the arteries bringing blood into the kidney, or the nephrons, or the coiled tube system, or other parts of the kidney. Some diseases attack several parts of the kidney at once. Kidney disease may involve one or both kidneys.

While there are several ways of grouping kidney diseases, the following are the major types:

1. Infections
Kidney infections are usually caused by bacteria. Most kidney infections are grouped under the name pyelonephritis. Kidney infection may result from infection of other parts of the urinary tract, or the blood may carry infection to the kidneys from other parts of the body. Infectious kidney diseases must be treated carefully. Inadequate treatment may mask the symptoms while the destructive process continues.

2. Hypersensitivity states
Normally, the body reacts to bacteria, viruses, and any other foreign matter by producing antibodies that attack and neutralize the foreign material, which is then passed harmlessly out of the body. In one of the most common kidney diseases, glomerulonephritis, it is thought that antibodies formed following a streptococcal infection of the throat or another part of the body are responsible, in some way not yet understood, for kidney damage. A number of other kidney diseases also appear to be caused by hypersensitivity states.

3. Birth defects and hereditary diseases
The exact number of children born with defects of the urinary tract is not known, but such disorders may be the most common type of birth defect. One of the more common of these is a narrowing of the ureter and urethra, which may cause damage—by restricting the flow—or prevent normal kidney development.

Some urinary-tract birth defects are serious and will cause difficulty, while others may have no noticeable effect. Many urinary-tract birth defects allow infections to develop very easily. It is especially important to detect these abnormalities, so that patients who have them can be watched closely for any sign of urinary-tract infections.

There are several kidney diseases that are inherited, the most common being polycystic kidneys. Here, cysts are present in the kidneys at birth and grow as the individual matures, eventually affecting kidney function.

4. Circulatory conditions
Cases of severe hypertension, or high blood pressure, which may cause or be caused by kidney disease, often result in kidney failure. The other circulatory problems related to kidney disease are not very common.

5. Tumors
Benign and malignant tumors may occur at any point along the urinary tract, including the kidney itself. Even benign tumors are dangerous, because they may obstruct the normal production and elimination of urine.

6. Metabolic diseases
Diabetes, gout, and other metabolic diseases usually involve the kidneys. Kidney stones and other obstructions, such as enlarged prostate glands, may stem from metabolic disturbances. Any obstruction of the urinary tract, if not relieved, may lead to destruction of the kidneys.

7. Injuries
In addition to injury due to blows, there are various substances such as dry-cleaning fluid and antifreeze that, if swallowed or inhaled, are poisonous to the kidneys and may seriously injure them.

FREQUENCY
Kidney disease occurs in all age groups. A large number of cases appear in persons between the ages of fifteen and fifty-four. An estimated 3,300,000 Americans harbor infectious organisms in their urinary tracts. A significant number of these persons will have no symptoms of their disease until kidney damage is far advanced. Kidney disease is unlike the majority of chronic diseases, because it so often disables during the middle, productive years of life. Because of this the social and economic impact of kidney diseases is much greater than mere numbers of cases show.

SYMPTOMS
Kidney disease may appear in either of two forms—acute or chronic. Acute kidney disease is sudden and abrupt in onset and is usually easily identified. Chronic kidney disease may be much more difficult to detect. More often than not there are no symptoms at all until irreversible damage has been done to the kidneys. Such cases are discovered only during physical examinations, which should include an analysis of a urine specimen. The urine specimen should be cultured for signs of infection. Symptoms that do appear

are many and varied, and many seem to indicate conditions other than kidney disease, especially stomach trouble.

A physician should be consulted immediately if there is:

1. Frequent urination.
2. Burning during urination.
3. Dark or bloody urine.
4. Facial swelling.
5. Pain in the small of the back.

Certain other more general symptoms, such as unexplained headaches or constant fatigue, may also be signs of kidney disease.

DIAGNOSIS

Because kidney damage can become quite severe while symptoms are absent or vague, several tests have been devised to help detect such damage.

Examination of a urine sample may reveal abnormal cells or a protein (albumin) not normally found. Blood tests can indicate inadequate removal of waste products by the kidneys. Chemical tests of many of the individual functions of the kidney are available and can help to pinpoint the location and amount of damage.

X-rays help in diagnosing certain types of kidney disease. Various dyes can be administered to patients that cast shadows on X-ray film, outlining the structures of the urinary tract or the vessels leading to the kidney. Sometimes a biopsy (a tiny bit of kidney tissue that has been removed for examination under a microscope) is necessary for an exact diagnosis.

TREATMENT

If kidney diseases are detected early in their course, many treatments are available. Kidney infections respond to medications such as antibiotics or sulfa drugs. It is very important that infections be adequately and completely treated to prevent their becoming chronic and progressively destructive. Some kidney diseases resulting from hypersensitivity can be treated with steroid drugs. Surgical correction of birth defects and obstructions can eliminate the pressure that builds up behind such blocks. Stones may pass unaided in the urine or may have to be removed surgically. For many persons who already have an irreversible impairment of their kidney function, close attention to diet and fluid intake may permit relatively normal lives.

In the past, the patient whose kidney disease had progressed, either undetected or despite treatment, to kidney failure, faced death. Now two developments of modern medical research can preserve many of these patients' lives.

The first of these is dialysis, which cleanses the blood of impurities and helps to restore normal chemical balance. One type of dialysis, peritoneal dialysis, uses the lining of the patient's own abdomen as a filter to remove waste products from the body. The second type of dialysis, hemodialysis, employs an artificial kidney machine for the same purpose. Either type of dialysis may be used for the patient with acute kidney failure — where the inability of the kidney to function is sudden and may be temporary.

Hemodialysis is also very effective in chronic kidney failure, the result of long-term, progressive kidney destruction. Patients on hemodialysis are usually treated at artificial kidney centers two or three times each week. Plastic tubes permanently implanted in blood vessels in a patient's arm or leg are attached to the artificial kidney, and the machine cleanses the blood of waste products, enabling patients who have lost kidney function to live and carry on almost all normal activities. Hemodialysis is very expensive, however. In an effort to lower the cost, the Public Health Services' National Center for Chronic Disease Control is currently engaged in development of new methods of hemodialysis, including the use of artificial kidneys at home. At the same time the Artificial Kidney Program of the National Institute of Arthritis and Metabolic Diseases is working to lower the cost and improve the efficiency of artificial kidneys and the other equipment used in hemodialysis.

The other new development is kidney transplantation. It is now possible for a surgeon to implant a kidney from one individual to another. The limiting factor in this is that the body's natural defense system may recognize the new kidney as foreign tissue and destroy it.

Much research is devoted to solving this problem of rejection in kidney transplants. Tissue cross matching—identifying persons with similar tissue characteristics, somewhat in the way blood-typing identifies similar blood characteristics—may provide a way of avoiding kidney rejection. If the body's defense mechanism can be overcome by drugs or other methods, the transplantation of a healthy kidney can mean return to a completely normal existence for patients whose kidneys have been destroyed.

kinesthetic sensations — the electrical impulses sent to the central nervous system by the nerves in muscles. When the muscle is working, the nerves transmit the impulses that help the central nervous system and brain to establish the body's balance and position.

knee — the hinge joint between the thigh and the lower leg. The knee joins the femur (or thighbone), the patella (kneecap bone), and the tibia (one of the two bones of the leg).
See joint.

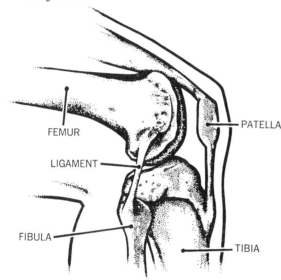

FEMUR

LIGAMENT

FIBULA

PATELLA

TIBIA

KNEE

knee — the patella
See knee.

Koch, Robert — German physician (1843-1910) whose pioneer work in bacteriology earned him the 1905 Nobel Prize.

His great contribution was his discovery that some bacteria cause diseases and that different bacteria cause different diseases.

Koplik's spots — small red spots with white centers that appear in the mouth before the appearance of the rash in measles. These spots are named for Henry Koplik (1858-1927), an American pediatrician.

K vitamin — *See Vitamin K.*

kwashiorkor — a syndrome or set of widely recognized symptoms caused by malnutrition, specifically a lack of protein and amino acids. The symptoms are slow or retarded growth, swelling, lack of resistance to disease, and diarrhea. In most cases, kwashiorkor can be cured by treating the patient (most cases occur among young children) with milk.

kyphosis — a condition in which the vertebral column (the spine) is abnormally curved in the chest area. This condition is sometimes referred to as hunchback.

I

labium — lips. Body tissues that have both inside and outside tissues.

labor — the process by which a child is delivered from his mother's body. Preparations for labor go on all during pregnancy. The muscles of the uterus tighten and relax. This process of tightening and then relaxing is called a contraction.

When labor begins, the contractions of the uterus become more and more frequent and intense. At first these contractions are fifteen or more minutes apart. The time between them gets shorter and shorter as labor progresses.

During pregnancy, the cervix (the narrow end of the uterus) softens and relaxes. By the time labor begins, it is thin and has opened to about one half to three quarters of an inch. A small amount of mucus is usually present in this opening as a sort of plug. As the baby is pushed against the cervix by the strong contractions of the uterus, this opening gradually gets larger until it is finally about four inches wide — big enough for the baby to pass through. As the cervix opens, the mucus plug comes loose and is discharged through the vagina. This usually means that labor will begin soon.

A sudden rush of water from the vagina means that the bag of waters surrounding the baby has broken. This may happen at the beginning of labor or not until just before the baby is born.

DURATION

The length of time spent in labor differs for every woman and for every pregnancy. Eight to fifteen hours of labor is an average for first children. Later babies may come more quickly, perhaps in four to eight hours. Women who have had a good diet and good care during pregnancy tend to have a shorter labor.

STAGES

Labor is divided into three stages. In the first stage, the contractions of the uterus stretch the opening at its lower end, the cervix. This allows the baby to move into the birth canal. In the second stage, the baby passes down through the birth canal and out through the vaginal opening. In the third stage, the placenta and membranes (the afterbirth) are loosened and expelled.

The first stage is the longest. During this stage, the contractions begin and grow increasingly frequent. The second stage, delivery, usually takes only an hour and a half to two hours with first babies. The strong muscles of the abdomen and the diaphragm begin to help the muscles of the uterus push the baby. The mother experiences a strong urge to push with each contraction.

The bony cavity in the center of the pelvis is normally filled with organs made of very soft tissues: the vagina, the uterus, the rectum, the bladder and the tube from the bladder, the urethra. During pregnancy the uterus and the bladder are pulled up out of the way into the abdomen. The tissues of other organs become softer, and the joints in the pelvic bones become more flexible.

During labor, the vagina stretches enough to allow the baby through, pressing the urethra and rectum flat against the walls of the bony cavity. The doctor often enlarges the exit by making a small cut, called an episiotomy, in the vaginal opening. This is done when the doctor feels the tissues might tear as the baby comes through the vagina. This cut heals better than a tear would. It is closed with a few stitches after the baby is born. An episiotomy is more likely to be necessary with first babies than with later babies. Some doctors do this routinely because the stitches give the pelvic organs more support.

The third stage of labor begins when the placenta starts to separate from its attachment to the lining of the uterus. In a short time, usually five minutes or less, the muscle wall of the uterus contracts once more, and the placenta and the membranes are expelled. There is usually a moderate amount of blood passed with the afterbirth from the place where the placenta was attached, but this bleeding soon becomes slight.

labyrinth — a complex of connecting canals and /or cavities, such as the inner ear.

lac — milk.

laceration — a wound that is torn, rather than cut. Lacerations have ragged, irregular edges and masses of torn or mashed tissue underneath. These wounds are usually made by blunt rather than sharp objects. A wound made by a dull knife, for instance, is more likely to be a laceration than an incision. Many of the wounds caused by accidents with machinery are lacerations, although they are often complicated by crushing of the tissues as well.

These wounds, in which the blood vessels are torn or mashed, do not bleed as freely as wounds produced by sharp cutting edges. Lacerations are frequently contaminated with dirt, grease, or other foreign matter that is ground into the tissues; they are therefore very likely to become infected.

lacrimal — of or pertaining to tears or the tear glands.

lactation — the production of milk in the breasts. True milk is not released for at least three days after the birth of a baby. Colostrum, the liquid secreted by the breasts during the first few days, is rich in protein and nourishes the baby until the milk is formed.

lactose — milk sugar. A simple sugar composed of glucose and galactose.

Laennec, Rene Theophile Hyacinthe — French physician (1781-1826) who invented the stethoscope. This device allowed physicians to listen to the sounds within the body, especially to the sounds of the heart and lungs, and to help determine the physical condition of those organs.

Landsteiner, Karl — Austrian-born physician (1868-1943) who won the Nobel Prize in 1930 for his discovery and description of blood groups or types. He was also one of the discoverers of the Rh factor in the blood.

In 1900 he discovered that all human blood is not alike. Landsteiner took blood from a number of persons, separated the red cells from the plasma, and placed the cells and plasma of each person in separate test tubes. Then he took the red blood cells of one person and mixed it with the plasma of another.

He found that the cells and plasma in some tubes remained mixed. In other tubes the cells separated from the plasma and settled to the bottom in a solid cluster or clump. By observing which plasma-cell combination clumped, he was able to divide his mixtures into four different groups or blood types: A, B, AB, and O.

In 1940 Dr. Landsteiner and Dr. Weiner of New York discovered the Rh factor in human blood. They found that about eighty-five percent of the population have this factor. People who have this factor in their blood are known as Rh-positive. The remaining fifteen percent of the population whose blood does not contain the Rh factor are known as Rh-negative.

See Rh factor.

lanolin — wool fat. Lanolin is obtained from the wool of sheep and is used as a base for many salves and ointments that are used on the surface of the skin.

laryngectomy — the surgical removal of the larynx. After this operation is performed, most patients can learn to speak again through a technique known as esophageal speech. This substitute speech is produced by expelling swallowed air from the esophagus. A well-trained and practical esophageal voice produces intelligible speech of surprisingly good quality. There are mechanical devices available for those patients who are unable to learn to use this type of speech.

See larynx.

laryngitis — an inflammation of the larynx (voice box). The primary symptoms of laryngitis are hoarseness and a changed (usually strained sounding) voice. Other symptoms may be a tickling in the throat, a sore throat, and a cough.

Laryngitis can be caused by a number of factors. It may follow an infection in the respiratory tract, or it may be a part of another disease such as syphilis or measles. Laryngitis may also be caused by abusing the voice, excessive smoking, breathing unclean air, etc. Additionally, laryngitis can be a symptom of a tumor.

Treatment depends on what is causing the laryngitis.

See larynx.

larynx — the passageway connecting the pharynx and trachea (windpipe). It produces the voice and consequently is also called the voice box.

The larynx is shaped like a tube. It has nine cartilages. One of these, the epiglottis, is responsible for covering the opening of the larynx when the mouth is in the process of swallowing. This closing or lid action prevents foreign material from entering the larynx and eventually reaching the lungs.

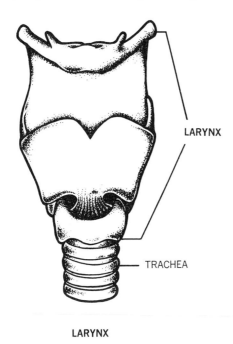

LARYNX

There are two pairs of folds in the larynx, but only the vocal folds (also called the true vocal cords) are involved in the production of vocal sound. The area between the vocal folds is known as the glottis.

Sound is produced when air, passing up out of the lungs through the glottis, causes a vibration in the vocal folds. The vibration is controlled by the de-

gree of tension in the folds. A whisper requires less tension than a shout does.

The sound coming from the larynx bears little resemblance to the vocal sounds normally associated with everyday speech. The sound produced in the larynx is filtered and amplified through other parts of the body, such as the mouth and nasal cavities.

The size of the larynx is about the same in children of both sexes. However, during puberty, the size of a male's larynx changes. In addition to growing larger, the vocal folds thicken and lengthen. This changes the pitch enough that a male's voice is generally deeper than a female's voice.

Lassa fever — a viral infection found in West Africa. Lassa fever causes very high fevers (up to 107°) and severe muscular pain. The fatality rate is high, because the virus kills faster than the body can defend itself.

laxative — any drug or agent that promotes excretion of solid wastes.

See purgative.

lead poisoning — a disease caused by the ingestion of substances containing lead. Studies indicate that children between one and three years of age are the most common victims, although older children also get the disease. Lead poisoning results in damage to the nervous system. The degree of damage is related to the amount and duration of exposure to lead. Once a child has the disease, unless his environment is changed, chances are very high that he will again be a victim.

Lead poisoning is caused by consumption over a period of time (three to six months) of paint or plaster containing lead. The condition is frequently associated with pica, which is an abnormal appetite for nonedible substances. Children left for long periods of time in their rooms or cribs, with no stimulation, may occupy themselves by biting on windowsills, eating paint flakes from walls or ceilings, or gouging the wall and eating the plaster.

In the early stages, the existence of lead poisoning is often without marked symptoms. There may be vague, nonspecific symptoms common in children, such as stomach pain, constipation, vomiting, irritability, and twitching. Unless a high level of suspicion for lead poisoning exists in the physician's mind, the diagnosis may not be recognized. As the disease progresses, the symptoms become stronger, and an elevated amount of lead is found in the blood and urine.

As the child continues to eat paint or plaster, lead levels in the blood, tissues, and bones build up. Therapy is directed at reducing the concentration of lead by using drugs that purge the body of the offending substances through the urinary tract.

Until about 1940 lead paint was frequently used on the interior and exterior of houses. Consequently, high-risk areas for lead poisoning are older dwellings, which often have several coats of paint containing lead on walls, woodwork, window-sills, etc.

Leeuwenhoek, Antonj Van — Dutch microscopist (1632-1723) who, among other contributions, discovered the interwoven structure of the muscle fibers of the heart.

leg — the part of the body between the knee and the ankle. Two bones form the leg: the tibia and the fibula.

lens — *See eye.*

leprosy — an infectious disease caused by the microorganism *Mycobacterium leprae*. It is not very contagious—only an insignificant percentage of the people who have spent their lives working with leprosy patients have ever contracted it. The method by which it is transmitted is not known. However, most of the cases in the United States are from the southernmost states in the eastern and central portions of the country.

There are two major types of leprosy: nodular and neural. In nodular leprosy there are masses of nodules that cause distortions in other tissues. In neural leprosy the nerves are affected, frequently producing a numbness and loss of feeling in the affected area; this in turn can result in loss of tissue and bone.

The prognosis for patients with leprosy depends to a certain extent on the type of leprosy—patients with neural leprosy generally respond better to treatment than do patients with nodular leprosy.

In the past, all patients were required by law to live in leprosy colonies such as the National Leprosarium in Louisiana. Today, however, many patients can live normal lives while under a doctor's care. Part of this change is because of remarkable medical progress in the treatment of leprosy. Just as important, however, is the acceptance, on the part of the general public, of the fact that leprosy is a disease rather than a curse. Leprosy as it is known today is not the same disease as the Biblical leprosy.

The treatment for leprosy is primarily chemotherapy (treatment by drugs). The sulfone-class drugs are used with good results for many patients, although it may take up to five years to effect a cure in some types of leprosy. Another drug in use is dapsone. Scientists are working on still other drugs.

leptospirosis — a bacterial infection. Leptospirosis is known by various names, such as swineherd's disease, mud fever, and autumnal fever. It is also called Weil's Disease, after the man who first described the disease. Once considered rare, today it is found in all parts of the world. It is spread to man from animals. There is little evidence that the infection can spread from one person to another.

Animal carriers of the leptospirosis bacteria include: cattle, swine, sheep, goats, horses, mules, dogs, cats, foxes, skunks, racoons, wildcats, mongooses, rats, mice, and bats.

Leptospirosis bacteria infect the kidneys of animals and are shed through their urine. People can get the disease by swimming in water or walking on moist soil that contains the infected urine. Most frequently, however, people get the disease either by handling a sick animal or by handling the kidney and other infected tissues of an animal that has had leptospirosis. This is why the disease is most prevalent among farmers and other workers who handle animals and animal products. The leptospirosis organism enters the human body through the nose, mouth, eyes, or through a break in the skin.

SYMPTOMS

The onset of the disease is sudden, with fever, headache, chills, muscle pains, and sometimes nausea and vomiting. Jaundice, skin rashes, blood in the urine, and a stiff neck are other common symptoms.

Because of the numerous and varied symptoms, it is sometimes hard to distinguish this disease from other diseases, including non-paralytic polio, mumps, meningitis, typhoid fever, undulant fever, and influenza.

Most cases are quite mild, and the patient recovers in one to two weeks. When the infection is severe, however, the kidney, liver, or heart may be damaged, and death can result.

The symptoms in animals are usually similar to

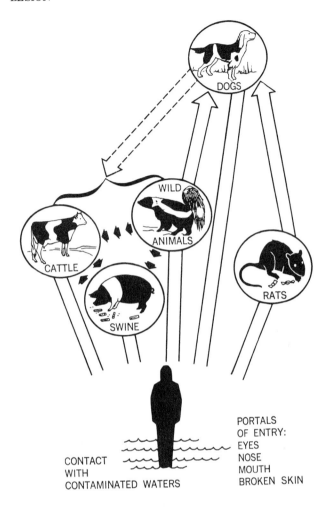

LEPTOSPIROSIS

leukemia — a fatal disease of the organs that manufacture blood, such as the lymph glands and bone marrow.

Normally, these organs manufacture only as many white and red blood cells as the body needs. In leukemia this blood formation gets out of control and there is a tremendous overproduction of white cells. The white cells do not mature, and they are not able to fight infection. The number of red cells is reduced, and the patient becomes anemic. The blood does not clot properly. Patients may thus die from infection, from hemorrhage, or from damage to vital organs.

The abnormal cells seen in leukemia resemble cancer cells in appearance and behavior. However, in leukemia the cells are present in the bone marrow and, in the majority of cases, in the blood, as well as in the tissues of the body. In other forms of cancer, the abnormal cells grow in the tissues only. Leukemia can develop at any age.

Scientists believe that several factors are involved in the development of leukemia. Recent studies show that radiation can produce the disease. Statistical surveys indicate that radiologists develop leukemia much more frequently than other people do. Also, an increased number of cases of leukemia has been found among those exposed to radioactive fallout from the atomic bomb blasts in Japan during World War II. These findings clearly establish radiation as one of the causes of human leukemia.

those in man but may be so slight that the illness is not detected. Infected dogs will sometimes continue to shed the leptospirosis organisms in their urine for a year or more after they have recovered from the disease. Therefore, people can be infected by an apparently healthy animal.

TREATMENT

If human infection is suspected, a physician should be called promptly and given a report of the patient's possible exposure to leptospirosis organisms. Although the best treatment for leptospirosis has not been clearly established, it is generally believed that certain antibiotic drugs, if given early, will shorten the course of the disease and lessen the severity of the symptoms.

lesion — any abnormal structural change in body tissues or organs.

SYMPTOMS

Leukemia can be chronic, acute, or subacute. There are two kinds of chronic leukemia. One begins in the bone marrow and the other in the lymphatic system. The bone-marrow type occurs most often in people thirty-five to forty-five years of age. The lymphatic type is found most frequently in those forty-five to fifty-four years of age. Chronic leukemia affects more men than women. It rarely occurs in children.

Chronic leukemia develops slowly, without warning. Many cases are discovered accidentally during examination for some other condition. Even after changes in the blood are noticed, several years may pass before significant symptoms appear in the body. One early change is an enlargement of the blood-forming organs, such as the spleen. As the spleen gets bigger, the patient may feel a sense of fullness or pain in the upper left side of the abdomen. Other symptoms may be sweating, skin eruptions, anemia, hemorrhages, nervousness, and loss of weight.

Acute leukemia most often affects children. It usually begins suddenly and progresses rapidly, often with a sore throat or other symptoms of a cold. The glands, spleen, and liver may enlarge rapidly. The child usually becomes pale and bruises easily. However, the beginning of acute leukemia can also develop slowly. In these cases pallor and bone pain are the main symptoms. Without treatment the patient lives only a short time—a few weeks or months.

Subacute leukemia has some of the characteristics of both chronic and acute leukemia. The course it follows is harder to predict.

Positive diagnosis of leukemia is made by microscopic study of the blood and bone marrow.

TREATMENT
Until recently there was little that could be done to change the course of acute leukemia. New hope has come with the use of certain drugs, with blood transfusions when necessary, and with antibiotics to help combat infections. While no cures have been reported, there have been encouraging temporary improvements with these new developments. Some patients are restored to apparently normal health for many months.

X-rays are widely used in the treatment of chronic leukemia, especially the type that originates in the bone marrow. It may relieve symptoms for a long time. Several drugs for treating chronic leukemia also have been found to give the same relief that X-ray treatment does.
See cancer.

leukocyte — a white blood cell.
See blood.

leukodermia — a condition in which there is a loss of skin pigment in certain areas of the body. The absence of pigment causes patches of very white skin.
See pigment, vitiligo.

leukoplakia — a condition, often caused by cigarette or pipe smoking, of white patches on the tongue, gums, or mucous membrane of the cheeks. When the irritant is removed, the patches usually disappear. However, the white patches can become malignant.

leukorrhea — a thick white or whitish discharge from the vagina.

levarterenol — one of the normal secretions of the adrenal glands. Levarterenol is also a prepared drug. It raises the blood pressure and is used to treat acute low blood pressure and shock.

lice — *See louse.*

ligament — a strong white band that helps to hold a bone in place. Ligaments extend from one bone to another and entirely around joints.

Ligaments are stretched or torn when a joint is forced to move beyond its normal turning point. This is called a sprain.
See sprain.

lightening — the time during the last month of pregnancy when the baby seems to be settling down or lowering himself in the mother's abdomen. It is more apparent with a first child. It means that the baby in the uterus is moving down a little into the bony canal of the pelvis to be in a better position when labor begins. This can sometimes happen so suddenly that it is startling.

limb — the general term for either an arm or a leg.

lingua — the tongue.

liniment — a liquid medicine that is applied to the surface of the skin. Liniments are usually oily.

linoleic acid — an important component of many of the unsaturated fats. It is widely found in oils from plants. A diet with a high linoleic acid content tends to lower the amount of cholesterol in the blood.

lipid — fat.

lipoprotein — a complex of fat and protein molecules.

Lister, Lord Joseph — British surgeon (1827-1912) who was the first to introduce antiseptic conditions to surgery and the operating room.

Before that time, a patient who needed surgery was in as much danger in the operating room as he was from his original illness. Lister started by using carbolic acid; later he used much weaker antiseptics that achieved the same purpose. He cleaned everything in the operating room that touched the patient. He even sprayed the air with carbolic acid. Finally he included carbolic acid in the patient's dressings. His discovery of the importance of antiseptic conditions did not gain immediate acceptance. However, today antiseptic operating rooms are one of the principle rules of surgery.

lithotomy — an operation to remove a stone from the bladder. The Hippocratic oath forbade physicians from performing this operation because it was supposed to be done by specialists. This is interpreted to mean that no physician should exceed the bounds of his capabilities or specialties.

litmus paper — a special, chemically prepared piece of paper that is used to test whether substances are acid or base. Acids turn blue litmus paper red; an alkali (base) will turn red litmus paper blue.

liver — the largest gland in the body. It is situated in the upper right part of the abdominal area below the diaphragm. The liver is composed of two major lobes: the right lobe and the left lobe. These lobes are divided by a cleft. The right lobe is made up of three sections: the right lobe proper, the quadrate lobe, and the caudate lobe. The liver is connected to the duodenum (the first part of the small intestine).

The liver secrets bile (a yellowish digestive juice) through the common bile duct into the duodenum. Bile is produced constantly. When

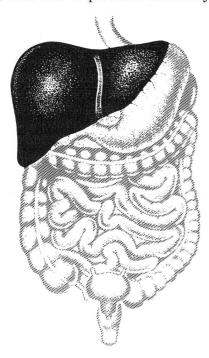

LIVER

the duodenum does not need it, the bile is secreted into the gallbladder, where it is stored until needed.

The liver performs many different functions. As mentioned above, it secrets bile. Additionally, the liver is involved in blood formation; in the production of clotting and anticoagulant agents; in storing proteins, fats, and other vital materials; and it is responsible for the neutralization of toxic substances.

lobectomy — a surgical operation to remove a lobe of the lung, liver, brain, etc.

local anesthetic — *See anesthesia, anesthetic.*

lochia — the discharge from the vagina that continues for a few weeks after childbirth. As the uterus grows smaller, clots of blood and tissue flow quite freely and contain a good deal of blood. The flow gradually subsides. At the end of the first week it has changed in color from bright red to dark red or brown. At the end of the second week it may be yellow or white, but it is not unusual for the dark discharge to persist for a while longer. Although this discharge from the vagina is often called menstruation, it is not.

lockjaw — *See tetanus.*

louse — a small parasitic insect. Lice are responsible for transmitting typhus fever, relapsing fever, and sometimes plague.

Three kinds of lice (the head louse, the body louse, and the pubic or crab louse) infest the human body. The names of the three types indicate the areas of the body on which each is usually found. Head and body lice look alike, but their habits are different. Lack of personal cleanliness is a common cause of infestation; however, any child or adult may inadvertently acquire an infestation by contact with infested people or articles.

While the lice themselves seldom cause serious trouble, the scratching they induce sometimes results in skin lesions and infections.

HEAD LOUSE

The head louse infests the hair of the head and causes itching and irritation of the scalp. A marked itching, particularly at the back of the head, which is the preferred nesting spot of this louse, should make one suspect its presence. Nits (or eggs) are usually abundant and can be easily detected. They are small, grayish bodies that first appear near the scalp but later are found on all parts of the hair. Although the head louse infests persons of all ages, children, and especially girls, because of their longer hair, are most apt to become infested.

BODY LOUSE

Unlike the head louse, the body louse does not ordinarily dwell on the body, but in the seams of undergarments and other clothing. Routine laundering or dry cleaning of clothing will, in large part, prevent louse infestation.

The louse feeds by sucking blood from the body, and it leaves minute blood specks on the skin, particularly around the neck, back, and abdomen or whatever part of the body is near clothing seams. The bites are irritating and cause severe itching. In long-standing cases, the skin becomes rough, red, and covered with scabs from scratching.

PUBIC OR CRAB LOUSE

The pubic or crab louse usually fastens itself to the hairs of the genital region, but is occasionally found in the eyebrows and in the hair of the armpits. Its nits look much like the nits of head lice and are glued to the hair. In feeding on the body, the pubic louse often leaves a tiny bluish or slate-colored stain just under the skin in the region of the chest, thighs, or abdomen. Severe itching is the characteristic symptom. Pubic louse infestations are especially common when people live or work under crowded conditions. They are acquired through personal contact—often with members of the opposite sex—or through contact with infested furniture or other articles.

LSD — lysergic acid diethylamide, a powerful man-made chemical usually referred to by its initials, LSD. It was first developed in 1938 from one of the ergot alkaloids. Ergot is a fungus that grows as a rust on rye, a common grain plant. LSD is so powerful that a single ounce is enough to provide 300,000 of the average doses.

Legally classed as a hallucinogen, a mind-affecting drug, LSD is noted mainly for producing strong and bizarre mental reactions in people and striking distortions in their physical senses — what and how they see, touch, smell, and hear.

Reasons given by some users for taking LSD include: "curiosity," "for kicks," "to understand myself better," or in quest of religious or philosophical insights.

Recent surveys and hospital reports show that the drug's popularity may be dropping, at least in some areas of the country, as its potential ill effects become better known.

Just how LSD works in the body is not yet known. It seems to affect the levels of certain chemicals in the brain and to produce changes in the brain's electrical activity.

Animal experiments with LSD suggest that the brain's normal filtering and screening-out process becomes blocked, causing it to become flooded with unselected sights and sounds.

Studies of chronic LSD users indicate that they continue to suffer from an overload of stimulation to their senses. Researchers believe this may explain the regular user's inability to think clearly and to concentrate on a goal.

EFFECTS

An average dose of LSD, amounting to a speck, has an effect that lasts for about eight to ten hours. Users take it in a sugar cube, a cracker, a cookie, or can lick it off a stamp or other object impregnated with the drug.

1. Physical

Physical effects of LSD are increased pulse and heart rate; a rise in blood pressure and temperature; dilated eye pupils; shaking of the hands and feet; cold, sweaty palms, a flushed face or paleness; shivering; chills with goose pimples; a wet mouth; irregular breathing; nausea; and loss of appetite.

The drug is not physically addicting as are the narcotics. That is, the body does not develop a physical need for LSD or physical sickness when it is withdrawn.

2. Psychological

People who use LSD say that it has a number of effects. The first effects, they indicate, are likely to be sudden changes in their physical senses. Walls may appear to move, colors seem stronger and more brilliant. Users are likely to "see" unusual patterns unfolding before them. Flat objects seem to stand out in three dimensions. Taste, smell, hearing, and touch seem more acute. One sensory impression may be translated or merged into another; for example, music may appear as a color, and colors may seem to have a taste.

One of the most confusing yet common reactions among users is the feeling of two strong and opposite emotions at the same time: they can feel both happy and sad at once, or depressed and elated, or relaxed and tense. Arms and legs may feel both heavy and light.

Users also report a sensation of losing the normal feeling of boundaries between body and space. This sometimes gives them the notion they can fly or float with ease.

Effects can be different at different times in the same individual. Researchers have found, even in carefully controlled studies, that responses to the drug cannot be predicted. For this reason, users refer to "good trips" or "bad trips" to describe their experience.

3. Thinking

Among LSD's other effects on the user is the loss of his sense of time. He does not know how much time is passing, but he does remain conscious. Scientists report that he can reason logically, up to a point, while undergoing the drug's effects. After the drug wears off, he usually remembers much of what happened to him. He may, for example, have become fascinated with an object in the room, like a chair or vase. On larger doses, he may feel mystical and report a sense of rebirth or new insights. But he is often unable to explain his experience to others. Many medical authorities feel that chronic or continued use of LSD changes values and impairs the user's powers of concentration and ability to think. This may lead to a tendency to "drop out" of society.

4. Creativity

Some users believe that if LSD can heighten their senses, it can also help them become more creative. However, studies of paintings, writings, and other works produced by drug users have failed to support this viewpoint. In many cases, works performed by people after they used LSD appeared to be noticeably poorer than before.

HAZARDS

Recent clinical reports on the illicit use of LSD have warned of definite dangers.

1. Panic

The user may grow frightened because he cannot "turn off" the drug's action. He may forget that a drug has changed his thinking and feeling and may fear that he is losing his mind.

2. "Flashbacks"

A flashback is a recurrence of some of the features of the LSD state days or months after the last dose. A flashback occurring without apparent cause can be very frightening and cause the user to belive that he is becoming psychotic. In some individuals this concern has caused fear and depression leading to suicide.

3. Accidental death

Because the LSD user may sometimes have paranoid feelings that he is invulnerable or even that he can fly, there have been cases of accidental death resulting from these beliefs. Users have been known to walk in front of moving cars or to attempt to fly from a high window, with disastrous consequences.

MENTAL ILLNESS

While there is some question whether LSD in itself can cause mental illness in a previously very stable individual, there is little doubt that LSD can play a role in bringing about acute and sometimes long-lasting mental illness in susceptible persons. Those most attracted to LSD in the hope that it will solve their problems or provide "instant insight" are often the individuals most susceptible to an LSD-precipitated breakdown.

YOUNG USERS

The strange sensations and clash of moods the drug causes can be frightening, even for a mature person. For young people who are still undergoing the process of emotional development and who may lack the resilience to maintain their mental equilibrium under LSD, the effects can be even more frightening and confusing. The young, growing brain is more vulnerable to all mind-altering drugs than the brain in which metabolic activity is stabilized.

BIRTH DEFECTS

A number of investigators have been studying the effects of LSD on chromosomes. These are the microscopic threads of matter in the nucleus of every cell; they carry genetic or hereditary information and guide reproduction. While some scientists have found these changes in the test tube, in animals and in man, other equally capable scientists have not. Whether LSD can cause birth defects remains an open question, and further studies are underway.

No conclusive or direct link has been found between LSD and chromosomal breaks, nor has it been found that such breaks cause birth defects. Nevertheless, until further research throws more light on the question, medical authorities warn that the drug must be considered a definite risk. Women of child-bearing age particularly are urged not to use it.

MEDICAL USES

The drug has been tested widely as a possible treatment for mental and emotional illnesses, including alcoholism and childhood autism. In studies so far it has failed to help the severely ill. However, under controlled conditions neurotics and alcoholics have made some improvements, according to investigators. The work is incomplete, but follow-up studies indicate that these improvements are not lasting. The drug is a valuable tool in biomedical research, but its therapeutic value appears limited at best.

LEGALITY

Because LSD is a dangerous drug when not used for research under medical supervision, it is closely regulated by the government. The law provides strict penalties for anyone who illegally produces, sells, or dispenses LSD. Possession of LSD is also illegal.

lumbago — a dull, nagging pain in the small of the back. This pain can be caused by a slipped vertebral disc, by strain, and by excessive nervous tension. The treatment depends on the cause.

lumbar — the small of the back.

lumen — the passageway inside a tubular organ. Vascular lumen is the passageway inside a blood vessel.

lungs — two cone-shaped bodies responsible for providing the body with air and with discharging certain waste products.

The lungs are soft, spongy, and elastic. The outside of each lung is covered by a closed sac called the pleura. The inner part of the lungs communicates freely with the outside air through the windpipe. The outside of the lungs is protected from air pressure by the walls of the chest cavity, creating a lessened pressure within the enveloping lung sac. The air pressure within the lungs expands them until they fill almost the entire chest cavity.

If any air gets through the chest wall, or if the lung is punctured so that air from the outside can communicate with the pleural sac, the lungs shrink because the air pressure is equalized outside and inside the chest cavity.

The lungs are not equal in size. The right lung has three lobes, and the left lung has two lobes. These lobes are closed systems, so that any one lobe can be removed without damage to the remaining lobes.

In passing to and from the lungs, air passes through the nose, throat, and the windpipe (trachea). In the nose the air is warmed and moistened. By means of the moist hairs and the moist mucous membrane of the nose, much of the dust is filtered out of inhaled air. Moreover, the sense of smell, which warns of the presence of some types of harmful gases, is situated in the nose. By the time air reaches the lungs it is much safer for them.

Large bronchial tubes (bronchi) leading from the windpipe carry the air that has been breathed in through the mouth and nose. These large tubes divide into smaller and smaller ones (bronchioles) until they are the size of fine threads. At the end of each small tube there is a cluster of tiny air sacs called alveoli. These air cells resemble a bunch of grapes, except they are many times smaller.

Around each air cell, which has very thin walls, is a fine network of small blood vessels or capillaries. The blood in these capillaries releases carbon dioxide and other waste matter brought from tissue activity all over the body. This takes place through the thin air-cell wall. In exchange, the blood takes on a supply of oxygen from the air breathed into the air cells. The discarded carbon dioxide and waste matter are removed from the air cells in the air that is breathed out of the lungs. This process is repeated about sixteen times every minute.

Breathing consists of two separate acts: inspiration and expiration. During inspiration, there is an enlargement of the chest cavity and a lowering of the pressure within the cavity. This is chiefly a muscular act: the ribs are raised, and the arch of the diaphragm falls and becomes flattened. The result of this activity is an increase in the capacity of the chest cavity and a partial vacuum that causes air to be drawn into the lungs.

Expiration requires only slight muscular action: the ribs fall to their normal position and the arch of the diaphragm rises. This results in a lessening of the chest cavity and an increase in the pressure within the cavity that forces air out of the lungs.

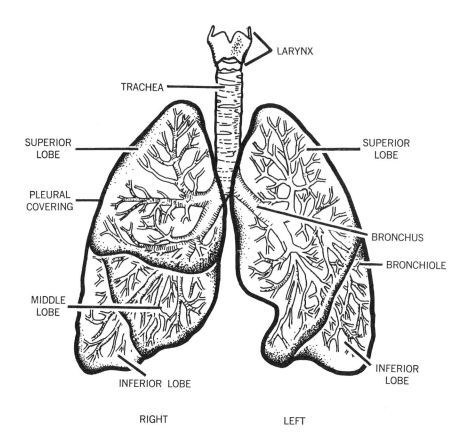

LARYNX

TRACHEA

SUPERIOR LOBE

SUPERIOR LOBE

PLEURAL COVERING

BRONCHUS

BRONCHIOLE

MIDDLE LOBE

INFERIOR LOBE

INFERIOR LOBE

RIGHT

LEFT

LUNGS

An average healthy man's lungs have the capacity to hold approximately five-thousand cubic centimeters of air. However, when his body is at rest, this same man may be inhaling and exhaling only five-hundred cubic centimeters of air at a time.

lupus vulgaris — a rare form of tuberculosis that attacks the skin, usually on the face. Lupus vulgaris begins with one or more brownish lesions. Subsequent lesions may appear differently. When the lesions heal, they leave disfiguring scars.

luteohormone — *See progesterone.*

luxation — dislocation.
See dislocation.

lymph — a nearly colorless liquid composed of excess tissue fluid and proteins and found in the lymph vessels and the lymph system of the body.
See lymph system.

lymph nodes — *See lymph system.*

lymphosarcoma — a cancer arising in any lymphatic tissue.

lymph system — a circulatory system of vessels, spaces, and nodes. The lymph system carries lymph, the almost-colorless fluid that bathes the body's cells. The system is important in the body's defense against infection.

The lymph nodes are small glands that act as filters for the lymph system. They remove bacteria, etc., from the lymph as it passes through the nodes. These nodes produce white blood cells and antibodies to help the body defend against infection. Lymph nodes are scattered throughout the body in clumps. The principal areas are the hand, neck, face, armpits, chest, abdomen, pelvic region, groin, and legs.

In addition to the lymph nodes, the lymph system also includes three other lymph organs. These organs are the spleen, the tonsils, and the thymus. Part of the function of the spleen is to produce white blood cells and to help the lymph nodes act as a filter. The tonsils and the thymus also manufacture white blood cells.

lysergic acid diethylamide — *See LSD.*

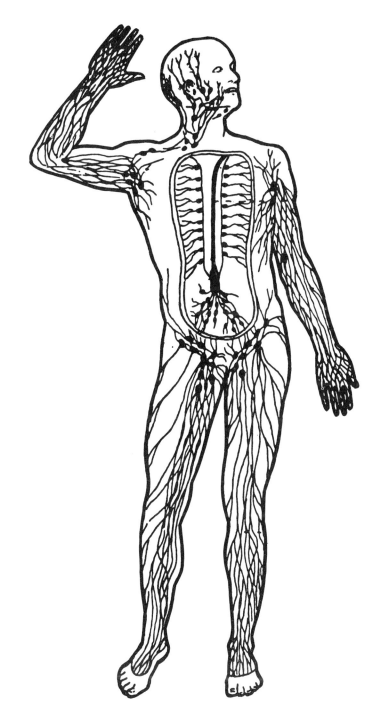

LYMPH SYSTEM

m

macule — an area or spot of discolored tissue (usually skin) that is not raised above the tissue that surrounds it.

maduromycosis — an infection that is caused by fungus. Maduromycosis usually affects the foot but may also be found in the hand and other body parts. The fungus generally enters the body through a wound. Maduromycosis is most frequently found in warm climates.

The fungus causes lesions and pus to form. The pus is discharged through dead tissue. If untreated, maduromycosis will destroy tissue and bone. Some forms of this disease, caused by specific molds, are treatable with penicillin and sulfonamides. However, other types will not respond to drugs, and in those cases the only treatment is amputation of the affected part.

An untreated case of maduromycosis can lead to death as a result of secondary infections.

magnesium — a mineral that is essential to the proper functioning of the body. Large amounts are found in the bones and the teeth. Among other functions, it plays an indispensable role in the body's use of food for energy.

Magnesium is found in goodly amounts in nuts, whole-grain products, dry beans, dry peas, and dark-green vegetables.

malabsorptive disease — an inability to digest and absorb food properly. This is frequently caused by the lack of a specific enzyme that is responsible for the digestion or absorption of a specific kind of food.

malaria — a communicable disease caused by tiny parasites that live in the blood.

The process by which malaria is transmitted requires one person already infected with malaria, one or more healthy people, and a female *Anopheles* mosquito. The cycle begins when this female mosquito bites the person who has malaria. The blood that is sucked into the mosquito's body contains the malaria parasites. The parasites develop into the infective stage within the insect's body. These parasites will develop over a two-week period. After this time any person the mosquito bites will become infected. This is because the mosquito injects the infective parasites at the same time it is sucking blood out of the person.

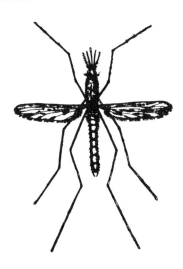

MALARIA CARRIER
(ANOPHELES MOSQUITO)

SYMPTOMS

About ten days to two weeks (although the incubation period can vary more than that) after being bitten, the infected person begins to exhibit the symptoms of malaria. The classic symptoms are a cycle of fever and chills, but they usually also include headache and nausea. Different varieties of malaria have different cycles. In one kind, the fever and chills occur every other day; in another type, they appear every third day; and others have different patterns.

During the active part of the cycle, the patient's fever may go so high that he is delirious. However, during the passive part of the cycle he may feel all right physically, although he is in a weakened condition.

TREATMENT

For years quinine was the best drug available for the treatment of malaria. Quinine has now been largely replaced by synthetic drugs, some of them developed during World Warr II, when quinine was in short supply. These synthetic drugs have proved to be more effective than quinine against all types of malaria. Two of the many drugs in use are chloroquine and primaquine.

PREVENTION

There are two ways to combat malaria: by killing parasites in the blood of infected persons, and by killing mosquitoes that transmit the disease.

Although malaria has been eradicated from the United States, it still constitutes one of the most serious public health problems in tropical and subtropical areas throughout the world.

An individual planning to travel in areas where malaria is still a problem is usually given drugs to protect him from the disease.

malignant — tending to produce death. In medical terms malignant refers primarily to cancer. A malignant tumor will grow relentlessly and eventually cause death unless it is removed. Conversely, a benign tumor is self-limited in its growth and is usually harmless.

malignant hypertension — a severe form of high blood pressure that runs a rapid course. It causes damage to the blood vessel walls in the kidneys, eyes, etc.
See hypertension.

malleus — one of the three tiny, linked bones in the middle ear. The malleus (also called the hammer) is the outer bone that is attached to the eardrum. The vibrations of the eardrum are passed on to the malleus. At the other end of the malleus is the second of the three middle ear bones, the incus. The vibrations of the malleus are moved along to the incus.

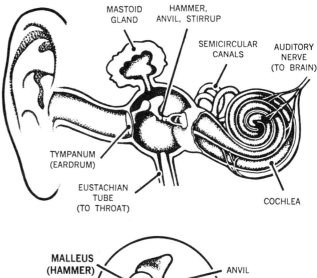

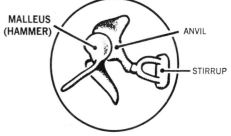

MALLEUS (HAMMER)

malnutrition — an impairment or risk of impairment to physical and mental health caused by failure to meet nutritional requirements. Malnutrition is the result of either the consumption of an insufficient quantity of food or of one or more essential nutrients. It may also be caused by faulty absorption or utilization of nutrients owing to physical or emotional causes.

In this country the most usual consequence of deficient diet is general undernutrition of a rather mild degree. As a rule, this is caused by a diet that is low in a number of essentials, and it develops when a person eats one food to excess and gets too little of other foods. The amount of iron, calcium, and other minerals may all be insufficient, or the diet may furnish insufficient vitamins. The consumption of protein may be inadequate in quantity, or in quality, or in both for

215

the best growth of muscles and other tissues. Malnutrition may also occur when the total food intake is not enough to supply the energy needed for bodily activities. A chronic disease or some particular physical defect may interfere with nutrition. Poor mental health, or simply unhappiness, may also be a factor. Such conditions may prevent a person from eating as much as he should or may interfere with his ability to utilize what he does eat. These situations usually result in a combination of mild symptoms of various diseases and in a general lack of well-being.

SPECIFIC MALNUTRITION

If there is a continuing deficiency in any of the substances essential to good nutrition, the body organs or tissues needing the largest amount of that material will suffer most. If there is a severe deficiency of any one of the dietary essentials, a specific deficiency disease is likely to result. Some of these diseases still occur among the most poorly fed children in this country, although they are much less common than formerly.

If the diet supplies too little of the iron, protein, and other materials needed for building red blood cells, the blood becomes deficient and the person is said to be anemic, or to have nutritional anemia.

If calcium, phosphorus, and vitamin D are not supplied in sufficient amounts, the bones become malnourished. If this happens to babies or young children, the bones tend to become soft and to bend easily. The disease called rickets may occur, and lasting deformities may result. In older children, a deficiency in calcium, phosphorus, and vitamin D will interfere with the normal growth of firm, strong bones.

A shortage of iodine in the diet is an important factor in the enlargement of the thyroid gland. The resulting condition is known as goiter.

Long-continued shortage of vitamin A results in night blindness, or inability to see in a dim light. An extreme lack of vitamin A may eventually cause a serious eye disease called xerophthalmia.

Inadequacy in the supply of thiamine (vitamin B_1) may cause impaired functioning of the digestive and nervous systems and eventually result in a disease called beriberi.

Deficiency in ascorbic acid (vitamin C) causes a disease known as scurvy. This condition may be mistaken for rheumatism and may occur at any age.

A deficiency of niacin (nicotinic acid) causes disturbances of the digestive tract, the nervous system, and the skin and may ultimately cause a disease called pellagra.

A lack of riboflavin (vitamin B_2) may result in a condition known as cheilosis, or "poor man's mouth." It may also cause lesions around the nose and eyes. These conditions are commonly found in association with pellagra.

malocclusion — a condition in which the upper and lower teeth do not meet evenly, resulting in an incorrect bit. An even bite is important for good speech and good nutrition.

Some types of malocclusion cannot be prevented because they are hereditary, but others can be avoided by early attention to a child's first teeth. Helping the child retain all his primary teeth as long as nature intended is one way to guide permanent teeth into their proper position.

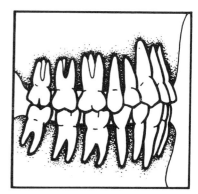

NORMAL BITE

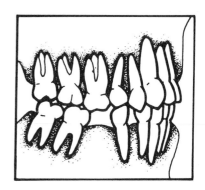

MALOCCLUSION

Frequently, when a primary tooth is prematurely lost, the adjacent existing teeth have nothing to hold them in line, and they tend to slide over into the empty space. This not only crowds the permanent tooth that eventually erupts into the gap, but it also starts a general movement of all the growing teeth in that area, resulting in malocclusion.

Malocclusion is considerably less frequent in cities that have fluoridated water. The baby teeth are retained and the permanent ones come in their proper places.

Malocclusion can be caused by childhood habits such as thumb-sucking; biting of the tongue, lips, or cheeks; or by mouth-breathing.

An uneven bite, caused by teeth that jut out too far or meet improperly, can be corrected by a specialist called an orthodontist. The realignment of the teeth may require braces and extraction of teeth.

Malpighi, Marcello — Italian anatomist (1628-1694) who, among other discoveries, demonstrated the existence of capillary connection between the arteries and veins in the lungs.

Malta fever — *See brucellosis.*

malunion — a condition in which a broken bone has healed improperly and the broken edges of the bone are not evenly matched together. Malunion occurs when the broken bone has not been properly set or has not been set at all. The condition is corrected by deliberately breaking the bone again and setting it properly.

mammary glands — *See breast.*

mandible — the large, horseshoe-shaped bone that forms the lower jaw. The mandible is attached to the rest of the face at two joints, each slightly in front of and below the ear.

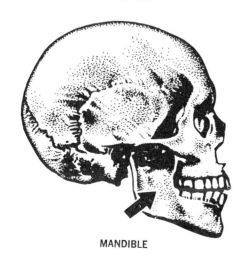

MANDIBLE

mania — an uncontrolled state of excitement exhibited in manic-depressive phychosis.
See manic-depressive psychosis.

manic-depressive psychosis — a very severe form of mental illness in which the patient alternates between mania (an uncontrolled state of excitement) and depression (a feeling of hopelessness).

Mantoux test — a simple skin test for detecting tuberculosis. It is one of the easiest and most effective methods for diagnosing tuberculosis.
See tuberculosis.

maple syrup urine disease — a defect in the metabolism of certain protein builders. This causes a "maple syrup" odor to urine; seizures; mental retardation; and early death. A special diet may be successful for prevention.

marihuana — a dried plant material from the Indian hemp plant *(Cannabis sativa)*. The plant grows wild in many parts of the world, including the United States, and is frequently cultivated for its commercial value in the production of fiber for rope, in birdseed, and for other purposes. In its drug use it is known by such names as "pot," "grass," "weed," "Mary Jane," and many others.

For use as a drug, the leaves and flowering tops of the plant are dried and crushed or broken into small fragments which are then typically rolled into thin, homemade cigarettes, often called "joints." It may also be smoked in small pipes and is occasionally incorporated into food and eaten. The smoke smells like burning rope or alfalfa. Because of its distinctive odor, users sometimes burn incense to mask the smell.

Marihuana varies greatly in strength, depending on where it is grown, whether it is wild or specifically cultivated for smoking or eating, and which portions of the plant actually go into the drug mixture. Marihuana is also sometimes adulterated with other materials such as the seeds and stems of the hemp plant, tea, catnip, or oregano, thus further reducing the strength of the resulting mixture.

Hashish ("hash") is the potent, dark-brown resin that is collected from the tops of high-quality cannabis. Because of the high concentration of resin, it is often five to six times stronger than the usual marihuana, although the active drug ingredients are the same. Basically, it is a much more concentrated form of the drug.

Tetrahydrocannabinol, or THC, is considered to be the basic active ingredient in marihuana and hashish. How much of this chemical is present determines the strength of the drug. Although various substances called THC have been sold illegally, the high cost and the difficulty of producing the material make it very unlikely that it is actually available illicitly. No samples of THC purchased on the black market so far have actually been found to be THC on chemical analysis.

Marihuana has been in widespread use for several thousand years, both for its intoxicating effects and for its presumed value as a medicine. As a medicine it has been used for such varied complaints as pain, cough, rheumatism, asthma, and migraine headaches. Other drugs have taken its place in modern medicine. At present it is no longer prescribed in the United States. Despite the fact that the drug is illegal in almost all countries, it has continued to be used for its intoxicating effects by many millions, especially in Asia and Africa.

Although estimates based on various surveys differ, it is generally conceded that the use of marihuana has sharply increased in the last few years, particularly among young people.

EFFECTS

When smoked, marihuana quickly enters the bloodstream and within minutes begins to affect the user's mood and thinking. The exact mechanisms of action and the alterations of cerebral metabolism are not well understood. Extensive research is currently underway to provide this basic information. Because it can cause hallucinations if used in very high doses, marihuana is technically classified as a mild hallucinogen. Despite several thousand years of use, less is presently known about the mode of action of this drug than is known about most other drugs in widespread use. Only in the last few years have the synthesis of THC and the development of methods to assay THC in marihuana made precision experiments possible.

1. Physical

The long-term physical effects of marihuana are not yet known. Extensive scientific research is currently underway to determine these effects. This research is based on both laboratory findings and research in countries where use has been widespread for many years.

The immediate physical effects on the user while smoking include reddening of the whites of the eyes, increased heartbeat, and coughing caused by the irritating effect of the smoke on the lungs. Users also report dryness of the mouth and throat. Reports of increased hunger and sleepiness are also common.

2. Psychological

The drug's effects on the emotions and senses vary widely, depending on such factors as the user's expectations, the circumstances of use and the strength and quantity of the drug used. Typically, time is distorted and seems much extended—five minutes may seem like an hour. Space may seem enlarged or otherwise distorted. Sounds and colors sometimes seem intensified. Thought frequently becomes dreamlike. The notion that one is thinking better is not unusual. Illusions (misinterpretation of sensations) are often reported. Hallucinations (experiencing nonexistent sensations) and delusions (false beliefs) are rare. The user frequently undergoes a kind of passive withdrawal accompanied by some degree of "high." The individual tends to withdraw into himself. Occasionally, uncontrollable laughter or crying may occur. While some users find the effects pleasant, other find them frightening or very unpleasant. Unfounded suspiciousness may occur, and this may be accompanied by marked fear or anxiety. Occasionally, such reactions may be sufficiently severe as to cause a susceptible individual to develop symptoms of panic, a paranoid state, or a temporary break with reality. Such effects may be more likely to occur in the youthful user whose personality is still in the process of rapid change.

Recent evidence has documented a loss of immediate recall and difficulty in thinking and speech owing to disorganization of recent memory. These have been found in experiments with single doses. The implications for the chronic marihuana user must await additional investigation.

3. Judgment

A person under the influence of marihuana may find it much harder to make decisions that require logical thinking. At the same time he may erroneously believe that his judgment is unimpaired or even that his mental functioning has been enhanced by the action of the drug. Performing any complex task requiring good reflexes and clear thinking may be impaired, making tasks such as driving particularly dangerous. Research is currently underway to determine more accurately the effects of varying quantities of marihuana on driving and other skilled activities.

4. Addiction

Authorities now think in terms of drug "dependence" rather than "addiction." Marihuana, which is not a narcotic, does not cause physical dependence as do heroin and other narcotics. This means that the body does not become dependent on continuing use of the drug. The body probably does not develop a tolerance to the drug, either, which would make larger and larger doses necessary to obtain the same effects. Withdrawal from marihuana used in ordinary amounts does not produce physical sickness.

A number of scientists think the drug can cause psychological dependence if taken regularly. All researchers agree that more knowledge of the long-term physical, personal, and social consequences of marihuana use is needed before national decisions about its legal status can be made.

marrow — the spongy, porous material found in the center of a bone. Until adulthood, bone marrow is red because it is actively producing red blood cells. When adulthood has been reached and there is no further growth, many bones no longer produce red blood cells. These bones then have a yellow bone marrow, which is largely composed of fat. However, because red blood cells constantly wear out and must be replaced, some of the bones in the body continue to have red bone marrow.

mastectomy — the surgical removal of a breast. The most common reason for this operation is cancer of the breast.

mastication — the process of chewing food to reduce it to the point where it can be comfortably swallowed. Mastication is the first of the digestive processes.

maxilla — the bone of the upper jaw. It supports the upper teeth and, together with the lower jaw bone, the mandible, composes the jaw.

measles — one of the most common of the childhood diseases. Community-wide epidemics of measles used to appear in the United States in two- or three-year cycles. Cases usually appear first among young school children, who then bring the disease home to their younger brothers and sisters. Measles was once such a common childhood disease that most children (more than ninety percent of them) had had it by the time they were fifteen years old. However, a vaccine for rubeola (measles) has been developed, and there is no longer any reason for a child or adult to have this disease.

CAUSE

The virus that causes measles is found in the secretions of the nose and throat of infected persons who discharge virus particles into the air when they talk, sneeze, or cough. People become infected by inhaling these virus particles. It is also possible to become infected with the virus by touching articles that have been in recent contact with an infected person's nose or mouth, such as handkerchiefs or clothes.

SYMPTOMS

The first symptoms suggest a severe cold. They include a runny nose; red, watery eyes; and a bad cough. Additionally, there are small red spots with white centers in the mouth, called Koplik's spots. These symptoms appear about ten to fourteen days after exposure to the infection. The patient may begin to run a temperature ranging from slightly above normal to as high as 103 or 104 degrees. About fourteen days after exposure, or four days after the cold symptoms, a blotchy red rash appears, first on the head and neck and later on other parts of the body. From five days to a week later this rash begins to fade.

The disease is contagious from four days before to five days after the appearance of the rash.

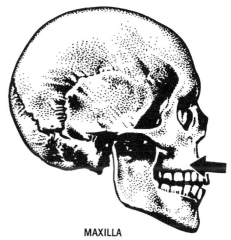

MAXILLA

TREATMENT

The treatment for measles consists primarily of keeping the patient comfortable and in comparative isolation. Isolation is important for two reasons: to keep the sick person from giving the disease to anyone else, and to protect the patient from other infections he might get from visitors.

During the time when the rash and fever are most severe, the patient should stay in bed and get as much rest as possible. He should drink plenty of water and other fluids, such as broth, fruit juices, and soft drinks.

Although it is not necessary to keep the room dark, there should be no strong light, because the disease makes the eyes very sensitive to brightness. Light will not damage the eyes, but it may cause discomfort.

Because of the possibility of ear complications, any patient complaining of an earache should consult a physician.

COMPLICATIONS

Measles can be dangerous because of the complications that can follow it. These include bronchopneumonia, middle-ear infection, and encephalitis. The encephalitis that occurs in about one out of every one thousand cases of measles often causes permanent brain damager, resulting in mental retardation.

PREVENTION

The only protection against this disease is immunization. Although infants usually have temporary immunity transferred to them by their mothers who have had the disease, this immunity gradually disappears after a baby becomes six to nine months old. All children should be vaccinated when they are twelve months old.

If an unvaccinated child is exposed to measles, his parents should immediately take him to a physician for a gamma globulin inoculation. The injection will modify the illness or prevent it altogether. This procedure is particularly important if the child is under two or three years old, because complications following measles are most likely to cause handicaps or even death when they strike this age group.

mecamylamine hydrochloride — a drug that blocks the transmission of nerve impulses at the nerve centers. Mecamylamine hydrochloride is one of the ganglionic blocking agents and may be used in the treatment of high blood pressure.

mediastinum — a term used to indicate the area between the lungs. It contains the heart, trachea, esophagus, etc. The area is also bordered by the sternum, the diaphragm, and the spine.

medicine — a general term for any drug.

medulla — a general term used to indicate the middle, central, or inner portion of a body part or organ.

medulla oblongata — the part of the brain that connects the brain and the spinal column. Located in the medulla oblongata are the nerve centers that control the beat of the heart, blood pressure, and the rate of respiration. An injury to this area of the brain can cause death, because it can disrupt so many vital functions.

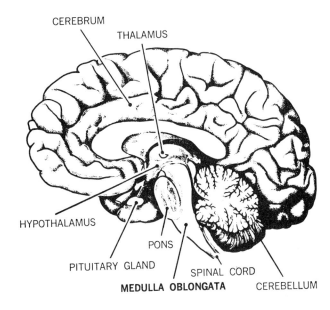

MEDULLA OBLONGATA

Meibomian glands — glands located near the upper and lower eyelids. They secrete an oily substance. If these glands become blocked, a cyst or small tumor may develop. These glands are named for Heinrich Meibom (1638-1700), a German anatomist.

melanin — the dark pigment that gives color to the skin, hair, and eyes.

melanoma — a skin tumor containing dark pigment.

melena — very dark bowel movements. This is usually an indication of internal bleeding.

membrane — any thin body tissue.

menarche — the time during puberty when a female's menstrual flow begins.

Ménière's disease — a disease (also known as Ménière's syndrome) that produces increased amounts of fluids in a portion of the inner ear. This causes head noises, nausea and dizziness, and hearing loss. The nausea and dizziness are caused by the disturbance of the delicate mechanism for maintaining balance, which is also located in the inner ear.

Ménière's disease may often be alleviated by medical or surgical treatment.

meninges — three layered membranes that cover and protect the brain and the spinal cord. The three layers are: the dura mater, the arachnoid, and the pia mater.

The dura mater is the outermost layer and is the toughest of the three membranes. Beneath the dura mater is the arachnoid, so named because it resembles a spider's web. Beneath the arachnoid, and closest to the brain, is the pia mater, a transparent membrane that actually touches the brain and spinal cord.

See meningitis.

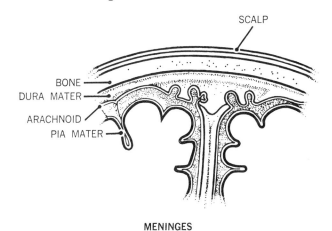

MENINGES

meningitis — an inflammation of the membranes covering the brain and spinal cord. It may be caused by any of several bacteria, viruses, or other microscopic organisms. A very serious form is caused by an organism called meningococcus. These bacteria may be present in the body with no effect, or they may cause serious illness. If meningococci reach the brain or spinal cord, they cause severe inflammation or meningitis. Without treatment, this disease is fatal in about half the cases; survivors may be left with disabilities such as deafness and paralysis.

CAUSE

Meningococci enter the body through the nose and mouth. They are spread by droplets sprayed into the air by sneezing and coughing or by direct contact. Usually, these bacteria stay in the nose and throat for a few days and then disappear without causing illness. During an epidemic, several thousand times more people carry and spread meningococci than become ill. Why most people do not get meningitis is unknown. Children are more susceptible than adults, but the disease can occur at any age. Meningococcal meningitis occurs most often in winter and spring. It is most common in temperate climates, but large epidemics have occured even in hot, dry regions.

When people live in crowded quarters—as in barracks or institutions—the bacteria can spread easily from one person to another. If one case develops, or the group has a healthy carrier, many people may get meningococci in their noses and throats, and some may become ill. This is often the way epidemics begin.

SYMPTOMS

Meningitis usually begins suddenly, with severe headache and stiffness and pains in the neck, back, and shoulders. Other symptoms are a high fever and often nausea and vomiting. A skin rash of tiny, bright-red spots frequently occurs. If these conditions appear, a physician should be consulted, because prompt treatment is essential.

A diagnosis of meningitis is confirmed by inserting a needle into the spinal column to withdraw fluid. This fluid is then analyzed.

TREATMENT

Antibiotics and sulfa drugs are effective in most cases of meningococcal meningitis. With early treatment, most patients get well quickly. A few deaths result from an overwhelming infection that defies even prompt treatment.

CONTROL

The control of meningitis epidemics depends on early recognition and immediate reporting of cases. It is important to follow the medical advice of a private physician or local health authority in caring for the patient and in the sanitary control of his immediate environment. Sometimes, to prevent an epidemic, physicians recommend that drugs be given to everyone who may have been exposed to the disease.

meningoccle — *See spina bifida.*

meningococcal meningitis — *See meningitis.*

meningomyelocele — *See spina bifida.*

menopause — the end of menstrual periods and, therefore, the end of childbearing years. It is also called the climacteric or "change of life."

The menopause usually occurs when a woman is between forty and fifty. It can occur earlier or later. It starts gradually and is recognized by the change in menstruation. The monthly flow becomes smaller in amount, then irregular, and finally ceases. Often, the time between periods becomes longer and longer—there may be a lapse of several months between them.

Before and during these changes in the monthly periods, certain symptoms may appear; e.g., hot or warm flushes, dizziness, weakness, nervousness, and insomnia. Many women have very mild symptoms; some have none at all; with a few, the discomfort is very severe.

The symptoms are caused by the disappearance of the female sex hormone that the ovaries produce. The same symptoms occur when the ovaries are removed surgically because of disease (surgical menopause). After a period of time ranging from a few months to a year or two, the body adjusts itself, and the symptoms disappear. While this adjustment is taking place, hot flushes, etc., can appear.

The menopause is not a complete change of life. The normal sex urges remain, and women retain their usual reaction to sex long after the menopause.

Medical treatment can be very successful in relieving symptoms of menopause. Medical care can help to correct nervousness and low spirits that often go along with menopause. Mental depression is not unusual at this time.

menses — the normal monthly blood loss during menstruation.

menstruation — the periodic shedding of the lining of the uterus.

About every twenty-eight days, midway between two menstrual cycles, changes take place in both the ovaries and the uterus. An ovary prepares to release one of its ova. At the same time, the lining of the uterus starts to grow. Tiny glands and blood vessels appear in the top half of this lining, and the whole of it becomes soft and velvety.

About fourteen days before the menstrual flow, a single ovum leaves one of the ovaries, stops for twenty-four hours at the entrance to a fallopian tube, then goes on through the tube into the uterus. If conception does not take place, the lining of the uterus then gradually stops growing and comes loose. As it loosens, the blood vessels that come away with it begin to bleed. This causes the menstrual flow of blood, which lasts several days. It carries away the unused top layer of the lining of the uterus and any other waste materials that may be present. As soon as this first menstrual period ends, preparation for another one begins. This cycle repeats itself, except during pregnancy, until the menopause.

mental illness — a mental or emotional disorder strong enough to interfere in a major or minor way with daily living.

The oldest records of human history show that there have always been people who suffered from mental illness. Such illness has existed in every kind of culture and civilization—from the most primitive to the most advanced.

For a long time the mentally ill were punished or, at best, neglected. They were thought to be possessed by demons, or "moonstruck," or to be less than human. Society put them out of sight and out of mind.

Today, society views the mentally ill as sick people who, like all sick people, need medical treatment.

It has been estimated, on the basis of certain surveys, that one in ten people in the United States is mentally ill. This refers to mental illness and emotional disorders in all forms—major and minor—and includes the many millions of people whose symptoms may be of a psychosomatic nature, as in ulcers or hypertension, or which may be as severe as a frank psychosis such as schizophrenia. The fact is, however, that no one knows how many people are mentally ill—partly because the boundaries between mental health and illness are as yet only dimly defined, and partly because many people with emotional disorders do not seek treatment.

TYPES

Mental disorders can be classified under four major headings: psychoses, neuroses, personality or character disorders, and psychosomatic diseases.

1. Psychoses

Psychoses (which the term "insanity" usually refers to) are generally characterized by strange feelings and behavior and by a distortion of reality. Psychoses are the most severe forms of mental illness. Patients with psychoses are called psychotics. In many instances, these patients are dangerous individuals—both to themselves and to other people. Frequently they must be hospitalized.

Some psychotic illnesses are caused by tumors of the brain, hardening of brain arteries because of age, or damage to brain tissue from alcohol or drugs. Psychotic illnesses that have a known physical cause are referred to as organic psychoses. In some cases, the mental illness can be cured or alleviated by removing the organic or physical cause. When no organic cause can be found, the mental illness is known as a functional psychosis. Patients with functional psychoses are treated with a variety of drugs, including tranquilizers.

Examples of psychoses are manic-depressive psychosis and schizophrenia.

2. Neuroses

The neuroses are less severe emotional disturbances, although in some cases thinking and judgment may be impaired. The trouble is mostly in the way a neurotic person feels—and often he feels very uncomfortable. Neurotics may be continually bothered by feelings of anxiety or depression, which use up their energies and fill them with nameless dread.

Neuroses take many forms. A housewife may be so neat that she gets upset if an ashtray is even an inch out of place; a man may worry so much about pleasing his boss that his nerves are always on edge. Other neurotic patterns may take the form of overeating to the point of obesity; sleepwalking; repeated hand-washing, touching objects or counting them; or irrational fears.

Most neurotics can be treated in a psychiatric clinic or under private professional care. Neurosis often has an up-and-down pattern; oc-

casionally the neurotic's anxiety becomes so great that he must be hospitalized, usually for only a brief period. But most neurotics are able to earn a living—although painfully and with effort; have a home life—although often a wretched one; and are seemingly normal in some activities—although abnormal in others. Relations with other people are often adversely affected.

3. Character of personaltiy disorders

Character or personality disorders are difficulties in adjustment that show themselves in the kind of disturbed behavior that is seen in the drug addict, the chronic alcoholic, or the delinquent. Usually the person with a character disorder does not feel great anxiety or guilt about his behavior, whereas most other emotionally ill persons with the same symptoms do. He behaves very much as if he does not care about the standards of conduct or achievement that are important to most people in our society. Irresponsibility and immaturity are often indications of this type of disorder.

At the least serious level, a person with a character disorder may be repeatedly discharged from jobs because he cannot make himself care enough about doing good work. A person with a more serious character disorder may cheat, steal, or lie; he may become an alcoholic, a drug addict, or a sexual deviate.

When a person engages in socially destructive acts without feeling any guilt about these acts, he is sometimes called a psychopath. No one knows for sure why the psychopath behaves as he does, but several reasons have been suggested. He may be a person who has not yet developed an adequate conscience; like a child he is impulsive, selfish, and shortsighted. He may have grown up in a group that did not have the same values as the large part of American society. It is often difficult to know whether an individual with a character disorder is emotionally ill or is healthy but antisocial.

4. Psychosomatic diseases

Psychosomatic diseases are those ailments in which the symptoms are primarily physical, although there may be a large emotional component. This type of emotional illness is understandable to anyone who has ever suffered from a headache after arguing with his employer or who has had diarrhea before taking an important examination. Included among the psychosomatic illnesses are asthma, peptic ulcer, colitis, hypertension, and certain types of arthritis.

The person suffering from a psychosomatic disorder may need psychological treatment, but he is also in need of medical treatment. He is very different from the hypochondriac who, although convinced that he is ill, actually has nothing organically wrong.

RECOVERY

As in all other illnesses, the sooner a diagnosis is made and treatment is begun, the better the chances are for recovery. The family physician, the teacher, the nurse, and others can often detect early signs of disorder and make appropriate referrals for help.

Even for those patients whose illness is sufficiently severe that they must be hospitalized, the outlook is increasingly hopeful. A recent survey of general hospitals with psychiatric services revealed an average length of stay of twenty days. Stays in state mental hospitals are usually longer but are still within the limits that give the family the expectation of the patient's improvement rather than years of dreary custodial care.

However, it should be kept in mind that mental illness is often chronic, although there are long periods of remission. A patient's ability to remain outside the hospital and stay well depends on several factors, including follow-up care in the community and understanding and acceptance from family, neighbors, friends, and fellow workers.

mental retardation — a condition of inadequately developed intelligence that significantly impairs the ability to learn and to adapt to the demands of society. Mental retardation is present at birth or develops during childhood and usually continues throughout life. More than two hundred specific causes of mental retardation have been identified. In approximately twenty to twenty-five percent of cases and cause is known. Among the known biological factors are hereditary factors, infections, nutritional deficiencies or toxic substances in the mother's system during pregnancy, and injuries. Lack of a healthful environment, including motivation, stimulation, and opportunity, is a large factor for many children.

Every year in the United States, approximately 126,000 infants are born whose mental development will never be normal. At present an estimated three percent of the population is mentally retarded.

A real increase in some types of mental retardation comes from modern discoveries in medical care. These have led to the survival of damaged or defective children who otherwise would die in infancy and to longer life for all who are retarded.

SYMPTOMS

Some mentally retarded children are behind in various stages of their development such as sitting up, crawling, walking, and talking.

Some are born with a combination of physical signs such as those in mongolism (Down's syndrome), which usually makes possible a diagnosis at birth. Other babies, born normal, develop jaundice in the first days of life. This warns the doctor that mental retardation may be threatening unless immediate steps are taken. A child with the enlarged head of hydrocephalus (excess fluid inside the skull) is in danger of mental retardation.

Other retarded children are, in all obvious ways, physically healthy and normal. Their mental retardation may not even be suspected until they enter school and cannot keep up with normal children.

The degree of mental retardation may range from mild to profound. In severe cases the condition is usually recognizable very early; when slight, it may require several years of observation to make the proper diagnosis. In terms of physical appearance, seventy-five percent of the retarded have the same characteristics as the rest of the population. On this basis alone only twenty-five percent are detectable through differences in head size, small stature, small hands, or slanted eyes. The overriding symptom of mental retardation is that the individual does not adapt or achieve in the same manner or degree as his contemporaries.

DEGREE

Mental retardation is classified on the basis of measured intelligence and adaptive behavior.

A person is said to be "profoundly" retarded if he is in need of constant care or supervision for survival. There is gross impairment in physical coordination and sensory development, and frequently the person is physically handicapped as well. People who are profoundly mentally retarded have an IQ of less than twenty.

A "severely" retarded individual has definitely retarded motor development as well as speech and language retardation. He is unable to learn reading and writing but is not completely dependent. He is capable to some useful work. Often, but not always, severely retarded people are also physically handicapped. Severe mental retardation indicates an IQ of between twenty and thirty-five.

People who are "moderately" retarded are slow in their development but are able to learn to care for themselves. Moderately retarded children are capable of being trained. However, as adults they still need to live and work in a sheltered and protected environment. An IQ of between thirty-six and fifty-one is indicative of moderate mental retardation.

A "mildly" retarded individual shows slow development. A mildly retarded child is capable of being educated within limits. As adults, with proper training, they can work in competitive employment. They are able to live independent lives. Mild mental retardation is shown by an IQ of between fifty-two and sixty-seven.

It should be noted that there are other ways of classifying mental retardation, and other IQ levels are used for these same classifications.

TREATMENT
The trend today is to encourage families to keep a retarded member at home unless his or her presence creates insurmountable difficulties for the parents or the brothers and sisters—or unless an institution can do more for the retarded person than can be done in his hime.

The retarded individual needs more medical checkups and advice than the normal person, since he may be more susceptible to infections. He also may feed poorly, have poor motor coordination, be underweight or overweight, lack normal eyesight, or be hard-of-hearing, and have speech and language problems.

If he has multiple handicaps, he requires more medical care than the average.

The retarded individual should be provided with as much education or training as he can profitably use. Plans begin with early training in the home and in preschool groups. They continue with special classes for the retarded in public or private schools and job-training for suitable employment.

PREVENTION
Genetic counseling, pregnancy before age forty, adequate prenatal care, family planning,

prevention of infection, control of metabolic diseases, discreet use of drugs during pregnancy, and good delivery techniques offer opportunities for prevention. Additional preventive opportunities are early detection of inborn errors of metabolism in the newborn, adequate immunization of the child, prevention of childhood accidents and accidental poisonings, and prevention of seizures caused by fever.

mercurial diuretic — one of various compounds of mercury commonly used to promote the elimination of water and sodium from the body through increased excretion of urine. A mercurial diuretic is sometimes used in congestive heart failure when tissues are waterlogged. Mercury in several different organic forms is used as a diuretic.
See diuretic.

mensentery — a membrane that attaches a body organ to a body wall. The term is usually used to indicate the peritoneal membrance that lines the abdominal cavity.

metabolism — a general term used to designate all chemical changes that occur to substances within the body. The rate of metabolism indicates how long the body takes to reduce a substance chemically into energy for use or storage.

metacarpus — the palm of the hand from the wrist to the fingers and thumb. There are five metacarpal bones. Each of these is connected with the wrist at one end. The other end is connected to the thumb or to one of the four fingers.

metaphase — the second stage in cell division.
See mitosis.

metastasis — the transfer of disease from one part of the body to another. In cancer, the new growths are characteristic of the original tumor.
See cancer.

methadone — a synthetic drug that can be given to a heroin addict to replace heroin. Methadone has the advantage of being less expensive and allowing the addict to maintain a normal life. However, methadone is also an addictive drug.
See heroin, heroin addiction.

methamphetamine — a stimulant, or a drug that stimulates the central nervous system. Methamphetamine is similar to amphetamine, but in many ways it is stronger. While methamphetamine does have important medical uses, it has become a drug of abuse, known as "speed" or "crystal."

See amphetamine.

microbe — *See microorganism.*

microorganism — any living organism that is too small to be seen by the naked eye. Microorganisms often cause diseases in animals and in man.

microscope — a piece of equipment that magnifies small objects, microorganisms, etc., many times. The magnification allows the investigator to identify microorganisms that are too small to be seen with the naked eye.

micturition — the passing of urine. Micturition is also called urination.

middle ear — *See ear.*

migraine — a severe, painful type of headache.

See headache.

milk — one of the most important of all foods. Babies begin life on a milk diet because it is so rich in important proteins, vitamins, etc. Milk is also important to growing children because of the amount of calcium it provides.

minerals — inorganic substances that are essential to the human body. Many different minerals are required by the body. They give strength and rigidity to certain body tissues and help with numerous vital functions.

Most of the hard tissues of the human body, such as bones and teeth, are composed in part of mineral elements. In the case of bones and teeth, relatively large amounts of calcium and phosphorus are needed to make up these structures, but the body also needs many other minerals, some in very minute quantities, to carry on its life processes. For instance, in order to function properly, muscles, nerves, and the heart must be constantly nourished by body fluids containing the correct proportion of minerals such as sodium, potassium, and calcium. Similarly, red blood cells cannot be formed or function properly unless sufficient iron is supplied to the body. The

consumption of small amounts of another mineral, fluorine, during the formative years prevents excessive tooth decay among young children and adolescents and during later life.

Altogether, about fifteen different mineral elements are required by the body, and all must be derived from food or drink. The minerals in which diets are most likely to be low, or deficient, are calcium, iron, iodine, and fluorine.

A well-balanced diet, especially one that contains adequate amounts of protein foods usually provides all the essential minerals in sufficient quantity to satisfy the body's requirements.

miosis — contraction.

1. An abnormal contraction of the pupil of the eye.

2. The phase in the course of a disease in which the symptoms begin to recede.

miscarriage — the birth of a baby at a time before it has developed enough to live in the outside world, usually before the fifth month of pregnancy. At least one pregnancy in ten terminates in miscarriage. About two-thirds of these occur in the first three months of pregnancy.

Miscarriages may be caused by factors other than abnormalities of the egg or infant. They may also be caused by glandular or nutritional problems. Miscarriage used to be blamed on a fall or a blow to the abdomen, but doctors now know that this is an exceedingly rare cause. The baby is protected within a sac of fluid in the uterus and usually escapes injury even in the event of a serious accident to the mother.

Slight bleeding may mean that a miscarriage is only threatening and that the baby may yet be saved. More severe bleeding, especially with cramps, usually means that a miscarriage is actually in progress.

See abortion.

mite — *See scabies.*

mitosis — the process of human cell division or reproduction. When a cell divides by mitosis, each of the two new cells has the same characteristics, and both are the same as the original cell.

STAGES

There are four stages in mitosis that are concerned with division. A fifth stage is the resting or interphase between cell division. Mitosis always begins with a cell in the interphase stage.

The first stage of change is called the prophase stage. During this stage, the chromosomes (which contain the hereditary factors or genes) duplicate themselves. During the resting stage, the cell contained forty-six chromosomes. After the prophase stage is complete, the same cell has ninety-two chromosomes—two complete sets of forty-six chromosomes.

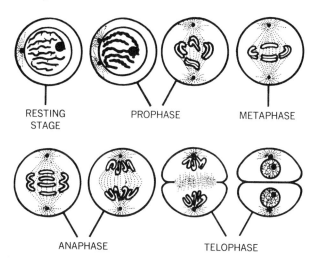

RESTING STAGE   PROPHASE   METAPHASE

ANAPHASE   TELOPHASE

MITOSIS

The next stage is known as metaphase. At this time the chromosomes line up at the center of the cell. The chromosomes then split up into two groups—each group is a complete set of chromosomes.

The third changing step in mitosis is anaphase. During this phase, each group of chromosomes moves to opposite poles of the original cell. When this stage is complete, the final stage, telophase, begins. A new cell wall forms in the center of the original cell. This new cell wall divides the original cell into two new cells, and the process is complete. Two new cells exist that are exact replicas of the original parent cell. The new cells are in the resting or interphase stage.
See chromosomes.

mitral insufficiency — an improper closing of the mitral valve between the upper and lower chambers in the left side of the heart. A mitral insufficiency allows a backflow of blood in the wrong direction. It is sometimes the result of scar tissue forming after a rheumatic fever infection.

mitral stenosis — a narrowing of the valve (called

the bicuspid or mitral valve) opening between the upper and the lower chambers in the left side of the heart. It is sometimes caused by scar tissue forming after a rheumatic fever infection.

mitral valve — a valve composed of two cusps or triangular segments. The mitral valve (also known as the bicuspid valve) is located between the upper and lower chambers in the left side of the heart.

mitral valvulotomy — an operation to widen the opening in the valve between the upper and lower chambers in the left side of the heart (mitral valve). It is usually performed when the valve opening is so narrowed that it is obstructing the flow of blood between the two chambers.

molars — the teeth that grind food. The first permanent teeth are the four "6-year" molars, one on each side of the upper and lower jaws. Appearing about the sixth year, behind the primary teeth, they are often mistaken for primary teeth.

The "6-year" molars are very important. They make it possible for the child to chew during the time the primary teeth are being replaced by permanent teeth. The position of the "6-year" molars largely determines the position of the other permanent teeth, which in turn influence the shape of the jaws and the child's appearance. If the "6-year" molars are lost, the shape of the jaw may be changed, and correction and alignment may later be required.

There are three sets of molars. The first set is the "6-year" molars. The second set erupts at the age of twelve or thirteen. The third and final set emerges between the ages of seventeen and twenty-one. These last molars are often referred to as the "wisdom teeth."

mole — a growth on the skin. Moles are usually pigmented and slightly raised skin blemishes.

molecule — the smallest unit into which a substance can be divided and still retain all its characteristic properties. One molecule of blood will react chemically the same way that a pint of blood will. However, if the molecule of blood is broken down any further, it is no longer blood and will react in different ways.

mongolism — *See Down's syndrome.*

monocular vision — a condition in which one eye is blind or one eye refuses to register images in coordination with the better eye.

mononucleosis — *See infectious mononucleosis.*

mono-unsaturated fat — a fat so constituted chemically that it is capable of absorbing additional hydrogen but not as much hydrogen as a polyunsaturated fat. These fats in the diet have little effect on the amount of cholesterol in the blood. One example is olive oil.
See cholesterol, polyunsaturated fat.

morbidity rate — the ratio of the number of cases of a disease to the number of healthy people in a given population during a specified period of time, such as a year. The term morbidity involves two separate concepts: incidence and prevalence.

Incidence is the number of new cases of a disease developing in a given population during a specified period of time.

Prevalence is the number of cases of a given disease existing in a given population at a specified moment of time.

morning sickness — a feeling of nausea that sometimes occurs during the first few months of pregnancy. Morning sickness is actually a poor name for the symptom, because the "sickness" is not confined to the morning hours.

moron — a term that was used to describe a certain level of mental retardation. This term has been replaced with a new type of classification system.
See mental retardation.

morphine — the most effective of all drugs in relieving pain. Properly used, it will relieve severe pain and assist in the prevention of shock.

Morphine, like all narcotics, is physically addictive. A patient taking morphine over a period of time develops a tolerance for the drug and requires larger and larger doses. There is also a danger of psychological dependency developing in the case of a patient using morphine over a period of time.

The size of the dose of morphine determines, to a certain extent, the degree of side effects present. As the level of the dose increases, so does the degree of the side effects. Morphine tends to make the patient drowsy, changes his mood (often to euphoria), produces constipation, and can cause nausea and vomiting.

Despite its drawbacks, morphine is still a very effective and useful drug. Although many synthetic drugs are used today in place of morphine, it remains an important drug, particularly in the treatment of pain in cases of terminal illnesses.

mosquito — a small flying insect.

Mosquitoes are found in almost every part of the world, at least during certain seasons. Their bites can cause intense discomfort, and when mosquitoes are present in great numbers, they seriously interfere with both work and recreation. In addition, mosquitoes carry several important diseases: malaria, encephalitis, yellow fever, dengue, and filariasis.

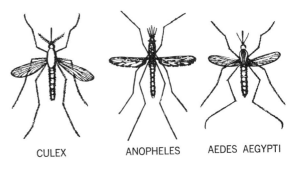

CULEX   ANOPHELES   AEDES AEGYPTI

MOSQUITO

When the mosquito pierces the skin and feeds on the blood of animals or people, it may become infected by disease organisms present in that blood. Subsequently, the mosquito may pass the infection on to other animals or people. Only female mosquitoes bite, and only certain species of mosquitoes carry disease. The *Anopheles* mosquitoes carry malaria, and several species, including common house mosquitoes (*Culex*), carry encephalitis. Also, *Aedes aegypti* carry urban yellow fever and dengue. Mosquito control activities of public health experts are directed toward eliminating certain disease-carrying species that may be present in a particular area. Widespread efforts to reduce numbers of *Anopheles* mosquitoes, for example, have helped to bring about eradication of malaria in the United States.

motion sickness — a feeling of nausea that may be accompanied by vomiting and which is caused by motion. Motion sickness is also known as travel sickness, car sickness, seasickness, etc. The motion does not have to be irregular; many people suffer from motion sickness while on a boat that is tied up at a dock—the perfectly regular motion of the waves rocking the boat can be as devastating as a bumpy airplane ride.

Motion sickness presents two problems. The first is the physical problem. Motion sickness is caused by an upset in the delicate balance mechanism of the inner ear. The parts of the inner ear that control balance (the semicircular canals and their appendages) have fluids in them. When the fluid moves, it touches small hairs, which in turn trigger nerve impulses to the brain. When the amount of motion and/or the kind of motion is sufficiently aggravating, the vomiting center of the brain is also triggered.

The second problem associated with motion sickness is a psychological one. The fear of flying can upset the stomach enough to cause motion sickness. Once a person has had motion sickness, whether from physical or psychological factors, he is prone to have motion sickness again. Thus, in addition to being afraid to travel, or actually having a disturbance in the balance mechanism, he also has to cope with his fear of motion sickness.

PREVENTION

Several drugs have been found to be very effective in preventing motion sickness. However, to get the best results, they should be taken some time before travel begins. Additionally, certain precautions can be taken to reduce the effects of travel.

Patients prone to motion sickness should sit in a place that produces the least motion: in the center of a plane or a ship. An effort should be made to avoid reading or other activities that give the brain visual signals that reinforce the nerve impulses from the inner ear. Neither food nor alcohol should be taken in excess. However, a moderate amount of alcohol can quiet fears, and travel on an empty stomach should always be avoided.

Temperature and stuffy air can be contributory factors in motion sickness. Cool, fresh air can help prevent this sickness.

mouth — the first part of the digestive system. The mouth is a cavity consisting of the hard palate and the teeth at the top, the cheeks as the side, the tongue and lower teeth as the floor, and the soft palate extending from the end of the hard palate to the pharynx.

The digestive functions of the mouth are mastication and lubrication. The teeth reduce food to manageable size. Saliva prepares the food to move easily down the rest of the digestive tract.

The mouth, an important part of speech, is also an alternate breathing passage.

mucous membrane — any membrane that secretes mucus.
See mucus.

mucus — a viscid, slippery fluid that moistens and protects body tissues. Mucus is secreted by mucous membranes.

multiple sclerosis — a chronic, progressive, degenerative disease of the central nervous system.

Multiple sclerosis is not contagious nor is it a mental disease. It is "multiple" in the sense that it produces multiple changes or lesions on the brain and spinal cord, which result in multiple effects in the body. More often multiple sclerosis attacks one area of the nervous system and later, after a period of improvement, the same area again or a different place. It is "sclerotic" because it leaves sclera or scars at the points where demyelination, the loss of the protective covering of the nerves, takes place.

For this reason, multiple sclerosis is known as a demyelinating disease. The fatty covering called "myelin," which normally protects and insulates the nerve fibers of the spinal cord and brain, disappears in scattered patches during multiples sclerosis. Without this myelin, body signals go wrong. Hence the characteristics of multiple sclerosis may include shaking or tremor, extreme weakness, and progressive paralysis.

Although the exact number of persons with multiple sclerosis is not known, it is among the leading neurologic ailments. Estimates are that about 500,000 Americans have multiple sclerosis or closely related diseases.

The ailment generally attacks people about twenty to forty years old, thus interfering with jobs and family life. In some studies, however, onset at age twenty or under was noted in twenty percent of patients.

SYMPTOMS
The symptoms usually appear gradually and

vary greatly from patient to patient. There may be visual disturbances, ranging from transitory blurring to double vision; slight weakness in the extremities; slurring of speech; and tremor. In some patients, the occasional and mild symptoms go on for years. In other patients, the symptoms are more severe, long-lasting, and come early in the course of the disease. The classic symptoms are tremor, double vision, and shimmering movements of the eyeball, called nystagmus.

A person with multiple sclerosis does not always have all these symptoms, and someone having one or more of these symptoms may not have multiple sclerosis. Moreover, many multiple sclerosis patients have remissions—periods of months or even years during which the symptoms disappear and the individual appears to be well.

No one knows why these improvements occur, but they may happen several times and can be followed by more severe symptoms. Thus, multiple sclerosis is a progressive disease.

In its early stages, however, multiple sclerosis is often difficult to diagnose. A physician diagnoses multiple sclerosis on the basis of the patient's history and clinical symptoms and signs. The average lag between onset of earliest symptoms and the diagnosis of multiple sclerosis has been about six years. Although the physician might suspect multiple sclerosis during a patient's first attack, quite frequently an additional attack or attacks must follow before the physician can be reasonably sure of a diagnosis of multiple sclerosis.

It is possible for the patient with multiple sclerosis to live for fifteen to twenty years after the diagnosis. The patient may die from some cause other than multiple sclerosis. As the disease progresses, the patient develops more severe symptoms and has shorter symptom-free periods. The weakness in his limbs may progress to paralysis, with complete loss of sensation and mobility. He may lose control of his bladder or have visual disturbances. His ability to get around becomes gradually diminished, and he may require a wheelchair or have to stay in bed. As the symptoms become more severe, reducing his ability to be mobile and care for himself, the patient may become depressed and bored. Whether as the result of the damage done to his nervous system or as the result of anxiety, he may be subject to fluctuations of mood. The "mood swing" is common. The patient may be on

top of the world one minute and depressed the next minute.

CAUSE

Many theories have been advanced as to what causes multiple sclerosis. These include alterations in the way the body uses foods, lack of food essentials such as traces of metals, a factor in climate, blood-vessel spasms, a genetic factor, toxins, viruses, and allergies. No theory has been verified. Perhaps several factors, some as yet undiscovered, are involved.

In the United States, multiple sclerosis is more common across the northern portions than in other parts of the nation. It is more frequently encountered in Canada and the northern countries of Europe than in the hot Mediterranean basin. Although multiple sclerosis does occur, though rarely, in hotter climates, no one knows why more cases are found in colder climates. Studies showed that the climate of the patient's childhood, not the climate where he lives when multiple sclerosis symptoms appear, contains an unidentified factor of cause. Once multiple sclerosis has occurred, there is no evidence that a move to a warm climate will control or cure it.

SYMPTOMS

Muscular dystrophy attacks persons of all ages. However, males are affected by muscular dystrophy from five to six times as often as females. The older the patient is when the disease begins, the more slowly, usually, does the disease progress. The only symptoms for years may be weak facial muscles that make the person unable to drink through a straw or to whistle. The weak face muscles give the individual a "flat smile" at the stage when he can no longer raise the corners of his mouth.

Many patients with muscular dystrophy eventually spend time in a wheelchair. In adults the ailment sometimes continues for twenty to thirty years or more. However, some become helpless within a few months.

Increasingly plump calf muscles (with fat replacing muscle fibers) make the child appear husky, but such muscles are abnormally weak. The arms begin to hang limply because the muscles in the shoulder girdle are weakening. Afflicted children rarely live to adulthood. In the last stages of muscular dystrophy, the affected muscles are often completely wasted, and the children are pitifully thin.

Pain rarely accompanies muscular dystrophy

in children. Also, the small muscles of the hand are often the last to be affected, so that patients can continue to use their fingers.

Muscular dystrophy is not contagious.

DIAGNOSIS

In some patients, the family doctor makes the diagnosis of muscular dystrophy from a clear-cut history, signs, and symptoms. In doubtful cases, he may refer his patient to a neurologist or to a clinic or research center. A significant number of patients with a diagnosis of possible muscular dystrophy are found to have a different ailment, at times one that can be treated.

Physicians are guided by the patient's medical history and any family history of muscular dystrophy. They observe the patient's movements and muscle reactions as part of a complete physical examination.

Laboratory tests include blood and urine examinations. Although no one test as yet provides proof of muscular dystrophy, certain chemical changes in the urine and blood of patients aid in the diagnosis of muscular dystrophy before body muscles become conspicuously wasted.

The diagnosis is sometimes made quite early after symptoms appear; at other times, years may pass before a positive diagnosis is possible.

Using a local anesthetic to prevent pain, a doctor sometimes takes a sample from a big muscle. Under the microscope, this "biopsy" tissue reveals any changes in the muscle fiber. The first biopsy for muscular dystrophy, performed in 1865, proved the presence of fat in the weakening muscles.

Also, a special kind of X-ray picture may show the fat in the muscle.

Another test sometimes used is called "electromyography," or EMG. The record of such a test is an electromyogram. The scientist inserts a fine needle-like electrode in the muscle. The individual bursts of electrical activity recorded from the muscle with muscular dystrophy are shorter and weaker than those from a healthy muscle. The EMG test helps the physician distinguish between diseases of muscle and diseases of nerve.

Further light on diagnosis of muscular dystrophy is coming from a research method called "tissue culture." A biopsy sample of living muscle is grown in a test tube, where changes in the behavior and appearance of the cells provide clues to the type of muscle disease.

TYPES

Some doctors subdivide muscular dystrophy into several different groups.

1. Childhood. (Other names are Duchenne or pseudohypertrophic.)

The label "pseudohypertrophic" refers to the "false" enlargement often associated with fat in the weakening muscles. Young boys, often around three years of age are affected much more frequently than girls.

2. Juvenile. (Other names include limb-girdle, or Erb, or Leyden-Mobius.)

This type sometimes begins in childhood but more often in the teens or twenties, with both sexes about equally affected. A slow muscle-wasting starts in the shoulder girdle (affecting use of the arms) or in the pelvic girdle (affecting the use of the legs). Pseudohypertrophy is uncommon in this type of muscular dystrophy.

3. Facio-scapulo-humeral. (Another name is Landouzy-Dejerine.)

Weakening starts in childhood or early adult life, in either sex. "Facio" refers to the face muscles, "scapulo" to the shoulder blade, and "humeral" to the upper arm. All these groups of muscles weaken slowly. Patients prepare to earn a living if possible, knowing they can expect to live to middle age.

Mixed types and rare types of muscular dystrophy also occur.

No classification is universally accepted today, even though the idea of a group of dystrophic diseases of muscles was published in 1891.

With a different approach, a group of specialists proposed these four main groups of the muscular dystrophies: severe generalized familial dystrophy and mild restricted muscular dystrophy, which are more usual; and progressive dystrophic ophthalmoplegia and dystrophia myotonica which are less usual.

TREATMENT

Although no cure has been discovered for muscular dystrophy, the general health can be helped by the family doctor or a neurologist.

Physical therapy often bolsters the delaying fight against weakness and crippling. However, it is expensive and does not cure muscular dystrophy. Sometimes the muscular dystrophy patient's doctor asks a physiatrist (doctor of physical medicine and rehabilitation) or a physical therapist to evaluate the patient. The doctor or such a specialist will know of any slings, braces, or other devices to help keep the weakening muscles useful.

"Frozen knees" or "bent and tight" knees are a risk, because the patient usually sits much of the day. Standing — with braces if necessary — exercises, and perhaps a cast for a few hours a day will delay or prevent this crippling and boost the general health. Other joints—the shoulder, for example—also need "range of motion" exercises because of this tendency to lose the ability to move normally.

Deep-breathing exercises help maintain healthy lungs. As the patient weakens, a proper corset may help to prevent slumping and spinal curvature and to maintain good lung space for breathing.

TREATMENT

Numerous treatments have been tested. Antibiotics, vitamins, various medicines, and low-fat diets have been tried. However, no specific drugs or forms of treatment have been widely accepted as consistently beneficial. General health considerations, such as obtaining plenty of rest, avoiding fatigue, and maintaining good nutrition, are especially important.

Many things can and are being done, however, for those with multiple sclerosis. Where physical therapy will be beneficial, physicians prescribe it for their patients. Doctors sometimes find they must encourage multiple sclerosis patients to maintain full range of motion in their arms and legs.

Rehabilitation helps some people, who have a remission of symptoms, to regain lost skills. Occupational therapy at home or elsewhere is useful for many patients, whatever their degree of disability.

There is considerable hope concerning multiple sclerosis today. More and more knowledge is being gathered as investigators dig deeper into its origins and behavior.

The multiple sclerosis patient today lives longer than was thought possible years ago. Many people with mild or even moderately severe cases can live normal lives and work regularly for years.

mumps — a highly contagious childhood disease caused by a virus. This virus is found in the saliva of infected persons and is spread by direct personal contact, through the droplets expelled by infected persons when they cough or sneeze, and possibly by using articles contaminated by them, such as their unwashed eating or drinking utensils.

Most cases of mumps occur during the winter and spring months and in children between the ages of five and fifteen. The disease is less frequent among adults. One attack usually makes a person immune for life.

In many cases the illness is so mild that it is not recognized or diagnosed. Ordinary cases in children are seldom serious. Sometimes the infection spreads to the reproductive glands or to the central nervous system. In general, the disease is more dangerous in teenagers and adults than in children.

SYMPTOMS

Signs of mumps appear between two and three weeks after exposure. The first sign is usually pain under one or both ears or under the chin. Often there is a fever, followed by swelling of one or more salivary glands—sometimes in the neck or throat, but usually just below and in front of the ears. Cases often start with chills, fever, headache, and loss of appetite for a day or two before the glands begin to swell. Most cases last about a week. A person with mumps is infectious from about a week before the glands start to swell until the swelling disappears.

TREATMENT

There is no specific treatment for mumps. The patient should stay in bed until the fever subsides. He should have plenty of liquids and a soft diet. Regular foods are difficult to swallow when the glands are enlarged, and highly spiced or acid foods may create pain.

murmur — an abnormal heart sound. It frequently sounds like fluid passing an obstruction. A murmur can be heard between the normal lub-dub heart sounds.

muscle — the tissue that is responsible for body movement. The fibers forming the muscles are bound together in bundles of different lengths, breadths, and thicknesses. Bundles of muscle tissue can shorten, lengthen, or thicken. This type of action makes possible the movements of various parts of the body.

There are two types of muscles. Voluntary muscles are those over which an individual can exert control, such as the muscles in the arms and legs. Involuntary muscles are those that an indi-

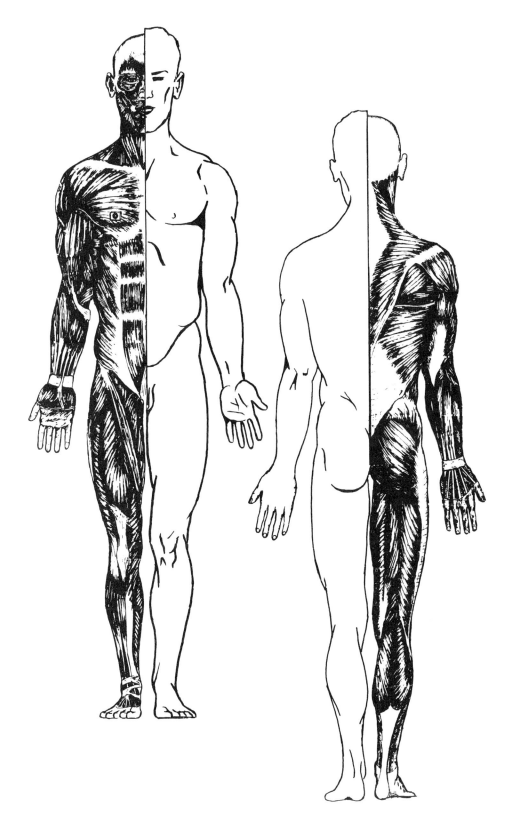

MUSCLE

vidual cannot control, such as the muscles of the heart and the muscles involved in digestion and breathing. Muscles are attached to bones by strong, fibrous cords called tendons. Tendons are not elastic, but the power of contraction or extension of the muscles to which they are attached causes the bones forming joints to move either by flexing or by extending.

The body has over six hundred muscles. Approximately forty percent of a male's weight is muscle. A female's weight is thirty-five percent muscle. The exact percentage depends on the physical condition of the individual. An athlete's weight will have a higher muscle percentage than that of an office worker.

muscular dystrophy — a group of diseases, often called the muscular dystrophies, that cause a progressive wasting and weakening of the muscles. Thus, it is known as progressive muscular dystrophy.

Muscular dystrophy weakens the voluntary muscles—the muscles on the outside of the body, such as the biceps of the arm. Unlike polio, the internal muscles, such as the diaphragm, are not affected by muscular dystrophy. Also unlike polio, it usually affects equally the muscles on both sides of the body, leading to symmetrical weakening and wasting.

For centuries, muscular dystrophy was confused with other wasting diseases. The problem was to distinguish muscular dystrophy, which is a specific muscle disease, from diseases where muscle-wasting is the result of the paralysis of a nerve, as in polio, or from various diseases of the bones and joints accompanied by wasting muscles.

In 1830 an Englishman wrote about his identification of some of the symptoms of muscular dystrophy. A French neurologist in 1850 published a description of the childhood form but still confused muscular dystrophy with another ailment. Not until 1891 was muscular dystrophy described as a clearly separate disease and given the name "progressive muscular dystrophy."

CAUSE
Muscular dystrophy has long been recognized as a disorder that often affects several people in one family. It is now well established that in most forms of muscular dystrophy an inherited characteristic coming from either parent is responsible. Scientists are searching for physical or chemical

abnormalities of the affected muscles that could explain the nature of this inheritance.

For example, in a research laboratory test in Florida, reported in 1961, proteins with an abnormal composition were found in muscle samples from patients with two types of muscular dystrophy. Such research progress adds to the hope that suitable treatment will be discovered for muscular dystrophy, since some other ailments caused by other inherited defects can be treated effectively by a special diet or medication.

Family problems increase as a child (especially a boy) with muscular dystrophy grows taller and sometimes heavier than the mother who has been lifting him. A wheelchair becomes essential but is expensive. An electrical or mechanical invalid-lift, also expensive, may be necessary to get the patient out of bed and into the wheelchair.

muscular rheumatism — *See fibrositis.*

myelin — the fatty covering that normally protects and insulates the nerve fibers of the spinal cord and brain.

A breakdown of myelin is the cause of difficulty in multiple sclerosis. Without myelin, body signals to and from the nerves cannot function properly.

myocardial infarction — the damaging or death of a part of the heart muscle. Myocardial infarction is caused by a reduction or a complete stoppage of the blood supply to that area of the heart. Myocardial infarction is also known as heart attack, coronary occlusion, coronary, and coronary thrombosis.

Acute myocardial infarction is the most frequent cardiac emergency. The incidence of myocardial infarction increases with advancing age, particularly after age fifty. The incidence is six times as high in males as in females.

CAUSE
Myocardial infarction is caused by the blocking or narrowing of a coronary artery by a clot. The underlying cause is arteriosclerotic heart disease. The death rate from myocardial infarction among smokers is nine times the death rate for nonsmokers. Most cases are unrelated to physical effort, with only about five percent occurring during heavy physical activity. About twenty percent of the attacks occur in sleep or when the patient is at rest. In a number of industries, it has

been found that the attack rate for myocardial infarction is significantly higher among sedentary employees than among those whose jobs require active and heavy physical activity.

SYMPTOMS

In about half of the cases, onset is preceded by a history of angina pectoris. There is sudden severe pain in the chest, often radiating to the left arm. It usually persists for several hours. There is a fall in blood pressure and also shock. The pain is accompanied by pallor, sweating, and shortness of breath.

TREATMENT

Recovery from myocardial infarction generally requires absolute bed rest for four to six weeks, morphine or other drugs for the relief of pain and apprehension, and an anticoagulant medication. The total treatment time averages three to four months.

Although eighty percent of patients with heart attacks survive the initial attack, sudden death is not an unusual occurrence during the first month. For the first thirty days the patient is acutely ill, requiring intensive medical and nursing care in a hospital. The crisis is usually passed in the third week, and the patient can be discharged about the sixth week.

For the younger patient, a heart attack may come at a time of life when his responsibilities to his family, employer, and community are the heaviest. Frequently, he has no history of cardiovascular disease. Abruptly, he finds himself seriously ill, completely dependent, fearful of death or a life of invalidism, and helplessly aware of his staggering responsibilities. In many diseases, the transition from self-sufficiency to dependency comes slowly, with automatic adjustments made along the way. For the heart-attack patient, the transition is cruelly abrupt. With each additional day of survival, the patient begins to realize that he is going to live, and some of his pessimism is usually replaced with optimism.

The cardiac patient differs from most other types of patients in that he has no obvious disability. The lack of visible signs of disability helps the patient resume previous relationships but, on the other hand, may make it harder for others to recognize the limitations imposed by the condition. Family members and others may become oversolicitous of the patient, refusing to let him do things for himself, thereby impeding his rehabilitation. Often the cardiac patient must quit

smoking and lose weight. Since eating and smoking have definite emotional components, patients attempting to stop smoking or to eat less require strong support from all quarters.

Most patients make a good recovery within two to six months, and about two-thirds of them return to the work they did previously. Employers are usually willing to make adjustments in conditions of work to accommodate the patient in his rehabilitation program. It should be remembered, however, that the patient has a damaged heart and the potential for another heart attack.

PREVENTION

Among some of the measures believed to reduce heart attacks are control of weight, elimination of smoking, regular exercise, diet selectivity, and medical supervision of related diseases, such as diabetes and hypertension.

myocardial insufficiency — an inability of the heart muscle (myocardium) to maintain normal circulation.
See congestive heart failure.

myocarditis — an inflammation of the heart muscle (myocardium).

myocardium — the muscular wall of the heart. The myocardium is the thickest of the three layers of the heart wall. It lies between the inner layer (endocardium) and the outer layer (epicardium).

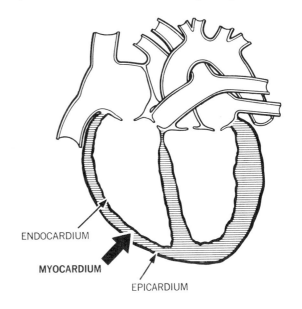

ENDOCARDIUM

MYOCARDIUM

EPICARDIUM

MYOCARDIUM

myopia — nearsightedness. In the nearsighted eye, distant objects produce a blurred image. This is usually caused by an abnormally long front-to-back diameter of the eye. Thus, the focal image is formed in front of the retina.

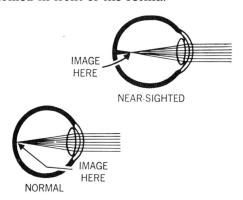

NEAR-SIGHTED

NORMAL

MYOPIA

Some cases of high myopia (where great correction is required) are progressive; they result from a disease rather than merely an error of refraction. Glasses may be unable to correct vision to normal range, and there may be destructive changes in various parts of the eye (choroid, retina, or vitreous body). High myopia tends to be accompanied by other changes that may be affected by strenuous physical activities.

myxedema — a form of cretinism occurring in adolescence or adulthood. The symptoms are similar—retardation, coarse hair, dry skin, and goiter. However, because it occurs after most growth has stopped, dwarfing is avoided. Like cretinism, myxedema is caused by a deficiency or a complete lack of thyroid hormone. Treatment consists of thyroid extract.

n

nails — a tough, dense modification of skin. Nails cover the ends of the fingers, thumbs, and toes. A nail grows out of its nail root. This root is embedded in the skin at the end of the nail closest to the body. The skin that covers the nail root and the sides of the nail is known as the nail wall. The tissue beneath the nail itself is referred to as the nail bed. The half-moon of white at the base of the nail is called the lunula.

The rate of growth of nails is subject to individual differences. However, an individual's fingernails usually grow twice as fast as his toenails.

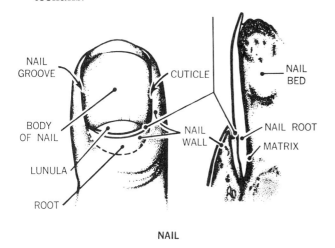

NAIL

nalorphine — a drug classified as a narcotic antagonist.

See narcotic antagonists.

nape — a nonmedical term indicating the external portion of the back of the neck.

narcolepsy — a condition characterized by overwhelming episodes of sleep during normal waking hours. A certain amount of muscle weakness is associated with the condition. The muscle weakness also comes and goes in spells but does not necessarily occur in connection with the sleeping spells.

Physicians usually treat narcolepsy with doses of amphetamines. The dosage is arranged so that it does not interfere with normal night sleep.

narcotic — an addictive drug that relieves pain and induces sleep. The narcotics, or opiates, include opium and its active components (such as morphine) and heroin, which is morphine that has been chemically altered to make it about six times stronger. Narcotics also include a series of synthetic chemicals that have a morphine-like action.

If a person has a tolerance for an opiate, he can usually function satisfactorily. This assumes that he is on a constant dosage level and that his body's reaction to the drug is minimal. It merely keeps him comfortable. This ability to perform, to stay awake and alert after being kept on a maintenance level has been demonstrated with the methadone maintenance treatment. An occasional person will be drowsy.

Generally, there is a feeling of relaxation and of being "high." This is accompanied by an "awayness," or pleasant, dreamlike state. As tolerance develops, however, the "high" is generally lost. An addict then requires the drug to avoid withdrawl sickness. In other words, at this point he is using the drug to feel normal.

237

Despite the inherent dangers of addiction, narcotics are extremely effective and important drugs.

See heroin, heroin addiction, morphine, withdrawal sickness.

narcotic antagonists — a class of drugs that partially reverse the effects of narcotic drugs. Narcotic antagonists are particularly important in the treatment of overdoses of narcotics.

An overdose of a narcotic depresses the respiratory reflex. The narcotic antagonists are extremely effective in rapidly restoring the respiratory rate to its normal level.

These drugs are also used in the detection of narcotic addiction. When a narcotic antagonist is given to a patient who is addicted to narcotics, the patient will exhibit the classical symptoms of withdrawal sickness.

See narcotic, withdrawal sickness.

naris — *See nostril.*

nasal cavity — the internal portion of the nose.
See nose.

nasopharynx — the upper part of the pharynx, which connects with the nose.
See pharynx.

nasus — *See nose.*

nates — the buttocks.
See buttocks.

Nathan's test — a test for tuberculosis. A special serum, with a dressing, is applied to the surface of the arm. The dressing is removed the next day. A positive reaction will appear within six days.

natural childbirth — a method of childbirth that requires the mother to be conscious and to cooperate actively with the processes of birth during labor and delivery. The expectant mother undergoes a program of education, exercise, and training (both physical and mental) in preparation for labor and delivery. The woman learns how to relax and to work in harmony with the contractions.

Because natural childbirth requires little or no medication, there is little or no anesthesia in the mother's system for the baby to absorb.

The decision as to whether or not to have a natural childbirth rests primarily with the woman. What is "natural" for one woman may not be natural for another.

natural immunity — the ability of a person to resist a disease without having had the disease and without being vaccinated against the disease. A natural immunity is based on the body's own defense and immunity system. The term is usually used to indicate an immunity to a disease that most people will contract when they are exposed to it.
See immunity.

nausea — a sensation that occurs before a person is going to vomit, or when he feels as if he might vomit. Nausea is a symptom rather than a disease. It may be caused by headaches, motion sickness, pregnancy, and radiation, as well as by an upset stomach. The treatment depends on the factor that is causing the nausea.

navel — the small scar in the middle or lower part of the abdomen. The navel is the remnant of the umbilical cord.
See umbilical cord.

nearsightedness — *See myopia.*

neck — the portion of the body that connects the head with the trunk of the body. The neck is very complicated because there are so many body organs and parts within it. Located within the neck are body parts such as the pharynx, esophagus, larynx, trachea, and the thyroid gland. Thus, the neck is a continuation of both the digestive tract and the respiratory system. The organs mentioned above, as well as a number of lymph nodes, are situated in the front of the neck.

The back of the neck consists of the spinal column. Within the spinal column are the spinal cord and a large number of nerves. Seven vertebrae form the beginning of the spinal column. These vertebrae, called the cervical vertebrae, are all located in the neck.

The first cervical vertebra is referred to as the atlas. The construction of the atlas allows the head to tilt up and down, or nod. The second of the cervical vertebrae is known as the axis. This vertebra permits the head to turn from side to side. The rotation of the head pivots on the axis.

When the spinal cord is cut or subjected to extreme pressure, paralysis of the body occurs below the site of the injury. Therefore, any serious injury to the back of the neck can lead to paralysis from the neck down.

See spinal cord, vertebra.

negative afterimage — the visual phenomenon that occurs after looking at a colored object and then at a white object. The afterimage will occur in the complimentary color. For example, after looking at a red ball and then directing the eyes to a piece of white paper, the eyes will "see" a green ball shape on the paper.

neonatal period — a term used to describe the first month of a baby's life.

neoplasm — any abnormal formation or growth. The term is usually used to indicate a tumor. The phrase "malignant neoplasm" is sometimes used to indicate cancer.

nephritis — an inflammation of the kidney.

See kidney.

nerve block — the anesthesia, or numbing, of an area of the body. This is accomplished by injecting the anesthesia in the vicinity of the region to be affected.

Nerve blocks are performed for a variety of reasons, including the relief of pain in facial neuralgia and for prevention of pain when a dentist is filling or extracting a tooth.

See anesthesia.

nerves — a collection or bundle of fibers (called neuron fibers) that are interconnected and pro-

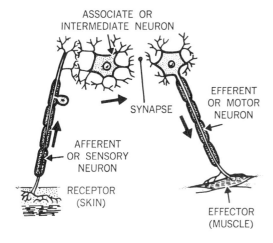

NERVE

tected by a sheath. The nerve cell itself has a nucleus, protoplasm, and a cell membrane. Projecting from the main cell body are many small fibers that have branches. These are called dendrites. One long fiber, called an axon, approaches (but never touches) the dendrites of the next nerve cell. The axon is covered by a white fatty substance that protects it.

There are three different types of nerves. Each type fulfills a slightly different function. A sensory nerve receives sensations and transmits them to the brain. A motor nerve transmits impulses from the brain to the muscles and glands. An associative nerve transmits impulses from sensory nerves to motor nerves.

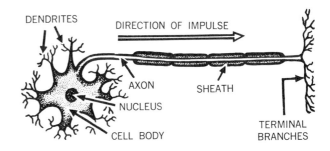

NERVE

The impulse moves from the dendrites, to the main cell body, to the axon. The impulse (which is actually a minute electrical charge) then jumps the space between the axon of one nerve cell and the dendrites of the next nerve cell. The small space between two nerves is called a synapse.

There are only eighty-six nerves in the entire body: twelve pairs of cranial nerves and thirty-one pairs of spinal nerves. All the remaining nerves in the body are only branches of the original eighty-six nerves.

See nervous system.

nervous system — the system that is responsible for keeping the various parts of the body and the organs controlling the body functions in touch with each other. The nervous system actually consists of two separate but interconnected and coordinated systems: the cerebrospinal system and the autonomic system.

CEREBROSPINAL SYSTEM

The cerebrospinal system consists of the brain and the spinal cord. The brain is a collection of nerve centers, each a central station for some part of the body—much like a central telephone station, with trunk lines or nerves connecting the parts of the body with their particular centers. Leaving the brain, these trunk nerves are bundled into the spinal cord, which passes down through the opening in the center of the backbone or spinal column, giving off branches to all parts and organs of the body.

Most of the nerves entering and leaving the spinal cord are either sensory nerves or motor nerves. Sensory nerves enter the cord conveying impressions of sensations, such as heat, cold, touch, and pain, from different parts of the body to the brain. Motor nerves leave the spinal cord conveying impulses from the brain to the muscles causing movement.

AUTONOMIC SYSTEM

The autonomic system is a series of nerve centers in the chest and abdominal cavity along the spinal column. Each of these nerve centers, although interconnected with the cerebrospinal system, presides over and controls vital organs and vital functions. This system is not under control of the will, but through it involuntary muscles are stimulated to act alike during periods of wakefulness and during periods of sleep. Thus, the heart beats, respiration continues, blood pressure is maintained, food is digested, and the excretory organs function without any conscious effort.

The autonomic nervous system consists of two sets of systems: the sympathetic nerves and the parasympathetic nerves. These two sets have opposite effects on the same body organs. For example, the parasympathetic nerves constrict the pupil of the eye; the sympathetic nerves dilate the pupil of the eye.

neuralgia — a painful disorder of one or more nerves. The nerve causing the pain is not necessarily damaged. Neuralgia usually causes sharp, fitful pains.

Facial neuralgia attacks persons over fifty years of age more frequently than it does younger people. In this disorder, excruciating pains flash intermittently across one side of the face. Sometimes a tingling of the skin warns that an attack is due. The spasms are usually "set off" by a draft of cold air or by swallowing, yawning, chewing, shaving, or similar activities. The pain can often be induced by pressing a sensitive "trigger point" along the nerve path. After a while, the painful flashes stop, only to appear again at any time

from hours to months later. If the condition is not relieved, the period between attacks becomes shorter and shorter, until pain is practically continuous.

Various infections or injuries of the nerve may cause neuralgia to strike other parts of the body. Sometimes the back of the neck, the eye, the lower back, or the chest may be involved. The symptoms may suggest other diseases. Sharp chest pains, for example, may suggest heart disease or pleurisy when they are actually caused by neuralgia. An experienced physician can identify true neuralgia.

In treating neuralgia, physicians use a variety of medicines. Some cases of neuralgia can be cured by an operation.

neuritis — a disorder of one or more nerves. Neuritis usually involves inflammation of a nerve or nerves and causes a constant, burning pain.

The disorder may be localized to one nerve or may involve many. Either type may result from injuries, poisons, infections, or chilling. The localized type is more common. The path of the nerve develops a burning sensation. The flesh may have a numb or "crawling" feeling. The skin is often reddened along the course of the nerve. The condition is not usually serious unless it is allowed to continue without treatment.

Sciatica is a localized neuritis of the sciatic nerve. This is the nerve that runs along the back of the leg.

A generalized neuritis is far more serious than a localized neuritis. It is often caused by prolonged illness, by exposure to chemicals such as lead or arsenic, or by alcoholism. Failure to eat and absorb enough food containing the B vitamins seems to be an important cause.

Usually the patient complains for several weeks of numbness, tingling in the fingers and feet, and of sensations of heat and cold. There may be a slight fever. After the initial symptoms, the patient experiences weakness and pain in the muscles. If untreated, he may lose all feeling in the "glove and stocking" areas of the arms and legs and develop paralysis. The untreated patient may eventually become bedridden.

Neuritis may occasionally be relieved by an operation to remove the cause (such as a tumor). A sound, carefully planned exercise program is often prescribed in addition to a variety of drugs.

neuroblastoma — a malignant tumor of the nervous

system; it is composed of immature nerve cells.

neurocirculatory asthenia — a complex of nervous and circulatory symptoms, often involving a sense of fatigue, dizziness, shortness of breath, rapid heartbeat, and nervousness. Neurocirculatory asthenia is also known as effort syndrome and soldier's heart.
See effort syndrome.

neurogenic — a term used to indicate anything that originates from within the nervous system.

neurosis — a functional nervous disease in which the personality remains more or less intact.
See mental illness.

neurosyphilis — syphilis that affects the central nervous system; that is, the brain, the meninges (the three layers that cover the brain), or the spinal cord. Neurosyphilis occurs when a patient who has syphilis does not get proper treatment—usually because he is not aware that he has it.
See syphilis.

nevi — relatively small benign growths on the skin. They are commonly referred to as moles, birthmarks, freckles, etc., depending on the consistency, color of pigmentation, and degree of elevation.

Some nevi have a tendency to become malignant. These are usually flat, dark moles that do not have hairs. Additionally, they are usually located in areas that receive constant friction from clothes, other skin, or foreign objects. Areas of special concern are the palms of the hands and the soles of the feet.

niacin — *See vitamin B.*

nicotine — a substance found in tobacco leaves. It has no medical uses and is an addictive substance. Although nicotine is very toxic, smokers develop a tolerance for it and can withstand much higher doses than nonsmokers can.

Nicotine affects the autonomic nervous system. It affects both the parasympathetic and the sympathetic nerves. Thus, the pupils of the eyes are first constricted and then dilated.

Niemann-Pick disease — a form of mental illness characterized by a defect of metabolism of fats.

This disease is inherited. The symptoms include a brownish discoloration of the skin and progressive blindness. Niemann-Pick disease, sometimes known as lipoid histiocytosis, often causes early death.

night blindness — *See nyctalopia.*

nipple — the dark, raised area of the breast that secretes milk.

nitrites — a group of chemical compounds, many of which cause dilation of the small blood vessels. These are called vasodilators. Amyl nitrite and sodium nitrite are examples of nitrites.

The importance of these compounds is that by dilating the blood vessels, they reduce the resistance to the flow of blood and consequently lower the blood pressure.

nitrogen mustard therapy — a treatment for cancer of the lymph glands.

nitroglycerin — a drug (one of the nitrites) that relaxes the muscles in the blood vessels. Nitroglycerin is used to relieve attacks of angina pectoris and spasm of the coronary arteries.

Nitroglycerin works by relaxing and dilating blood vessels. This allows blood to flow more easily through the vessels, and consequently lowers the blood pressure and reduces the work load of the heart muscle.

Nitroglycerin is probably the best and most widely used drug for the relief of pain in angina attacks. It is taken in tablet form, either under the tongue (where it quickly dissolves) or chewed. Nitroglycerin will not do its job if it is simply swallowed in tablet form. Most patients experience total cessation of pain within two minutes.

nitroglycerin poisoning — mild nitroglycerin poisoning frequently occurs among men who handle explosives that are high in nitroglycerin content. Some persons are highly susceptible to nitroglycerin and should never handle or be around explosives containing it.

The symptoms of nitroglycerin poisoning are a queer, full sensation of the head; giddiness; headache in the frontal region and extending to the back of the head and neck with increasing severity; irregular pulse; dilation of the pupils of the eyes; pain in the front of the chest; muscular weakness; nausea and vomiting; loss of consciousness; and convulsions in extreme cases.

nitrous oxide — a colorless gas that is the oldest of the inhaled gas anesthetics. "Laughing gas," as it is also known, was first made by Priestley in 1776.
See anesthetics.

nocturnal emission — the involuntary ejaculation of semen during sleep.

node — a term used to indicate a small swelling that is hard or solid to the touch.

nodule — *See node.*

noradrenaline — *See norepinephrine.*

norepinephrine — a hormone secreted by the adrenal glands. Norepinephrine produces a rise in blood pressure by constricting the small blood vessels. As a synthesized drug, norepinephrine is sometimes used in the treatment of shock.

normal — a term used to indicate something that falls within a regular or established pattern. The concept of normalcy is a very difficult one in medicine. What is normal for one person is not necessarily normal for another person.

Physicians refer to certain reactions to certain drugs as normal reactions. This means that most people have these reactions. For example, most people experience a certain amount of pain relief from aspirin. That is the normal reaction. However, some people are allergic to aspirin and their response to it may include an upset stomach or a rash, as well as more violent reactions. When compared with the average reaction, theirs is not normal, but their body is reacting normally for them.

Another example is the range of individual differences in body temperature. Normal, or average, body temperature is 98.6°F. when taken orally. Anything below that is called subnormal; anything above that is referred to as a fever. However, there are people whose temperature is normally (for them) 98°F. or even lower. They are perfectly healthy, but their temperature is not normal. When people like this report a temperature of 98.6°F., they are usually running a fever, even though their temperature is normal for most people.

An experienced physician is always aware of individual differences. He uses the concept of normal as a yardstick to compare an individual's reactions, not as a rule to which all patients must adhere. One of the reasons medicine is considered to be an art as well as a science is the degree to which these individual differences affect diagnosis and treatment.

normotensive — any condition characterized by normal blood pressure.

nose — the part of the face that contains the sense of smell. The nose, or nasus, is also a very important part of the respiratory system.

The nose is composed of two nostrils that are divided by a nasal septum (made of bone and cartilage). Farther in are a group of scroll-shaped bones referred to as the conchae or the turbinates. All the interior surfaces of the nose (including the conchae) are covered by mucous membranes. The surface of the mucous membranes is covered with tiny hairs called cilia. Several small openings in the nasal cavities lead to the sinuses. The sinuses help to adjust the pressure within the nose.

Air enters the nose filled with small particles, bacteria, etc. The cilia on the mucous membranes act as filters, preventing foreign matter from entering the lungs. The mucous membranes secrete a thick fluid called mucus which also helps to stop foreign matter from going any farther in the respiratory system. Additionally, the mucus and the mucous membranes warm and moisten the incoming air. This is particularly important on cold, dry days. People who breathe through their mouths are losing the protection the nose gives to the respiratory system.

Located within the nose are nerve endings of the olfactory nerves. This pair of cranial nerves is responsible for the sense of smell. When the nose is congested with mucus (as happens during a cold), the mucus covers the nerve endings, causing a reduction in the ability to detect odors. The sensations of smell and taste are closely related. Thus, when there is a loss of the sense of smell, the sense of taste will also be affected, although not necessarily to the same degree.

The nose plays an important role in the production of intelligible speech. The sounds emerging from the larynx (voice box) are very crude. They are refined by passing up through the nose and the sinuses (as well as through the mouth). When the nose is congested, the sound of the voice changes, usually becoming considerably deeper.
See sinus.

nosebleed — bleeding through the nose. Nosebleeds are usually caused by the rupture of one or more of the small blood vessels in the nose. The rupture itself can be caused by sneezing, a foreign object in the nose (including a finger), etc.

nose drops — medicine taken in liquid form through the nose. Nose drops are usually used to help clear the sinus passages and allow free breathing.

nostril — one of the pair of outside openings to the nose.
See nose.

notifiable disease — a disease that a patient or his physician must report to health authorities. Diseases are classified as notifiable because they can cause serious epidemics or because health authorities need statistics about them.

notochord — the first supportive structure of an embryo. In humans, the notochord is an immature spinal column. As the human embryo grows, the notochord is replaced by the real spinal column.

novocain — a trade name for procaine.
See procaine.

nucleus — a specialized portion of the protoplasm of cells. The nucleus contains the chromosomes and is responsible for coordinating cell activities.
See chromosome.

nullipara — a term used to indicate a woman who has not yet given birth to a live child. A woman who has had a miscarriage or whose child is stillborn is considered to be a nullipara until she has produced a live birth.

numbness — a condition in which an area of the body is insensitive when touched. Numbness can be caused by disease, malfunctioning body parts, etc. Numbness can also be artificially induced by drugs to relieve existing pain or to prevent pain during a surgical or dental procedure.

The sensation of touch and external pressure is transmitted by nerves. When the nerves are damaged or blocked (as by an anesthetic), the brain does not receive the proper information from the affected nerves.

The term numbness is usually used to indicate a loss of surface and subsurface feeling. This can be very dangerous, because part of the body's warning system is lost. Thus, if a patient with a numb finger is burned, he may not realize it until the deep nerves are affected. By the time the deep nerves are alerted, very serious damage may have been sustained.
See nerve, nervous system.

nurse — an individual specially trained in the care and handling of sick people.

nursing — *See breast-feeding.*

nutrition — the combination of processes by which a living organism receives and utilizes the materials necessary for the maintenance of its functions and for the growth and renewal of its components.

From simple one-celled plants to highly complex human beings, all living things need food. Food is necessary to support growth, to repair constantly wearing tissues, and to supply energy for physical activity. Unless the food consumed supplies all the elements required for normal life processes, the human body cannot operate at peak efficiency for very long. If an essential nutrient is missing from the diet over long periods of time, deficiency diseases such as rickets, scurvy, or certain anemias may develop.

Everyone needs the same nutrients throughout life but in different amounts. Proportionately greater amounts are required for the growth of a body than just for its upkeep. Boys and men need more energy and nutrients than girls and women. Large people need more than small people. Active people require more food energy than inactive ones. People recovering from illness need more than healthy people.

The nutrients in food that are necessary for good health can be divided into certain groups —proteins, carbohydrates, fats, vitamins, minerals, and water. Most common foods consist of combinations of the above. Foods that are good sources of one food element usually also contribute other essential elements as well, but no one food supplies all needed nutrients in sufficient amounts. For good nutrition all essential food elements must work together. Therefore, well-balanced nutrition calls for a well-chosen variety of foods.

Proteins make up the basic material of each body cell. They are the main constituents of the muscles and most lean tissues of the body. Proteins are required in the daily diet for growth, maintenance, and repair of tissues, as well as for many other body processes.

The carbohydrates (starches and sugars) serve as sources of energy for the human body: to do external and internal work, and to maintain body temperature. Carbohydrates are the most economical sources of body energy.

Fats are primarily a source of food energy, and in this respect they are more than twice as "rich" as carbohydrates or proteins.

The vitamins are compounds that are essential in very small amounts for the proper utilization of foods and for healthy functioning of the human body.

Most of the hard tissues of the human body, such as bones and teeth, are composed in part of mineral elements. The body also needs minerals, some in very minute quantities, to carry on various life processes.

Water is an important nutrient without which the normal life processes cannot take place.

Good nutrition is just as important for older people as it is for infants and growing teenagers. However, some of the nutritional requirements do change in elderly people. Usually, less physical work is performed in advanced age, and therefore the body's requirement for calories is lower. Dietary calories that are not used are stored in the form of body fat, and many persons who continue the richer diet of their physically more active days may become too heavy. This is the main reason why fewer carbohydrates and less fat are needed in the food of the aged.

See carbohydrates, fats, minerals, proteins, etc.

nyctalopia — the inability to see at night or in a low-light level. Nyctalopia is also known as night blindness.

The ability of the eye to see at night or in a dark room depends on the rods in the retina. The rods transmit black, white, and gray impulses. When the rods are not functioning properly, there is no low-light vision (color- and bright-light vision are not affected by the rods).

Nyctalopia is caused by a lack of rhodopsin, a substance formed from vitamin A. Night blindness can also be an inherited condition.

nystagmus — an abnormality of the eye characterized by rapid, involuntary, jerky movements of the eyeball. These movements may be horizontal, vertical, rotary, or mixed. Nystagmus is usually associated with congenital diseases but may develop as a result of constant exposure to poor lighting. The vision may be impaired because the eyes cannot remain still long enough to focus on an object.

obesity — a bodily condition in which there is an excess of fat in relation to other body components. The condition is presumed to exist when an individual is twenty percent or more over normal weight. This is a general guide. A diagnosis should be made by a physician.

Obesity is a common condition, especially in middle life. Conservative estimates indicate that about twenty million people weigh more than ten percent over normal weight. Obesity occurs with about equal frequency in young adults of both sexes, with more women becoming overweight after age thirty. It has a tendency to occur among members of the same families and is thought to be more prevalent among individuals at the lower end of the social, educational, and economic scale.

There was a time when overweight was considered a sign of prosperity and abundance. Plumpness spoke well for a person, for it indicated a comfortable position in life. However, it is now known that the fat person is not necessarily well-nourished. Excessive body weight puts an undue strain on the heart, and in predisposed individuals it encourages the emergence of latent diabetes. Obesity also increases the liability to a number of diseases, such as high blood pressure and hardening of the arteries and, as a rule, tends to shorten the life-span.

Obesity is caused by a persistent caloric intake that exceeds the energy output needs of the body. Causation is a complex problem, but current knowledge includes such factors as heredity, emotions, culture, diet, and lack of exercise.

In advanced cases, there may be fatigue; short-ness of breath; and aching of the back, legs, knees, and feet. Excoriation and infection of the skin beneath the rolls of fat occurs. At a later date, signs of hypertension, heart failure, respiratory failure, arthritis, and diabetes may develop.

TREATMENT

Reduced to simple terms, the successful treatment of obesity involves achieving a balance between diet and exercise. The attainment of this balance is a complex affair requiring the best efforts of the patient and the therapist. Treatment should be undertaken only under the supervision of a physician. Increased physical activity should not be sporadic but should become an integral and comfortable part of the patient's life. In establishing a diet, emphasis should be placed on nutritional adequacy and on the amount and type of food eaten. The fact that the excess of just 100 calories (a small chocolate bar contains 155 calories) a day will add up to 3,000 calories a month, or almost a pound of body weight, indicates the intricacy of the balance required in diet and exercise. Over a year, this will amount to a weight gain of ten pounds. On the other hand, a deficit of 500 calories per day will result in the loss of approximately one pound per week. The rate of weight loss should be controlled and under ordinary circumstances should not exceed two pounds per week. Drugs, formula diets, and fads involving food or exercise may result in short-term weight losses, but over a long period, these generally prove ineffective, with the patient returning to his original weight.

245

In the American culture, where fat people are considered to be unattractive, obesity represents an aesthetic problem, and therefore a psychological one. The more immediate gains of improved personal appearance, better social acceptance, greater physical fitness, and the feeling of well-being play a more important role in motivating people to lose weight than the more remote concerns of lessened morbidity and improved longevity.

Weight reduction may be very difficult for the patient and frustrating for the therapist. Reassurance, ego support, and reinforcement of the goals established by the therapist and patient are important techniques in working with the obese patient. For some obese people, overeating may be the most satisfactory way for them to meet life's stresses and strains. If this is the case, it may be futile and even undesirable to encourage this type of person to curtail his eating unless a substitute method is developed for handling his emotional problems.

The role of exercise in weight reduction is subject to a great deal of misunderstanding. There is a widespread misbelief that exercise consumes very few calories and that an increase in appetite automatically follows an increase in exercise; conversely, there is widespread misbelief that reduction in food intake automatically follows the reduction of physical activity.

Exercise should be regular and daily, not sporadic. The life pattern should be reorganized so that some form of exercise becomes an integral part of daily living. The alternate to exercise is persistent hunger, which, as a weight-control technique, is doomed to failure. There should also be an understanding of the caloric "burn off" rate of various types of exercise. For example, a 160-pound man uses 350 calories an hour when he walks at the rate of four miles per hour. He uses 300 calories an hour when he plays golf and 500 calories or more an hour in a game of tennis.

PREVENTION

Experience has demonstrated that some success is attained in weight reduction in persons who have become obese as adults. However, it has been found to be most difficult to reduce adults who have been obese throughout adolescence or since childhood. The major effort in prevention should be directed toward preventing children and adolescents with familial tendencies toward obesity from becoming obese by emphasizing to them desirable food and exercise habits. In women, excessive weight is most apt to occur after age twenty, during pregnancy, and after menopause. Men tend to gain weight between twenty-five years of age and old age. Both sexes tend to gain weight after they have quit smoking cigarettes, or when accident or illness suddenly immobilizes them. Preventive measures are especially applicable at these times.

See nutrition, overweight.

obstetrician — a doctor whose specialty is the care and treatment of women from pregancy through labor and delivery.

See labor, pregnancy.

obstetrics — the branch of medicine that deals with pregnancy, labor, and delivery.

obstruction — a term indicating the blockage of a body vessel. Obstructions can occur in any body vessel. They can be very serious, and, if they occur in certain places, they can be fatal. For example, a child who swallows something solid may find his trachea obstructed or blocked. Unless the object is removed or an alternate breathing passage is made (tracheostomy), the child may die from lack of air.

A blood clot formed in another part of the body may be carried to one of the arteries of the brain, where it obstructs the further flow of blood and causes a stroke.

Obstructions may be caused by foreign objects, by blood clots, by naturally formed "stones" (such as gallstones), and by tumors (benign or malignant).

occipital — of or pertaining to the back of the head or cranium. The occipital region is called the occiput.

occiput — *See occipital.*

oleaginous — a term used to indicate that a substance is oily or greasy.

olfactory nerve — the cranial nerve that transmits the sense of smell from the nose to the brain.

omagra — gout that occurs in the shoulder.

See gout.

oncology — the branch of medicine that is concerned with tumors.

onyx — the technical term for a fingernail or a toenail.
See nails.

onyxis — an ingrown nail. This occurs more frequently to the toenails than to the fingernails. The friction and pressure of shoes may cause the skin surrounding the nail to grow over the side of the nail.

open-heart surgery — surgery performed on the open heart while the bloodstream is diverted through a heart-lung machine. This machine pumps and oxygenates the blood in lieu of the action of the heart and lungs during the operation.

Open-heart surgery is performed to replace or correct damaged or diseased sections of the heart.

open wound — any break in the skin. When the skin is unbroken, it affords protection from most infections, bacteria, or germs. However, when the skin is broken, no matter how slight the break, germs may enter, and an infection may develop. Any wound where the skin is broken should receive prompt medical attention, and only sterile objects should be in contact with any open wounds. If germ life has been carried into an open wound by the object causing the break in the skin, nature attempts to wash out the germs by the flow of blood; but some types of wounds do not bleed freely.

Statistics indicate that about one open wound in every twenty shows evidence of infection, and, where open wounds do not receive early first aid or medical care, the rate of infection is nearly doubled.

A break in the skin may range from a pin puncture or scratch to an extensive cut, tear, or mash. An open wound may be only the surface evidence of a more serious injury to deeper structures, such as fractures, particularly in head injuries involving fracture of the skull. In first aid, open wounds are divided into four classifications: abrasions, incised wounds, lacerated wounds, and punctured wounds.
See abrasions, incisions, lacerations, punctures.

ophthalmia — an acute inflammation of the eye or the conjunctiva.
See conjunctivitis.

opuate — *See narcotic.*

opium — the powder produced by drying the seeds of *Papaver somniferum,* the poppy plant that grows in the Near East.

Raw opium has been used as a pain-killer for thousands of years. It has also been used in the treatment of dysentery. However, not until the early part of the nineteenth century were the potent derivatives of opium isolated: morphine in 1803, codeine in 1832, and papaverine in 1848.

Opium and its derivatives are narcotics or pain-reducers. They are physically and sometimes psychologically addictive. Despite the dangers inherent in their use, the opium derivatives are the most effective narcotic agents known to man.
See morphine, narcotic.

optic nerve — the nerve that transmits sight impulses from the retina of the eye to the brain.

oral — of or pertaining to the mouth.

oral ulcerations — *See aphthous stomatitis, canker, erythema multiforme, pemphigus.*

orchis — *See testis.*

orchitis — the inflammation of a testis. Orchitis is frequently caused by a venereal disease. The testis is swollen and painful.
See testis.

organ — any separate body part such as the heart, liver, etc. The term organ is usually used to indicate an internal body part.

organic heart disease — a heart disease that is caused by some structural abnormality in the heart or circulatory system.

organism — any living animal or plant.

orgasm — the climax of sexual intercourse.

orifice — the opening to any body part.

orthodontics — the branch of dentistry that deals with uneven bites, or malocclusion. The correction of these problems may necessitate wearing metal braces or a bite plate in order to push or pull the teeth into proper position. Occasionally one or more teeth may have to be removed.
See malocclusion.

orthodontist — a dentist whose specialty is correcting uneven bites, or malocclusion.
See malocclusion, orthodontics.

orthopedics — the branch of surgery that deals with the bones and the joints.

oscillometer — an instrument that measures the changes in magnitude of the pulsations in the arteries. The oscillometer is especially useful in studying the circulation in the periphery of the body.
See artery.

osmosis — the diffusion (or movement) of a fluid through a membrane from an area of higher pressure to an area of lower pressure. The membranes through which osmosis can take place are called semipermeable membranes. These semipermeable membranes allow fluids and small molecules to pass through them, but they block the passage of larger molecules. Thus, these membranes act as a sieve.

In the human body, cell membranes are semipermeable and permit this diffusion. Oxygen, blood, and digested nutrients pass through cells by osmosis, providing energy for growth and replacement as well as for regular life processes. Blood is pumped under pressure from the heart to the large arteries. From the arteries, blood passes into even smaller blood vessels until it reaches the smallest blood vessels, called capillaries. By the time blood reaches the capillaries, the pressure has been considerably reduced. However, the pressure of the blood in the capillaries is still greater than the fluid in the cells. Hence, through the process of osmosis, blood in the capillaries enters the individual cells.

The movement of fluids, waste material, etc. through the body tissues is a result of osmosis. Waste materials are removed from the blood in the kidneys through this same process.

osteitis — an inflammation of one or more bones.

osteoarthritis — a degenerative joint disease. Osteoarthritis seems to be caused by a combination of aging, irritation of the joints, and normal wear and tear. It is far commoner than rheumatoid arthritis, but, as a rule, it is less damaging. Older people are more likely to have osteoarthritis than are younger people.

Chronic irritation of the joints is the main con-tributing factor. This may result from over-weight, poor posture, injury, or strain from one's occupation or recreation.

The primary characteristic of osteoarthritis is degeneration of joint cartilage. This becomes soft and wears unevenly. In some areas it may wear away completely, exposing the underlying bone. Thickening of the ends of the bones may also occur. The remainder of the body is seldom affected. Except in some cases that involve the hip joints or knees, the disease seldom causes serious deformity or crippling.

Common symptoms are pain, aches, and stiffness. Pain is usually experienced when certain joints are used, especially finger joints and those that bear the body's weight. Enlargement of the fingers at the last joint often occurs. Although permanent, enlargements (nodes) of this type seldom lead to disability.

No specific cure for osteoarthritis is known. However, a number different treatments are available for the relief of pain and the partial remission of the disease.
See arthritis.

osteomyelitis — a serious bone inflammation caused by a pus-producing microorganism. When osteomyelitis is not treated, the infection spreads throughout the marrow of the bone.

Osteomyelitis can occur after a bone has been fractured and one of the broken ends of the bone pierces the skin. The open end of the bone may then be exposed to microorganisms capable of causing this infection. Before the discovery of antibiotics, osteomyelitis was often caused by a serious infection in another part of the body that spread to the bone or bones. Today, most infections are cured before they can enter the blood-stream and attack the bones.

The symptoms of osteomyelitis are sudden pain in the bone and an elevated temperature. Treatment consists of chemotherapy—usually penicillin when the diagnosis is made before the infection spreads too far into the bone marrow. If the infection has spread, drainage of the affected bone may be needed in addition to the drugs. When the infection is severe, parts of the bone may have to be removed.

osteoporosis — a disorder that causes a gradual decrease in both the amount and strength of bone tissue. In osteoporotic patients there is a gradual thinning-out of individual bones, which become less dense, or more porous, and tend to lose their normal strength.

The bones usually involved first in osteoporosis are those of the spine and pelvis. Ordinarily, the disease thins individual bones of the spine, which are then compressed by the weight of the body and eventually reach the point of outright fracture and collapse. At any stage of osteoporosis the patient may have chronic low-back pain. As the disease advances, the patient's back becomes deformed, the patient grows progressively shorter, and capacity for physical activity becomes more and more limited. Also as the disease progresses, other bones become thinned, particularly those of the legs and arms.

Because the affected bones are weak and porous, often breaking under even minor stress, the disease is responsible for many of the fractures experienced by elderly people. Osteoporosis is often the real cause of the numerous broken hips that hospitalize so many older people for long periods and which, in many cases, begin their physical decline. This disease is one of the major causes of physical disability in old age, especially in women. In this respect, it ranks closely behind arthritis.

The vast majority of osteoporosis cases are found in people who are over sixty years of age. Women who have passed the menopause are especially vulnerable and comprise more than sixty percent of all cases. The processes leading to the disease begin during the thirties and forties, however, and it is occasionally seen in middle-aged people.

Recent surveys have shown that three out of every ten women over the age of fifty who have sought medical care for any reason have osteoporosis. Of men over sixty-five years of age who have seen physicians, one-fifth suffer from this disorder.

CAUSE

Living bone is composed essentially of two elements: a soft framework made of protein; and calcium salts deposited in and on this protein mold, which turn it into stony, hard tissue. In the normal adult, the skeleton constantly and systematically rebuilds itself. Old bone is continually reabsorbed by the body, and new bone is produced to replace it. This tearing-down and building-up is normal for human bone at all ages, from the period of growth during the first twenty years throughout life.

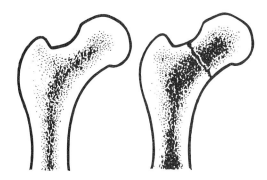

OSTEOPOROSIS

In the regeneration of bone, formation of the protein mold is stimulated by certain hormones—chemical substances produced by endocrine glands to control the activities of other organs. Normally, after menopause and in old age there is a decrease in the body's production of male and female hormones. This decrease is thought to interfere with the regeneration of new bone in older persons, and so is believed responsible in part for the progressive loss of bone substance in osteoporosis, since the normal tearing-down of existing bone continues.

Another important factor in osteoporosis seems to be the long-term balance between intake and loss of calcium in the individual. During the normal process of continual tearing-down and building-up of bone, about one-seventh of the skeleton's calcium is lost and replaced every year. All adults constantly lose varying amounts of calcium in the urine and by way of the intestine. These daily losses must be replaced with new calcium from food and drink. If, over a period of years, the amount of calcium in the diet is insufficient, the skeleton is likely to be lacking in calcium—the major component of bone's strength. It has therefore been suggested that another factor leading to osteoporosis, in addition to the hormonal decline of old age, is a chronic, many years' shortage of dietary calcium. This is especially likely in those people whose daily calcium requirement is higher than usual, either because of excessive loss of calcium via the kidneys or because of failure of the body to absorb adequate calcium from the diet.

A third possible factor is lack of exercise. A normal degree of activity, far from harming healthy bone, helps to strengthen points of wear with strong new bone matter. During the years of vigorous physical activity, the bones that are used most remain most strongly mineralized.

249

As they age, most people become less active physically. In old age, as the physical demands on the skeleton decrease (due to increased periods of rest), there is a lack of stimulation to maintain calcium in the body areas of stress and wear. As loss of calcium continues, there is a slow and gradual, but nevertheless constant, thinning of the bones (owing to their decreased use).

SYMPTOMS
With the exception of occasional low-back pain, osteoporotic bones are neither painful nor tender until they have become so weak that a sudden strain results in their breaking. Aside from collapse of bones of the spine (vertebrae), the most common site of fracture is in the neck of the thigh bone (femur). This results in excruciating pain in the hip region, inability to move the upper leg or bear weight on the hip, and, in many cases, a shortening of the leg on the affected side.

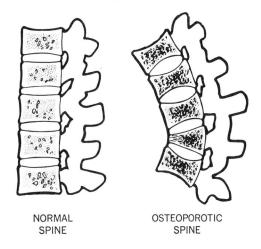

NORMAL
SPINE

OSTEOPOROTIC
SPINE

OSTEOPOROSIS

DIAGNOSIS
Because osteoporosis is such a common condition among women past fifty, its presence in such patients should always be suspected by physicians. A positive diagnosis is usually made on the basis of X-ray examinations of the involved bones. Specific chemical tests of the blood, however, are needed to confirm suspicion of osteoporosis and to rule out other bone diseases. Examination of a small specimen of bone, usually taken from the hip, and of the bone marrow is sometimes useful in making a conclusive diagnosis of osteoporosis.

TREATMENT
Treatment of osteoporosis varies with the conditions of individual cases. In general, to encourage bone mineralization, the patient is given a planned diet rich in calcium and protein. Sometimes vitamin D is also prescribed. If a major change in diet is not practical, the patient's usual meals are supplemented with calcium salts in the form of tablets. In addition, the physician may prescribe a mixture of hormones to encourage regeneration of the protein mold of the bones. The patient is encouraged to engage in physical activity (within the limits of his or her ability) because prolonged immobilization and extensive chair and bed rest tend to increase thinning of the bones.

When the condition also involves bone fractures, early treatment is concentrated on relief of pain and repair of the injury. Braces and other supports, a limited period of bed rest, and, occasionally, surgery may be required. Here too, the patient is given a relatively high-calcium, high-protein diet.

Osteoporosis should be considered a lifelong disease, requiring long follow-up care. In some patients, no matter how appropriate the prescribed treatment and how faithfully it is followed, no permanent improvement may occur, and the condition may even grow worse. However, current research suggests that many patients can expect to improve and return to a reasonably comfortable life, even though this process may require months and years.

PREVENTION
The symptoms and complications of osteoporosis may be severe. A serious attempt to prevent this disorder should be made by everyone. The most rational preventive measure is a reasonable calcium intake throughout life, with special attention to a high dietary calcium supply from age forty on. Physicians often recommend that the daily diet include milk (or skim milk) and milk products (cheeses and ice cream, for example). Shellfish, canned sardines, salmon (with bones), and green vegetables and meat, the latter for its protein content, are also advised. With adequate calcium, physical activity and regular exercise will tend to prevent the loss of minerals from the bones, which results from lack of activity.

otitis media — an infection of the middle ear, frequently caused by the spread of bacterial infection from the throat. When pus forms and settles in the middle ear cavity, it may cause a hearing loss. However, if the infection is properly treated, the loss is likely to be temporary.

Otitis media is the most common cause of childhood hearing loss. Among people in their twenties and thirties, it is a major cause of hearing loss.

Some of the diseases that can cause otitis media include measles, mumps, and scarlet fever, as well as flu and the common cold.

otolaryngologist — a physician who specializes in the care and treatment of the ears, nose, and throat. The initials of ear, nose, and throat—ENT—are an alternate name for an otolaryngologist.

otologist — a physician whose specialty is the diagnosis and treatment of the ear and ear problems.

otosclerosis — a condition in which deposits or new bone forms between the stapes bone and the oval window in the middle ear. This can restrict or immobilize the lever action. It does not usually cause trouble, but in about one out of every ten cases, the deposits or new bone growth anchors the stapes and prevents this tiny bone from properly transmitting sound waves to the inner ear.

TREATMENT

Surgery for hearing losses caused by otosclerosis was tried as long ago as 1876 and in some cases was successful. Many developments were necessary, though, before it could be widely used.

Operations with sterile techniques, antibiotics, and other means of preventing or controlling infection have provided one great advance. Another has been the operating microscope, which, by enlarging objects as much as sixty times, enables the ear surgeon to see clearly what is occurring in the tiny space within which he works. Important, also, has been the information gained from laboratory study of ear structures and from work with animals.

Today, a stapedectomy is the most commonly performed type of operation for otosclerosis. In this operation, the stapes is removed and replaced with a metal wire. The wire performs the job of the stapes (sound conduction). Sometimes the oval window is covered with a bit of fat taken from the ear lobe (although other substances are also used).

A general anesthetic is often used. However, when a local anesthetic is used, the patient ex-

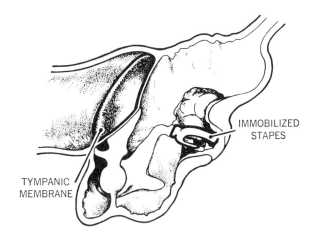

TYMPANIC MEMBRANE

IMMOBILIZED STAPES

OTOSCLEROSIS

periences a return to almost normal hearing on the operating table. The immediate improvement on the operating table is frequently followed by temporarily poorer hearing for two weeks to a month. Sometimes sounds are distorted for even longer.

The stapedectomy operation is now reported to benefit about ninety-five percent of suitable otosclerosis patients. However, many years must pass before doctors can be sure that the improvement will last indefinitely.

Earlier operations, still occasionally performed on otosclerosis patients, include mobilizing (freeing) the stapes, and fenestration, which involves opening a new window between the middle and inner ear.

See ear, hearing, oval window, stapes.

outer ear — the part of the ear that includes the external ear and the external auditory canal. The auditory canal terminates at a tightly stretched

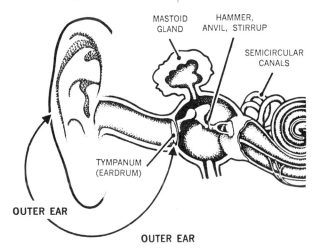

MASTOID GLAND

HAMMER, ANVIL, STIRRUP

SEMICIRCULAR CANALS

TYMPANUM (EARDRUM)

OUTER EAR

OUTER EAR

membrane called the eardrum. The primary purpose of the outer ear is to act as a funnel for sound on its way to the eardrum, where it produces vibrations of the eardrum.

outpatient — a patient who is receiving treatment at a hospital but who does not require hospitalization. Physical therapy and X-ray treatment are two examples of treatment often received by outpatients.

ova — the female sex cells or eggs that are produced in the ovary. The singular of ova is ovum.

oval window — an opening in the wall of the bone housing the inner ear. The oval window is the connection between the middle ear and the inner ear. The flat end of the stapes (called the footplate) fits into the oval window. As sound comes through the middle ear (in the form of vibrations), the footplate at the inner end of the stapes moves in and out of the oval window at the same rate that the eardrum is vibrating.

See stapes.

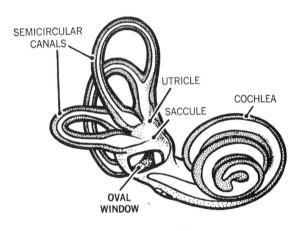

OVAL WINDOW

ovaries — the two small female organs that produce ova, the female sex cells or eggs. An ovary is about the size and shape of an almond. The ovaries are located at the outer end of the fallopian tubes—one to the right and one to the left.

Each ovary contains about 300,000 ova. Out of this large supply, only about 400 actually reach maturity during a woman's life. Of these 400, only a few are finally fertilized and go on to become human beings.

About every twenty-eight days, midway between two menstrual cycles (about fourteen days

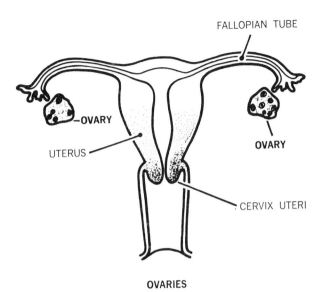

OVARIES

before the menstrual flow), a single ovum leaves one of the ovaries. The two ovaries alternate: one month the ovum is released from the right ovary; the next month an ovum is released from the left ovary. This cycle repeats itself, except during pregnancies, until the menopause, when the childbearing part of a woman's life comes to an end.

See fallopian tubes.

overdose — taking more of a drug or drugs than the body can safely handle. An overdose of some kinds of drugs can kill the patient by depressing the central nervous system or the respiratory system so much that breathing ceases.

An overdose can occur by accident, such as when a child gets into the medicine cabinet. It can also happen when an addict takes a stronger dose than his body will tolerate.

Overdoses may be deliberate, as in the case of a potential suicide attempt. Depending on what drug was taken and the length of time between the overdose and the time the patient receives treatment, an overdose may or may not be fatal. Doctors treat overdosed patients in several different ways; again treatment depends on the exact drug that caused the overdose. The stomach may have to be emptied or pumped out, or an antagonist drug may be needed to reverse the effects of the original drug.

overweight — a condition in which the body weight is more than it should be. The term overweight is used as a middle ground between correct body weight and obesity (a condition in which the body weight is approximately twenty percent or more over normal or correct body weight).

All other explanations to the contrary, the most frequent and important cause of overweight is the consumption of more food than is needed, coupled with too little physical exercise.

Being overweight is not healthy; however, it is especially serious in people with heart problems. People with heart disease cannot afford to be overweight, because excess weight increases the burden on an already overtaxed heart. This is particularly true of the person who has had a heart attack, who has congestive heart failure, or who has high blood pressure. Many physicians consider weight control a basic part of treatment for heart disease.

TREATMENT

There are no miracle shortcuts for losing weight safely except eating fewer high-calorie foods and simultaneously getting more exercise. A good reducing diet is one that cuts down on total calories consumed but does not cut out any dietary essentials. Naturally, there is no place for candy, rich desserts and gravies, extra pats of butter, alcoholic beverages, potato chips, nuts, soft drinks, or between-meal snacks in the diet of a person who wants to lose weight.

A reducing diet that is used for a limited time only is quite useless. In many cases the individual, after his limited objective is achieved, will backslide and revert to his old food pattern, with the result that his temporary weight loss is soon wiped out. Some fad diets can cause trouble by placing an additional burden on the heart. It takes a permanent, lifelong change in food habits to achieve permanent results.

People who are overweight should ask their physician for a prescribed diet that will fit their needs.

See obesity.

ovum — *See ova.*

Oxygen — a gas composing about twenty percent of the air in the atmosphere. It is the most essential requirement for life. While man can exist for a week or more without food and for several days without water, he can only live for minutes without oxygen.

A normal healthy adult male body holds approximately two quarts of oxygen. That is enough to last about four minutes. After that length of time, there will be damage to the body tissues. The first tissues that are damaged are the brain cells. With every second that passes, the damage becomes more extensive and there is less and less chance of recovery.

A person who has stopped breathing (or whose oxygen supply has been curtailed) is in immediate, critical danger. Life is dependent on oxygen, which is breathed into the lungs and then carried by the blood to every body cell. Because body cells cannot store oxygen and the blood can hold only a limited amount of oxygen, death will result from a continued lack of breathing.

The primary job of oxygen in the body is to help oxidize (or burn) food. This oxidization process turns food into energy that can be used immediately or stored for later use.

Because of the vital importance of bringing oxygen into the body, artificial respiration should be applied at once when breathing has ceased. Artificial respiration keeps oxygen moving in and out of the lungs (and consequently throughout the body) until the patient's own breathing pattern is restored.

See artificial respiration, lungs.

oxytocin — a hormone secreted by the posterior lobe of the pituitary gland. Oxytocin causes the muscles of the uterus to contract. This hormone also helps the breast release milk.

See hormone, pituitary gland.

ozone — a form of oxygen. Under ordinary conditions it is a colorless or pale-blue gas and has a characteristic pungent odor. In high concentrations it is extremely flammable, and in liquid form it becomes a dangerous explosive.

As a strong oxidizing agent, ozone has many uses. Its greatest use is in the suppression of mold and bacterial growth, such as in the treatment of drinking-water supplies and industrial wastes, and the sterilizing of food products. Other uses of ozone include the rapid aging of wood; the aging of liquor; rapid drying of varnishes and printing ink; production of peroxides; bleaching of oils, waxes, textiles, and papers; and deodorizing of feathers.

Despite its usefulness, ozone is acutely and chronically toxic to humans. Workers in enclosed spaces where ozone is produced or used should be on guard against the potential hazards to which they may be accidentally exposed.

OZONE POISONING

Even in low concentrations, inhaled ozone may cause dryness of the mouth, throat irritation, coughing, headaches, and pressure or pain in the chest, followed by difficulty in breathing. Varying in individuals, and depending on the concentration of ozone and the period of exposure, ozone can produce many other injuries. It impairs the sense of smell, disguises other odors with a continuous odor of ozone, alters taste sensation, and reduces the ability to think. Ozone also depresses the nervous system, thus slowing the heart and respiration and producing drowsiness and sleep.

Exposure to relatively small concentrations for an hour can cause a serious cough and fatigue. Exposure to sufficient quantities for two hours results in a marked reduction in the capacity of the lungs. Exposure for four hours can cause the lungs to fill with fluid and start bleeding. Inhaled in concentrations not acutely injurious, ozone may bring on, hasten, or increase the severity of diseases of the respiratory tract. It is a special hazard to people who already have heart or respiratory problems. Exposure to high concentrations of ozone, or continuous exposure, can cause death.

The injured patient should be removed from exposure immediately. He should lie down, remaining at rest until he can be seen by a physician. In cases of acute exposure, the examining physician may hospitalize the patient until the danger of severe lung damage or possibly pneumonia has passed. When small amounts of ozone are inhaled, the symptoms usually disappear after the patient is removed from exposure. The patient should be examined by a physician, but frequently no treatment is required.

p

pacemaker — a small mass of specialized cells in the right upper chamber of the heart. These cells are responsible for the electrical impulses that initiate the contractions of the heart. The natural pacemaker is also called the sinoatrial node or the S-A node of Keith-Flack.

The term pacemaker, or, more exactly, electric cardiac pacemaker, or electric pacemaker, is also applied to an electrical device that can be substituted for a defective natural pacemaker. The artificial pacemaker controls the beat of the heart by a series of rhythmic electrical discharges that replace the missing natural electrical impulses.

If the electrodes that deliver the discharges to the heart are placed on the outside of the chest, the device is called an external pacemaker. If the electrodes are placed within the chest wall, it is called an internal pacemaker. An internal pacemaker is surgically implanted in the chest. It is a self-contained unit, requiring only periodic battery changes.

pain — an elementary sensation of physical suffering. The sensation of pain is part of the protective system of the body. Pain serves as a warning of bodily damage, disease, or malfunction.

For example, when a finger is burned, the pain provides a warning to the body. The body responds by removing the injured finger from the source of the burn. When the body experiences pain and there is no apparent external cause, the pain itself is a warning to consult a physician. Frequently, there is no visible manifestation of the source of the pain—such as a burn or a wound. The lack of physical evidence indicates the possibility of disease or malfunction.

Although the pain of a wound is usually restricted to the vicinity of the wound, the sensation includes areas other than the wounded locality. Following the original wound, the damaged nerves send electrical impulses to the brain. In turn, the brain (actually the cerebral cortex) refers or projects the sensation of pain to the damaged part. Pain that follows an unpleasant stimulus to the skin surface (as in a pinch or a slap) is usually fairly strong, very localized, and follows the onset of the stimulus rather quickly. If no serious or permanent damage has been done, the pain recedes rapidly once the source of the pain has been removed.

However, pain that results from a disease or disorders does not respond this way. When nerves in the vicinity of internal organs are warning the brain that there is trouble in their area, the brain does not necessarily send the pain sensation to the same exact location. Instead of being localized, the pain may appear in a region that is connected to the original source only through the nervous system. Thus, heart pain from angina pectoris may appear over a large area of the chest, and, additionally, a painful sensation may occur in the left arm. This sensation is called referred pain.

Pain or the sensation of pain occurs in the brain. Consequently, if there is no brain, or if the brain is depressed by drugs (as by a general anesthetic) or by injury, there is no sensation of pain. Naturally, once the brain returns to normal, the sensation of pain returns. At the same time, if the nerves do not send a warning to the brain, the brain cannot initiate the pain sensation. In repairing a relatively minor laceration, a physician may use a local anesthetic. This depresses the affected nerves. Consequently, these nerves do not inform the brain of the injury, and no pain is felt until the local anesthetic wears off and the nerves resume their normal functioning powers.

Some pain has no physical (internal or external) basis. This pain is said to be psychogenic or psychosomatic. This type of pain—as intense as if it were caused by a physical stimulus—is caused by emotional disorders.

Another type of pain, known as neurogenic, can be very confusing, because, like psychogenic pain, it mimics pain from a physical stimulus. Unlike psychosomatic pain, neurogenic pain has a physical basis, although not necessarily in the painful area. Neurogenic pain results from an improper functioning of one or more of the nerves.

The concept of pain as it affects individuals is a difficult one. The same physical stimulus applied to several patients results in different reactions. Although, in all probability, the pain felt by each will be similar, their reactions may differ greatly. The concept of pain tolerance really refers to an individual's ability to experience pain quietly. For example, a child who receives an injection will normally cry and make quite a fuss. An adult receiving the same injection will usually accept it quietly. While the pain sensation is equivalent, the ability to tolerate it or to control the reaction to it differs considerably. Similarly, a person who must have injections on a regular basis becomes accustomed to accepting the pain sensation, although the pain is still present. There is, however, one important difference. The person who periodically experiences the same level of pain knows what to expect. He prepares himself for it. However, sudden, unexpected pain will provoke a stronger reaction, although not necessarily a more painful one.

This ability to accept pain quietly is part of what is known as the pain threshold. The threshold is different for each individual and may vary within an individual, depending on the type of pain involved. Much of pain tolerance depends on early training.

Severe pain can be fatal. One of the body's reactions to unbearable pain is shock, a condition in which the circulation of the blood is seriously disturbed. Other symptoms of pain include nausea, perspiration, and a feeling of faintness. Painkillers are used to reduce the body's reactions and thus prevent shock. Some of these, usually the strongest ones, affect the central nervous system. Other medicines control the pain at the point of injury.

See anesthetics, nerve.

palate — the roof or top of the mouth. It acts as a partition between the mouth and the nasal cavity. The palate is divided into two major parts: the hard palate and the soft palate.

The hard palate is primarily bone that is covered by membrane. It assists in chewing and swallowing.

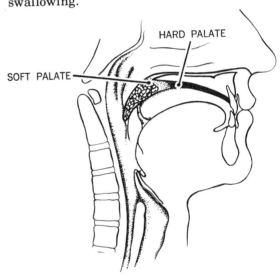

PALATE (HARD & SOFT)

The soft palate is located beyond the hard palate. It begins at about the place where the teeth end. It is composed of a muscle that is covered by membrane. A projectile from the soft palate, the urula points down towards the throat. When food or liquid is swallowed, part of the soft palate moves to protect the nasopharynx by covering it. This motion forces the swallowed material into the digestive tract instead of the respiratory system.

See cleft palate.

palpitation — a fluttering of the heart or an abnormal rate or rhythm of the heartbeat that is experienced by the patient himself.

palsy — *See paralysis.*

pancarditis — an inflammation of the whole heart, including the inner layer (myocardium), and the outer sac (pericardium).

pancreas — a large elongated gland lying behind the stomach. The digestive juices of the pancreas (amylase, proteinases, and lipase) are secreted through the pancreatic duct into the duodenum. These enzymes act on all types of foods. Pancreatic amylase converts starch into the complex sugar called maltose. The proteinases reduce proteins. Lipase converts fats to fatty acids and glycerol.

The pancreas also contains special groups of cells, the islands of Langerhans, that secrete the hormone known as insulin. This hormone is needed for the proper utilization of sugar by the body tissues. Insulin enters the blood directly. It does not go by way of the intestinal tract as do the pancreatic enzymes.

See diabetes.

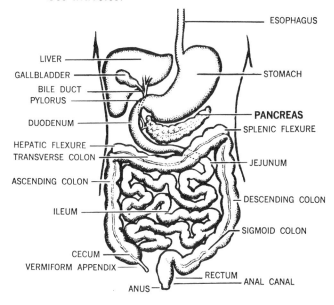

PANCREAS

pandemic — the spread of an infectious disease over a wide area. A pandemic is larger than an epidemic. The term is usually restricted to diseases that spread over all or almost all the world. Outbreaks of influenza have been pandemic.

papaverine — a drug derived from opium. Papaverine is a muscle relaxant. However, its use has declined because of the discovery of other agents that, while not more effective, have fewer serious side effects.

papillary muscles — small bundles of muscles in the wall of the lower chambers of the heart to which

the cords leading to the cusps of the valves (chordae tendineae) are attached. When the valves are closed, these muscles contract and tighten the cords that hold the valve firmly shut.

papilloma — a tumor, such as a wart, that occurs in the skin or the lining of internal organs.

Pap smear — a technique developed chiefly by Dr. George N. Papanicolaou (1883-1962) that involves the microscopic examination of cells collected from the vagina. These cells are shed from the uterus into the vagina as part of the normal life process.

The Pap smear is an excellent technique for the early detection of cancer of the uterine cervix, or neck of the womb. In fact, the Pap smear is one of the major reasons for the decrease in deaths from cancer of the uterine cervix.

Gynecologists now routinely do a Pap smear as part of the annual examination of female patients.

paraldehyde — a drug that acts as a sedative and hypnotic.

See sedative.

paralysis — the inability of a normally mobile body part to move. Paralysis may occur to voluntary muscles (such as those in the arm) or to involuntary muscles (such as the heart muscle or breathing muscles). This condition may result from disease, malfunctioning, or from foreign substances such as poisons. Paralysis almost always involves the nerves in the affected area. For whatever reason, the electrical impulse is not being carried properly through the nervous system.

Some types of paralysis are only temporary and end when the cause is removed; others are permanent.

Paralysis is also known as palsy.

paranoia — a type of mental illness in which the patient has delusions. These delusions frequently take the form of fears. That is, the patient is afraid that there is some sort of conspiracy against him. Paranoia is one of the more severe forms of mental illness.

paraplegia — the loss of both motion and sensation in the legs and lower part of the body. This condition is the result of a disease or injury to the spinal column. Among the diseases capable of causing paraplegia are poliomyelitis, muscular dystrophy, multiple sclerosis, and tumors of the spinal cord. Principal traumatic (or accidental) causes include birth injuries, automobile accidents, airplane crashes, gunshot or shrapnel wounds, and falls or injuries in industry and sports.

The loss of motion and sensation occurs from the site of the disease or damage to the spinal cord downward. Additionally, there may be a loss of normal control of the bowels and bladder.

parasite — any organism that lives off another organism.

parasympathetic nervous system — a subdivision of the autonomic or involuntary nervous system. Stimulation of the various parasympathetic nerves causes the pupils of the eyes to contract, the heart to beat more slowly, and produces other nonvoluntary reactions.
See nervous system.

parathyroid glands — small, round bodies, usually four in number, located just behind the thyroid gland. The hormone they secrete, parathormone, regulates the calcium and phosphorus content of the blood and bones. The amount of calcium is important in certain tissue activities such as bone formation, maintenance of normal muscular excitability, and milk production in the nursing mother.

Diminished function or removal of the parathyroid glands results in a low calcium level in the blood. In extreme cases death occurs; it is preceded by strong contractions of the muscles and by convulsions.

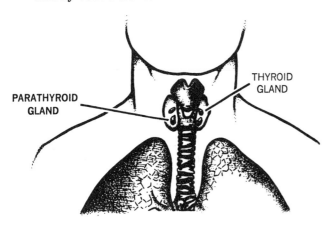

PARATHYROID GLAND
THYROID GLAND

PARATHYROID GLAND

paregoric—a drug derived from opium. Paregoric is also called camphorated opium tincture. Paregoric was used primarily in the treatment of children. However, its use has diminished in recent years.
See opium.

parietal — a term that refers to the walls of a body cavity.

parietal pericardium — a thin membrane sac that surrounds the heart and roots of the great vessels. It is the outer layer of the pericardium.

Parkinson's disease — a slowly progressive disorder of the central nervous system. It is characterized by tremor in muscles that are at rest, and by stiffness and slowness of movement.

CAUSE
The exact cause of the disease in most cases is unknown. Among the known causative factors are: arteriosclerosis, cerebral vascular accidents, head injuries, syphilis, toxic agents, and drugs.

Many research people are convinced that part of the basal ganglia is the brain center for much of the tremor and stiffness of Parkinson's disease.

Parkinson's disease is slightly more common in men than women and generally occurs between ages fifty and sixty. Surveys indicate that there are about 300,000 cases in the United States and that 25,000 to 43,000 new cases can be expected each year. According to present estimates, about one out of every forty persons now living will develop Parkinsonism. There is some evidence that heredity plays a role in this disease.

SYMPTOMS
An extreme variability characterizes the rate of development of this disease. For some, the onset of symptoms is mild, such as a slight tremor and stiffness on one side that does not impair functioning. For others the symptoms are marked, and within months of the onset the patient requires total care. There is a typical general appearance of the patient with Parkinson's disease: masklike and waxen features, rhythmic tremor of the fingers, stooped posture, and a gait in which the patient walks as if he were about to fall on his face.

There may be drooling or a blank facial expression. This results from the loss of semiautomatic movements such as swallowing saliva and the movement of facial muscles.

The typical patient with Parkinson's disease is usually in his fifth or sixth decade. The disease is insidious and slowly progressive, lasting from five to twenty years. It may not be incapacitating for several years, permitting the patient to remain active and employed. It is important to the patient's well-being that he continue to be as active as possible. Continuation of employment is possible, especially if the patient's occupation is more intellectual than manual. The patient may have difficulty in writing, dressing himself, maintaining his balance, and turning around quickly.

Unlike some neurological diseases, Parkinson's disease seldom impairs the patient's mental ability. Sight or hearing is not affected, nor is there paralysis of the limbs or loss of control of bowels or bladder. In later stages of the disease there may be slurring of speech and some incapacity. Because of the tremor, patients may require additional rest.

HISTORY

As far back as Biblical times, "shaking palsy" was known. In the second century A.D., Galen, a Greek physician and medical writer who worked in Rome described the shaking palsy. Its history is foggy until the 17th century, when a few physicians wrote about its tremor or rigidity. Several conditions with tremor were confused with this disorder, and rigidity without tremor sometimes was not recognized as the same disease.

In 1817, an important study of this was published. The author was Dr. James Parkinson, a London physician with a keenly observing mind. So carefully did Dr. Parkinson, in his "Essay on the Shaking Palsy", distinguish this disease from others that his "Essay" is reprinted in some recent books. His words describe many of today's cases:

"Involuntary tremulous motion, with lessened muscular power in parts not in action and even when supported; with a propensity to bend the trunk forward and to pass from a walking to running pace: the senses and intellects being uninjured."

TYPES

For many years, textbooks classified Parkinson's disease as "postencephalitic " (following attacks of encephalitis), "arteriosclerotic" (associated with arteriosclerosis), or "idiopathic" (unknown causes). A newer classification distinguishes six categories:

1. Parkinson's disease (technically, paralysis agitans or idiopathic Parkinsonism).
2. Postencephalitic Parkinsonism.
3. Other central nervous system disease with some Parkinsonian features.
4. Symptomatic pseudo-Parkinsonism.
5. Essential tremor (essential, like idiopathic, means of unknown cause).
6. Other dyskinesias. In dyskinesia, "dys" means "difficult" or "faulty," and "kinesia" means "motion."

TREATMENT

There is no cure for Parkinson's disease, but three kinds of treatment will help relieve symptoms. These are medication, physical therapy, and surgery. Stress and anxiety should be avoided as well as excitement, which causes the tremor to become worse.

1. Medication

Because no one perfect medicine has yet been discovered, treatment must always be under continued direction from the patient's doctor. He seeks the best combination of medicines and the best amounts for the needs of each individual. He watches for bothersome side effects that limit the use of medicines and switches varieties as necessary. Patients must be aware of advertised medicines and any form of quackery.

2. Physical therapy

Physical therapy offers exercises of various types including stretching, which help the patient preserve as much function as the disease allows in his individual case. Physical therapy and exercises are helpful in controlling rigidity and preventing contractures that could be painful. The Parkinson patient must be responsible for his part in carrying out the exercise program for the rest of his life. The patient profits greatly from the consistent guidance best given by a physical therapist.

3. Surgery

Surgery is a treatment, not a cure, and is suitable only in carefully selected cases. Since 1937 surgery for Parkinson's disease has shown active progress although there were scattered attempts at surgery as early as 1909. The early surgery for the ailment could at best substitute a paralysis for a heavy tremor. But rarely would a Parkinson patient prefer partial paralysis to tremor.

Dating from 1942, a small lesion (a destroyed or inactivated area) has been precisely created in suspect areas on one side of the brain. (This surgery is performed only in carefully selected cases.) The trembling or the stiffness on the opposite side has stopped, with no apparent paralysis, and with restoration of normal use. Surgeons have used several methods to make such a lesion.

These include electrocoagulation: the extremely high-frequency sound waves called "ultrasonics"; a clever miniature knife; freezing; a drop of a chemical for temporary effect, or absolute alcohol for permanent change.

Time will tell how long the improvement brought about by various types of surgery will last and how useful it will be to the patient. Meanwhile, the younger Parkinson patient, with symptoms principally on one side and in good mental and emotional health; seems to be the carefully selected type of case who appears to have benefited by such surgery.

parotid gland — the largest of the salivary glands. It is located near the ear.
See saliva, salivary glands.

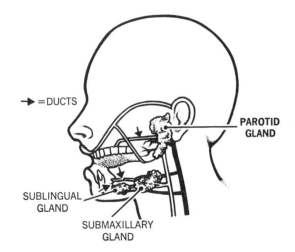

PAROTID GLAND

paroxysm — a sudden onset or intensification of one or more symptoms.

paroxysmal tachycardia — a period of rapid heart beats that begins and ends suddenly.

parrot fever — *See psittacosis.*

Pasteurella tularensis — the causative agent of tularemia.
See tularemia.

Pasteur, Louis — French chemist and bacteriologist (1822-1895) whose work with fermentation led to the process of pasteurization of milk.

Pasteur is also famous for his work with anthrax and rabies. He continued Edward Jenner's work and showed that dead or weak forms of bacteria and viruses can produce protective reactions against later exposure to stronger forms of the same bacteria or viruses.

patella — the knee cap.
See knee, knee cap.

patent ductus arteriosus — a congenital heart defect. A small duct between the artery leaving the left side of the heart (the aorta) and the artery leaving the right side of the heart (the pulmonary artery) which normally closes soon after birth, remains open. As a result of this duct's failure to close, blood from both sides of the heart is pumped into the pulmonary artery and into the lungs. This defect is sometimes called simply patent (or open) ductus.
See congenital heart defects.

patent foramen ovale — a type of congenital heart defect. An oval hole between the left and right upper chambers of the heart, which normally closes shortly after birth, remains open.

pathogenesis — the chain of events leading to the development of a disease.

pathognomonic — a symptom that is so specific or so characteristic of a particular disease or disorder that a definite diagnosis is possible from its presence.

pathology — the study of the essential nature of disease and of the structural and functional changes it causes.

Pathology is important in determining the cause of sudden or unexplained deaths. However, a pathologist, although he works with tissue that is no longer alive, is frequently an important part of a surgical team. When a surgeon is operating to remove a tumor, it is the pathologist who tests a small piece of the tumor to determine whether the tumor is benign or malignant. This can often be accomplished while the patient is on the operating table and can help avoid the necessity for two operations.

Pavlov, Ivan Petrovitch — Russian physiologist (1849-1936) who is best remembered for his work with conditioned or learned reflexes. This work was done with dogs. Pavlov conditioned the dogs to expect food every time a bell was rung. This was accomplished by ringing the bell just before the animal was fed. After the animal was trained, it salivated (the natural reaction to food) whenever the bell rang. At the time, Pavlov was actually studying the digestive glands—work for which he won the Nobel Prize for Medicine in 1907. However, his work on conditioned reflexes proved to be an important contribution to the study and practice of psychology.

pectoral — of or pertaining to the chest.

pediatrician — a doctor whose specialty is the care and treatment of children. The practice of pediatrics is one of the few specialties in which the physician's practice is limited by the age of his patients.

The impression a pediatrician makes on a child is very important. If the child is afraid of the pediatrician, he may harbor a lifelong fear of doctors and thus avoid seeing a doctor for problems that can be cured in the early stages.

pediculosis — infestation of the scalp or hairy parts of the body or of clothing with lice. Lice are transmitted by direct contact with infected persons or their personal possessions, particularly clothing or infected bedding. The symptoms of pediculosis are inflammation of the skin, itching, and white eggs (nits) on the hair. The treatment consists of dusting the body and clothing (especially along the seams) with a specially prescribed powder.

See louse.

pellagra — a type of malnutrition caused by a deficiency of niacin, one of the B vitamins.

See malnutrition.

pelvic examination — an internal examination of the vagina, cervix, and uterus.

pelvis — the basin-shaped bony structure at the lower portion of the trunk. It is located between the movable vertebrae of the spinal column, which it supports, and the lower limbs, upon which it rests. It forms the floor of the abdominal cavity and provides deep sockets into which the heads of the thigh bones fit. The pelvis is composed of four bones: two lower bones of the backbone and the wing-shaped hip bones on either side.

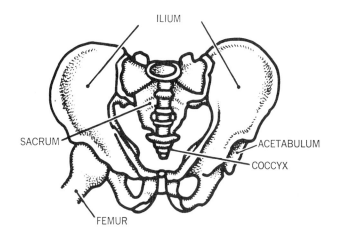

PELVIS

The exact shape of the pelvis differs between men and women. The male pelvis is narrower and more compact than the female pelvis. The male pelvis is designed for strength and speed; the female pelvis is designed to support pregnancies.

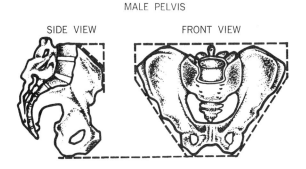

MALE PELVIS

SIDE VIEW   FRONT VIEW

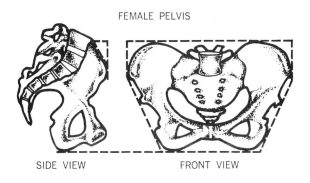

FEMALE PELVIS

SIDE VIEW   FRONT VIEW

PELVIS

The upper outer edges of the pelvis form the area known as the hip. A person whose weight is normal for his height will be able to feel the edges of the pelvis.

pemphigus — one of the most severe and rare types of oral ulcerations. It is a recurrent disease involving the mouth and skin. There are three forms of this disease: pemphigus vulgaris, pemphigus vegetans, and pemphigus conjunctivae. The most common type that involves the mouth is pemphigus vulgaris. This form of the disease can be either acute and malignant or chronic and benign.

Middle-aged people, those forty to seventy years of age, and persons of Mediterranean origins are the most frequent victims, although the number of cases is very small. The cause of the disease and why it attacks these particular groups are unsolved mysteries.

SYMPTOMS

The onset of pemphigus is insidious. At first the blisters are not painful. The patient feels a sensation of dryness in his mouth and a slight pain or discomfort when eating hot or spicy food. He may also have difficulty swallowing. Next, bullae — large blisters — form on the lips, tongue, cheek, palate, or gums. Often these blisters are not seen, because they break easily, leaving a reddish erosion with ragged edges. It is after they break that the blisters become very itchy and painful. Salivation increases and is often tinged with blood.

In about three-fourths of the cases of pemphigus, blisters form first in the mouth. Lesions on the skin may not appear for several months, and sometimes they never appear. When they do appear, they form over the entire body—face, trunk, arms, and legs. These blisters are thin-walled and translucent and are filled with a yellow fluid. When they break, they form a foul, yellow membrane.

Another characteristic symptom is "Nikolsky's sign"—the top layer of skin can be rubbed off with slight pressure.

In the early stages of the acute form of the disease, there may be periods of remission, with complete healing of the sores. Later, with each attack the blisters and following erosions gradually become larger, until the whole mouth is involved. Eating and drinking become extremely painful. The skin, covered with large blisters, has the appearance of a severe burn.

Acute pemphigus runs a rapid course. Mortality is high. About half the patients succumb to the continual loss of body fluid through the breaking blisters, as well as to strain, malnutrition, and final involvement of the vital organs.

The prognosis of chronic pemphigus vulgaris is much more hopeful. This form of the disease may last for years, causing only minor discomfort to the patient. The blisters are more "tense." They do not break easily, and they tend to heal well.

TREATMENT

Treatment of pemphigus can only be palliative, because there is no known cure for this disease. Cortisone has been used to alleviate symptoms, and penicillin has been used to prevent secondary infection. Mild mouthwashes can help relieve pain in the mouth. Since the cause is unknown, treatment can be directed only to the manifestation of the disease.

penicillin — an extremely important antibiotic. It was first discovered by Fleming in 1928. Although it was discovered by accident, Fleming did try a few experiments with it. The results of his experiments were not very promising. Later investigators determined that the poor results Fleming achieved were brought about by the crudeness and impurity of the penicillin with which he was working.

In 1939 Fleming's work was continued by a group of researchers in England. Their results were very encouraging. However, the war effort in England restricted the amount of research, experimentation, and, most importantly, production possible in England at the time. Researchers in the United States continued the work. By 1943 enough penicillin had been produced for experimental use.

Penicillin, like all antibiotics, is manufactured or made from living organisms. In the beginning penicillin was very difficult and expensive to produce. The amount of time needed to produce even small amounts necessitated the effective use of every gram. The supply was so small that it was necessary to extract the traces of penicillin found in the urine of patients receiving penicillin treatment. By the end of the 1940's new production techniques were available. These new techniques vastly increased the availability and at the same time reduced the cost of the drug.

Penicillin is produced from a mold called *Penicillium notatum*. Today there are many forms of penicillin, including different varieties of semisynthetic penicillins. Although some microorganisms have developed a resistance to the effects of penicillin, it is still one of the most widely used of all the antibiotics in the treatment of infection.

The drug is used in the treatment of streptococcal and staphylococcal infections. More specifically, penicillin is the first choice in treating diseases such as scarlet fever, meningitis, gonorrhea, syphilis, pneumonia, etc.

See antibiotics.

penicillinase — a drug employed in the treatment of penicillin reactions.

penis — the male sex organ. It is composed of three cylindrical bodies of spongy, cavernous tissue bound together by connective tissue and loosely covered by a layer of skin. Two of the bodies, corpora cavernosa, lie side by side. The third, corpora spongiosum, lies in the groove between the other two.

The dilated end of the corpora spongiosum is known as the glans penis. The cavernous tissue becomes greatly distended with blood during sexual excitement. This causes the erection of the penis. The penile portion of the urethra passes through the corpora spongiosum.

The loose skin of the penis folds back on itself, thus forming a prepuce, or foreskin, and covers the glans. This foreskin is frequently removed surgically (circumcision) to prevent irritation and to facilitate cleanliness.

pepsin — an enzyme that helps to digest protein. Pepsin originates in the stomach.

peptic ulcer — a noncancerous, crater-like sore (called an erosion) in the wall of the stomach or intestine. This ulcer erodes through the thin, inner mucous membrane lining and into the deeper muscular wall of the stomach or intestine. Peptic ulcers occur only in those regions of the gastrointestinal tract that are bathed by the digestive juices secreted by the stomach. These digestive juices contain hydrochloric acid and a protein-digesting enzyme called pepsin; hence the name "peptic ulcer."

Almost all peptic ulcers occur either in the stomach itself or in the small intestine just below the stomach. Those in the first portion of the intestine, the duodenum, are called duodenal ulcers, and those in the stomach are called gastric ulcers. In the United States duodenal ulcers are about eight times more common than gastric ulcers.

Ulcers of the stomach or duodenum may occur from infancy to old age but are most frequent after the age of twenty. People in their thirties, forties, and fifties are slightly more prone to develop ulcers than those in the older age groups, but an ulcer may be more serious in an elderly patient. Both men and women develop ulcers, but in this country they occur more frequently in men. Recent statistics, however, indicate that peptic ulcer disease is increasing among women.

According to popular belief, ulcers occur typically in the striving executive who is exposed to the chronic stress of responsibility. Medical experience, however, has shown this belief to be only partly true. Peptic ulcers occur with equal frequency in men in all walks of life. Salesmen, corporation executives, construction laborers, and bus drivers have about the same statistical chance of developing ulcers. However, the notion that anxiety and stress help cause ulcers is certainly true, and the person who is under continuous strain, no matter what his or her station in life, is the person who is most likely to develop an ulcer.

HEREDITY
Statistics suggest that a person who has one or more family members with ulcers is slightly more prone to develop an ulcer than someone from a family having no ulcer patients. In many cases this may be because of the anxiety-ridden environment in such a family.

The hereditary factors, if any, leading to ulcer formation are not understood, but the tendency for ulcers to "run in families" is much less pronounced than in many other diseases, such as diabetes or gout. It is very possible that a person who has close blood relatives with ulcers will never develop one himself.

CAUSES
The hydrochloric acid and pepsin secreted by the stomach bring about the digestion of meat and other proteins as they reach the stomach. In the normal person the mucous membrane lining of the stomach and duodenal wall is resistant to this digestive mixture, and no ulcers develop. In some people, however, this resistance breaks down, and an ulcer forms. There are, then, two

263

factors important in the formation of an ulcer: the amount of acid and pepsin secreted by the stomach, and the ability of the intestinal wall to resist erosion by this mixture.

Doctors agree that of these factors, secretion of too much acid and pepsin is by far the more important. The great majority of people with duodenal ulcers and some with gastric ulcers secrete much more acid than the normal person. Perhaps in the other individuals with ulcers there is a lowered resistance to normal amounts of acid. In any case the excessive secretion of acid appears to be the important factor and is the one that can be altered medically.

The large middle portion of the stomach, called the body of the stomach, is lined with cells that produce acid and pepsin. There are two important triggers that stimulate these cells to secrete more acid. The first trigger mechanism involves a large nerve (the vagus nerve) connecting the brain to the stomach. When a person is hungry, sees or smells food, or becomes anxious and upset, impulses coming down this nerve cause acid and pepsin to pour out from the cells into the stomach cavity.

The second trigger to acid-secretion is the presence of food itself in the lower part of the stomach and the duodenum. When food comes in contact with the lower portion of the stomach, this portion of the organ secretes a hormone-like substance into the bloodstream. This substance (gastrin) in turn stimulates the stomach to secrete additional acid. Although the food, by stimulating gastrin secretion, causes more acid to be secreted, it absorbs and neutralizes much of the acid and pepsin. The overall effect of most foods is protection of the stomach and duodenal wall.

It is easy to see why a person who is tense most of the time can develop an ulcer. His stomach will secrete acid not only at mealtime, because of the stimulation of food, but on and off throughout the day whenever he is tense. On these occasions his stomach and duodenum will not be protected from the corrosive action of the digestive juices by the presence of food.

Some specific foods and many drugs can greatly increase the amount of acid and may also be directly irritating to the stomach and duodenal wall. Alcohol, coffee, and aspirin are notorious examples of this type of irritant.

SYMPTOMS

The most common, almost universal, symptom of peptic ulcer is pain. As the stomach empties itself of food, undiluted acid comes in contact with the ulcer, thus causing the discomfort. This pain is usually steady and may feel like a "gnawing" or "burning" in the stomach. It often seems to be located in a small area of the abdomen, usually somewhere between the navel and the lower end of the breastbone. It appears from thirty minutes to two hours after a meal and is usually relieved by eating more food or taking antacids. In some ulcer patients pain of this type occurs off and on for many years.

DIAGNOSIS

When a patient describes his pain as similar to that above, the physician naturally suspects an ulcer. To prove that an ulcer is causing the trouble, he may have the patient swallow a thick, chalky liquid containing barium, which will show up on an X-ray film. The stomach and duodenum are outlined on X-ray pictures taken from various angles, and an ulcer crater may be seen filled with the barium.

Occasionally, pain similar to ulcer pain can be produced by diseases of other organs in the abdomen and chest, and the physician must perform other examinations and tests to rule out the possibility of these.

TREATMENT

In general, the treatment of ulcers by a physician is directed toward decreasing the amount of acid or irritants that reach the ulcer and interfere with the normal healing process. Proper diet; emphasis on frequent, small feedings; the use of antacids and drugs; and relief of nervous tension are important ways of accomplishing this.

1. Diet

The degree of restriction in the diets of ulcer patients varies greatly. A newly discovered ulcer that is causing only moderate discomfort may heal if the patient eliminates only alcohol, coffee, and other irritating food; cuts down on smoking (another stimulus to stomach secretions); and eats a few crackers or drinks some milk when he feels pain. However, a patient with a long-standing, complicated ulcer may have to eat only milk and crackers on an hourly schedule until improvement takes place.

In most people with ulcers, however, a very strict diet can be avoided. For example, meat and well-chewed raw vegetables may be allowed if the patient is doing well and these foods do not obviously cause him pain. In general, ulcer patients are instructed to take an antacid, milk, or a soft food when they feel pain, and they should eat some type of food every two hours during the day. This tends to absorb and neutralize the corrosive stomach secretions. Every person with an active ulcer should strictly avoid alcohol, coffee, heavily spiced food, excessive smoking, and irritating drugs such as aspirin.

Medical opinion varies as to the effect of cigarettes on ulcers, but smokers do have a slightly higher rate of gastric ulcer than do nonsmokers.

2. Antacids and drugs

Antacids are medications that absorb and neutralize hydrochloric acid in the stomach. There are over 500 types on the market, and the physician can usually find one that is not unpleasant for the patient to take. Some people with ulcers take these at regular intervals; others take them only when they feel pain.

A physician may also prescribe belladonna or a similar drug to block the passage of acid-stimulating impulses down the vagus nerve to the stomach.

3. Reduction of worry and tension

This is the most important but sometimes the most difficult part of the management of an ulcer.

It is known that severe or prolonged tension can be a causative factor in ulcer disease. The person who develops an ulcer may often be overly conscientious or one who, by trying to build his self-esteem, takes on more jobs and responsibility than time or ability allow. All human beings are different, however, and the situations that create tension in some do not seem to bother others. In one person the stress of a job that is too demanding may lead to an ulcer; in another, anger and anxiety experienced in a difficult family situation may be the important factor.

The patient and his physician should work together to help the patient understand the stress factors of his life and to remedy them. Occasionally, mild sedatives or tranquilizers may be used to help the patient relax. In some cases a vacation from work or family, a change of job, or even hospitalization for rest may be necessary.

4. Surgery

In the vast majority of cases if enough attention is paid to diet, antacids, and relief of nervous tension, the ulcers will heal. In some patients, however, more extensive measures must be taken. In general, these are also directed toward reducing the amount of acid secreted by the stomach.

There are several operations for ulcers. One type of operation involves the removal of varying portions of the lower stomach that secrete the acid-stimulating gastrin. This type of operation also removes parts of the stomach that actively secrete acid and pepsin. Another type of operation involves cutting the nerve (vagus) that stimulates the stomach to produce its secretion. Quite often both procedures are used in the same patient.

Most people get along well following these operations, but occasionally a patient cannot digest large meals or may have difficulty with too rapid "dumping" of the stomach contents into the lower intestinal tract.

COMPLICATIONS

In addition to pain, ulcer patients often experience the following more-serious complications:

1. Narrowing and obstruction

Ulcers in the duodenum or in the narrow section where the stomach meets the duodenum may become inflamed and swollen or scarred and may cause the intestinal opening to become narrow or closed. This intestinal obstruction keeps food from passing from the stomach, and the patient vomits his meals or may constantly regurgitate the secretions of the stomach. Surgery may be necessary to correct this.

2. Hemorrhage

As the ulcer erodes into the muscular portion of the intestinal wall, it damages blood vessels there and may cause bleeding. If the damaged blood vessels are small, the blood oozes out slowly and over a long period of time, and the patient may become anemic. However, if the ulcer causes damage to a large blood vessel in the stomach or duodenal wall, the hemorrhage into the intestine is more rapid and potentially very dangerous. The patient may feel light-headed, or faint, or he may collapse suddenly. Without prompt medical attention, usually consisting of transfusion and possibly surgery, he may bleed to death internally. In some cases of bleeding ulcers the stool is stained tarry-black by the digested blood.

3. Perforation

Occasionally, an ulcer will erode all the way through the wall of the stomach or duodenum, and partially digested food and bacteria from the digestive tract will spill into the sterile abdominal cavity and result in peritonitis. A sudden perforation causes severe pain throughout much of the abdomen. Perforations are a medical emergency and require hospitalization and, usually, corrective surgery.

percussion — tapping the body as an aid in diagnosing the condition of the parts beneath the area being tapped. The sounds that the tapping makes are indicative of the condition of the internal organs. Percussion is used in much the same manner as one taps on a barrel to detect its fullness.

perennial hay fever — *See hay fever*.

pericarditis — an inflammation of the thin membrane sac (pericardium) that surrounds the heart.

periodontal disease — a disorder affecting the tissues and membranes surrounding the teeth.

There are several types of periodontal disease. In its early stages the most common type takes the form of gingivitis, or inflammation of the gums. This condition may develop into periodontitis (sometimes called pyorrhea), the chronic, destructive stage of the disease. It usually affects people over twenty-five years of age.

A major cause of periodontal disease is tartar, or calculus, that forms along the gums. This results in swelling and inflammation. As the disease progresses, the gums become more inflamed and pull away from the teeth, creating pockets between the gums and the teeth. Germs and food particles become wedged in these pockets, create more inflammation, and set up a vicious circle.

As the disease worsens, the inflammation spreads, the pockets deepen, and pus forms in them. The infected gums ulcerate and bleed, and tissue damage increases. In the final stages, the bone that supports the teeth is attacked and destroyed. Unless the person receives treatment, the teeth loosen and eventually come out.

This final stage, the deterioration of the bone to which the teeth are anchored, has provided evidence of periodontal disease in ancient times. Examination of the skulls of early man, of Egyptian mummies, and even of Indians who inhabited this country before Columbus' time has revealed bone destruction typical of pyorrhea.

CAUSES

Many factors are believed to contribute in some way to the development of periodontal disease. The two chief culprits are debris and tartar. Debris commonly starts as soft particles of food remaining in the teeth; these gradually become adherent bacterial masses called plaque. They can be removed by the process of thorough brushing and other cleansing. Tartar, or calculus, is the crust-like material formed by deposition of calcium and phosphate from saliva in neglected plaque. Unfortunately, tartar is not removed by simple brushing. Here the dentist's tools for scaling and cleaning are needed at regular intervals.

Aging also seems to have an undefined effect on the gums, since periodontal diseases affect more people in later years. However, the practice of good oral hygiene, started early in life, can largely avert this disorder in most people, even into old age.

Thus, it is evident that good oral hygiene is an effective preventive of periodontal disease and holds clues to its cause. But there are still many questions to be answered.

Other elements associated in one way or another with the development of this condition include malocclusion, or bad alignment of the teeth; bruxism, or grinding of the teeth; and loss of teeth, which causes remaining teeth to drift out of position. Irritation of the gums, caused by worn fillings, sharp edges of decayed teeth, and ill-fitting dentures, or mechanical injury, may also lead to eventual periodontal disease. Poor nutrition, deficient in proteins and certain minerals and vitamins, is believed to contribute to the weakening of oral tissues. A person who breathes through his mouth instead of his nose, who is a lip-biter, or who unduly presses his tongue against his teeth is more likely to develop peridontal disease.

TREATMENT

Once periodontal disease has begun treatment will depend on the stage of the disease. If it has not progressed far, treatment may consist only of removing hardened tartar from around and under the gums. If pockets have formed between the teeth and gums, they must often be removed surgically to prevent further impaction of food.

In its final stages, periodontal disease attacks the underlying tissue that supports the teeth. Treatment at this stage may involve bone and reconstructive surgery. It is estimated that at least half of the cases of the disease have bone deformities that must be corrected to allow complete and successful treatment.

periodontitis — *See periodontal disease.*

peripheral nervous system — the part of the central nervous system that is composed of the twelve pairs of cranial nerves and thirty-one pairs of spinal nerves stemming from the brain and the spinal cord, respectively.

The cranial nerves include voluntary fibers going to the eye muscles, the salivary glands, the heart, the smooth muscles of the lungs, and the intestinal tract. The spinal nerves send fibers to all muscles of the trunk and extremities, the involuntary fibers going to smooth muscles and glands of the gastrointestinal tract, genitourinary system, and cardiovascular system.

See cranial nerves, spinal nerves.

peripheral resistance — the resistance offered by the arterioles (small arteries) and capillaries to the flow of blood from the arteries to the veins. An increase in peripheral resistance causes a rise in blood pressure.

peristalsis — a term used to describe a wavelike movement. Food moves down and through the digestive system by peristalsis. The actual movement is caused by a series of timed contractions that push the food onward.

peritoneum — the smooth, transparent membrane that lines the abdominal cavity and part of the pelvic region. The peritoneum allows the organs in the area to move against each other with little or no friction.

peritonitis — an inflammation of the peritoneum. Peritonitis is caused by microorganisms that infect the peritoneum. This may follow a perforated ulcer, a ruptured appendix, an unsterile operation, or an abdominal wound, for instance. The chief symptoms are intense pain and tenderness. Peritonitis can be very serious if not treated promptly with antibiotics.

pernicious anemia — a form of chronic anemia characterized by disturbances of the gastrointestinal and neurological systems.

The disease is more common in the north temperate zones of Europe and the United States. While occurring in all races, pernicious anemia is more common among blond, blue-eyed people, such as natives of the British Isles and Scandinavian countries. Usually, patients are over thirty-five years of age. Males and females are affected equally. Heredity seems to play some role, since about twenty percent of cases have some family history of the disease.

CAUSE
The exact cause of pernicious anemia is unknown. The disease is the result of a deficiency in the gastric juices that permit the body to absorb vitamin B_{12}. The lack of B_{12} causes premature death of red blood cells, thereby reducing the capacity of the blood to carry oxygen to the tissues.

SYMPTOMS
The onset of anemia is insidious. Depending on the stage of the disease, a patient may have the following symptoms: loss of appetite, fatigue, lassitude, pallor, faintness, jaundice, sore tongue and mouth, diarrhea, digestive disturbances, depression and irritability that may ultimately lead to a psychosis, numbness and tinglihg of the fingers, other neurological deficits, and shortness of breath on exertion.

TREATMENT
Pernicious anemia cannot be cured. It is controlled by adequate diet and injection of vitamin B_{12} every week. Lifelong treatment is required if neurological crippling is to be prevented.

For the patient with pernicious anemia, continuous therapy is essential in order to prevent such complications as numbness in the extremities and an unsteady gait. Since some patients may have difficulty in walking, they should be protected from falls. They also have lost their normal resistance to infection and should be protected from people who have any type of infection. Pernicious anemia cannot be controlled by diet alone nor by taking medication by mouth. Injections are preferred by most physicians in order to ensure that the vitamin B_{12} is absorbed and is not destroyed in the stomach.

PREVENTION
No speecific steps can be taken to prevent pernicious anemia. Early and continuous medical care, however, will prevent the disabling effects of this disease. Since all anemias have an underlying cause, treatment prior to establishing the exact cause may serve to mask such diseases as

cancer, cirrhosis, uremia, hypothyroidism, arthritis, infections, and certain poisons. People should be warned against taking medications containing vitamins or iron without medical advice.

personality disorders — *See mental illness.*

perspiration — *See sweating.*

pertussis — *See whooping cough.*

pesticides — substances used to kill pests. The pests may be weeds, insects, rats and mice, algae, nematodes (worms), and other destructive forms of life. Pesticides that are used only for killing insects are called insecticides.

Killing garden pests, ridding homes of insects or rodents, and defleaing or delousing pets are common household uses of pesticides.

Guarding people's health and protecting fruits, vegetables, and forests are well-known commercial, agricultural, and governmental uses of pesticides.

Attacking specific diseases through organized programs and insect-and rodent-control was among the earliest and most important use of pest-killers. Scientists have been studying the benefits to be gained from using pesticides and the most effective methods of using them for disease control. At the same time they have been determining whether these poisons, plus the methods of using them, present significant dangers to man and his environment.

The fact that in our country today we are in such good control of once-feared diseases such as malaria, yellow fever, typhus, and plague is in part because of the use of pesticides against the insects and rodents that transmit these diseases to man.

HAZARDS
Improperly used, pesticides can and do cause illness and even death to human beings. To avoid improper use, it is very important that anyone who uses a pesticide understands its purpose and properties.

It is most essential to understand that pesticides, by necessity, are poisons. However, there is a great variation between the different compounds in use as pesticides with regard to their toxic hazard. A few materials are dangerous in the relatively small amounts that spraymen en-

counter by skin contact and by breathing during their work. However, most compounds have not produced occupational poisoning. Accidental ingestion (swallowing) has been responsible for most of the deaths from pesticides.

In addition to fear of accidental exposure, there is concern about possible long-term effects of pesticide contamination that may remain in the environment and—through air, soil, food, and water—may eventually adversely affect living things. The possible danger here is in inhaling or ingesting dangerous amounts through air, water, or food. This is why the Food and Drug Administration sets limits on the amount of pesticide residue that may safely remain on food crops at harvest and also polices our food supply to enforce these limits.

petit mal — *See epilepsy.*

phantom limb — the sensation of feeling in a limb that has been amputated. This phenomenon is caused by the stimulation of nerves in the remaining part of the limb that had continued into the amputated part.

pharmacology — the science that deals with the study of drugs in all its aspects. Scientists who work in this field are responsible for testing drugs to determine their proper uses, the dangers, and the correct dosage levels.

pharmacopoeia — an official listing of drugs and drug standards. In this country, the U.S.P. (United States Pharmacopeia) is the legally accepted standard text.

pharmacy — the science of preparing and dispensing drugs.

pharynx — the tubular passage that connects the nose, mouth, larynx, and esophagus. The pharynx is part of both the respiratory tract and the digestive system. It has a lining of mucous membranes that allows easy passage of both food and air.

The part of the pharynx that connects with the nose is called the nasopharynx. The connection is at the back of the nose above the soft palate. The oropharynx, the juncture of the mouth and the pharynx, is between the soft palate and the epiglottis. The laryngopharynx is the portion of the pharynx between the epiglottis and the esophagus. The pharynx begins to narrow below the epiglottis and becomes the esophagus.

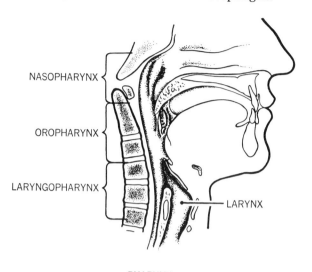

NASOPHARYNX

OROPHARYNX

LARYNGOPHARYNX

LARYNX

PHARYNX

phenobarbital — one of the slow-acting barbiturates. Phenobarbital is an anticonvulsant and is used as such in the treatment of epilepsy. It is also used to treat patients suffering from angina pectoris.

See barbiturates.

phenol — a strong antiseptic. Phenol, also known as carbolic acid, was first used as an antiseptic by Lister in 1867. Phenol is not used very frequently today. Other substances (some of them phenol derivatives) are less toxic and more effective.

See antiseptic.

phenylbutazone — a drug used in the treatment of arthritis and related disorders, such as gout and osteoarthritis. Phenylbutazone is very effective in treating many cases of these conditions. However, phenylbutazone can have many serious side effects (vomiting, diarrhea, insomnia, edema, anemia, etc). Consequently, the drug is often used as a last resort, and even then it is used with great care.

phenylketonuria — a disorder that can, if undetected and untreated, cause convulsions and severe mental retardation. Phenylketonuria, or PKU, is characterized by a "musty" smell to urine. The cause is an inborn (or congenital) lack of an enzyme, phenylalanine hydroxylase. The lack of this enzyme can be detected by a simple test at birth.

If the test is positive for PKU, a diet with reduced amounts of phenylalanine is started to try to prevent brain damage.

phlebitis — the inflammation of a vein. This often occurs in the leg and usually involves the formation of a blood clot in the inflamed vein. The danger of phlebitis is that the blood clot will move from the affected vein to another area of the body where it can cause more damage. If the blood clot reaches the heart or brain, it may cause death.

The usual treatment is to immobilize the affected region by putting the patient to bed. At the same time, the patient is frequently given an anticoagulant drug to help dissolve the blood clot.

phobia — any unnatural, unwarranted, or abnormal fear.

physical fitness — a measure of the body's strength, stamina, and flexibility. It is a reflection of the ability to work with vigor and pleasure, without undue fatigue, with energy left over for enjoying hobbies and recreational activities, and for meeting unforeseen emergencies. Physical fitness is important for mental health as well as for physical health. It requires proper nutrition, adequate rest and relaxation, good sleeping habits, good health practices, and especially adequate physical exercise.

The human body contains more than six hundred muscles; overall, the body is more than half muscle. Muscles make possible every overt motion. They also push food along the digestive tract, suck air into the lungs, and tighten blood vessels to raise blood pressure when more pressure is needed to meet an emergency. The heart itself is a muscular pump. Muscles are meant to be used. When they are not used, or are not used enough, they deteriorate.

An obvious effect of regular exercise is the firming of flabby muscles. In addition, research indicates that exercise produces beneficial changes in the functioning of internal organs — especially the heart, lungs, and circulatory system. The heartbeat becomes stronger and steadier, breathing becomes deeper, and circulation improves.

Research lists these benefits experienced by people who, after a prolonged period of sedentary living, have undertaken a systematic conditioning program:

1. Increased strength, endurance, and coordination.

2. Increased joint flexibility.

3. Reduction of minor aches, pains, stiffness, and soreness.

4. Correction of remediable postural defects.

5. Improvement in general appearance.

6. Increased efficiency with reduced expenditure of energy in performing both physical and mental tasks.

7. Improved ability to relax and to reduce tension voluntarily.

8. Reduction of chronic fatigue.

physical therapy — the treatment of disease by physical means. Physical therapy includes the use of heat, cold, water, light, electricity, manipulation, massage, exercise, and mechanical devices. This type of treatment is also known as physiotherapy.

physiotherapy — *See physical therapy.*

pia mater — the transparent membrane that covers the brain and spinal column. The pia mater is the innermost of the three membrane layers that cover the brain and which are collectively referred to as the meninges.
See meninges.

picric acid — a substance used in the treatment of minor burns.

piles — *See hemorrhoids.*

pimples — *See acne, comedo.*

pinkeye — *See conjunctivitis.*

pinpoint vision — a defect of the eye in which there is vision in the center of the eye only, with no visual field at all. Pinpoint vision is also called central vision or direct vision.

pinworms — small, round worms that live in the lower digestive tract of human beings. The female worm is about ¼ inch long; the male is much shorter.

The worms are most common in children. However, all the members of a family, adults as well as children, may become infected when a child brings home the pinworm infection he has acquired from playmates. Families in all economic circumstances can be affected, because the infective eggs are easily spread, and the parasite has a simple life cycle.

Pinworms enter the body when pinworm eggs are swallowed. The eggs hatch in the stomach, and the larvae pass through the small intestine into the large intestine. They remain there until they develop into adult worms, probably within five to six weeks. The female worms are then ready to deposit their eggs. They migrate down the rectum and out of the anus, where they deposit their eggs in the folds of skin surrounding the anus. After expelling many thousands of eggs, the female worm shrivels up and dies. The male worms may also migrate out of the anus and die. The migration and egg-laying usually occur at night, from a half hour to several hours after the person has gone to bed. In the case of heavy infections, migration may occur during the day, especially during periods of rest or relaxation. In the moist folds of the skin each egg develops to the infective stage in five to seven hours. The cycle of infection (or reinfection of the same individual) is completed when the infective eggs are swallowed.

Of the thousands of eggs expelled by each female pinworm, many may get on the fingers, especially if the victim has scratched himself. This is the most usual way for a person to be reinfected, and it can result in continual introduction of new worms into the body. The spread of eggs to other individuals is brought about when the sticky-coated eggs are scattered on bed linen and personal clothing, towels, tubs, faucet handles, washbowls, doorknobs, furniture, and even food. In confined rooms infected linen and clothing, when shaken, will throw many eggs into the air, where they may be inhaled or swallowed by persons exposed to the contaminated air.

SYMPTOMS

A sensation varying in intensity from a very mild tickling to severe itching or pain usually occurs when migrating female worms are on the anus or the surrounding skin. In women and girls, migrating worms may enter the vulva and vagina, frequently causing a vaginal discharge. Infected children sometimes have dark circles under the eyes and are pale. Restlessness, sleeplessness, loss of appetite, loss of weight, and sometimes nausea and vomiting occur. Infected children are apt to be irritable, hard to manage, and inattentive at school.

DIAGNOSIS

Diagnosis of pinworm infection is based on finding the female worm or the pinworm eggs. Worms may be detected at the anal opening of a child or adult at night by separating the buttocks and directing a light on the opening. If this method fails, giving a shallow enema may bring out worms. If pinworm infection is suspected but the worms cannot be found by these methods, further diagnostic tests can be performed by a laboratory. A physician or nurse can explain how to pick up pinworm eggs with a special cellulose tape slide or swab that can be obtained from most public health laboratories. Since the worms migrate and deposit eggs erratically, it may be necessary to make a swab on four or five consecutive nights before the presence of pinworms can be ruled out as a cause of the symptoms.

Since eggs of the pinworm are not usually deposited in the intestinal tract, stool examination cannot be relied on for diagnosis.

TREATMENT

Treatment should be in the hands of a physician. All infected persons in a household should be treated at the same time, so that all sources of infection can be eliminated at once. In addition to the medicine given to eradicate the worms, a physician will recommend the use of one of a number of soothing ointments or creams that can be smeared on the buttocks around the anus to relieve the itching and irritation that accompany the infection.

pituitary gland — a small, pea-sized gland located at the base of the brain. The pituitary gland controls all the other endocrine glands in the body. It is divided into two lobes: an anterior and a posterior lobe.

ANTERIOR LOBE

The anterior lobe plays the master role. Many different functions are attributable to its secretions.

1. Growth hormone influences skeletal growth. Disease of the gland may cause giantism (overgrowth), dwarfism (undergrowth), or acromegaly (a disease in which the hands, feet, and lower jaw enlarge).

2. Thyrotropic hormone influences the thyroid gland, stimulating the thyroid to secrete its hormone.

3. Gonadotropic hormone influences the gonads (the female ovaries and the male testi-

cles). This hormone is essential for normal development and functioning of the reproductive system.

4. Adrenocorticotropic hormone (ACTH) is related to the activity of the cortex of the adrenal glands. The removal of the pituitary gland leads to the rapid atrophy of this portion of the adrenal glands.

5. Hormones are secreted by the anterior lobe of the pituitary gland that contribute to the proper functioning of the parathyroid glands and to the pancreas, although the exact mode of action is not yet understood.

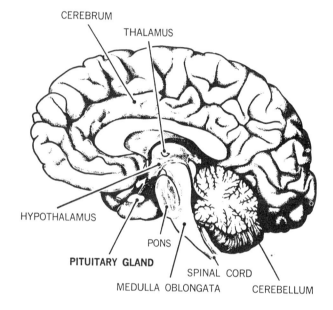

PITUITARY GLAND

POSTERIOR LOBE

The posterior lobe of the pituitary gland produces at least three secretions: antidiuretic hormone (ADH), which inhibits the excretion of water by the kidneys; vasopressin (pituitrin), which stimulates the contraction of smooth muscles; and oxytocin (pitocin), which specifically stimulates contraction of the muscles of the uterus (particularly following delivery).

When ADH is not produced in adequate amounts, urine volume can increase from ten to fifteen times the normal daily volume. This condition is called diabetes insipidus.

See endocrine glands.

placebo — a harmless, inactive substance given to patients in controlled tests. The placebo helps the researcher to evaluate the effectiveness of the real drug by guarding against any psychological effects or reactions to the idea of the medication.

In many experiments, half the patients will be given the test drug and half will be given a placebo. The patients are not told whether they are taking the real drug or the placebo. The results are then tabulated to see if there is any difference. In a double-blind experiment neither the patients nor the physician are aware of who is getting the real drug.

placenta — a disk-shaped organ that grows in the lining of the uterus after a fertilized egg has attached itself to the wall of the uterus. The placenta is slightly raised and covered by a transparent membrane. Blood from the mother circulates in it, as does blood from the fetus (baby).

Blood from the fetus flows in and out through two arteries and a vein. These arteries and the vein are encased in the umbilical cord, which attaches to the surface of the placenta at one end and to the baby's navel at the other end. The waste products of the fetus are carried through the blood vessels of the umbilical cord into the placenta, where they are exchanged for oxygen and nutrients from the mother. The vein in the cord carries these materials back to the baby. The main purpose of the placenta is to make possible this interchange.

Once the baby is born, the placenta is no longer needed. After birth the placenta starts to separate from its attachment to the lining of the uterus. In a short time, usually five minutes or less, the muscle wall of the uterus contracts once more, and the placenta and the membranes are expelled from the body. There is often a moderate amount of blood passed with the afterbirth (as the placenta and membranes are then called) from the place where the placenta was attached to the uterus, but this soon tapers off.

plague — an acute, highly infectious disease caused by *Pasteurella pestis*. The microorganism is generally carried by rodents and transmitted to humans by fleas. There are two major types of plague: bubonic plague and pneumonic plague. Pneumonic plague attacks the lungs; bubonic plague causes buboes, or swollen lymph glands.

Historically, plague has been referred to as the Black Death. Two of the most famous epidemics of plague occurred during the fourteenth and seventeenth centuries. In 1347 the great European plague started in Constantinople. Within three years it had swept through Europe. It is estimated that one half of the entire population of Europe died during the epidemic. In 1665 there was a devastating epidemic of plague in London. Approximately 75,000 people died from the disease.

There have been no recent plague epidemics; however, the disease has not been completely eradicated.

plantar warts — *See wart.*

plaque — any patch or accumulation. Plaques play a major role in atherosclerosis, or hardening of the arteries, and in tooth decay and periodontal disease.

ARTERIAL

The exact way an artery "hardens" is one of the major unsolved problems of medical science and the subject of hundreds of research studies. For some reason still not clearly understood, fat-like substances build up on the inside walls of the arteries. They gradually accumulate and form thick deposits called plaques. These deposits both roughen the artery's normally smooth inner lining and narrow the channel for blood flow, making it more difficult for enough blood to get through.

DENTAL

Plaque is also a significant factor in tooth decay and periodontal disease. Certain types of bacteria found in most people's mouths are able to attach themselves to the teeth and then grow and multiply into increasingly larger bacterial colonies called plaque.

This type of plaque is difficult to see even on the exposed surfaces of the teeth, because it is colorless and transparent. It usually has to be stained to be seen. However, sometimes plaque accumulates so heavily that, even without staining, it can be seen as whitish mats on and around the teeth.

Once plaque is established on the teeth, more bacteria lodge in the sticky plaque and reproduce. Many of these bacteria also act on sugars to produce acids that attack the tooth enamel. Once the enamel is dissolved by acid, bacteria from the plaque actually invade the underlying dentin to continue the destruction of the tooth.

See atherosclerosis, dental caries, periodontal disease.

plasma — the cell-free liquid portion of uncoagulated blood. It is different from serum, which is the fluid portion of the blood obtained after coagulation.
See blood.

plaster of paris — a chemical substance used to make hard casts for the immobilization of injured body parts. Plaster of paris is a dry powder that, when mixed with water and then allowed to dry, forms a firm mold. The wet plaster of paris is applied to bandages, which are then rolled around the affected body part. Because plaster of paris dries into such a hard substance, any area that is to be put into a cast is first covered by soft padding.

plastic surgery — a special branch of surgery that is concerned with correcting disfigurements. Plastic surgery includes purely cosmetic surgery, such as restructuring unattractive noses. However, plastic surgery is also concerned with the reduction of scar tissue. This can be extremely important, because large scars (as from extensive burns) can cause a loss of mobility.

The major aim of the plastic surgeon is to reduce the amount of the scar tissue to the smallest possible size. This is frequently achieved by hiding the scar within natural wrinkles.

platelets — *See blood.*

pleura — the two-layered membrane that surrounds and protects the lungs. The pleura is divided into two parts. One pleura encloses the right lung; the other encloses the left lung. The two layers of the pleura are separated by only a thin layer of fluid.

pleurisy — an inflammation of the pleura, the membrane that covers the lungs. The most common cause or pleurisy is infection, either viral or bacterial.

Dry pleurisy is the easiest type of pleurisy to diagnose. There is sudden pain, usually during respiration. The pain is caused by the friction that results when the two layers of the pleura rub together. In cases of dry pleurisy, the protective fluid between the two pleura layers is partially replaced by a sticky substance known as fibrin. Dry pleurisy is not contagious, although the underlying cause may be. It is treated by any drugs needed to stop the infection and by bed rest. Frequently, drugs are not needed at all.

Serofibrinous pleurisy, or pleurisy with effusion, is caused by an excess accumulation of fluid between the two layers of the pleura. Treatment may include the withdrawal of the excess fluid through a long needle inserted into the space between the pleura layers.

Empyema is a type of pleurisy in which fluid containing pus infiltrates the area between the pleura membranes. This is by far the most serious type of pleurisy. It must be treated with antibiotics. Complications resulting from empyema include meningitis, pericarditis, and endocarditis.

plexus — a network of nerves, veins, or lymph vessels in a particular area, such as the solar plexus in the upper abdomen.

Plummer-Vinson syndrome — a wasting-away of the mucous membranes of the mouth, pharynx, and esophagus. This syndrome is caused by deficiencies in the diet and frequently precedes cancer of the mouth. It is common among women in Sweden and apparently accounts for their unusually high incidence of mouth cancer.

pneumoconiosis — a chronic lung disease caused by the inhalation of dust and other foreign particles. There are various forms of this disease, caused by such irritants as asbestos. These foreign particles damage the lungs and reduce their capacity.

pneumonia — a general term for infection of the lungs. It can be caused by different kinds of bacteria or virus or by the presence of foreign matter such as fatty droplets of liquids that have been inhaled. Frequently, the symptoms of pneumonia include high fever, chills, vomiting, and a cough. Difficult, rapid breathing is another symptom.

Pneumonia begins when the microbes or the foreign matter that has entered the lungs sets up an inflammation. As part of the inflammation, fluid rushes into the lungs. When the cause of the disease is a virus or bacteria, the fluid is used by the invading organisms as a culture, or growth media. When the cause is foreign matter, the fluid provides a growing place for any organisms already present in the lungs or respiratory system.

TYPES

Pneumonia can be classified by the causative agent or by the location of the infection. Thus, bronchopneumonia is pneumonia that affects the alveoli (a cluster of tiny air sacs) of the lungs closest to the bronchi (bronchial tubes). The phrase lobar pneumonia indicates that an entire lobe is involved. Lobular pneumonia is patchy or scattered throughout parts of a lobe.

Pneumococcal pneumonia is caused by the pneumococci bacteria. This type of pneumonia is contagious. It is a lobar pneumonia; that is, it attacks an entire lobe. The bacteria usually reach the lungs by means of the respiratory tract. In fact, pneumococcal pneumonia can often be traced to an infection in the upper respiratory tract. Other bacteria, such as staphylococci, can also cause pneumonia.

Virus pneumonia is the term usually used to indicate pneumonia from unknown causes. Aspiration pneumonia is caused by foreign substances in the lungs. It is one of the usual types of pneumonia that occur following an operation. Another type of postoperative pneumonia is called hypostatic pneumonia. Hypostatic pneumonia attacks patients whose lungs are already congested.

TREATMENT

The treatment of pneumonia depends on the kind of pneumonia and, more specifically, on the cause. The pneumonias are usually treated with antibiotics, sometimes with cough medicines, and frequently with bed rest.

See lungs.

poison — any substance that causes bodily disturbance, injury, or death by chemical rather than mechanical means. It would be almost impossible to list all poisons, because a great many substances are harmless if used in the proper way but are poisonous if used in the wrong way or in the wrong amount. For instance, nearly all drugs and medicines are potentially both beneficial and poisonous; the effect is determined by the method of use and by the amount taken into the body. Such things as alcohol, coffee, and tobacco are actually poisonous substances for which the human body has certain tolerances; poisoning results if these tolerances are exceeded. Powdered glass, needles, metal splinters, and other foreign bodies are damaging when applied to or introduced into the body, but they are not classified as poisons, because their action is mechanical rather than chemical.

The action of a poison depends on several factors. The action will be more severe if a large dose is taken, because more of the poison will be absorbed in a short period of time. The toxicity of substances varies greatly — a few drops of one poison might be immediately fatal, while another poison might not be harmful unless taken by the tablespoonful. The age and body weight of the victim should also be considered. Infants, young children, and very old people are more likely to be killed by small doses of poison. In general, the less a person weighs, the smaller will be the fatal dose. Another factor that influences the action of poisons taken by mouth is the condition of the stomach; poisons taken on an empty stomach will act much more quickly (and therefore more violently) than those taken when the stomach is full.

The action of any poison is dependent, also, on the tolerance that the individual has for the particular substance. Some people seem to have a natural resistance to the action of certain poisons; others are so highly sensitive to them that even a small amount, such as might be given in a medicine, produces toxic effects. Habit is sometimes a factor to consider — drug addicts can tolerate doses of the habit-forming drugs that might kill the average person. The effectiveness of a poison also depends on the general health of the victim.

The physical state of the poisonous substance also determines its effectiveness. Gases are absorbed more quickly than liquids, and liquids are absorbed more quickly than solids. Related to this is the fact that the way in which a poison enters the body determines to some extent the speed and effectiveness with which it acts. In general, inhaled poisons are likely to work most quickly, injected poisons next, and poisons taken by mouth more slowly. Poisoning by skin contact usually occurs quite slowly over an extended period of time. Also, some substances are poisonous when taken in one way but not when taken in another; for example, snake venom may cause death when injected (as by a snakebite) but may be relatively harmless if swallowed.

GENERAL SYMPTOMS

It is often very difficult to recognize a case of poisoning. Most poisons do not give rise to symptoms that are sufficiently uniform or characteristic to provide a sure means of identification. Many poisons cause symptoms that are so similar to those of various diseases that they cannot be readily distinguished.

In addition to these difficulties, there is the fact

that the symptoms vary according to the amount of poison taken and the length of time it has been in the system. There may be several fairly distinct degrees or stages of poisoning, and the symptoms may be different in each stage.

However, there are some general signs that might indicate that a person has been poisoned. Intense pain frequently follows poisoning. Nausea and vomiting may occur. The victim may become delirious, or he may collapse and become unconscious. Poisoning by caustic acids, alkalis, phenols, and metallic salts is likely to cause corrosion, swelling, and bleaching of the skin, mouth, and throat. Brown or black stains on the skin or mucous membranes may be indicative of iodine poisoning; yellow stains may be caused by nitric acid and picric acid. Some poisons turn the urine red, dark green, bright yellow, or black; any unusual color may be an indication of poisoning. Many substances cause the victim's breath to have a peculiar odor.

In almost all cases of acute poisoning, the victim is likely to have considerable trouble in breathing. Some poisons characteristically cause paralysis; others cause convulsions. Some poisons cause the pupils of the eye to contract (become smaller) and others cause them to dilate (become larger). The skin may be flushed or pale, or perhaps bluish in color. Shock is always present in cases of acute poisoning.

CAUSES

Poisoning occurs in a variety of ways. Sometimes it is the result of attempted suicide or homicide. Frequently, it is accidental — a person takes an overdose of medicine, or by mistake takes some poisonous substance such as lye, iodine, or arsenic. Poisoning may be caused by the continuous use of a substance that is not dangerous if taken for a short time but which is cumulative in effect — that is, the poison is not eliminated from the body as quickly as it is absorbed. Poisoning also occurs from overexposure to industrial materials such as ammonia, gasoline (and, in fact, all petroleum products), lead salts, mercury, and many others as well as from exposure to various toxic by-products of industrial processes. The venom of some snakes, spiders, and scorpions causes poisoning.

TYPES

There are four ways that poisons can enter the body.

1. Ingestion

Poisons may be swallowed intentionally or by mistake. These poisons are usually assigned to one of several different categories, according to their effects on the body. Corrosives are substances that rapidly destroy or decompose the body tissues they contact. Examples of corrosive poisons are acids, phenols, and alkalis.

Irritants are substances that do not directly destroy the body tissues but cause inflammation in the area of contact. Examples of irritant poisons are arsenic, zinc sulfate, and potassium nitrate.

Depressants are substances that depress the nervous system. Examples are morphine and its derivatives, barbiturates, and alcohol.

Excitants are substances such as strychnine and camphor, which stimulate the nervous system.

2. Inhalation

Poisons may be inhaled in the form of noxious dusts, gases, fumes, or mists. Poisonous gases are made as by-products of certain operations or processes, such as exhaust fumes from internal combustion engines. Carbon monoxide, gasoline vapors, carbon dioxide, and ammonia are examples of poisons that can be inhaled.

3. Skin contact

Many inorganic and organic substances, in the form of gases, fumes, mists, liquids, and dusts, cause poisoning when they come in contact with the skin. Except in a few instances, poisonings that result from skin contact do not progress rapidly but manifest themselves gradually after continued exposure to the agents causing them. Lead, mercury, gasoline, and carbon tetrachloride are examples of substances that can cause poisoning by skin contact.

4. Injected poisons

Many poisons may enter the body through breaks in the skin. Infected wounds, drugs injected hypodermically, bites of rabid animals, and the bites of poisonous snakes and insects are examples of injected poisons.

TREATMENT

The treatment for poisonings depends to a large degree on the exact causative agent. Thus, not all corrosive poisonings are treated the same way. Another important factor is the length of time between the poisoning and the beginning of treatment. Some poisons work so quickly that the

patient may die before effective treatment can be given. All cases of poisoning require immediate attention by a physician. However, if a physician cannot be reached immediately, the correct first aid procedures should not be delayed.
See individual causative agents.

poison ivy — a poisonous plant. It grows in the form of climbing vines, shrubs that trail on the ground, and erect shrubbery growing without support.

The leaves vary in length from one to four inches. They are green and glossy in summer; in the spring and fall they are red or russet. The fruit is white and waxy and resembles mistletoe. Although poison ivy assumes many forms and displays seasonal changes in leaf coloring, it has one constant characteristic that makes it easy to recognize: the leaves always grow in clusters of three.

CAUSE
The irritating substance in poison ivy is the oily sap in the leaves, flowers, fruit, stem, bark, and roots. The plant is poisonous even after long drying, but is particularly irritating in the spring and early summer when it is full of sap.

Most cases of ivy poisoning are caused by direct contact with the plant. Some are caused by handling clothing, garden implements, and pets that have been contaminated by the oily sap. People differ in their sensitivity to poison ivy. Some are so sensitive that exposure to smoke from a brush fire containing poison ivy will cause inflammation of the skin. Too many people become poisoned because they have not learned to recognize poison ivy; they walk through it, brush against it, and gather its attractive foliage. Usually, they transfer part of the irritant from their hands to their faces and other parts of their bodies. Serious and distressing cases of poisoning in the mouth and rectum have resulted when children and others eat the leaves and fruit from this poisonous plant.

SYMPTOMS
The first symptom noticed after ivy poisoning is a burning and itching sensation. This is followed by a rash and swelling and probably by small or large blisters. The length of time elapsing between contact with poison ivy and the first symptoms varies from a few hours to seven days.

TREATMENT
If there are large blisters or severe inflamma-

tion, or if the inflammation is on the face or genitals, the help of a physician is needed to relieve discomfort and guard against secondary infections.

Stubborn cases that do not respond to proper treatment may be caused by repeated contact with contaminated clothing. Any suspected garments should be dry-cleaned or washed with plenty of soap.

When there are only a few small blisters on the hands, arms, or legs, they can often be treated at home. Any one of the following methods may be used for relief: wet compresses with boric acid solution, starch-solution baths, or calamine lotion.

PREVENTION
Obviously, the best prevention is to avoid contact with the poison ivy plant. However, when contact has been made, the patient should wash the affected skin area as soon as possible several times and rinse in running water after each sudsing. This should remove or make less irritating any oil that has not already penetrated the skin.

poison oak — a poisonous plant that is similar to poison ivy.
See poison ivy.

poison sumac — a poisonous plant that is similar to poison ivy.
See poison ivy.

polio — *See poliomyelitis.*

poliomyelitis — a disease caused by any one of three closely related viruses. This disease used to be fairly common in the United States, particularly in the summer. It was so common that during the first half of the twentieth century there were many epidemics of the disease. However, the use of the Salk and the Sabin vaccines has drastically reduced the number of new cases. These vaccines have been so effective that there have been no poliomyelitis epidemics since 1966.

Poliomyelitis is best known as a disease that causes paralysis. However, only the most severe form of polio (as poliomyelitis is sometimes called) causes lasting paralysis. The great majority of cases result in no lasting paralysis.

The virus causing poliomyelitis enters the body through the respiratory system. The virus attacks the cells in the central nervous system.

The exact method by which the virus cells move from the respiratory system to the central nervous system is not known.

TYPES

There are two ways that polio can affect an individual patient. These two types are referred to as the minor and the major illnesses.

1. Minor illness

In this form, poliomyelitis can be so mild that the patient may be entirely unaware of any infection. When symptoms are present in the minor illness, they are usually limited to vague complaints. Typical symptoms are headache, slight temperature elevation, sore throat, and upset stomach. These complaints generally disappear from one to three days after they appear.

2. Major illness

This form of polio is more serious and can result in permanent paralysis (although permanent paralysis occurs in only a small percentage of the major illness). The major illness may be preceded by the minor illness. When this happens, the patient will have the vague complaints of the minor illness. The symptoms disappear for a few days, and then the symptoms of the major illness appear. However, most cases of the major illness do not begin this way.

The major illness usually begins with pain in the muscles, a stiff neck, an elevated temperature, and headache. Depending on the severity of the case, paralysis may follow the initial symptoms. The paralysis is caused by the damage done to the central nervous system. If the virus has not destroyed too many cells, the paralysis will not be permanent, although temporary weakness may follow the paralysis.

TREATMENT

To date, no drugs have been found that are effective in treating poliomyelitis once the disease has begun. Physicians usually prescribe bed rest and, in severe cases, hospitalization.

PREVENTION

There are two types of vaccines to prevent polio. The first of these was developed by Jonas Salk (born 1914). It is administered by injection, usually in three separate shots for the three different poliomyelitis viruses. The second vaccine was developed by Albert Sabin (born 1906). The Sabin vaccine is an oral vaccine, also generally administered in three different doses. Because it was so frequently given to school children on a sugar cube, the Sabin vaccine has been nicknamed the sugar-cube vaccine.

polycythemia — an abnormal condition of the blood. Polycythemia is characterized by an excessive number of red blood cells.

polygraph — an instrument for simultaneously recording several different pulsations. The polygraph was first used as a tool in diagnosis. Today its use is primarily in the field of law enforcement, where it is referred to as a "lie detector."

polyp — a mass, or small stemlike growth, of swollen mucous membrane projecting into a body cavity such as the nose or the intestines.

polyunsaturated fat — a fat so constituted chemically that it is capable of absorbing additional hydrogen. These fats are usually liquid oils of vegetable origin, such as corn oil or safflower oil. A diet with a high polyunsaturated fat content tends to lower the amount of cholesterol in the blood. These fats are sometimes substituted for saturated fat in a diet in an effort to lessen the hazard of fatty deposits in the blood vessels.
See cholesterol.

pons — the part of the brain that connects the cerebrum and cerebellum with the medulla (medulla oblongata). The pons is shaped like an oval.

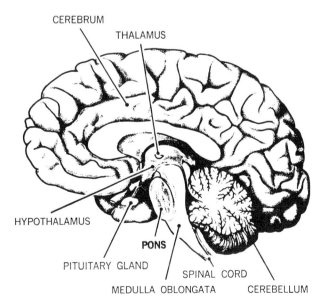

PONS

277

Nerve impulses that originate in the cerebellum and cerebrum pass through the pons on the way to the rest of the body. Nerve impulses originating elsewhere in the body pass through the pons on the way to the cerebrum and cerebellum. Additionally, the pons is the source of several of the cranial nerves.

See cranial nerves.

popliteal — of or pertaining to the back of the knee.

post — a prefix indicating an event occurring after another event or a body organ or part that is located behind another organ or part.

posture — the position of the body. Good posture is the correct alignment of the body and all body parts when standing, sitting, lying down, or in any phase of activity.

Good posture helps to conserve energy, promotes the efficient use of muscles, and avoids back strain and fatigue.

pregnancy — the condition of a woman between the conception of a child and the time she begins labor to deliver the child. There are numerous tests for pregnancy. Some of these tests can determine a pregnancy as early as one week after conception.

DURATION

The average time from conception to birth is about 266 days. It is almost impossible to know exactly when conception has occurred. Consequently, doctors rely on the fact that most babies are born about 280 days after the beginning of the mother's last normal menstrual period. Another method of calculating when the baby is due is to count back three months from the first day of the last normal menstrual period and then add seven days. Regardless of the way the due date is determined, only about one in twelve babies is actually born on the exact day indicated. The birth date may vary from one to two weeks before or after the expected date. Occasionally, the birth

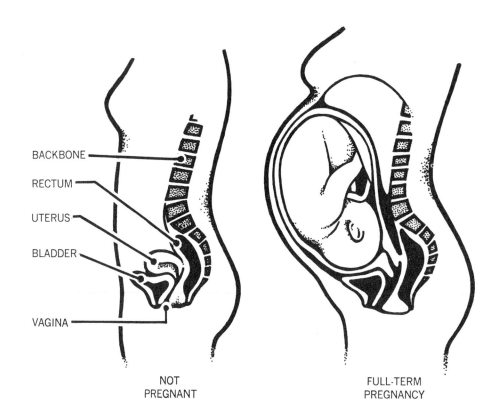

BACKBONE

RECTUM

UTERUS

BLADDER

VAGINA

NOT
PREGNANT

FULL-TERM
PREGNANCY

PREGNANCY

will be even further away from the expected date. Individual differences account for most of this wide variation. However, other factors, such as the health of the mother, can cause the length of a pregnancy to vary.

NOURISHMENT

Women who are properly nourished are less likely to encounter some of the complications of pregnancy. They usually recover more quickly after their babies are born and produce milk of good quality for breast-feeding. As a rule, their babies are healthier and physically better prepared for life.

Most physicians do not want an expectant mother to gain more than fifteen to twenty-five pounds if her weight was previously normal. Basically, the pregnant woman should eat the same amount of food as before, with emphasis on a higher protein intake and less fat and carbohydrate foods. Proteins are essential to maintain her body and to permit the child to grow and develop.

Milk taken daily provides calcium for the infant's bones and teeth and prevents calcium loss on the part of the mother. Iron-rich foods are needed to provide iron for the infant's and mother's blood.

prelingual deafness — the total or near-total loss of hearing that occurs before normal speech habits have been established.

The lack of meaningful hearing during infancy and early childhood (when speech develops) has drastic effects on the development of both speech and language. Normally, speech develops as a direct result of hearing. Speech is both a way of making the sounds that are called words and a system of symbols that stand for something. Language is the system of symbols that uses words to represent objects, actions, ideas, and meanings.

The small child who cannot hear is doubly handicapped. He has difficulty acquiring the meanings for which language stands as well as difficulty in talking.

premature baby — a baby whose weight is less than five and a half pounds at birth. The premature baby usually has not had a full nine months to develop, although it is possible for a premature baby to be a full-term baby.

CAUSES

Premature births occur in only about ten per-

cent of all births that go beyond the fifth month. The causes of premature birth are varied and, in some cases, cannot be determined. No one knows for sure what triggers the muscles of the uterus to begin labor contractions. What is known, however, is that the health (both physical and mental) of the mother can play a large role in premature birth. For example, early birth can be caused by syphilis, toxemia, and other serious health problems.

The birth of a premature baby is ordinarily not a great problem among healthy, well-nourished mothers. Those who are malnourished or who suffer from some chronic illness are more susceptible. Premature birth occurs more frequently in twin pregnancies than in single births. Usually, in these circumstances, these babies are relatively mature in spite of their small size. They may be expected to do better than a single baby of the same size.

SPECIAL CARE

A premature baby is placed in an incubator until his body is ready to adjust to life in the outside world. Temperature and humidity are carefully controlled in the incubator. Extra oxygen can be supplied if it is needed. Special precautions are taken to keep infection away from the baby when he is fed or changed.

How long a premature infant stays in the hospital depends on his progress. A baby who weighs almost five and a half pounds at birth may need very little special care. The smaller ones are usually kept in the hospital until they weigh at least five pounds and show in other ways that they are strong enough to get along without hospital care.

The premature baby loses weight after birth, just as full-term babies usually do, but it may take him a longer time to regain the loss. Once he makes up the loss, however, the premature baby frequently grows quite rapidly.

prenatal — an event or problem that occurs before birth.

presbycusis — a hearing impairment associated with aging. Presbycusis is generally first noticed after sixty years of age.

The higher tones frequently begin to fade during the thirties and continue to fade as the years go by. However, the tones necessary to understand speech may show no great change for decades. Unless something besides age is interfering, many people are in their seventies before they notice that their hearing is less acute. Some people never have any noticeable loss.

Presbycusis was once believed to be caused by disintegration of the cells in the cochlea of the inner ear. Now, however, research has shown that changes with aging of the brain appear to be primarily responsible for this type of hearing loss.

presbyopia — farsightedness. A condition in which the eyes have difficulty focusing on close objects.
See farsightedness, hyperopia.

prescription — a written directive for a specific medicine or medicines. The prescription tells the pharmacist what the medicine is or what it is made from and gives directions for the proper dosage, which the pharmacist transfers to the label. Additionally, the prescription usually advises the pharmacist how many times the patient may have refills without speaking to the doctor again.

When a physician writes a prescription for a patient he bases his decisions (what drug, how frequently the drug or medicine should be taken, etc.) on the individual patient, his symptoms, and his past history. Consequently, the prescription for one patient may not be the same as the prescription for another patient even if the two have the exact same symptoms.

prescription drug — any drug or medicine that is not sold without a prescription from a doctor. These drugs are usually stronger or have more side effects than over-the-counter drugs, which can be bought and sold without a doctor's prescription.

pressor — a substance that raises the blood pressure and accelerates the heartbeat. The term is also used to denote certain nerve fibers that produce a rise in blood pressure when they are stimulated.
See blood pressure.

pressure point — a place where a main artery lies near the skin surface and over a bone. Pressure points are very important in controlling hemorrhage, particularly when blood is escaping from a major blood vessel.

The objective of applying pressure to a pressure point is to compress the artery against the bone, thus shutting off the flow of blood from the heart to the wound. There are twenty-two pressure points on the body, eleven on each side.

prevalence — the number of cases of a given disease existing in a given population at a specified moment of time.
See incidence.

prickly heat — a rash that looks like little pimples or blisters. In many parts of the country, prickly heat is a more-or-less constant nuisance in the summer — especially to babies. The rash commonly appears in the folds of the neck and shoulders, but it may spread downward and into the creases of the legs of fat babies.

primaquine — a drug used in the treatment of malaria.
See malaria.

primary herpes — *See herpes simplex.*

primary hypertension — an elevated blood pressure that is not caused by kidney or other evident disease. Primary hypertension is also called essential hypertension and is more commonly known as high blood pressure.
See blood pressure, hypertension.

primipara — a term used to indicate that a woman has already given birth to at least one child.

procaine — a drug used as a local anesthetic. Procaine, better known as novocaine, was synthesized in 1905 by Einhorn. Procaine is probably the most popular of all local anesthetics. It has a wide variety of uses, including local anesthesia in dentistry.
See anesthetics.

procaine amide — a drug that is sometimes used to treat abnormal rhythms of the heartbeat.

proctoscope — an instrument used to examine the rectum.

progesterone — an important female hormone. Progesterone is secreted by the corpus luteum (the yellow body that is the remainder of the follicle from which an ovum grows).

Progesterone, also called luteohormone, is responsible for the growth of the lining of the uterus and for menstruation. When an ovum is

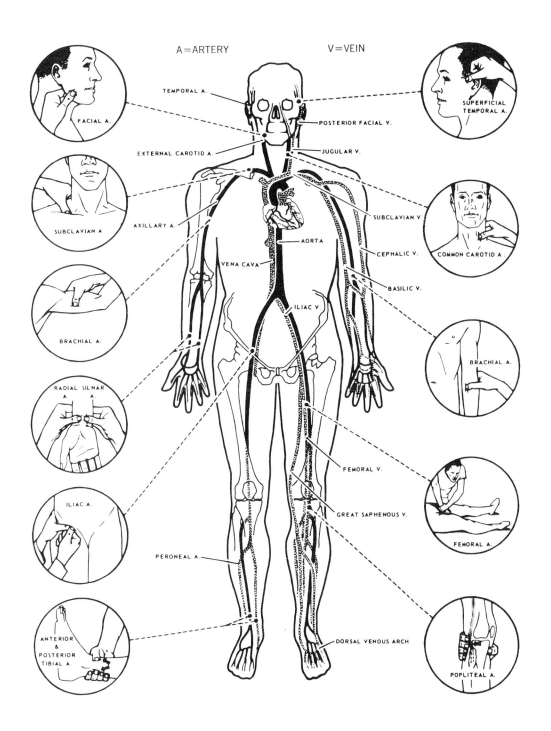

A=ARTERY   V=VEIN

PRESSURE POINTS

not fertilized, the corpus luteum is sloughed off and the secretion of progesterone is slowed. Menstruation follows. Conversely, when the ovum is fertilized, the corpus luteum continues to secrete progesterone. The hormone stimulates the continued growth of the uterus lining, providing a place for the embryo to grow.

Additionally, progesterone stimulates the mammary glands (breasts) during pregnancy to prepare them for the production of milk.

See hormone.

prognosis — the attending physician's estimation of the probable course, length of time, and lasting effects (if any) of a patient's disease or condition. The physician bases his estimation on his knowledge of the patient, the patient's individual history, and the symptoms and nature of the particular disease or condition.

prophylaxis — any treatment that prevents a disease or condition. The prophylaxis for some diseases, such as smallpox, is a vaccination that confers immunity to the disease. The preventative treatment for other diseases may be drugs or simply a return to good health habits.

prostate gland — a gland, about the size of a chestnut, that is part of the male reproductive system. It lies just below the urinary bladder and surrounds the first inch or so of the urethra, the canal that carries urine from the bladder. The secretion of the prostate provides part of the fluid that is produced during the male reproductive activity. Not all the gland's functions are fully understood.

PROSTATE CANCER

Prostate cancer causes few deaths among men under forty. But after age fifty-five it becomes the third highest cause of cancer deaths among men, and after age seventy-five it is the main cause.

1. Symptoms

Any sort of continuing urinary difficulty may be a symptom of prostate cancer. Such difficulties include a weak or interrupted flow of urine, the need to urinate frequently (especially at night), inability to urinate, difficulty in starting urination, blood in the urine, a flow that is not easily stopped, and painful or burning urination.

These symptoms may occur when a malignant tumor partly obstructs the neck of the bladder,

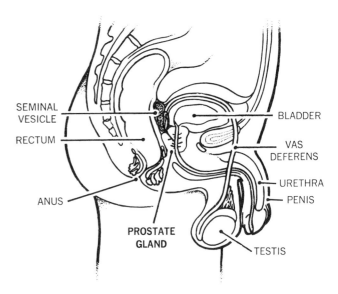

PROSTATE GLAND

but more often they result from a noncancerous enlargement called benign prostatic hypertrophy (or BPH). More than half of the men in the United States over fifty suffer from BPH, which often requires surgical removal of part or all of the gland. Only a physician can tell if the symptoms are caused by a benign or malignant enlargement or by other illnesses.

Pain in the pelvis, lower back, or upper thighs may also be a sign of prostate cancer. Sometimes such pain is the first or major symptom.

2. Diagnosis

The only procedure that determines conclusively whether a tumor is malignant is a biopsy — the removal of a small piece of tissue for examination under a microscope. This simple surgical procedure may be done through a special needle under local or general anesthetic. The tissue sample may also be removed as part of surgery to relieve obstruction of the urinary canal, which often occurs when benign prostatic hypertrophy or a malignant prostatic tumor encroaches on the canal. The biopsy may be part of surgery that exposes the prostate area completely and can be followed by removal of the entire prostate, if necessary.

3. Treatment

When the cancer is confined to the prostate gland, the patient can usually be treated successfully by surgical removal of the gland.

When cancer extends beyond the prostate, it can usually be checked by controlling the body's production of androgens, the male hormones essential for the prostate's growth. Control can be accomplished by orchiectomy, which is the removal of the testes, the major source of androgens. It can also be effected by the administration of synthetic female hormones, the estrogens, to prevent the manufacture of androgens by the testes and perhaps counteract the action of the androgens.

Frequently, both methods are used separately or together, they usually bring about striking improvement — shrinking of the tumor, relief of symptoms, and a greatly improved feeling of well-being that lasts several months to several years or more. Sometimes estrogens or orchiectomy are used when cancer seems to be confined to the prostate — as a precaution in case the tumor has spread without evidence.

Radioactive gold or phosphate is sometimes injected into the tumor area to destroy as many cancer cells as possible. Also, some form of the hormone cortisone is sometimes administered later in the course of the disease; the cortisone helps suppress the action of the adrenal glands, which may also contribute to the body's production of androgens.

prosthesis — the replacement of a missing body part with an artificial substitute. A prosthetic may be used for cosmetic purposes, as for example, the use of a "glass" eye; or a prosthetic may be needed to allow the patient a return to a relatively normal life. This is the case with an artificial leg, which allows the patient more mobility than a wheelchair or crutches would permit.

prostigmine test — a test for pregnancy. This test requires that the woman be given prostigmine. If the woman is pregnant, there will be no reaction. If the woman is not pregnant, the prostigmine will cause her to menstruate. The prostigmine test is usually limited to women who have already missed one menstrual period.

protein — the basic substance of every cell in the body. Proteins are the main constituents of the muscles and most lean tissues of the body. All life requires protein. It is the chief tissue-builder.

Proteins are required in the daily diet for growth, maintenance, and repair of tissues, as well as for many other body processes. These other processes include the formation of hemoglobin (the blood protein that carries oxygen to the cells and carries carbon dioxide away from the cells) and the production of antibodies (the substances that help the body fight infection).

After foods are eaten, the proteins are broken down (digested) into amino acids, which are then rearranged to form the many special and distinct proteins in the body. Any extra food proteins not utilized in this specialized fashion are used as a source of energy.

Among the many different amino acids, eight are called "essential," since body tissues cannot manufacture them; these essential amino acids must be furnished in the diet. The amino acid makeup of a food protein determines its nutritive value. Those proteins that supply all the essential amino acids in about the same proportions they are needed by the body rate highest in value. Foods that provide good amounts of these top-ranking proteins meet the body's needs best. Generally, these are foods of animal origin — meat, fish, poultry, eggs, and milk.

protoplasm — the semisolid, colorless material that is the physical material of life. Protoplasm assumes a wide variety of shapes and densities. For example, the soft body layer generally referred to as fat is protoplasm, but the hard material of bones is also protoplasm.

protraction — the act of moving a part forward. The term is frequently used to describe the forward motions of the lower jaw and the clavicle.

proximal — a term indicating nearer or closer. It is the opposite of distal.

psittacosis — a type of pneumonia caused by a virus. Psittacosis, also known as parrot fever, is carried by parrots, pigeons, parakeets, etc. People become infected with psittacosis when they inhale the nasal secretions from an infected animal. It is also possible to become infected from the animal's excretions, by being bitten by an infected animal, etc.

The symptoms of psittacosis are elevated temperature; headache; a dry, persistant cough; and chills. Parrot fever can be very dangerous. In serious cases, the disease may last for a month or more. Fatalities from serious cases can run as high as one in five.

Treatment for psittacosis is similar to treatment for pneumonia. Bed rest is very important, and antibiotics are usually used.

psoriasis — a fairly common skin disease. Psoriasis is characterized by thickened, reddish patches of skin covered with heavy, whitish scales. Although not painful, the scaly sores may be disfiguring.

Normally, the outer layer of skin, or epidermis, reproduces itself about once a month. As new cells form, the old surface skin is shed unobtrusively in the form of tiny flakes. In psoriatic skin, however, the production of new cells is speeded up, and the diseased skin reproduces itself every three or four days. This faster growth produces imperfectly formed cells that are shed from the diseased areas in large numbers, thus accounting for the asbestos-like scales of the disease.

This abnormal process does not allow for the formation of normal protective surface layers of skin — layers that usually act as a barrier against the environment, and which prevent loss of vital tissue substances through the skin. Lack of this protective barrier further encourages the formation and shedding of psoriatic scales, which are about ninety percent protein; thus, severe cases result in a great daily loss of this essential constituent of body tissue.

Although psoriasis may occur anytime, it is most common between the ages of fifteen and thirty-five, is rare in infancy, and afflicts males and females with equal frequency. There tends to be a higher than average percentage of cases among fair-skinned peoples, particularly those in nontropical areas. Psoriasis is not a contagious disease and cannot be caught from or given to others.

It is estimated that more than four million Americans have psoriasis, making it one of the most common single skin diseases in this country.

CAUSE

The cause of psoriasis is unknown. There is some evidence that the disease may be hereditary, but this has not yet been proved conclusively. Body chemistry disturbances have been suspected, possibly acting as trigger mechanisms in persons whose inherited traits make them more susceptible to the disease. There is also the influence of hormones, since the disease will often clear temporarily during a pregnancy. It is also known that periods of emotional disturbances or stress will aggravate psoriasis.

SYMPTOMS

Psoriasis usually begins gradually, but may come on suddenly. The individual's general health is rarely affected. Small, bright-red spots appear, often on the scalp, the elbows or knees, or the lower part of the back, although any part of the skin may be affected. The initial spots may be only the size of a pinhead. Soon, the affected area may be covered with sticky-dry scales in thin layers that, when peeled off, reveal a smooth, moist surface studded with tiny, bleeding points. The spots may increase in size and may combine to form larger and larger patches, some of which produce irregular, sometimes bizarre, patterns as they spread.

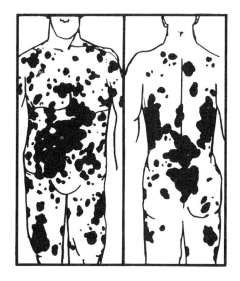

PSORIASIS

Affected spots often appear at the exact site of a minor injury to the skin, such as a cut, burn, or bruise. Attacks may be mild or severe, and the sores may clear up or recur abruptly for no apparent reason. One of the more usual features of the disease, however, is its frequent recurrence throughout a lifetime. In many instances, the disease improves in the summer months following exposure to sunlight and recurs in the winter, sometimes with renewed vigor. A few cases, however, will worsen in the summer, a fact that further complicates the search for the cause of psoriasis.

Affected spots on the face are usually small and are not generally located near the ears, eyes, mouth, or nose. The nails may sometimes show changes in the form of speckling, punctures, and depressions.

Psoriasis is not easy to diagnose. It may often be confused with several other skin disorders.

TREATMENT

Although no cure now exists for psoriasis, many beneficial treatments are available. The method of treatment depends on the area of the body that is affected, the stage of development of the disease, and the response to medication. Modern therapy strives to slow down the rapid growth of cells characteristic of psoriasis in order to allow time for a protective layer of skin to form.

The simplest forms of treatment are advisable initially. Physicians often recommend daily removal of scales with soap and water, followed by application of a lubricant. Mild cases of psoriasis that develop rapidly also often heal rapidly, although the condition may worsen without proper care.

When the scalp is affected, a solution containing sulfur and salicylic acid may be applied daily, and the hair may require shampooing several times each week. Salicylic acid aids in removing the scales, while sulfur is believed to promote healing.

When more intensive treatment is needed, one of the safest and most satisfactory remedies is one that has been used for many years — a combination of coal-tar ointments and ultraviolet radiation. This form of treatment, particularly for patients in whom large areas of skin are affected, may be performed best in a hospital over a period of several weeks and is generally most effective.

Significant progress in the treatment of advanced psoriasis has been achieved in recent years through local applications or local injection of steroid drugs. In the former method the drugs are applied in the form of creams or ointments and then covered with a plastic film for one or two days. Equally beneficial results have been obtained by injecting steroid drug preparations, notably triamcinolone, into the site of the affected spots.

Two types of drugs taken by mouth are effective in treating extensive, persistent psoriasis: the steroids and certain antimetabolic drugs. These drugs are methods of last resort and are used only for severe cases. They are potentially dangerous when taken orally, and, frequently, a severe flare-up of the disease occurs after they are discontinued.

Most cases of psoriasis can be effectively controlled through diligent use of medication. Many patients with mild forms of the disease, however, do not take the time necessary to carry out the required treatment procedures. A more severe case of psoriasis may actually respond better to treatment, because the patient works harder at treating it. Clearing is usually incomplete, but the disease sometimes disappears for many months and even years. More often, however, psoriasis comes and goes at intervals.

psychiatrist — a medical doctor whose specialty is the care and treatment of patients with mental disorders.

psychiatry — the branch of medicine that deals with mental disorders.

psychologist — a person who has had special training in the field of psychology. A psychologist is usually a person with a doctorate in psychology.

psychology — the branch of science that deals with the mind, behavior, and related subjects.

psychomotor epilepsy — *See epilepsy.*

psychosis — a severe, specific mental disorder that has a characteristic origin, course, and symptoms. Psychosis is the most severe form of mental illness. People who are psychotic (suffering from psychosis) have lost contact with reality.
See mental illness.

psychosomatic — a term pertaining to the influence of the mind, emotions, fears, etc. upon the functions of the body, especially in relation to diseases and physical disorders.
See mental illness.

psychotherapy — the treatment of disorders by the use of means such as persuasion, suggestion, educational techniques, lay or religious counseling, or help from a psychologist or psychiatrist.

puberty — the period of time during which the body reaches full sexual maturity. Puberty usually begins in the early teens and is completed within one to three years. However, puberty is subject to very wide individual differences. Thus, puberty may begin earlier or later and may last a long or a relatively short time.

Puberty is a time of intense problems for some young people. Aside from sociological causes, hormonal imbalance is common. This imbalance can result in a great deal of unhappiness. In general, once puberty has been completed the hormones are balanced again, and most of the problems they have caused are eased if not resolved.

The beginning of puberty (which can be identified with the growth of the secondary sex characteristics) is controlled by the pituitary gland.

See pituitary gland, secondary sex characteristics.

pulmonary — of or pertaining to the lungs.

pulmonary artery — the large artery that conveys unoxygenated blood from the lower right chamber of the heart to the lungs. This is the only artery in the body that carries unoxygenated blood; all the others carry oxygenated blood to the body.

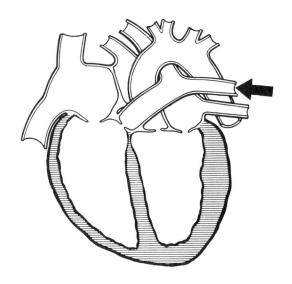

PULMONARY ARTERY

pulmonary circulation — the circulation of the blood through the lungs. The flow is from the right lower chamber of the heart (called the right ventricle) through the lungs, back to the left upper chamber of the heart (called the left atrium).

pulmonary valve — a valve formed by three cup-shaped membranes at the junction of the pulmonary artery and the right lower chamber of the heart (right ventricle). When the lower chamber contracts, the pulmonary valve opens and the blood is forced into the artery leading to the lungs. When the chamber relaxes, the valve is

closed and prevents the blood from flowing backward into the right ventricle.

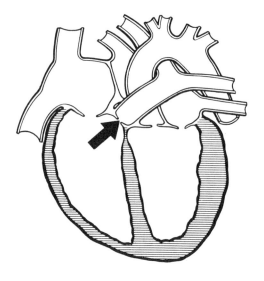

PULMONARY VALVE

pulmonary veins — four veins (two from each lung) that conduct oxygenated blood from the lungs into the left upper chamber of the heart (called the left atrium).

pulse — the expansion and contraction of an artery that may be felt with the finger. The pulse count (number of contractions per minute) is a reflection of the heartbeat. The pulse may be felt in many different areas of the body. However, most physicians prefer to take a pulse count on the inside of the wrist. The phrase "a racing pulse" means that the heart is beating or contracting faster than normal.

The heart of the normal adult contracts approximately seventy-two times per minute when the body is at rest. Consequently, the pulse rate will be seventy-two for the average adult at rest. Factors affecting the pulse (or heartbeat) include emotions, physical activity, and general health.

pulse pressure — the difference between the blood pressure in the arteries when the heart is in contraction (systole) and when it is in relaxation (diastole).

See blood pressure.

pulsus alternans — a pulse in which there is a regular alternation of weak and strong beats.

See pulse.

punctures — wounds that are caused by objects that penetrate some distance into the tissues while leaving a relatively small surface opening. Puncture wounds are produced by pointed instruments such as needles, splinters, nails, and pieces of wire. As a rule, small puncture wounds do not bleed freely; however, large puncture wounds may cause severe internal bleeding.

Most of the articles causing punctured wounds are full of germs. Thus, the infection-causing germs are often driven deep into the wounded tissues. The small openings and the relatively few number of blood vessels that are cut prevent free external bleeding. This in turn heightens the danger of infection.

pupil — the opening of the iris in the eye. The pupil is the site where light rays actually enter the eye. The size of the pupil varies greatly. In bright light, the pupil shrinks so that only a small portion of the available light enters the eye. In dim light or at night, the pupil opens to admit all of the available light. When the pupil is small, it is said to be contracted; when it is large, it is said to be dilated.

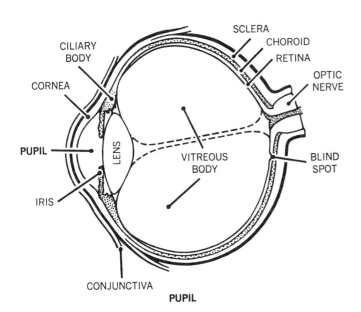

PUPIL

The pupil appears as the black circle in the middle of the eye. Depending on the size of the pupil at any given moment, there will appear to be more or less color to the eye. That is, the size of the iris seems to depend on the degree of pupil dilation. Actually, the size of the pupil is controlled by the muscles of the iris.

purgative — a drug used to help relieve constipation. *See cathartic, constipation.*

Purkinje fibers — the specialized fibers that form a network in the walls of the lower chambers of the heart. These fibers are believed to be involved in conducting electrical impulses to the muscular walls of the two lower chambers (ventricles). In turn, the electrical impulses are responsible for the contractions of the heart.

pus — a collection of dead tissue and white blood cells suspended in a fluid. The fluid may be very watery, or it may be in a semisolid state. Pus is a product of the inflammation process.

pustule — a small skin elevation that is filled with pus.

pyelitis — an infection of the renal pelvis, the receptacle between the kidney and the ureter. Symptoms may include fever, vomiting, loss of appetite, and cloudy or smoky urine. A positive diagnosis is based on an examination of the urine.

Pyelitis is more common in females than in males, perhaps because the female urethral tract is shorter and infection can reach the kidney more readily.

pyloric stenosis — an obstruction in the digestive system. The condition is most common in newborn babies. The obstruction is located where the opening of the stomach leads into the intestines. Pyloric stenosis is frequently a congenital condition.

The condition is characterized by frequent vomiting so forceful that the regurgitated milk lands some distance from the baby's body. This violent vomiting is caused by the unnaturally narrowed opening leading from the stomach to the intestines. The narrowing is caused by a thick, tight wall that blocks the free passage of food between the stomach and the intestines.

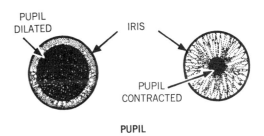

PUPIL

Pyloric stenosis can sometimes be treated with drugs that relax the muscular wall. More frequently, however, an operation is needed to relieve the obstruction.

pyorrhea — the chronic, destructive stage of periodontal disease. Pyorrhea attacks the underlying tissue that supports the teeth.
See periodontal disease.

q

Q fever — a disease caused by microorganisms called rickettsiae. These microorganisms are classified as being between bacteria and viruses. The symptoms include an elevated temperature and respiratory involvement. Q fever is usually treated with broad-spectrum antibiotics.

quack — any person who pretends to be a physician or who purports to have medical knowledge (almost always for sale) that he does not have. Quacks prey on people who are looking for quick or inexpensive cures. The quack rarely cures, and he almost inevitably provides "treatment" until his patient's money runs out or the patient dies of the disease.

quadriplegia — a condition in which all four of the patient's extremities are paralyzed. The condition is frequently the result of a diseased or damaged spinal column.

quadruplets — a pregnancy that results in the birth of four babies. Quadruplets are quite rare. They are usually fraternal rather than identical. This means that an ovary has released four cells instead of one, or that both ovaries have released cells. In this case, each baby has its own placenta and bag of waters.

quarantine — a method used to prevent the spread of communicable diseases. Isolation or quarantine of infected persons and susceptible contacts is one of the oldest procedures in public health. This procedure has many shortcomings in respect to its effectiveness in controlling the spread of infec-

tion. It is used much less frequently than in the past.

Isolation of patients with a communicable disease, while removing a source of infection from the environment, overlooks other sources such as "missed" cases, atypical cases, and healthy people who are carriers of the infection.

Additionally, quarantine is not effective in some communicable diseases. These are diseases in which the patient is contagious (capable of passing on the infection) before he shows any signs or symptoms of the disease.

quartan fever — a type of malaria in which the patient has malarial symptoms every fourth day (counting the day the symptoms occur as the first day.)
See malaria.

quinidine — a drug that is occasionally used to treat abnormal rhythms of the heartbeat.

quinine — a bitter-tasting drug that was used to treat the chills and fever of malaria. It is also used to suppress attacks of the disease.

Quinine is made from the bark of the chinchona tree that grows in the Andes Mountains. The Indians of that region were the first to use the bark as a medicine. Spanish missionaries were probably responsible for bringing it to Europe in the early part of the seventeenth century. In 1820 chemists learned how to extract the pure drug from the bark. In 1944 it was made artificially in the laboratory.

For centuries, quinine was virtually the only

drug used in the prevention and treatment of malaria. Today, however, it has largely been replaced by other drugs that are more effective and have fewer side effects.

See malaria.

quinsy — the development of an abscess in the vicinity of the tonsils. The abscess is a complication of tonsillitis; the infection spreads from the tonsils. Quinsy causes severe pain, especially when the patient opens his mouth. The disease is treated with antibiotics. Occasionally, the abscess has to be drained. The removal of the tonsils usually prevents reoccurrence of the abscess.

See tonsilitis.

r

rabbit fever — *See tularemia.*

rabies — an infectious disease that affects the nervous system, including the brain and spinal cord, of animals and man. Once it develops, it is almost invariably fatal.

Rabies is caused by a virus that is present in the saliva of infected animals. The virus is usually transmitted by a bite. However, it can also be transmitted when the saliva of an infected animal comes in contact with a fresh wound or with the thin mucous membrane of the lips or nose. The virus does not penetrate normal, unbroken skin.

All warm-blooded animals, including man, are susceptible to rabies. However, the disease is principally one of biting animals such as dogs, skunks, foxes, wolves, cats, and coyotes. Bats have become increasingly important as natural spreaders of rabies, as have the biting type of animals mentioned above. Rabies is present in all parts of the United States. It is one of the most widespread diseases known: rabies is found in the Arctic as well as in the temperate and tropical countries of the world. It occurs in animals during any season of the year. Many cases are reported in farm livestock such as cows, horses, hogs, and sheep. These animals generally contract the disease from the bites of infected dogs, cats, or wild animals such as skunks and foxes. During the past decade the incidence of rabies in skunks, foxes, and bats has soared, and many people have been attacked by these rabid wild animals.

INCUBATION PERIOD
The period from the time infection enters the body until the virus reaches the brain and produces symptoms is known as the incubation period. In humans this interval varies from fourteen days to a year or more, the average being twenty to sixty days.

The length of the incubation period is influenced by the location and the severity of the bite wound through which the virus enters the body. Bites of the head, neck, hands, and other exposed areas are likely to produce symptoms most rapidly.

SYMPTOMS
There are two clinical types of the disease in dogs and other animals. One is called furious rabies, the other is called dumb rabies.

1. *Furious type*
One of the first symptoms is the changed disposition of the animal. A previously playful dog becomes sullen, prefers to be alone, and refuses food. A day or so later it grows unnaturally restless. It may lie down intermittently, only to repeat its restless movements. Restraint increases its nervousness and irritation. It may attack without warning. As the disease progresses, the dog snarls viciously, barks and growls at imaginary objects, and may chase and bite other animals with which it had previously lived in harmony. If free, it may wander long distances from home, biting as it goes, until it drops and dies from paralysis or exhaustion. The furious type also is observed in other animals, including cats, foxes, cattle, swine, skunks, horses, and wildcats.

2. *Dumb type*
This type is more difficult to recognize. The

symptoms of excitement and irritability are absent or so slight as to be unrecognized. The progress of the disease is more rapid than in the furious type, and death from paralysis usually occurs within two or three days from the onset of the disease. The paralysis is frequently first noted in the lower jaw, and the appearance and choking of the animal may lead to the belief that the dog has a bone in its throat. Any attempt to relieve the animal is dangerous, because it may result in infectious saliva getting into some skin wound. The choking or throat paralysis may be observed in all animals that are susceptible to rabies. It is especially dangerous in cattle and horses, because farmers or attendants often attempt to remove the object that is thought to be the cause of the choking. In this way the person attempting to assist the animal may injure himself unknowingly and hence allow infected saliva to enter the wound.

TREATMENT

Once symptoms have developed, the disease cannot be cured. The major aim of treatment, therefore, is the prevention of the disease after the patient has been bitten.

Any animal may have rabies. Consequently, authorities suggest that any animal that bites an individual be considered rabid until proven otherwise. All animal bites require immediate attention by a physician. Every effort must be made to catch the animal alive. The animal is then placed in confinement for a specified period of time so that it can be observed for the possible symptoms and development of rabies.

In all cases where the animal is known to be rabid, or when it cannot be caught and examined and there is even a slight suspicion of rabies, a series of injections, known as the Pasteur treatment, must be given as soon as possible.

The Pasteur treatment requires a series of daily injections (lasting from fourteen to twenty-one days) of a rabies vaccine. As the name implies, this treatment was discovered by Louis Pasteur. Although the vaccine is very effective if given promptly, it is useless if begun after the symptoms appear.

rachischisis — *See spina bifida.*

radiation — a charge of energy thrown off by atoms. Radiation can take many different forms. The earth is bombarded every day by radiation in the form of cosmic rays from the sun. Chest X-rays send powerful rays through the body. Powerful radiations are frequently used in the treatment of cancer. Nuclear explosions produce another type of radiation.

See radiation sickness, X-ray.

radiation sickness — the result of an overdose of or exposure to a source of radiation. This condition is usually the result of accidents in nuclear laboratories or of a nuclear explosion.

Radiation sickness is caused by the destruction of body cells, especially the blood-forming cells. The symptoms of an overdose of radiation are nausea, vomiting, and fatigue. The symptoms generally do not appear immediately. The amount of time that elapses between the overexposure and the onset of symptoms depends on the exact amount of radiation received. The larger the dose, the faster the symptoms appear.

The treatment depends on the severity of the exposure. In some cases, the patient will recover spontaneously; in others, blood transfusions or bone-marrow transplants are needed. In extremely severe cases, radiation sickness may cause death.

radium — an intensely radioactive metallic element. It is found in minute quantities in uranium and other similar minerals. The radioactivity of radium is a result of the disintegration of the atom.

radius — one of the two bones of the lower arm. When the arm is hanging straight down and the palm is facing forward, the radius is the bone farthest from the body. Because of the way the two bones are connected, the radius and the ulna (the other lower arm bone) cross over each other when the wrist is turned.

rales — abnormal respiratory or breathing sounds. Rales may be moist or dry, depending on the fluid in the air passages.

rash — an eruption on the skin or "breaking out" of the skin. Rashes are usually pink or red in color. A rash is a symptom of some sort of problem rather than a separate disease.

rauwolfia — a drug consisting of the powdered whole root of the plant *Rauwolfia serpentina.* Rauwolfia lowers the blood pressure and slows the heart rate. This drug is sometimes used in the treatment of hypertension, or high blood pressure. It is classified as an antihypertensive agent.

raw milk — milk that has not been pasteurized.

reaction — a local or generalized physical response to a form of medication. Many vaccines produce reactions. These may include slight fever, tenderness, redness, and swelling around the area where the vaccine was injected.

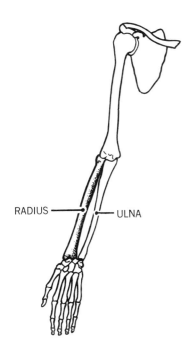

RADIUS

receptor — a nerve ending that is sensitive to stimuli. There are five kinds of receptors. The most important—touch—are bare nerve endings located next to hairs. The other receptors are for heat, cold, pressure, and pain.

The receptors for pain are naked nerve filaments. These are the most numerous. They are also the only kind present in the deeper tissue, although stimulation of these usually causes the pain to be referred to a skin area.

Nerve endings for touch, pressure, heat, cold, and pain are widely distributed in the skin and mucous membranes; those for pain and pressure are also located in other parts of the body. The receptors for these senses, however, are unevenly distributed. For example, the skin of the back possesses relatively few touch and pressure receptors, while the fingertips have a great many such receptors. The skin of the face has relatively few cold receptors, and mucous membranes have few heat receptors.

recovery room — the room into which most patients are moved immediately following surgery. In the recovery room, the patient is carefully watched. Blood pressure and other tests are made frequently (these special tests depend on the particular type of operation the patient has had). In most hospitals, the patient is kept in the recovery room until the major effects of the anesthesia have worn off and the patient begins to regain consciousness. Sometimes the patient remains in the recovery room until he is fully conscious.

rectal examination — an examination of the rectum. The physician inserts a gloved finger into the rectum. Through the thin wall of the rectum the physician can also feel the position and size of other body organs that are located in the same area.
See rectum.

rectum — the last five inches (approximately) of the large intestine that lead into the anal canal. It follows the contour of the sacrum and the coccyx until it curves back into the short anal canal.

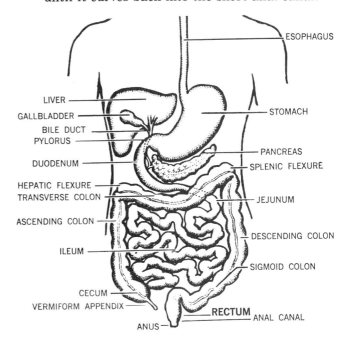

RECTUM

recuperation — the process or the period during which a patient recovers his health following an illness.

red blood cells — the oxygen-carrying cells of the blood.
See blood.

reduction — the physical act of placing a body part back into its proper position. When a bone is fractured, it usually has to be reduced—put back into place. The term is also used to describe the treatment sometimes needed for a serious hernia.

referred pain — *See pain.*

reflex — an involuntary response to a stimulus. A reflex is produced when sensations that are received by a sensory nerve are brought to the spinal cord and the impulse is transferred to a motor nerve. An impulse is then sent out to a muscle or gland. That impulse produces the action. The path these impulses take and the arrangement of these nerves is called a simple reflex arc. The action that is produced is called a reflex action.

A good example of a reflex action is what happens when a person touches a hot stove. After the hand comes in contact with the heat, it is jerked away without thinking. No action on the part of the brain is required.

refraction — a test made by an eye specialist to determine the distortion of vision in the eye.

regurgitation — the backward flow of a semiliquid or a liquid in the body. The term is usually applied to the backward movement of undigested food from the stomach (vomiting) or to the backward flow of blood through a defective valve.

rehabilitation — the return of a person who has been disabled by accident or disease to the maximum attainable physical, mental, emotional, social, and economic usefulness.

Depending on the severity of the disability, rehabilitation may require the aid of a physical therapist, a psychologist or psychiatrist, a social worker, or a clergyman, in addition to the services of the attending physician.

relaxant — any drug or agent that promotes a reduction in tension.

remission — a diminution or abatement of the symptoms of a disease. The term is also used to indicate the period during which this occurs.

Remissions can last for very long periods of time, but they can also be very short-lived. The patient may be entirely free of symptoms and the disease may appear to have disappeared; or the remission may be only partial, with the patient experiencing relief from only some of the symptoms.

renal — of or pertaining to the kidney or kidneys.

renal circulation — the circulation of the blood through the kidneys. As the blood flows through the kidneys, waste products, certain chemical elements, and water are removed from it.
See kidney.

renal disease — any disease of the kidney that results in a general impairment of function. Damage to the kidneys cannot be repaired. As the efficiency of these organs decreases, toxins build up in the blood.

renal hypertension — high blood pressure that is caused by damage to or disease of the kidneys.

renal pelvis — the cavity in the middle of a kidney; it is the upper end of the ureter.
See kidney, ureter.

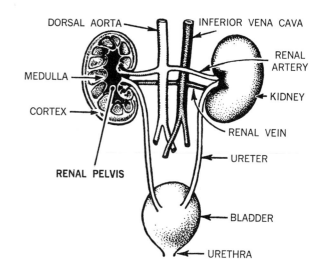

RENAL PELVIS

rennin — a prominent component of gastric juices during infancy. It helps to coagulate milk protein. It is doubtful that it is present in the adult stomach.

reserpine — one of the organic substances found in the root of the plant *Rauwolfia serpentina*. Reserpine lowers the blood pressure, slows the heart rate, and has a sedative effect.

respiration — the act of drawing air into the lungs and forcing carbon dioxide out of the lungs. In a normal healthy adult, respiration occurs about sixteen times a minute or 23,040 times a day.

Complete respiration includes not only the exchange of oxygen and carbon dioxide, but also the exchange that takes place between the capillaries and the peripheral tissues of the body.

REGULATION

The rhythmical movements of breathing are controlled by the respiratory center in the medulla oblongata of the brain. Nerves from the medulla come down through the neck to the chest wall and the diaphragm. The nerve to the diaphragm is called the phrenic nerve; the one to the larynx is the vagus nerve; and those to the muscles of the thorax are the intercostals.

The respiratory center is stimulated by the chemical changes in the internal fluid environment. The most important chemical influence is carbon dioxide. With increased bodily activity there is a consequent increase in the production of carbon dioxide and an increase in its content in the blood. Under such circumstances, the respiratory center responds by stimulating the nerves controlling respiratory movements. The respiratory rate is thus increased, and the body rids itself of the excessive carbon dioxide.

The respiratory center also has nerve connections with higher centers in the brain. Through them, the rate of respiratory exchange may be altered by emotional stimuli such as fright. Shallow breathing, sighing, and sobbing are examples of altered respiratory rate brought about by emotional stimuli. Physical stimulations of the body can also cause alterations; for example, splashing cold water on the face or the chest, or submersion into cold water, will cause deep, gasping respiration.

The muscles of respiration normally act automatically. The respiratory cycle consists of inspiration (breathing air into the lungs), expiration (breathing air out of the lungs), and rest (an interval between breaths). Normal respiration is fourteen to eighteen (average of sixteen) cycles per minute.

CAPACITY

When filled to capacity, the lungs hold about six liters of air (the average for a twenty-three-year-old male weighing 160 pounds, in a resting position). Only one half of one liter of this total volume enters and leaves the lungs at each natural respiration. This is known as tidal air. The volume of air that can be taken in by a maximum inspiratory effort (this is over and above tidal air) is called the inspiratory reserve. The volume of air that can be expelled by the strongest possible expiratory effort after the tidal air has been allowed to escape naturally is called the expiratory reserve. The sum total of the tidal air and the inspiratory and expiratory reserves is known as the vital capacity. The volume of air remaining in the lungs after the strongest possible expiration is referred to as the residual air.

respiratory infections — infections that attack parts of the respiratory system or the entire respiratory system. These infections can be as simple as the common cold or as complicated and dangerous as pneumonia.

Because the entire respiratory system is interconnected, respiratory infections that begin in the upper respiratory tract have a tendency to spread into the lower respiratory tract.

respiratory system — the parts of the body that together are responsible for bringing air into the lungs and for expelling carbon dioxide from the body.

The system of passageways that conducts air to the lungs is composed of the nasal cavity or the mouth, the pharynx, the larynx, the trachea, and the bronchi. These are discussed under separate entries.

resuscitation — *See artificial respiration.*

retention — the act or process of keeping something in place or retaining something within the body. The term is frequently used to indicate a lack of ability in the bladder to release or expel the urine it has collected. The term may also indicate that the body is retaining too much fluid in the individual cells.

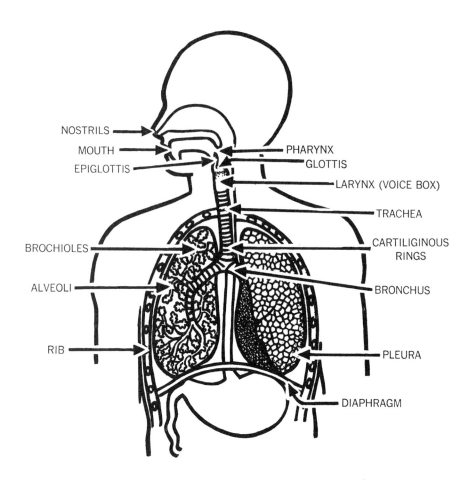

NOSTRILS

MOUTH

EPIGLOTTIS

PHARYNX

GLOTTIS

LARYNX (VOICE BOX)

TRACHEA

BROCHIOLES

CARTILIGINOUS RINGS

ALVEOLI

BRONCHUS

RIB

PLEURA

DIAPHRAGM

RESPIRATORY SYSTEM

retina — the light-receptive layer of the back of the eye. The retina is the terminal end of the optic nerve. It forms the lining of the eyeball.

retinitis — an inflammation of the retina. Retinitis is characterized by an impairment of vision and a distortion of sight.

retinitis pigmentosa — a disease, frequently hereditary, marked by progressive pigmentation and deterioration of the retina and disturbance of its nerve elements.

retroversion — the term used to indicate that a body part has tipped or been displaced backwards.

rhesus factor — *See Rh factor*.

rheumatic fever — a disease, usually occuring in childhood, that may follow a few weeks after a

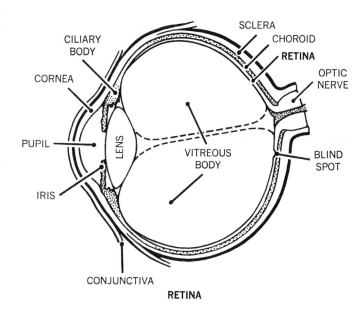

CILIARY BODY

SCLERA

CHOROID

RETINA

CORNEA

OPTIC NERVE

PUPIL

LENS

VITREOUS BODY

BLIND SPOT

IRIS

CONJUNCTIVA

RETINA

streptococcal infection. In some cases, the infection affects the heart and may result in permanent, structural damage to the muscle valves and to the lining of the heart.

Rheumatic fever is most prevalent in the Rocky Mountain region, New England, and the north and central states. Its occurrence is lowest in the south and southwest. The onset, seasonal in nature, is highest during late winter and early spring, and it is lowest during summer and early fall. While all ages are susceptible, this disease rarely occurs in children under five years of age. It is most common in children six to twelve years old. It is a significant cause of death for children six to ten years of age. For unknown reasons, rheumatic fever is declining in the United States, both as a disease and as a cause of death.

CAUSE

There are a number of different kinds of streptococcal germs; however, it is believed that only one of these, hemolytic group A streptococcus, is the usual cause of rheumatic fever.

Although the precise cause of rheumatic fever is unknown, it is generally believed to be the result of a previous streptococcal infection. Approximately one to three per cent of those individuals with an upper respiratory infection caused by hemolytic group A streptococcus develop rheumatic fever. Poverty, overcrowding, mulnutrition, dampness, and poor housing predispose children to streptococcal infections and therefore to rheumatic fever.

The streptococcal infection is contagious, but rheumatic fever is not. Scientists do not know why some people develop rheumatic fever after a streptococcal infection while others do not.

SYMPTOMS

The onset may be abrupt and dramatic, or it may begin insidiously, with many bouts of the disease going unrecognized. Generally, there is a history of a child who recently had an upper respiratory infection, sore throat, tonsillitis, or scarlet fever. It may be characterized by fever; sore, swollen joints; a skin rash; involuntary twitching; or small nodes under the skin.

TYPES

Rheumatic fever may have several forms. It gets its name from the more usual form in which there is fever along with pain and swelling in the joints. The pain and swelling are likely to move about from one joint to another. The child may be very sick and uncomfortable. With some children, however, rheumatic fever is so mild that it may not be noticed at all.

Another form of rheumatic fever is chorea, or St. Vitus dance. In chorea the child may develop jerky movements of the face, arms, and legs. These movements are especially noticeable when he tries to feed or dress himself or to pick up something. He may have crying spells for no known reason. Attacks of chorea may come and go and often last for a long time.

TREATMENT

The treatment for rheumatic fever is usually limited to bed rest. This gives the child's natural strength a chance to combat his illness. It is often necessary for the child to be in a hospital. The first attack may be over in a few weeks, or it may last for months. Then the patient must continue to rest in bed until the doctor is sure the active stage is over. This is essential, even though the child may look well and feel fine. Depending on the intensity of his illness, the patient may require bed rest for from two weeks to more than six months.

PREVENTION

Rheumatic fever can be prevented by early diagnosis and adequate therapy for all streptococcal infections. The streptococcal disease can be identified by laboratory evaluation of throat cultures and can be treated with antibiotics. Penicillin and certain other antibiotics are effective destroyers of the streptococcus germ. Used promptly, according to the doctor's orders, whenever a sore throat or tonsillitis strikes, they can usually prevent the first attack of rheumatic fever.

Anyone who has had rheumatic fever is more likely to have it again. His heart may have escaped damage from a first attack but can be injured by a later one. The child who has had one attack of rheumatic fever should be protected as much as possible from contracting a "strep" infection from his family friends, or schoolmates who may have sore throats.

For patients known to have had earlier bouts with rheumatic fever, emphasis is placed on the prevention of streptococcal infections through the daily use of prophylactic penicillin without interruption until well into adult life. For patients allergic to penicillin, sulfa drugs or erythromycin are used as a prophylaxis.

rheumatic heart disease — the damage done to the heart, particularly the heart valves, by one or more attacks of rheumatic fever. The valves are sometimes so scarred that they do not open and close normally.

rheumatism — a group of chronic illnesses that attack the joints, muscular tendons, ligaments, bursae, etc. Although the rheumatic diseases have been studied for many years, the cause or causes are still unknown. Some cases follow sprains, infection, or joint injury, but this is the exception rather than the rule.

Many scientists suspect viruses or bacteria, but no one has found a "rheumatic germ". Other scientists suspect allergy, the nervous system, or the hormones. Still others suspect a disorder of the metabolic system (the body's means of using food as fuel to carry on life).

It is known, however, that emotional shock can bring on an attack of rheumatism. Attacks often follow changes in the weather. These may not be causes, but they could be triggers that set off an underlying condition.

Rheumatic diseases affect children as well as adults and elderly people. The most common form of rheumatism is rheumatoid arthritis, or arthritis. Approximately one-third of all cases of rheumatism are actually arthritis. Other forms of rheumatism are osteoarthritis, gout, and fibrositis.

See arthritis, fibrositis, gout, osteoarthritis.

rheumatoid arthritis — *See arthritis.*

Rh factor — a substance that is found in the blood cells of approximately eighty-five percent of all humans. The eighty-five percent of the population who have the Rh factor in their blood are known as Rh positive. The remaining fifteen percent whose blood does not contain the Rh factor are known as Rh negative. The type of blood a person has (A, B, AB, or O) has nothing to do with the Rh factor. Like blood groups, the Rh factor is inherited and never changes.

DISCOVERY

The Rh factor was discovered in 1940 by Dr. Landsteiner and Dr. Weiner. In working on

another problem, they had injected the blood of Rhesus monkeys into rabbits. The rabbits' blood developed antibodies to the Rhesus monkeys' blood. The scientists then took the rabbit serum containing Rh antibodies (named for the Rhesus monkeys) and tested it against human red cells from many different people. They found that about eighty-five percent of the human red-cell samples were agglutinated (made to clump or cluster together) by the immune rabbit serum, and about fifteen percent were not. In other words, the blood of most people contains a substance, or factor, that is similar to the antigen (which causes the antibody to develop) in the monkeys' blood.

IMPORTANCE

There are two situations in which the absence of the Rh factor can cause trouble.

1. *Blood transfusion*

Rh positive blood can never be given to an Rh negative person, even if they both have the same blood type or group. The first transfusion may cause no trouble, but, by the time a second transfusion is given, there may be enough antibodies against the Rh positive cells to cause an antigen-antibody reaction. This reaction can be as severe as if the transfused blood belonged to a different group.

2. *Pregnancy*

When both father and mother are Rh positive or when both are Rh negative, there is no danger. However, complications may arise if the mother's blood is Rh negative and the father's is Rh positive. If the child inherits its father's Rh positive blood, the unborn baby's blood may enter the mother's circulatory system and give rise to antibodies. These, in turn, may enter the baby's bloodstream and attack its red blood cells. The mother's blood is not affected; only the red blood cells of the baby are destroyed.

Ordinarily, the first baby who causes this reaction in the mother will not be affected by the mother's antibodies. However, if the mother has already developed these substances before her first pregnancy as a result of a transfusion with Rh positive blood, even the first baby might be affected by the antibodies. This rarely occurs, however, because great care is taken to check for the Rh factor before giving a blood transfusion.

This problem does not always occur. Many Rh negative mothers have healthy Rh positive babies. About thirteen percent of all marriages are between Rh negative women and Rh positive men. Among the babies born to this group, only about one in twenty-five will have a dangerous reaction. Furthermore, there is rarely any danger to the first child.

However, when the problem does occur, the destruction of red cells in the baby may lead to a condition called hemolytic disease of the newborn, or erythroblastosis fetalis. The first signs are severe anemia and a failing heart. If the baby survives these disorders, a destructive form of jaundice called kernicterus may occur within forty-eight hours of birth. This afflicts an estimated 2,000 newborn babies every year in the United States. About half of these babies die; the other half usually live with permanent brain damage, accounting for about one-tenth of the cases of cerebral palsy.

Danger to the Rh positive baby has been greatly reduced in recent years. The doctor can tell by means of a blood test whether the mother is Rh negative. If so, he can test the father's blood to see whether he is Rh positive — to determine whether there is any risk to the child. Then, during pregnancy, he can test the mother's blood for evidence of Rh antibodies. Finally, even if the mother's Rh antibodies should attack the baby's red cells before birth, an exchange transfusion of Rh negative blood given immediately will save the baby from damage.

rhinitis — an inflammation of the mucous membrane that lines the nose. It is frequently the result of an allergy.
See allergy.

rhodopsin — a red pigment located in the rods of the eye. When light hits the rhodopsin, it stimulates the rods and allows vision. When there is a lack of rhodopsin, the result is a condition called night blindness.

rhonchus — a rattling sound in the throat caused by partial obstruction. Rhonchus may also be an abnormal respiratory sound in the bronchial tubes.

rib — one of a pair of bones located in the chest. There are twelve pairs of ribs. They form a series of curved bones that support the chest wall. In the back they join the thoracic vertebrae; in the front, each rib terminates with cartilage.

The first seven ribs are attached to the sternum, or breastbone, and are called true ribs. The eighth, ninth, and tenth pair of ribs are united by their cartilage to the cartilage of the seventh rib. These three pairs are known as the false ribs. The last two pairs are open in the front and are referred to as the floating ribs.

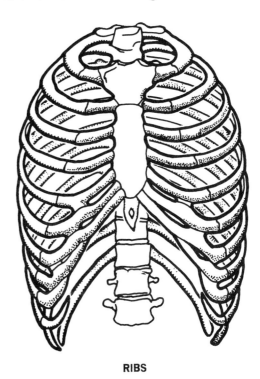

RIBS

riboflavin — *See vitamin A.*

ribonucleic acid — *See RNA*

ribosomes — large particles containing RNA. Ribosomes are found in the cytoplasm of a cell.
See RNA.

rickets — a bone condition caused by a lack of or a deficiency of vitamin D. Without the proper amount of vitamin D, the bones tend to bend and become distorted.

rigor mortis — the stiffening of the body that occurs from a few minutes to several hours after death. When the body dies, there is an accumulation of waste products because of the cessation of circulation. This causes the muscle cells to become firm and rigid.

ringworm — a group of four communicable diseases

that are caused by fungus growth on the surface of the body. The four are ringworm of the feet (athlete's foot), ringworm of the nails, ringworm of the body, and ringworm of the scalp.

RINGWORM OF THE FEET

The most common of the fungus diseases that attack the skin is ringworm of the feet, more commonly known as "athlete's foot." Athlete's foot develops on a person's feet when the fungus, which may be present but causes no trouble on some feet, begins to grow and to multiply. This fungus grows best in moist, warm, poorly ventilated places, such as on skin between toes that stay damp with perspiration.

The symptoms of infection are: itching, cracking or scaling of the skin, and sometimes small blisters that contain a watery fluid. If the disease continues without treatment, there can be larger blisters and raw places on the skin that resemble the effects of poison ivy.

RINGWORM OF THE NAILS

Ringworm of the nails occurs when the fungus grows in or under the nails. The fungus growth can penetrate the nail, causing it to become thickened and misshapen, discolored, chalky, pitted, grooved, and brittle. This is the most stubborn form of ringworm infection.

RINGWORM OF THE BODY

Ringworm of the body is spread by contact with infected persons or by touching their clothing and other contaminated articles. Unlike athlete's foot, which is transmitted only from person to person, ringworm of the body can be spread to people by cats, dogs, and other animals that have ringworms.

Indication of infection is usually in the form of one to four flat, ring-shaped sores that may be dry or scaly, or crusted and moist. As the sores enlarge, the center of the ring frequently clears and leaves apparently normal skin. Ringworm of the body can be transmitted from one person to another or from animals to persons as long as the sores remain on the skin.

RINGWORM OF THE SCALP

Ringworm of the scalp is another skin disease that can be spread from person to person or from animals to people. Children are more likely to develop the infection than are adults, but the disease can occur at any age.

Clothing contaminated by an infected pet or person; barber's unsterilized tools; back of theater seats; toilet articles, including combs and brushes — all these are possible sources of the fungus. Because one kind of fungus that causes ringworm of the scalp is commonly present in the soil around barnyards, contact with infected pets or farm animals can cause infection.

Scalp ringworm generally begins in the form of a small pimple or sore, then spreads into a ring-like shape to leave an area of scaly baldness that may be permanent. Infected hairs become brittle and break easily.

Riolan, Jean — French physician (1577-1657) and Dean of the Faculty of Medicine at Paris. Riolan was a staunch adherent to the old classical theory of anatomy. He was one of the most active opponents of William Harvey, who discovered the circulation of the blood.
See Harvey, William.

RNA — single-strand molecules of a type of nucleic acid. RNA is the abbreviation for ribonucleic acid.

The RNA molecules are formed in the nucleus according to the blueprint of DNA (deoxyribonucleic acid). They then proceed into the cytoplasm and, with the help of other RNA molecules, assemble cellular building blocks (the amino acids into operational proteins such as enzymes.
See DNA.

Rocky Mountain spotted fever — an acute infectious disease transmitted to man through the bite of an infected tick. Ticks are small, insect-like creatures about a quarter of an inch in length. They dwell chiefly in uncleared land, brush, and woods. They are usually brownish in color and, when fully grown, have eight tiny legs that enable them to move with great speed and lightness.

Rocky Mountain spotted fever was originally believed to be limited to the Rocky Mountain region of the United States (hence its name) but has since been found to occur in forty-four of the fifty states. The illness is most prevalent in spring and summer, when ticks are most active.

Not all ticks are infected. In even the most heavily tick-infected areas (such as certain sections of Montana), it has been estimated that only one tick in three hundred is infected and able to transmit Rocky Mountain spotted fever.

When ticks get on a person, they crawl about

for some time before selecting a place to bite. Having selected a spot, they attach themselves to feed in such a way that they are difficult to remove. Even after attaching themselves and starting to feed, ticks sometimes do not transmit the germ for as long as four to six hours. This gives a person time to discover the ticks and remove them before infection can take place.

Ticks can move so lightly and rapidly that they frequently cannot be felt on the body. Even after they have attached themselves to a particular spot, their bite is painless and may easily go unnoticed. As they begin to feed, however, they gradually become engorged and swell, so that after several hours they are about the size of a jelly bean.

SYMPTOMS

Once a person has been bitten by an infected tick and has contracted spotted fever, the first symptoms will appear in from four to twelve days after the bite or smear. The attack of spotted fever, which may come on suddenly, is characterized by a chill, rapid rise in temperature, severe headache, restlessness, and insomnia. About three to four days after the fever begins, a pinkish skin rash appears. The individual spots are small and distinct. The rash usually breaks out first on the arms and legs, especially around the wrists and ankles. Later, it may spread over the entire body, including the face, the palms, and the soles of the feet. The patient suffers chiefly from headache. He is often restless and may become delirious. Rocky Mountain spotted fever is a serious, acute illness. A doctor should be called at the first appearance of symptoms.

TREATMENT

The danger of death from Rocky Mountain spotted fever has been radically reduced by the use of broad-spectrum antibiotics.

PREVENTION

There is a vaccine for the prevention of Rocky Mountain spotted fever. Before the discovery of effective drugs for treating the disease, vaccination was strongly urged for children and adults who spent a lot of time outdoors in tick-infested areas. However, since these drugs have proved so effective in treating the disease, vaccination is specifically recommended only for those who live in heavily infested areas or whose occupation or hobby takes them frequently into areas where they will be greatly exposed to ticks.

The vaccine is usually given in three injections at intervals of seven to ten days. A yearly booster dose consisting of a single injection is given if exposure occurs each year. The vaccine commonly causes discomfort similar to that experienced by patients vaccinated against typhoid fever.

Most ticks are harmless. However, since there is no way of knowing by looking at it whether a particular tick is infected, it is wise to treat each tick as though it might be capable of transmitting the disease. Anyone exposed to ticks should be examined carefully at least once a day, especially during the season when ticks are most prevalent. Children playing outdoors during the season should be inspected twice a day from top to toe. All clothing should be removed and a careful search made; special attention should be given to the hairy parts of the body and the back of the neck. Campers, picnickers, fishermen, and others whose occupations or hobbies take them into tick-infested areas should examine themselves in similar fashion. If these precautions are taken, ticks may be discovered and removed before they have time to cause any harm.

See ticks.

Roentgen, Wilhelm Konrad — German physicist (1845-1923) who discovered the principles of X-rays.

See X-ray.

root canal — a small canal within the root of a tooth. Tiny blood vessels and nerves extend from the pulp chamber of the tooth, through the canal, to the end of the root. At the end of the root canal these small blood vessels and nerves join larger blood vessels and nerves.

See tooth.

roseola — a communicable disease that usually affects young children between six months and three years of age. Roseola is characterized by a high fever (103°-105°) that lasts for three or four days. The elevated temperature rapidly returns to normal after that time, and a rash or large, pink blotches appear on the skin. There is no specific treatment for roseola, although a child may need treatment if he convulses from the high fever.

Roseola is also known as infantile roseola or roseola infantum.

roughage — indigestible food material, such as celery. These foods provide a certain amount of bulk that aids in the proper functioning of the intestines.

roundworm — an intestinal parasite.

rubella — *See German measles.*

rubeola — *See measles.*

rule of nine — a method of determining the extent of burns.
See burns.

rupture — the tearing open or bursting of a body part. This may be caused by inflammation, disease, or by excessive pressure (internal or external).
See hernia.

S

Sabin, Albert Bruce — American research scientist (born in 1906) who developed the oral vaccine for poliomyelitis in 1955.
    See poliomyelitis.

sac — a body organ or part that is shaped like a bag, pouch, or pocket.

saccule — one of two small sacs located in the inner ear. With the other sac — the utricle — it helps the semicircular canals establish a sense of balance in the body.
    See semicircular canals.

sacroiliac — the joint or junction between the sacrum and the ilium. The sacrum is the last part of the spinal column (with the exception of the coccyx). The ilium is one of the wing-shaped bones that help form the pelvis.

sacrum — the part of the vertebral column (spinal column) formed by the fusion of five false vertebrae. It is roughly triangular in shape. The sacrum is joined on each side with the hip bone or pelvis. This is the last part of the vertebral column before the coccyx and, with the coccyx, it forms the rear wall of the pelvis.

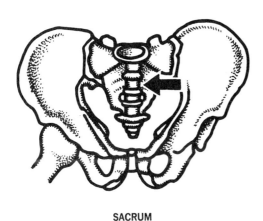

SACRUM

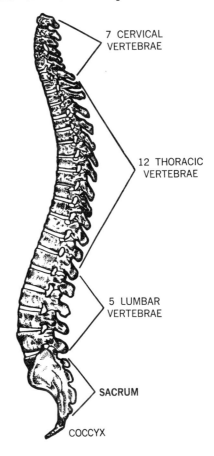

7 CERVICAL VERTEBRAE

12 THORACIC VERTEBRAE

5 LUMBAR VERTEBRAE

SACRUM

COCCYX

SACRUM

St. Vitus' dance — a disease of the central nervous system that is usually found as a complication of rheumatic fever. St. Vitus' dance is also known as Sydenham's chorea.

The primary symptom of this disease is manifest through involuntary, uncontrollable movements throughout the body. St. Vitus' dance is rarely fatal and usually disappears in two or three months. No cause is known, and the only treatment is bed rest.

See reumatic fever.

salicylates — a class of drugs that have analgesic, antipyretic, and anti-inflammatory effects. The salicylates are used for the relief of pain and fever in cases of headache, gout, rheumatic fever, and a wide variety of other nonspecific problems. The best known drug in this class is acetylsalicylic acid, or aspirin.

saliva — a fluid secreted into the mouth by the salivary glands (parotid, submaxillary, and sublingual). Saliva is used to moisten food, make food easier to chew, and to lubricate the food mass to aid in swallowing. It contains one principal enzyme, ptyalin. This enzyme initiates the digestion of starches, breaking them into the complex sugar, maltose.

salivary glands — three pairs of glands, located in the vicinity of the mouth, that secrete saliva. One half of each of the pairs is located on either side of the face. The largest of these pairs are known as the parotid glands. Each of the parotid glands is situated slightly in front of the ears. The second pair, the sublingual glands, are located under the tongue. The submaxillary glands the third pair, are found under the edge or indentation of the lower jaw.

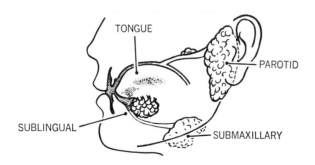

SALIVARY GLANDS

These glands are controlled by one pair of the twelve cranial nerves. The parasympathetic nervous system stimulates these glands and causes them to create and secrete saliva. This happens when food is present in the mouth, when there is an anticipation of food, or when there is an odor of food present. Additionally, certain other sensations can cause the secretion of saliva.

See saliva.

Salk, Jonas E. — American research scientist (born 1914) who first discovered a vaccine for poliomyelitis. The Salk vaccine, invented in 1953, was given as an injection.

See poliomyelitis.

Salmonella — a type of bacteria.

See salmonellosis.

salmonellosis — an infection caused by the Salmonella bacteria. This infection is a type of food poisoning. It is caused by eating food that is not prepared or preserved properly, allowing the Salmonella bacteria to grow and multiply in it. Proper cooking eliminates the bacteria, and proper storage prevents its growth.

The symptoms often include severe pain in the stomach, nausea, headache, an elevated temperature, and diarrhea. Certain types of salmonellosis closely resemble typhoid fever.

Salmonellosis frequently occurs in large groups who have eaten the same foods. Epidemics of salmonellosis have occurred in nursing homes and colleges. Treatment may require the use of antibiotics.

salt — sodium chloride (common table salt) or the combination of an acid and a base.

See sodium chloride.

S-A node — see sinoatrial node.

saphenous vein — a vein originating in the foot. It extends up the inside of the leg and thigh to join the femoral vein in the upper thigh. This vein is sometimes used at the ankle for intravenous injections.

sarcoma — one of the two main classes of cancer. A sarcoma is a cancer that develops in the connective or supportive tissues of the body, such as in the bones. The other main class is carcinoma, a

cancer that develops in the lining or covering tissues of organs.
See cancer.

saturated fat — a fat so constituted chemically that it is not capable of absorbing any more hydrogen. Saturated fats are usually the solid fats of animal origin, such as the fats in milk, butter, meat, etc. A diet high in saturated-fat content tends to raise or increase the amount of cholesterol in the blood. Sometimes these fats are restricted in the diet in an effort to lessen the hazard of fatty deposits (plaques) in the blood vessels.
See cholesterol.

scabies — a raised, zigzag track or furrow near the surface of the skin that is caused by mites. They cause intense itching and sometimes allergic reactions.

Because of their small size (only about one-fiftieth of an inch long), most species of mites go unnoticed by man. They are actually among the most numerous and varied animals on earth. Mites are not insects. They are actually related to ticks and spiders.

Although some types of mites carry disease from person to person, the parasitic mite that causes scabies (sometimes referred to as "The Itch") does not. This type of mite burrows barely beneath the skin, where it feeds and lays its eggs. This can cause great discomfort. Scratching is of very little use and may actually create skin infections.

Scabies occurs most often in the webbing between the fingers and around the wrists, but it can also appear elsewhere on the body.

SPREAD

Mites travel from person to person through handshaking, close physical contact, and from bedclothes. Scabies often spreads through a family and occasionally through an entire institution that houses many people. During times of upheaval caused by natural disasters and war, the incidence of this disease increases.

Differing only slightly from the mites that cause scabies in humans is a second type that causes the disease in dogs, cats, horses, and other domestic animals. People sometimes become infected with this second type through close contact with animals, such as by riding a horse or holding a puppy.

TREATMENT

Treatment consists of using a pesticide that is effective against the mites and safe for use on the human body. It is usually dispensed in a vanishing cream rather than as a powder or dust.

scalds — injuries caused by contact with hot solutions, hot vapors, or steam. Burns and scalds are essentially the same type of heat injury and are usually treated the same way.
See burn.

scalp — the part of the head on which hair grows. The scalp is tough, very thin, and is not as elastic as other skin areas.

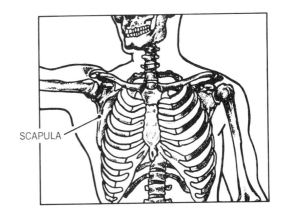

SCAPULA (FRONT VIEW)

scalpula — a triangular-shaped bone that is situated in the upper part of the back. It forms the rear portion of the shoulder girdle. One of its corners forms a part of the shoulder joint, joining with the humerus.

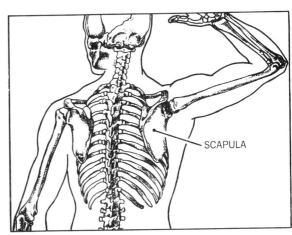

SCAPULA (BACK VIEW)

scar — tissue that forms following the destruction of normal tissue. Scar tissue is not elastic; it will neither stretch nor contract. Small scars usually cause few problems (with the exception of scars in certain areas of the heart). However, scar tissue that covers a large amount of surface area can effectively immobilize movement in the affected parts. Thus, when a large portion of the normal skin around the elbow has been replaced with scar tissue, the patient may be unable to bend the affected elbow because the scar tissue will not stretch.

The formation of scar tissue depends on the amount of damage, particularly the depth of the injury. A wound or burn that removes the first layer of skin (the epidermis) will usually not leave a scar. However, when the next layer of skin (the dermis) is penetrated, scar tissue will almost always form. Scars can be caused by diseases such as chickenpox; smallpox; and rheumatic fever, which can scar heart valves. They may also be caused by burns, cuts, open fractures, and by surgery.

When extensive areas of the body are covered with scar tissue, it is sometimes necessary to replace the scar tissue with skin grafts from another area of the body.

One branch of medicine, plastic surgery, deals with the problem of replacing or reducing scar tissue.

scarlatina — *See scarlet fever.*

scarlet fever — a common communicable disease of childhood. Scarlet fever, also known as scarlatina, is often a complication of rheumatic fever. Like rheumatic fever, it is caused by streptococcus.

The symptoms of this disease are sore throat, vomiting, and a rapid rise in temperature. A fine rash usually appears on the body and limbs. Bed rest and antibiotics are used to treat scarlet fever.

Schick test — a test that reveals an individual's susceptibility or immunity to diphtheria. The Schick test is used only when an individual has been exposed to diphtheria. When the results of the test are positive (indicating that the person is susceptible), it is necessary to give the individual passive immunity at once in order to prevent the disease.

See diphtheria, immunity.

schistosomiasis — a disease caused by the Schistosoma parasite. These microorganisms enter the body through the skin. They usually attack the lower digestive tract (small intestine, colon, and rectum) and the urinary system (primarily the bladder). The disease is found in places such as Africa, Egypt, and South America.

schizophrenia — a form of mental illness. The most striking symptom of schizophrenia is the patient's withdrawal from reality.

See mental illness.

sciatica — a localized neuritis (an inflammation of one or more nerves) of the sciatic nerve (the nerve of the back of the leg). It may occur without apparent cause, or it may result from arthritis or from an infection. The pain often extends from the hip to the toes, usually of just one leg. The skin sensation may be disturbed. In some types of sciatica, if the course is not checked, the muscles in the calf may begin to waste away and the foot may become bent.

sciatic nerve — the nerve that extends down the back of the leg.

sclera — the firm, fibrous, outer membrane of the eye. The sclera forms a protective layer for the sensitive inner eye. It is white in color, with the exception of the transparent segment that covers the cornea.

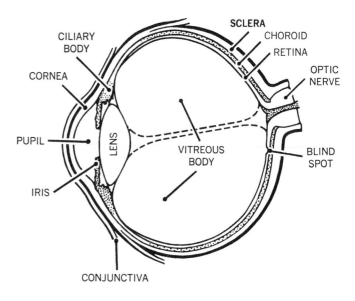

SCLERA

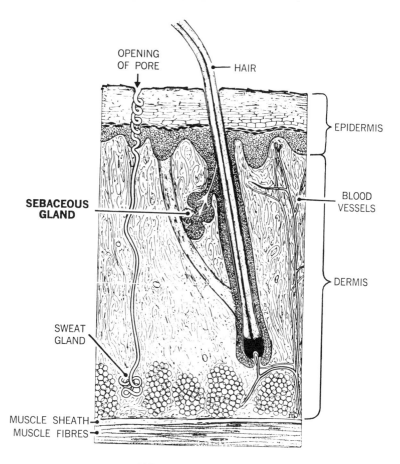

OPENING OF PORE

HAIR

EPIDERMIS

BLOOD VESSELS

SEBACEOUS GLAND

DERMIS

SWEAT GLAND

MUSCLE SHEATH
MUSCLE FIBRES

SEBACEOUS GLAND

scleritis — an inflammation of the sclera of the eye. It may exist alone or may involve the cornea, iris, or choroid.

sclerosis — a hardening or thickening of body tissue. Sclerosis is often caused by an accumulation of fibrous tissue, but there are other causes.
See atherosclerosis, multiple sclerosis.

scrotum — a loose pouch of skin that contains the testes and parts of the spermatic cord. Immediately beneath the skin of the scrotum is a thin layer of muscular fibers that can contract to draw the testes closer to the body. These fibers can also relax to allow the testes to hang farther from the body.

A temperature that is lower than that of the rest of the body is necessary for the proper growth of sperm cells. The muscular activity of the scrotum acts effectively to regulate the environmental temperature of the testes.
See spermatic cord, testes.

scurvy — a condition that results from a deficiency of vitamin C. The major symptoms are bleeding (especially of the gums) and pain in the joints. The treatment involves increased amounts of vitamin C.

sea sickness — *See motion sickness.*

seasonal hay fever — *See hay fever.*

sebaceous cyst — *See wen.*

sebaceous glands — glands that are associated with the hair follicles. They secrete oil (sebum) into the hair follicles near the surfaces of the skin.
See sebum.

seborrhea — a condition in which the sebaceous glands are malfunctioning. In seborrhea the sebaceous glands are overactive, secreting an excess of sebum. The sebum forms greasy scales.
See sebaceous gland, sebum.

sebum — an oily or greasy substance secreted by the sebaceous glands. Sebum keeps the hair from becoming dry or brittle and forms a protective film on the skin that limits the evaporation and the absorption of water.

See sebaceous glands.

secondary hypertension — an elevated blood pressure that is caused by (and therefore secondary to) certain specific diseases or infections.

secretin — a hormone produced in the small intestine. Secretin stimulates the pancreas and the liver. It is secreted when the stomach empties its contents into the small intestine.

secretion — the name of the process of releasing a substance formed in a gland and the general term applied to the substance that is released.

See gland, hormone, etc.

sedative — a drug that depresses the activity of the central nervous system, thus producing a calming effect.

Sedative drugs are manufactured for medical purposes to reduce tension and anxiety, to treat certain psychosomatic disorders, and to induce sleep. Certain sedatives are used in the treatment of epilepsy.

The barbiturates, made from barbituric acid, are by far the largest group of sedatives. Barbiturates, especially the short-acting ones, may lead to heavy abuse.

On the street, the sedatives are called "goofballs," "sleepers," and "downers." They appear in a variety of colored capsules or tablets. Seconals are called "red devils." Nembutals are "yellow jackets," Tuinals are "rainbows," and Amytal capsules are "blue angels."

Besides the barbiturates, other sedatives that may be abused include glutethimide (Doriden); chloral hydrate; bromides; and certain minor tranquilizers, such as meprobamate (Miltown, Equanil), and chlordiazepoxide (Librium).

See barbiturate.

seizure — an epileptic attack. It may include total or partial loss of consciousness and convulsive muscular movements such as twitching, thrashing, jerking, biting, etc.

A seizure is the result of an abnormal release of energy within the brain. While there is no clear cause for all seizures, they can sometimes be caused by great nervous tension; a sudden noise; or by a bright, flickering light. This happens most frequently when an epileptic is not taking the proper medication or has discontinued the use of his medication.

Nothing can be done to stop an attack once it has started. Ordinarily, the seizure will be over in a few minutes. While the seizure itself is not dangerous, the patient may injure himself as he thrashes around. Care should be taken to prevent this from happening by clearing the area in the immediate vicinity of the patient who is experiencing a seizure.

semen — the fluid composed of spermatozoa (sperm cells) and secretions from the seminal vesicles and prostate gland. Semen is discharged as the ejaculate during sexual intercourse. There are millions of sperm cells in the semen of each ejaculation.

semicircular canals — three small tubes located in each ear. These canals are situated in the inner ear slightly above the cochlea. Although the semicircular canals are found in the ear, their purpose is to help the body balance itself.

The inside of each canal is covered with small, hairlike cells called cristae. The canals are partially filled with fluid. Changes in the position of the head cause movement of the fluid within these organs. The movement of the fluid triggers the cristae, which then send a signal to the brain. This impulse is relayed along a branch of the acoustic or auditory nerve.

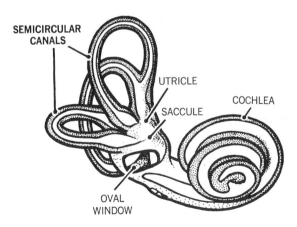

SEMICIRCULAR CANALS

semilunar valves — cup-shaped valves. The aortic

valve at the entrance to the aorta and the pulmonary valve at the entrance to the pulmonary artery are semilunar valves. They consist of three cup-shaped flaps that prevent the backward flow of blood.

seminal fluid — *See semen.*

seminal vesicles — two pouches that are situated (in the male) between the bladder and the rectum. They secrete and store a fluid to be added to the secretion of the testes at the time of ejaculation.

sensation — a physical or mental feeling that is the result of the body's reaction to the stimulation of one or more nerves.

sensori-neural loss — *See ear.*

sepsis — a type of poisoning that results from infection. The infection is caused by bacteria and the toxins they produce.

septal defects — *See congenital heart defects.*

septicemia — the invasion of the blood by toxin produced by bacteria. Septicemia is commonly referred to as blood poisoning.

septum — a division or partition between and within a body area. In the heart, a muscular wall divides the left and right upper chambers. This wall is called the atrial or interatrial septum. Also in the heart, a muscular wall divides the left and right lower chambers. This is the ventricular or interventricular septum.

The nasal cavity is divided into a right and left side by a partition referred to as the nasal septum.

sequestra — small fragments of bone that have lost their blood supply as a result of trauma (during extraction of a tooth) or as a result of infection. They tend to work loose from the bone and, like foreign bodies, are slowly forced out through the gums.

serotonin — a naturally occurring compound that is found mainly in the gastrointestinal tract and in lesser amounts in the blood. Serotonin has a stimulating effect on the circulatory system.

serous membranes — lining tissues of the body that are moistened by a fluid resembling the serum of the blood. Serous membranes are found in the form of moistened coverings of the lungs, heart, brain, spinal cord, and organs contained in the abdominal cavity.

serum — a clear, pale-yellow liquid. It is the fluid portion of the blood that remains after the cellular elements have been removed by coagulation. Serum is different from plasma, which is the cell-free liquid portion of uncoagulated blood.

Servetus, Michael — the Spanish physician (1509-1553) who discovered the circulation of the blood through the lungs. He was burned at the stake in Geneva because of his religious doctrines.

sesamoid bone — a bone that develops within a tendon. One example of a sesamoid bone is the patella or kneecap. This is a small, oval-shaped bone overlying the knee joint.

sex hormones — the hormones that control and stimulate the growth of the secondary sex characteristics. The two major types of sex hormones are estrogens, which produce female characteristics; and androgens, which produce male characteristics. Every person has both male and female sex hormones. The difference is primarily one of the degree or amount of the hormones.

An imbalance of the sex hormones can cause the appearance of some secondary sex characteristics in the wrong sex. Too much androgen can cause male secondary sex characteristics in the female; too much estrogen can cause female characteristics in the male.

sex-linked characteristics — *See genetics.*

shingles — *See herpes zoster.*

shivering — a series of tremors or trembling of the body. Shivering is an involuntary action of voluntary muscles. It is one of the methods the body uses for the maintenance of normal body temperature. It can be brought on by an elevated body temperature or by an exposure to extreme cold.

shock — a condition in which the circulation of the body is seriously disturbed.

Some degree of shock follows all injuries. It may be slight and almost unnoticed, lasting only a moment, or it may be severe enough to cause death. Shock is often the cause of death in cases of burns, hemorrhage, poisoning, fractures, and other serious injuries. It may occur immediately following the injury, or it may begin several hours later. Even if it does not occur immediately, it is a real danger.

DEVELOPMENT

When an injury occurs, the patient is usually aware of only the specific part of his body that has been injured. In reality, the body as a whole has been injured, and the body as a whole attempts to recover from the injury. A series of changes takes place, designed to restore the body to its normal, healthy condition.

Sometimes, however, the changes that occur may in themselves cause further damage to the body. To some extent this is what happens in shock. When a person is injured, the blood flow in his entire body is disturbed. To overcome this difficulty, the heart beats faster, and the blood vessels near the skin and in the arms and legs contract, thus sending most of the available blood supply to the vital organs of the body and to the nerve centers in the brain, which control all vital functions.

While this is happening, the other body cells do not receive enough blood and therefore do not get enough oxygen or food. The blood vessels, like the rest of the body, suffer from this lack, and eventually they lose their ability to contract. When this happens, the vital organs and the brain do not receive enough blood either, and the condition of shock becomes worse and worse. If this situation continues, the damage becomes so extensive that recovery is impossible. In less-severe cases, prompt first aid treatment for shock may make the difference between life and death. In mild cases of shock, recovery usually occurs naturally and rather quickly.

CAUSES

Serious shock occurs as a result of serious injury to any part of the body. Crush injuries, fractures, burns, poisoning, and prolonged bleeding are very likely to cause serious shock. An interruption of breathing, from whatever cause, is almost always followed by severe shock. In short, any damage to the body is accompanied by or followed by some degree of shock.

There are a number of factors that affect the seriousness of shock. Age, for example, is often a determining factor, since very young children and very old people do not usually have as much resistance to shock as young or middle-aged adults. Pain can produce shock or can increase its severity. People who have been starved, deprived of water, or exposed to extremes of cold or heat go into shock very easily. Excessive fatigue can increase the severity of shock. As a general rule, people who have any kind of chronic sickness are likely to go into shock more easily than healthy people. In addition to these factors, there are some unexplained differences between individuals in regard to their resistance to shock — an injury that might cause only mild shock in one person could cause serious, perhaps fatal, shock in another.

SYMPTOMS

A person who is going into shock may show quite a few signs or symptoms. However, signs of shock do not always appear at the time of the injury — indeed, in many very serious cases they may not appear until hours later.

The symptoms shown by a person suffering from shock are directly or indirectly caused by

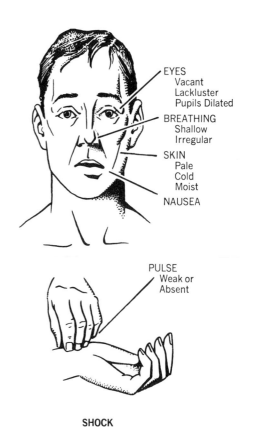

EYES
Vacant
Lackluster
Pupils Dilated

BREATHING
Shallow
Irregular

SKIN
Pale
Cold
Moist

NAUSEA

PULSE
Weak or
Absent

SHOCK

the fact that the circulation of the blood is disturbed. The pulse is weak and rapid. Breathing is likely to be shallow, rapid, and irregular, because the poor circulation of the blood affects the breathing center in the brain. The temperature near the surface of the body is lowered because of the poor blood flow; consequently, the face, arms, and legs feel cold to the touch. Sweating is likely to be very noticeable. A person in shock is usually very pale, but in some cases there may be a bluish or reddish color to the skin. The pupils of the eyes are usually dilated (enlarged).

If the patient is conscious, he may complain of thirst. He may have a feeling of weakness, faintness, or dizziness. He may feel nauseated. Also, he may be very restless and feel frightened and anxious. As shock deepens, these signs gradually disappear, and he becomes less and less responsive to what is going on around him. Even pain may not arouse him. Finally, he may become unconscious.

PREVENTION AND TREATMENT

In attempting to prevent shock or in the treatment of shock, the retention of body heat, the proper positioning of the body, and the relief of pain are crucial.

1. *Heat*

Heat is important in the treatment of shock to the extent that the injured person's body heat must be conserved. Exposure to cold, with resulting loss of body heat, can cause shock to develop or to become worse. While it is important to keep the patient warm, it is just as important to avoid overheating the patient. When the patient is too warm, there is a tendency to lose body fluids by sweating. This also brings the blood closer to the surface, thus defeating the body's own effort to supply blood to vital organs.

2. *Position*

The best position to use for the prevention or treatment of shock is one that encourages the flow of blood to the brain and to the heart. If the patient is lying down and his head is on a level with or lower than his feet, the flow of blood to and from the overworked heart is greatly aided. By taking advantage of gravity, the blood in the dilated and engorged blood vessels in the abdominal cavity tends to drain back to the heart. This increases the amount of blood reaching the heart and relieves part of the strain on the heart caused by its attempt to supply all parts of the body with the required amount of blood. Never permit a patient in a state of shock to sit up; the additional strain on the circulation and heart can greatly increase the state of shock.

3. *Relief of pain*

A long-accepted but false generalization is that all extensive injuries are associated with severe pain and that the more extensive the injury, the worse the pain. In reality, severe and even fatal injuries may be considerably less painful than a mashed fingertip, which can cause agony.

Another generalization is that with similar injuries everyone experiences the same amount of pain. This, too, is incorrect. Some feel pain far more severely than others. Also, those who would not be in much pain from a wound when rested, relaxed, and confident might experience severe pain from the same wound if exhausted, tense, and fearful. Persons in shock tend to feel less pain. However, pain, unless relieved, may cause or increase shock.

Relief of pain can often be accomplished without the use of drugs. This relief may be as simple as loosening tight clothing. Sometimes pain can be relieved by furnishing adequate support for an injury. Fractures of bones in which the surrounding tissue swells rapidly are extremely painful when left unsupported. Adequate immobilization of fractures not only relieves pain but prevents further tissue-damage and shock.

shock treatment — *See electroconvulsive therapy.*

shoulder — the joint that attaches the upper extremity, the arm, to the body. The shoulder consists of the clavicle, the scapula, and the humerus.

The clavicle (collar bone) forms the front portion of the shoulder girdle. It lies in a horizontal position just above the first rib. The inner end of the clavicle is round and is attached to the sternum. Its outer edge is flattened and is fixed to the scapula.

The scapula (shoulder blade) is a triangular bone located in the upper part of the back. It forms the rear portion of the shoulder. Its lateral corner forms a part of the shoulder joint, joining with the humerus.

The humerus is the bone of the arm, joining the scapula to form the shoulder joint. A rounded portion of this bone fits into a recess of the scapula.

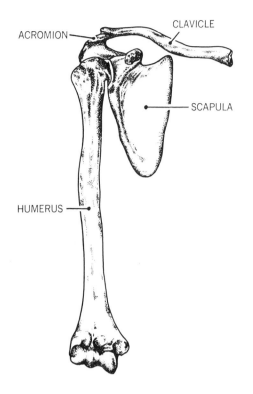

ACROMION

CLAVICLE

SCAPULA

HUMERUS

SHOULDER

shunt — a passage between two blood vessels or between the two sides of the heart where an opening exists in the wall that normally separates them. In surgery, a shunt is an operation to form a passage between blood vessels to divert blood from one part of the body to another.

sickle cell anemia — a chronic disorder of the blood characterized by red blood cells that are sickle or crescent-shaped.

Sickle cell anemia is an inherited disease. It occurs when an altered type of hemoglobin is present in red blood cells. Hemoglobin is the substance in the red blood cells that enables them to carry oxygen throughout the body. In sickle cell anemia, the red blood cells take on a sickle-shaped form, thus giving the disease its name.

The changes in the red blood cells lead to a variety of symptoms. The most prominent are periodic attacks of acute pain (called sickle-cell crises), anemia with weakness, jaundice, and leg ulcers. The disease process often causes lowered resistance to infectious diseases.

Sickle-cell anemia, like another somewhat similar disease, thalassemia, is one of a group of blood disorders that is inherited from parents. The parents may not actually have either of these diseases but merely carry the defective trait for one of them. Such a "carrier" can pass this trait to his children but does not necessarily show any symptoms himself. Just as thalassemia appears to be limited to Caucasians, sickle cell anemia has been found so far only in Blacks. Sickle cell anemia is not an infectious disease and cannot be caught from others by contact.

Dr. Linus Pauling, the distinguished scientist and sickle-cell expert, who discovered the abnormal hemoglobin molecule that causes red blood cells to sickle, estimates that about two out of twenty-five American Blacks carry the sickle-cell trait, while the full disease occurs about once in 400 births. When both the mother and father carry the defective sickle-cell trait, the statistical probability is that one in four children may be born with sickle cell anemia, two in four may be born carriers like their parents, and one child in four may be born neither diseased nor a carrier. If only one parent carries the sickle-cell trait, as is probably more often the case, the child will be either a carrier or normal, with a one-in-two chance of being normal.

Apparently, sickle cell anemia is a consequence of a protective mechanism against another disease, malaria. Studies in Africa and the Mediterranean basin, where malaria has long been a problem, have shown that people with sickle-cell hemoglobin are less susceptible to lethal malaria than are normal individuals. As a result, in these areas, where malaria has been taking its toll of the population for generations, many people have sickle-cell hemoglobin because they are descended from "trait-carrying" ancestors who survived malaria. In other words, the higher early death rate among individuals without the trait limited the number of offspring without the trait. In the United States and other areas where malaria is under control, sickle-cell hemoglobin is no longer useful.

CAUSE

The cause of sickle cell anemia was discovered a few years ago, when the disorder was identified as a "molecular disease." Scientists found then that this disease was caused by a change in the molecular structure of hemoglobin in red blood cells.

The difference in structure causes the red blood cells to twist into the shape of a sickle. With their shape changed, the sickled blood cells cannot pass freely through many of the very small blood vessels. Frequently, the twisted cells pile up, causing blood clots that block the flow of blood to the local tissues. The sickled cells are also destroyed by natural body processes more rapidly than are normal cells.

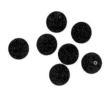

NORMAL CELLS

SICKEL-SHAPED CELLS

SICKLE CELL ANEMIA

SYMPTOMS

People with sickle cell anemia show the usual symptoms of severe anemia. They are often poorly developed and have a short trunk with long arms and legs. Many patients are moderately jaundiced, the whites of their eyes turning greenish-yellow. Chronic "punched-out" looking ulcers often appear about the ankles, along with a pallor in the palms of the hands, lips, nail beds, and tissue linings of the mouth. Severe pain in the abdomen and in the knees, elbows, and other joints is experienced from time to time in almost all patients with the disease.

In more-severe cases, other symptoms include weakness, headache, dizziness, ringing in the ears, and spots before the eyes. Patients are sometimes drowsy, irritable, and behave oddly. Some patients become used to their chronic anemia and in spite of some weakness can carry on daily activities except during painful episodes. In carriers of the disease trait, the symptoms and anemia are absent except under circumstances of unusual stress, such as high-altitude airplane flights, for example, where a moderate lack of oxygen may cause abdominal pain, nausea, and vomiting.

Sickle cell anemia is difficult to identify, be-

cause the symptoms are similar to those found in other diseases, such as abdominal and nerve disorders and rheumatic fever. Blood tests must be made to determine whether the red blood cells are sickling. Even then, the presence of some sickled cells alone, without the symptoms, only indicates the presence of the sickle-cell trait.

TREATMENT

Medical science has no cure for sickle-cell anemia. Nevertheless, many of the symptoms can be relieved to some extent. Much use is made of pain-killing drugs during an attack of severe pain, fever, and shock. Some physicians use ice packs that are placed on the joints to help prevent the "clumping" of sickled blood cells. The ice packs also tend to maintain the local circulation. Other doctors suggest blood transfusions and bed rest to help relieve painful attacks. These attacks last from four to seven days.

New blood tests make it easier to detect carriers of sickle-cell anemia. In view of this, physicians sometimes warn carriers who are considering marriage of the risk that their children may be born with the disease.

Patients with the full disease, as well as carriers, are advised against high altitudes and unpressurized airplanes or any situation that might cause a moderate lack of oxygen. A lowered amount of oxygen may lead to a sickling crisis, with accompanying abdominal pain, nausea, and vomiting.

The degree of anemia in patients may increase and decrease but the anemia never disappears completely except in extremely rare cases. Death of sickle-cell anemia patients can result from infections, heart or kidney failure, or from damage to a vital organ because of lack of oxygen. Some patients with the full disease die at an early age and, until recently, most patients have not lived beyond forty years. Today, however, the life-span of these patients has been increased considerably through treatment of infections with antibiotic drugs.

side effect — an effect that is aside from or in addition to the desired effect. Side effects occur as a result of taking medicines or other kinds of treatments.

Because the chemical balance of the body is so delicate, almost any drug is capable of upsetting it to some degree. Side effects are the physical (although sometimes mental) manifestations of the change in the body's chemical balance. The range of side effects is enormous. Some drugs cause no more than a slight side effect that the patient does not even notice. However, other drugs can cause headaches, upset the stomach, and change the mood of the patient. In addition, certain drugs can have very serious, even fatal, side effects.

sight — the ability to see objects clearly. This is accomplished (at different distances) by reflex or automatic changing of the thickness of the lens of the eye and of the diameter of the pupil to bring an object into focus.

The eye is like a camera. The pupil in front allows the entrance of light, and the retina in the back of the eyeball receives the image. The nerve endings for the sense of sight are tiny rods and cones standing on end, side by side, in the retina. They are very sensitive and very close together. By a complex chemical reaction, these small organs act like the film in a camera, recording the picture for the brain. The optic nerve conveys the impulses from the retina to the visual area of the brain, where the visual image is consciously perceived.

The muscles controlling the movement of the eyeball provide for focusing of both eyes on one spot at the same time. If it were not for the fine adjustment provided by these muscles, each eye would focus on a different spot, resulting in a dual or blurred image being perceived by the brain.

sign — any objective evidence of disease.
See symptom.

sinoatrial node — a small mass of specialized cells in the right upper chamber of the heart that give rise to the electrical impulses that initiate contractions of the heart. The sinoatrial node is also called the pacemaker.

sinus — a general term used to indicate a body cavity. The sinuses that people commonly refer to are technically called the paranasal sinuses. These are air spaces in the bones of the skull that drain into the nasal cavity. They are lined with mucous membranes that continue into the nose.

There are four pairs of paranasal sinuses: maxillary, frontal, ethmoid, and sphenoidals. The maxillary sinuses are located under the eyes in the vicinity of the upper cheek. The frontal sinuses are situated over the eyebrows. The eth-

moid sinuses (actually a collection of air cells) are found in the space between the nose and the eye socket. The sphenoidal sinuses are located in back of the nasal cavity.

The paranasal sinuses add resonance to the voice, help to maintain the proper pressure within the nasal cavity and produce mucus.

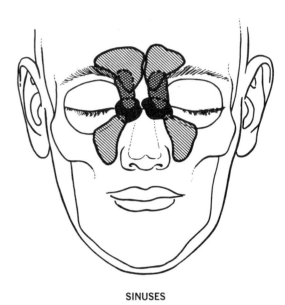

SINUSES

sinuses of Valsalva — three pouches in the wall of the aorta (the main artery leading from the left lower chamber of the heart) located behind the three cup-shaped membranes of the aortic valve.

sinusitis — an infection of the lining of the paranasal sinuses, which are the air spaces in the bones of the head and face. These hollows are connected with the nose by small openings; the mucous membrane or lining of the nose is continuous with the lining of the sinuses. Thus, infection of the nose can travel rapidly to the sinuses.

The air spaces that most commonly become infected are those above the eyes, between and behind the eyes, and in the cheek bones below the eyes.

Inflammation of the nasal passages, usually caused by a cold, may close the sinuses, interfering with drainage and trapping air in the cavity. If a sinus is closed for any length of time, the air in it is absorbed and a vacuum forms, causing severe pain. When inflammation of the lining of a sinus blocks the air space and drainage, pus or other secretions that have formed may press on the sinus wall, also causing intense pain.

CAUSE

Sinus trouble can be caused in a number of ways. Among the most frequent are infections of the nose and throat, such as the common cold, influenza, measles, scarlet fever, and whooping cough. Allergies, enlarged adenoids, or other nasal obstructions also may cause sinusitis.

Blowing the nose violently, diving, or swimming with the nose under water, all may force infectious material into the sinuses. Frequent use of sprays, oils, and antiseptics in the nose may injure the mucous membrane and bring on sinus trouble.

People who work outdoors are less likely to have sinus infections than those who work in crowded rooms where the air is hot and dry, cold and damp, or full or irritating vapors or dust.

SYMPTOMS

Although sinusitis is common among men, women, and children of all ages, many persons who believe they have sinus trouble actually do not. While symptoms vary from person to person, there are certain fairly general warning signs.

Usually there is headache or pain over the infected sinus. There may be pain in the cheek, upper teeth, or elsewhere in the head. The forehead may be tender to pressure. The nasal passages often are dry and clogged because of the swollen membrane and lack of drainage. There may be a discharge of pus from the nose, or a dripping from the back of the nose into the throat. Sometimes the sense of smell is partially lost. Other symptoms may be fever; cough; swelling of the cheeks, eyelids, or forehead; general fatigue; and aching.

An acute infection of the sinuses may clear up or it may develop into chronic sinus trouble. Sometimes a chronic case shows few symptoms except susceptibility to frequent and prolonged colds. But persistent, uncured sinusitis may lead to diseases such as bronchitis, mastoid infection, and arthritis.

TREATMENT

Medicines are often prescribed to shrink the swollen membranes, lessen the discharge, and get rid of the focus of infection. There are a number of valuable drugs for the treatment of sinus infection, and new ones are being constantly developed.

Pain from sinusitis (although not the infection itself) is sometimes relieved by putting a hot-water bottle; hot, wet compresses; or an electric pad over the inflamed part. In severe cases even medical treatment fails to cure sinusitis, and an operation may be necessary to open the sinus and allow it to drain.

sitz bath — a hot bath used in the treatment of rectal or pelvic conditions. The water level is high enough to cover the patient's hips. The temperature of the water is usually 110°F., and the patient remains in the sitz bath for about twenty minutes.

skeleton — the bony framework of the body. This framework supports and gives shape to the body. It protects vital organs; affords attachment for tendons, muscles, and ligaments; and forms joints that allow muscular movement.

The adult human skeleton is composed of 206 distinct bones. These are classified according to shape as long bones, short bones, flat bones, and irregular bones. The skeleton is divided into four major parts: the head, trunk, pelvis, and extremities.

HEAD

The head is composed of twenty-two bones. Eight of these are closely united to form a bony case (the skull) that encloses the brain. Fourteen other bones are part of the formation of the face. The only moveable bone in the head is the lower jaw.

TRUNK

The trunk is made up of fifty-six bones. The spinal column, or backbone, of an adult consists of twenty-six segments, called vertebrae. These are joined by strong ligaments to form a flexible column that encloses the spinal cord.

The chest is formed by twenty-four ribs, twelve on each side. These are attached in the back to vertebrae or segments of the spinal column. The seven upper ribs are attached in front to the breastbone by means of cartilage. The next three ribs are attached in front by a common cartilage to the seventh rib above instead of to the breastbone. The lowest two ribs, known as floating ribs, have no attachments in front.

PELVIS

The pelvis is the basin-shaped, bony structure at the lower portion of the trunk. It is situated between the movable vertebrae of the spinal column, which it supports, and the lower limbs, upon which it rests. The pelvis is composed of four

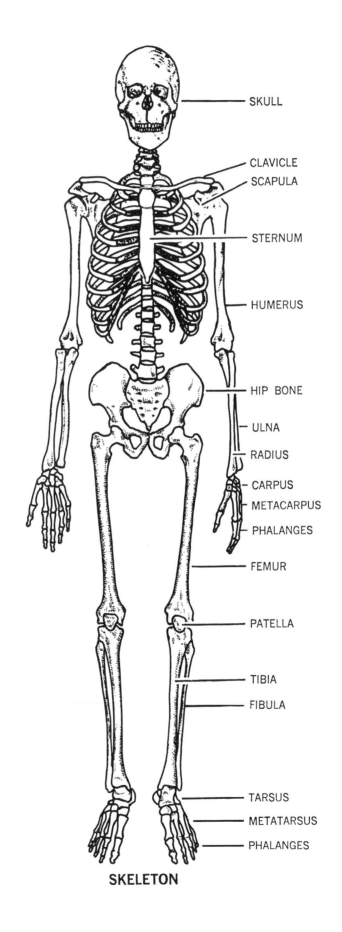

SKULL

CLAVICLE
SCAPULA

STERNUM

HUMERUS

HIP BONE

ULNA

RADIUS

CARPUS

METACARPUS

PHALANGES

FEMUR

PATELLA

TIBIA

FIBULA

TARSUS

METATARSUS

PHALANGES

SKELETON

bones: the two lower bones of the spinal column and the winged-shaped hip bones on either side. It forms the floor of the abdominal cavity and provides deep sockets into which the heads of the thighbones fit.

EXTREMITIES

Each upper extremity consists of thirty-two bones. The collarbone or clavicle (a long bone, the inner end of which is connected to the breastbone or sternum and the outer end to the shoulder blade or scapula at the shoulder joint) lies just in front of and above the first rib. The shoulder blade or scapula (a flat, triangular bone) lies at the upper and outer part of the back of the chest and forms part of the shoulder joint. The arm bone (humerus) extends from the shoulder to the elbow. The two bones of the lower arm or forearm (ulna and radius) extend from the elbow to the wrist. There are eight bones of the wrist that form the heel of the hand. The palm consists of five bones. There are fourteen bones of the fingers (two in the thumb and three in each finger).

Each of the lower extremities consists of thirty bones. The thighbone, or femur, is the longest and strongest bone in the body. It extends from the hip joint to the knee. The upper end of the thighbone is rounded to fit into the socket in the pelvis; the lower end broadens out to help form the knee joint. The kneecap (the patella) is a flat, triangular bone located in front of the knee joint. Two bones in the leg extend from the knee joint to the ankle. They are the tibia and the fibula. There are seven bones of the ankle that form the back of the foot. Five long bones form the front of the foot. The toes are composed of a total of fourteen bones.

skin — the protective covering of the body. The skin covers almost every visible part of the human body. Even the hair and nails are outgrowths from it. The skin protects the underlying structures, preventing bacteria from penetrating into them and protecting them from injury and from drying. It contains nerves that transmit the sensations of touch, heat, cold, pain, and pressure. It

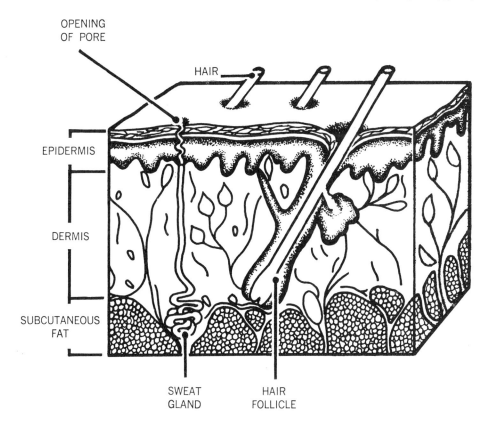

OPENING OF PORE

HAIR

EPIDERMIS

DERMIS

SUBCUTANEOUS FAT

SWEAT GLAND

HAIR FOLLICLE

SKIN

helps dispose of body wastes. The skin also plays an important role in the regulation of body temperature by acting as a large, radiating surface that allows the sweat glands to cool the body through the evaporation of sweat.

The skin is composed of two main layers. These are the outer layer, or epidermis; and the inner layer, or dermis, which is referred to as true skin. The outer layers of the epidermis are flat and lifeless. They resemble dry, clear, overlapping scales. This scaly layer, if unbroken, is able to block the passage of almost every known variety of disease germ. However, its protective powers are reduced if the skin is not cleaned regularly.

Normally, the outer layer of skin (the epidermis) reproduces itself about once a month. As new cells form, the old surface skin is shed unobtrusively in the form of tiny flakes. The newly formed cells are responsible for pushing the older cells outward. The nearer they approach the surface, the drier or more scalelike they become. It is because of this constant activity of the deeper cells of the epidermis that any injury to the skin, if it goes no deeper than its outer layer, is repaired in a few days and leaves no scar. Among these deeper cells are special cells containing pigment, the color and quantity of which are the chief factors in determining the complexion.

The dermis has nerve endings for touch, heat, cold, and pain, as well as motor nerves leading to the blood vessels. Also located in the dermis are the sebaceous glands, the sweat glands, and the hair follicles.

skin allergies — an allergy that is caused when certain substances come into contact with the skin. The symptoms may be a simple itching or may become a skin eruption that oozes, crusts, and scales.
See allergy.

skull — the bony framework that encases the brain. The skull is divided into two parts: the cranium and the face. There are twenty-two bones in the skull; eight of them form the cranium, and fourteen form the face.

CRANIAL BONES
These bones are firmly united and fit snugly together. The lines between the bones where the adjacent bones meet are called sutures. The most important bones are the frontal bone that forms the forehead, contains the frontal sinuses, and

helps form the eye socket and the nasal cavity; the two parietal bones that form the roof of the skull on each side; and the occipital bone that forms the back or base of the skull. The occipital bone contains a large opening, the foramen magnum, which permits passage of the spinal cord from the cranium into the spinal canal formed by the vertebrae.

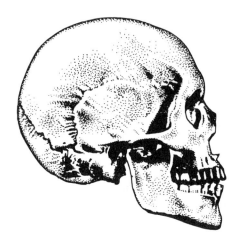

SKULL

FACIAL BONES
Of the fourteen bones of the face, the major bones are the two maxillary bones that form the upper jaw, the walls of the nose, and a portion of the eye socket. In each of these there is a large cavity, the maxillary sinus. The mandible is a loose bone that forms the lower jaw. It is shaped somewhat like a horseshoe and is the only bone in the skull that is movable.

sleep — a periodic state of rest during which consciousness and bodily activity are diminished. It is usually considered as a period in which constructive processes build up and repair the body.

Certain changes take place in the body during sleep. Respiration is slowed, less blood is sent to the brain, and greater amounts of blood go to the extremities during sleep periods. Digestion continues, but at a slower rate. The temperature of the body may drop somewhat, and the action of the heart is slowed.

sleeping sickness — *See trypanosomiasis.*

sling — a piece of material that is used to support injuries of the shoulder, arm, elbow, forearm, wrist, hand, or fingers. The sling is looped around the neck, and the arm is placed between the edges.

slipped disk — a vertebral disk that has slipped or been displaced. The vertebral disks are pads composed of a type of cartilage and are situated between the vertebrae of the spinal column. Their main purpose is to protect the spinal cord (and ultimately the brain) from damage by acting as a cushion when the body is bumped.

A disk can slip out of position when too much strain is placed on it. This happens most frequently when a person attempts to lift a heavy weight from the wrong postural position. The disk moves from its natural location into the area where there are many nerves running through the spinal column. The pain associated with a slipped disk is caused by the pressure exerted by the disk against a nerve.

The treatment for this condition may be bed rest, manipulation of the area to return the disk to its proper place, or a surgical operation.

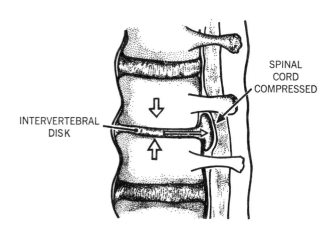

SPINAL CORD COMPRESSED

INTERVERTEBRAL DISK

SLIPPED DISK

small intestines — *See intestine.*

smallpox — a very serious infectious disease. Before the discovery of vaccination, smallpox swept back and forth over every continent. It was one of the most dreaded diseases in the world. It killed at least a fourth of its victims and left the survivors scarred, pitted, and often blind. Yet, even in the Middle Ages it was known that smallpox was "catching," and that the sick gave it to the well. Consequently, the victims were sometimes shunned and left to die alone or to get well as best they could.

Smallpox still exists in many countries and kills and disfigures the unvaccinated just as it did centuries ago.

CAUSE

Smallpox is caused by a virus. It is spread by the secretions from the mouth and nose of the patient and by material from his pox and scabs. Transmission of the disease can be through direct contact with the patient or from handling articles that have been recently soiled by him. The infection usually moves through the air only as far as a cough or sneeze can spray secretions from the mouth or nose. A patient can give the disease to others before the rash appears, all during his illness, and until the scabs and crusts on the eruptions have disappeared.

SYMPTOMS

The average incubation period is fourteen days but it can be shorter or a few days longer.

The first symptoms are not always the same. Usually, there is fever and headache and often aches and pains in the body and limbs. In most cases, the rash appears later. There may be only a few skin lesions, or there may be so many that they run together. They appear first on the face and then spread to the arms and other parts of the body and can occur in the mouth, nose, vagina, and eyes. The sores form crusts that fall off within ten to forty days.

TREATMENT

The illness varies greatly in severity. In severe cases there is deep pitting or scarring; in mild cases there may be none at all. There is no known cure for smallpox. Medical care is aimed at relieving the patient's discomfort, preventing complications, and stopping the spread of the disease to other people.

PREVENTION

Of all the contagious diseases, smallpox is one of the easiest to prevent. A successful vaccination, recent enough to give protection, is all that is necessary. In fact, if all people were properly vaccinated, this disease could be stamped out completely.

The first effort to control smallpox through immunization began in 1715, when an attempt was made to induce a mild form of smallpox in order to produce an immunity to the naturally spread disease. This was achieved, in many cases, through a direct arm-to-arm inoculation—a procedure that too often proved dangerous. Vaccination was discovered in 1796 by an English country physician, Dr. Edward Jenner, who proved through carefully planned experiments that the milder disease, cowpox, protected against small-pox.

To be assured of protection, the vaccination must show a visible reaction or "take." If a vaccination does not show this reaction, it may mean that it was improperly performed or that the vaccine had lost its potency because of age or inadequate refrigeration.

smell — one of the most primitive of the senses. Odor is perceived when the mucous membrane in the upper nose is stimulated. The olfactory nerve (one of the cranial nerves) conveys the sense of smell to the olfactory center in the brain.

The sense of smell is not as well developed in man as it is in animals.

snakebite — the body's physical reaction to the venom injected by the bite of a snake.

Two kinds of poisonous snakes, the Crotalidae and the Elapidae, are present in the United States. The Crotalidae (frequently called the "pit viper" family) are abundant and include the true rattlesnakes, the pygmy rattlers, copperheads, and water moccasins. The Elapidae family has only one representative—the coral snake. The venom of the Crotalidae is hemotoxic (poisonous to the blood). The venom of the Elapidae (coral, cobra, and kraits) contains a highly potent neurotoxin (poisonous to nerve tissues). In addition, some snake venom contains other toxins.

SYMPTOMS

The first symptoms of bites by poisonous snakes are a feeling of stinging pain in the immediate area of the bite and rapid swelling and discoloration. The part becomes painful, and, as the poison enters the system through the venous circulation, more symptoms develop.

The bite from the Crotalidae (pit vipers) may produce the following symptoms:

1. Tissue swelling at the site of the bite and gradually spreading to surrounding areas. Swelling occurs between three to five minutes following the bite, but may continue for as long as an hour and be so severe as to burst the skin.

2. Severe pain at the site of the bite.

3. Escape of blood from the capillaries. Accumulation of blood in the tissues may cause severe pain.

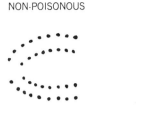

NON-POISONOUS

POISONOUS

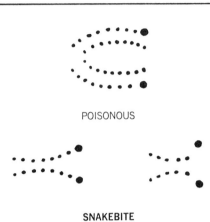

SNAKEBITE

4. Severe headache and thirst.

5. Bleeding from some of the internal organs into the intestines and the excretory tract. Blood in the urine or stool may be evidence of such internal bleeding.

The bite from the Elapidae (coral, cobra, and krait) may produce the following symptoms:

1. Irregular heartbeat, followed by generalized weakness and exhaustion, ending in shock.

2. Severe headache and dizziness, as well as mental disturbances such as incoherent speech, stupor, mental confusion, and, possibly, unconsciousness. Extreme pain is not characteristic.

3. Muscular incoordination, such as inability to reach for and pick up an object or to move from place to place; sometimes muscle spasms and twitching.

4. Difficult or labored breathing and even respiratory paralysis.

5. Numbness and tingling of the skin, particularly of the lips and soles of the feet.

6. Chills, fever, and excessive sweating.

7. Nausea, vomiting, and diarrhea.

TREATMENT

Antivenom serums have been developed to neutralize or combat the poisons of different types of snakes. It is important, however, to have a proper identification of the type of snake in order to administer the proper antivenom. This can be accomplished by killing the snake, so that qualified persons can identify it, or by examining the fang impressions the bite leaves in the skin.

The primary rule of first aid in snakebite cases is to keep the patient calm. It is also very important to immobilize the affected part and to position it below the level of the heart. A snakebite victim who becomes overly excited or who runs for help is only speeding the flow of the venom throughout his body.

When the bite is on the arm or leg, a tourniquet should be placed two to four inches closer to the heart than the site of the bite. It should be tight enough to stop the flow of blood in the veins but not in the arteries. Every twenty minutes the tourniquet should be released for thirty seconds to allow fresh blood to enter the extremity.

If more than an hour is going to elapse before antivenom can be injected, the bite should be carefully incised and suctioned. Two cuts (each not more than one-half-inch long and one-quarter-inch deep) should be made with a sharp, sterile instrument. The cuts should be made over the fang marks, lengthwise over the arm or leg. Suction can then be performed by a suction cup or by mouth (but only if there are no open sores in the mouth). The suction should be continued for thirty minutes. The sooner suction is started, the better. If as much as an hour has passed since the bite was inflicted, incision and suction should not be used.

sneeze — a forced expulsion of air through the nose and the mouth. Sneezing is an involuntary action that is caused by the irritation of membranes in the nose.

socket — a hollow area in a bone. The socket receives the rounded or semiround area at the end of another bone. The socket and the round end that fits into it form a joint. However, not all sockets are parts of joints. For example, the two sockets above the cheekbones are not joints. They are the space into which the eyeball fits.

sodium — a mineral that is essential to life. It is found in nearly all plant and animal tissue. Table salt (sodium chloride) is almost half sodium. Excess sodium that is retained in the body holds water with it. This causes an accumulation of fluids (edema) that often shows up as swelling in the feet, ankles, legs, or some other part of the body. In some types of heart or kidney diseases the amount of sodium intake must be restricted.

sodium pentothol — *See sodium thiopental.*

sodium thiopental — one of the most widely used of all general anesthetics. Sodium thiopental (also called sodium pentothol) is injected into the patient (as opposed to inhaled anesthetics, such as ether). It takes effect very quickly. However, sodium thiopental usually does not produce enough pain relief to be used by itself. Consequently, it is frequently used in conjunction with another anesthetic. The sodium thiopental is used to put the patient to sleep; the other anesthetic is used to deepen the level of unconsciousness.

See anesthetics.

solar plexus — a network of sympathetic nerves located in the abdomen behind the stomach.

spasm — an involuntary muscle contraction. Spasms usually occur in a series.

speech — the verbal expression of thoughts. Speech is controlled by the coordinated action of several nerve functions. The speech center is located deep in the brain. From the speech center, nerve impulses are directed to the larynx. This organ contains folds of mucous membranes called vocal cords. When air is forced from the lungs, past these folds, certain sounds are produced, and, in conjunction with the movements of the throat, lips, tongue, and teeth, articulate speech results.

The sound that emerges from the vocal cords is very crude; in fact, it is usually not comprehensible. The parts of the head already mentioned, plus the sinus cavities, add resonance and clarity to the sound, refining it to the point where it can be clearly recognized as individual words.

Speech is learned through imitation. Children learn to speak clearly and distinctly by imitating the words they hear other people speak. When a child cannot hear, he retains the ability to speak. However, he has nothing to imitate. Therefore, deaf children must be taught how to use their mouths, tongues, etc., in order to produce understandable speech.

sperm — *See spermatozoa.*

spermatic cord — a part of the male reproductive

321

system. There are two spermatic cords, each of which suspends and supplies a testis. These cords are formed by the ductus deferens, arteries, veins, lymphatics, and nerves bound together by connective tissue. The spermatic cords extend into the scrotum to suspend the testes.

spermatozoa — the male sex cells. They are often referred to as sperm. Spermatozoa are much smaller than the female sex cells, or ova. They move by lashing their long, slender tails. Spermatozoa are produced in the testes and are ejaculated in the seminal fluid.

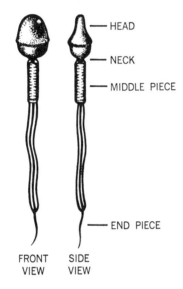

HEAD

NECK

MIDDLE PIECE

END PIECE

FRONT VIEW   SIDE VIEW

SPERMATOZOA

sphincter — a muscular ring. There are several of these rings in the body, including two in the stomach, one in the rectum, and one in the urethra. They serve the purpose of controlling the flow of fluids and solids into and out of the organs to which they are attached.

sphygomanometer — an instrument for measuring blood pressure in the arteries.

spina bifida — a birth defect of the nervous system. The words spina bifida literally mean "cleft spine." Every infant's backbone, while developing in the mother, remains open until about the twelfth week of the mother's pregnancy. In spina bifida, one or more of the individual bones of the back (vertebrae) fail to close completely, leaving a cleft or defect in the spinal canal.

There is no known cause of spina bifida.

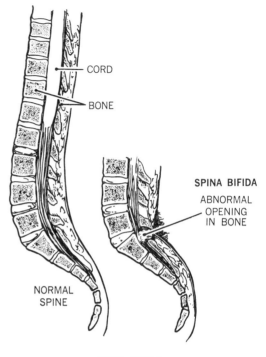

CORD

BONE

SPINA BIFIDA
ABNORMAL OPENING IN BONE

NORMAL SPINE

SPINA BIFIDA

SYMPTOMS

In its slightest form, called spina bifida occulta, the abnormality causes no symptoms at all and may never be discovered. However, sometimes an X-ray of the spine that is taken for some other purpose reveals a small, unclosed portion of the spinal canal. A depression or dimple in the backbone over the defect or a tuft of hair can also lead to the discovery of this harmless type of spina bifida.

Mild or serious symptoms appear in some of the forms of spina bifida. In these cases, a sac protrudes from the backbone, usually at the lower end of the spine. The sac can be as small as a nut or as large as a grapefruit. Sometimes the sac is completely covered with skin, but in other cases the nerve tissue is exposed.

When the sac contains some of the coverings (meninges) of the spinal cord, the ailment is called a meningocele. In more complicated cases, called a meningomyelocele, the coverings and some of the spinal cord have slipped through the bony opening as a sac. In these cases, the sac usually contains some spinal fluid.

Since the sac most commonly contains portions of the lower end of the spinal cord, it is the legs of the patient that are most likely to be affected. In mild forms, the only difficulty might be weak muscles and inadequate skin sensation. If the

322

injury to the spinal cord is more serious, the patient could have leg paralysis and no skin sensation on the legs. Even in relatively mild spina bifida, bladder control is likely to be a troublesome complication.

Such symptoms are ordinarily present from the time of birth. However, symptoms may not develop until adolescence. Rapid growth of the body at this time may overstretch the shortened nerves, leading to a progressive weakness.

COMPLICATIONS

Serious complications often occur. Where there is a large sac, especially one with a thin surface, friction from the baby's movements or clothing is likely to make the tissues raw. Infection of the spinal cord and brain coverings can result. In former days, meningitis frequently was a fatal complication.

Another common complication results from disturbances of the spinal fluid that ordinarily bathes the brain and spinal cord. In patients with meningocele, abnormal collections of fluid may take place not only in the spinal sac but also in the cavities within the brain. When an abnormal amount of fluid collects within the skull, an enlargement of the head, called hydrocephalus, can occur.

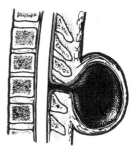

SPINA BIFIDA WITH MENINGOCELE

TREATMENT

In the slightest cases of spina bifida, no treatment is required. The moderate cases require judgment as to whether surgery is advisable. Surgery prevents worsening of the condition in some instances but cannnot restore the lost functions. In those extreme cases where the sac of spina bifida breaks or appears about to break, immediate surgery becomes essential if the patient's condition permits.

Surgeons have operated on spina bifida patients of all ages, beginning from a few hours after birth. Where hydrocephalus is or threatens to be a complication, surgery to shunt the extra fluid away from the brain is saving many patients whose condition would have been hopeless a few years ago. Investigators are developing and testing a variety of drugs with the goal of controlling hydrocephalus without surgery.

Infections can be a serious complication, whether in the bladder, the brain, or the spinal cord. Antibiotics are saving many patients with infections.

Because of the paralysis of some muscles in the legs, it is quite common for patients with spina bifida to develop stiffening of the joints and actual abnormalities of posture of the legs and feet. It is important from an early age that a child with spina bifida should have any necessary orthopedic measures to prevent such "contractures."

The family doctor, the orthopedic specialist, or the physiatrist (doctor of physical medicine and rehabilitation) frequently prescribes corrective shoes, braces, crutches, or other devices. These help the patient to make the most effective use of the weakened muscles and to prevent the extremity from being maintained in an improper or awkward position. Crippling from "frozen" ankles, knees, or hips can often be prevented by "range-of-motion" exercises. Some doctors order these started three or four times daily when the baby is a couple of days old. The goal is to keep joints movable and leg muscles from shortening (contracture). In some instances, operations for the transfer of tendons to restore proper muscle balance are helpful.

Persons with spina bifida occulta ordinarily live normal lives. Some of those with moderate symptoms of spina bifida may have a shortened lifespan. Because of modern surgical and medical progress, even babies born with severe spina bifida have an improved chance to survive.

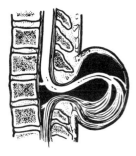

SPINA BIFIDA WITH MENINGOMYELOCELE

spinal column — a series of bones in the back. The spinal column, or vertebral column, consists of twenty-four moveable or true vertebrae, the sacrum, and the coccyx. It is divided into five regions: cervical (neck), thoracic (chest), lumbar (lower back), sacral and coccygeal (both in the pelvis). The spinal column encloses and protects the spinal cord.

See spinal cord, vertebra.

spinal cord — a part of the central nervous system. It joins the medulla oblongata of the brain and extends from the atlas (the first cervical vertebra) to the lower border of the first lumbar vertebra, where it tapers off to a point.

The cord is surrounded by the bony walls of the vertebral canal (the hollow space within the spinal column). It is enclosed in three protective membranes and is suspended in a fluid solution. The spinal cord does not fill the vertebral canal, nor does it extend the full length of the canal. The nerve roots arising from the lumbar and sacral regions must pass some distance down the canal before making their exit.

In a cross section, the cut surface shows white and gray areas. The white substance is composed almost entirely of nerve fibers and surrounds the gray substance, which is composed of fibers and nerve-cell bodies. The spinal nerves move in pairs (thirty-one pairs) from the spinal cord. They leave the vertebral canal through the spaces between adjacent vertebrae. These nerves are then distributed to all parts of the body.

The spinal cord may be thought of as an electric cable containing many wires (nerves) connecting the parts of the body to each other and to the brain. Sensations received by a sensory nerve are brought to the spinal cord, and the impulse is transferred either to the brain or to a motor nerve.

spinal nerves — the thirty-one pairs of nerves that start in the spinal cord and leave the spinal column through the spaces between the vertebrae. The thirty-one pairs include eight cervical, twelve thoracic, five lumbar, five sacral, and one coccygeal nerves.

Spinal nerves contain all types of sensory and motor fibers of both the voluntary and autonomic nervous systems.

spine — any bony spur. The term spine is also used to refer to the spinal column.

See spinal column, vertebra.

spirits of ammonia — a fluid solution containing ammonia and alcohol. Spirits of ammonia (or aromatic ammonia spirit) is used to stimulate the respiratory system. Its vapor can be inhaled, or it can be diluted in water and given by mouth.

spleen — a body organ that is composed of lymphoid tissue and is located in the upper left part of the abdominal cavity. The spleen lies under the diaphragm and is protected by the lower portion of the rib cage. It is roughly oval in shape and extremely variable in size. The weight range can be from three-and-one-half to nine ounces in the average adult male.

Placed in the course of the bloodstream by the splenic artery, the spleen acts as a filter and as a reservoir of blood. During the course of a day, the entire volume of blood repeatedly circulates through it. While much of its function remains somewhat obscure, it is known to serve three purposes: the final disposition of old and damaged red blood cells, the storage of blood, and the production of lymph cells and possibly some white blood cells.

Old or damaged red blood cells apparently are destroyed in the spleen. Iron from the hemoglobin (the oxygen-carrying part of the red blood cells) that is released in this way becomes available for the formation of new red blood cells, and the remainder is used for conversion into bile pigments. The spleen stores a small portion of the iron and converts a minor portion into bile pigments. The principal portion of storage and conversion is performed by other body organs.

Large numbers of red blood cells can be stored in the body of the spleen. The spleen itself can dilate (or expand) considerably to accommodate a relatively large volume of the blood. The cells and blood volume can be discharged into the bloodstream during the stress of excitement or exercise. The injection of epinephrine has the same effect.

The third function is in many respects the most obscure. It is definitely understood that lymph cells in large numbers and possible other white blood cells are produced by the spleen. However, other functions influencing the development or life-span of the red blood cells and platelets are not clearly defined. Because it produces lymph cells, which in turn produce immune substances, the spleen may be considered to play a role in the body's defense against infection.

Because the spleen has so many blood vessels,

rupture can result in a rapidly fatal hemorrhage or in a slower bleeding that may eventually endanger life. A blow to the lower left chest or abdomen occasionally results in a split or tear in the spleen. Under conditions of great enlargement, when the outer surface is stretched very thin, rupture may occur from a very slight blow.

The spleen is not essential to life, because its functions are also performed by other organs and tissues. Thus, the spleen can be removed without causing permanent damage.

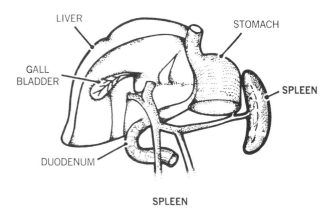

SPLEEN

splint — any stiff material that can be used to support and protect injured parts such as fractures, dislocations, or suspected broken bones. A splint prevents movement at the point of the fracture (or injury) and at the nearest joint.

spondylitis — an inflammation of one or more of the vertebrae of the spinal column.

sprain — an injury to the ligaments that support a joint. A sprain usually involves a momentary dislocation, with the bone slipping back into place of its own accord. A sprain is caused by the violent wrenching or twisting of the joint beyond its normal limits of movement. Although any joint may be sprained, sprains of the ankle, wrist, knee, and finger are most common.

Tearing of the supporting ligaments is probably the most serious part of a sprain, but there is also a considerable amount of damage to the blood vessels and other soft tissues that surround the joint. When the blood vessels are damaged, quite a lot of blood escapes into the joint itself and into the tissues. This causes the severe pain and marked swelling that are characteristic of a sprain.

Sprains range from minor injuries, causing pain or discomfort for only a few hours, to severe cases,

where tearing of the tissues requires many weeks of medical care before normal use of the joint is restored.

spring hay fever — *See hay fever.*

stapedectomy — an operation to correct a hearing loss that has been caused by otosclerosis. In this condition the stapes (one of the three little bones in the middle ear) is frozen into position and thus fails to vibrate properly. The stapedectomy operation removes the stapes and replaces it with a piece of wire or other material.
See otosclerosis.

stapes — the innermost bone of the middle ear chamber. The stapes (also called the stirrup because of its shape) is the smallest bone in the human body. It is connected to the incus (also known as the anvil). The stapes fits into the oval window between the middle ear and the inner ear. When the stapes moves (as a result of sound vibrations), fluid in the inner ear carries the vibrations into the canal of the cochlea.

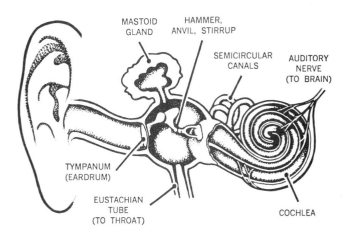

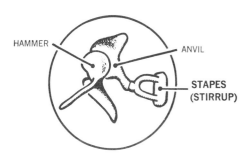

STAPES (STIRRUP)

staphylococcus — a bacterium that is round or spherical and occurs in bunches or clusters. Infections that are caused by these microorganisms tend to be concentrated in one area, such as a boil.

starch — a form of carbohydrate.
See carbohydrate.

stasis — a stoppage or a slackening of the blood flow.

stenosis — a narrowing of an opening. Mitral stenosis, aortic stenosis, etc., means that the valve indicated has become narrowed so that it does not function normally.

sterile — a condition in which no living germs or microorganisms are present. This is accomplished by extreme heat or by the use of strong chemicals.

The term sterile is also used to indicate the lack of ability to reproduce. This has nothing to do with the physical ability to have sexual intercourse. In the man, it means a lack of sperm cells; in the female, a lack of ova.

sterilization — the process of making some thing or some place sterile by removing or killing existing microorganisms. It is also the process of rendering an individual incapable of reproducing. This may be done in the male by a vasectomy and in the female by tying the fallopian tubes. Other means of sterilization include castration and hysterectomy.
See sterile.

sternum — a bone situated in the middle of the upper part of the chest wall in front of the spinal column. The sternum (also known as the breastbone) is connected with both clavicles (collarbones) and with the cartilages of the first seven pairs of ribs.

steroids — a collective term for a group of chemically similar compounds. Steroids are produced by the body (in the cortex of the adrenal gland) and have been synthesized. These compounds affect a variety of body functions. The salt and water balance, the ability of the body to meet conditions of stress, and the ability to resist infection are all affected by steroids.

stethoscope — an instrument used to listen to sounds within the body.

stimulants — drugs that stimulate the central nervous system. They induce a transient sense of well-being, self-confidence and alertness. They are used to combat fatigue, curb appetite, and reduce mild depression. The stimulants include drugs such as cocaine, amphetamine, dextroamphetamine, and methamphetamine.

Research has shown that these compounds resemble the natural body hormones ephinephrine and norepinephrine. As a result of this similarity, these drugs can act directly by mimicking the natural hormones in their effects on nerve endings. They can also act indirectly by causing increased release of the natural hormone. Consequently, these drugs stimulate the areas of the nervous system that regulate blood pressure, heart, respiratory, and metabolic rates, all of which are increased. Appetite is markedly decreased, and the senses are hyperalert. The body behaves as if it were under emergency life conditions.
See amphetamine, cocaine.

stimulus — any physical force or phenomenon that occurs outside of the body but which causes any type of response or reaction within the body.

stirrup — *See stapes.*

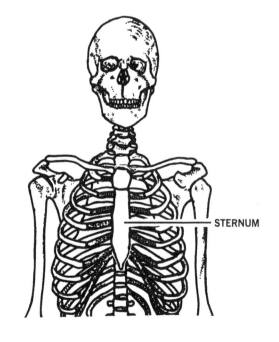

STERNUM

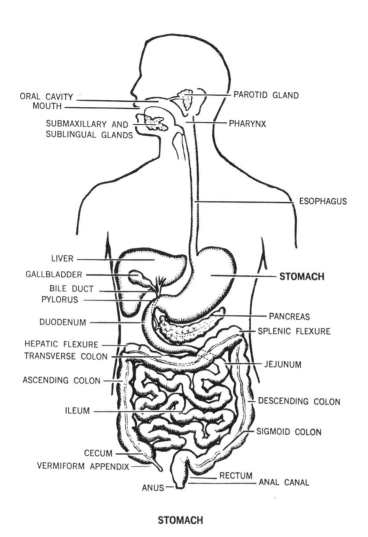

ORAL CAVITY
MOUTH
SUBMAXILLARY AND
SUBLINGUAL GLANDS
PAROTID GLAND
PHARYNX
ESOPHAGUS
LIVER
GALLBLADDER
BILE DUCT
PYLORUS
DUODENUM
HEPATIC FLEXURE
TRANSVERSE COLON
ASCENDING COLON
ILEUM
CECUM
VERMIFORM APPENDIX
ANUS
STOMACH
PANCREAS
SPLENIC FLEXURE
JEJUNUM
DESCENDING COLON
SIGMOID COLON
RECTUM
ANAL CANAL

STOMACH

Stokes-Adams syndrome — sudden attacks of unconsciousness. The attacks sometimes include convulsions. Stokes-Adams syndrome may accompany a heart block.

stomach — one of the primary organs of the digestive system. The stomach connects the lower end of the esophagus and the first portion of the small intestine, the duodenum. It lies in the upper left part of the abdomen. Muscular rings, or sphincters, at each end of the stomach form valves to close off the stomach. This prevents the contents from escaping (in either direction). The sphincter at the esophageal end is called the cardiac sphincter; the one at the duodenal end is known as the pyloric sphincter.

The stomach acts as an initial storehouse for swallowed material and as an aid in the chemical breakdown (or digestion) of food substances. Small glands in the wall of the stomach secrete gastric juice, the principal components of which are hydrochloric acid and pepsinogen.

Hydrochloric acid activates pepsin from pepsinogen, tends to kill bacteria that enter the stomach, inhibits the digestive action of ptyalin (an enzyme secreted in the mouth), and helps to regulate the opening and closing of the pyloric sphincter. The action of pepsin is confined to protein, which it splits into simpler forms.

The food contents of the stomach and the gastric secretions are mixed by muscular contractions of the stomach wall. When the food is sufficiently prepared to leave the stomach, it enters the small intestine in a semiliquid form called chyme.

CANCER
For the past several decades, stomach cancer has been occurring less and less frequently in the United States. Today only about six percent of all

cancer deaths can be attributed to cancer of the stomach, as compared with twenty percent twenty years ago.

Although it has been suggested that excessive consumption of alcoholic beverages, habitual drinking of very hot or very cold liquids, and the use of chewing tobacco might cause stomach cancer, there is no scientific proof that any of these factors is involved.

There has been speculation as to the role diet plays in the development of cancer of the stomach. Many experts consider it significant that stomach cancer has been on the decrease during the same time in which great changes in food habits have taken place in the United States. In the past fifty years the consumption of citrus fruits and lettuce has greatly increased. At the same time, the consumption of potatoes, wheat flour, and cabbage has decreased. In high-income diets, larger amounts of beef, milk, and green vegetables have also been introduced. Cancer investigators believe that diet must be at least partially responsible for the downward trend in the incidence of stomach cancer in this country.

It has been suggested that methods of preparing or preserving food may be as important as the foods themselves. For example, a relationship has been suggested between the high rate of stomach cancer in rural Iceland and the practice of eating smoked meat and fish kept in smokehouses for long periods. However, studies have not provided any conclusive findings on what relationship, if any, the process of smoking food has to the development of stomach cancer.

It has long been suggested that cancer of the stomach "runs in families." Several studies have shown that close relatives of stomach-cancer patients are two or three times as likely to develop the disease as are other persons. This increased risk, however, may be caused more by a shared environment than by any inherited susceptibility.

1. Symptoms

The first symptoms of stomach cancer are much like those of less-serious digestive illnesses. Vague digestive discomfort, aggravated by eating, and a distaste for food ordinarily well tolerated are complaints voiced by patients with a variety of diseases, including stomach cancer.

Other symptoms of stomach cancer — blood in the stools or vomiting, rapid weight loss, and pain — are of such a dramatic nature that they are not likely to be ignored. However, by the time these symptoms begin, a malignant tumor may have been present for as long as twenty months. It may have started to spread to the adjacent lymph glands and to other organs such as the liver or lungs.

2. Diagnosis

A thorough physical examination for stomach cancer includes laboratory tests such as a red and white blood-cell count and analysis of the acidity of the stomach contents. Anemia (a condition characterized by a reduction in the number of red blood cells) and achlorhydria (the absence of hydrochloric acid from the gastric secretion) are often found in patients who have or who later develop stomach cancer.

The most important of all diagnostic methods is X-ray examination. The patient swallows a dose of a barium salt. This fills the stomach with a substance through which the X-rays cannot pass. After an appropriate interval the radiologist observes the flow of barium under the fluoroscope. X-rays of various areas of the stomach are taken from several different angles, with the patient in various positions. An experienced radiologist can recognize abnormalities in the outline of the stomach as they show up in the barium X-ray and fluoroscopy.

3. Treatment

The only successful treatment for cancer of the stomach is prompt, surgical removal of the malignant tumor. This operation involves the removal of a part or all of the stomach, depending on the location of the malignancy. Sometimes parts of other abdominal organs, such as the spleen and pancreas, are removed if they are in the immediate neighborhood of the tumor and are believed to be affected.

Substitute stomachs have sometimes been constructed from segments of the colon or the small intestine, but many surgeons no longer follow this procedure. Any postoperative difficulties in digestion can largely be prevented by a diet low in carbohydrates and high in protein and fat, with several small meals daily instead of the usual three.

Survival from stomach cancer is related to the disease's stage at the time treatment begins.

stomatitis — an inflammation of the lining of the mouth, tongue, or gums.
See aphtohous stomatitis.

strabismus — a deviation of the eye that the patient cannot overcome. Strabismus is often referred to as crossed eyes. This condition requires treatment by a specialist, because crossed eyes do not cure themselves.

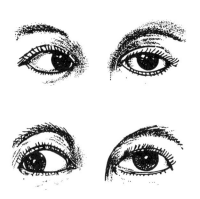

STRABISMUS

strain — an injury caused by the forcible overstretching or tearing of a muscle or a tendon. Strains are caused by lifting excessively heavy loads, by sudden or violent movements, or by any other action that pulls the muscles beyond their normal limits.

The symptoms of a strain are pain, lameness or stiffness (sometimes involving knotting of the muscles), moderate swelling at the site of injury, and discoloration caused by the escape of blood from injured blood vessels into the tissues. The treatment for a strain is usually limited to rest, elevation of the injured part, and the application of cold compresses or an ice bag.

strangulation — the forced stoppage of a flow of oxygen or of blood. When strangulation involves oxygen, the usual cause is a blockage occurring within the respiratory system. When strangulation involves the flow of blood, the cause is often a body organ that has shifted or been forced out of place and which is caught and held in an improper position.

streptococcus — a bacterium that is round or spherical and occurs in chains. Infections caused by these microorganisms tend to involve a widespread problem within the body.

streptomycin — an antibiotic drug discovered during World War II. Streptomycin was an important addition to the previously established an-

tibiotic drugs because it attacked certain types of microorganisms against which penicillin was not effective. Today streptomycin is used in the treatment of tuberculosis. It is also used to treat tularemia, peritonitis, etc. Streptomycin can cause many different side effects. These range from an allergic reaction to hearing loss.

stroke — a sudden interruption of the blood supply to a part of the brain, caused by the obstruction or rupture of an artery. A stroke is also called a cerebrovascular accident, apoplexy, or an apoplectic stroke.

The cells of the brain require a good blood supply in order to work properly, more so than most other cells in the body. Blood flow to and from the brain is by way of a complex network of blood vessels — arteries and veins. The main arteries of the brain branch off into smaller and smaller branches that carry blood to every part of the brain.

If anything happens to reduce significantly or to stop the flow of blood to any part of the brain, that part will not function properly; this may cause weakness or numbness or loss of sensation or of movement in some part of the body. The decrease or loss of function depends on the extent of damage. The part of the body affected depends on the area of the brain involved and is usually on the side of the body opposite to the affected side of the brain.

SYMPTOMS
A stroke can occur while a person is awake or asleep. If it happens while he is awake, he may suddenly fall to the floor because of paralysis of one of his legs, or he may suddenly become unconscious. If the stroke occurs while the patient is asleep, he may be found unconscious, or he may fall as he attempts to get out of bed. In about half of all stroke cases, the patient experiences some difficulty with his speech.

CAUSE
There are five important ways in which a stroke may occur.

1. *Hemorrhage (bleeding)*
The wall of an artery of the brain may break, permitting blood to escape and thus damage the surrounding brain tissue.

2. *Thrombosis (clot formation)*
A clot of blood may form in an artery of the

brain and may stop the flow of blood to the part of the brain supplied by the clot-plugged artery.

3. *Embolism (blocking of a vessel by a clot floating in the bloodstream)*

A clot from a diseased heart or, less commonly, from elsewhere in the body may be pumped to the brain and stop up one of the brain's arteries.

4. *Compression (pressure)*

A tumor, swollen brain tissue, or a large clot from another vessel may press on a vessel of the brain and stop its flow of blood.

5. *Spasm (tightening and closing down of the walls of an artery)*

An artery of the brain may constrict and thus reduce the flow of blood to an area of the brain. If the spasm is of short duration, permanent damage does not necessarily occur.

There are a number of causes for the five different ways in which the circulation of blood to the brain may be disturbed. These include defects of the vessels that may develop before birth, physical injury, infections of the blood vessels, general infections, blood diseases, heart disease, hardening of the arteries, and high blood pressure.

TREATMENT AND REHABILITATION

Most cases of stroke are not fatal. Some patients recover from a stroke within a few weeks or months; in others, varying degrees of paralysis of an arm and leg and some difficulty in speech may persist. This paralysis of the arm and leg and the lower part of the face on one side is known as hemiplegia (half stroke, or paralysis of one side of the body).

When a person has had a stroke, a physician should be called immediately. The doctor will advise whether the patient should be treated at home or taken to a hospital. In past years there was very little that doctors could do for patients who had strokes. Today, however, there is a much more hopeful attitude, even though present knowledge does not ensure recovery of every stroke patient. Physicians have several methods of treatment to help patients immediately after a stroke has occurred.

Very soon after the stroke has occurred (often within twenty-four hours), treatment should be started to help restore use of the affected arm and leg. This begins with assisted movements of the arm and leg. Within a few days the patient is encouraged to move his own arm and leg. He is gradually encouraged to sit up, then to stand, and finally to walk. The physician may also prescribe a brace or support.

If there is difficulty in speech, retraining should begin early. When the difficulty is great, the help of a speech therapist is desirable. The greatest disability occurs among patients who have suffered damage to the speech centers of their brains (aphasia). Their ability to communicate with others is impaired. The patient may be able to understand what is said to him, although he may not be able to speak. The speech-retraining process is often long and difficult.

PREVENTION

With present knowledge it is not possible to prevent the majority of strokes and other cases of cerebral vascular disease. However, some of the conditions causing cerebral vascular disease can be treated. Such treatment may help prevent strokes. High blood pressure is one of the major diseases associated with strokes, although the exact relationship is not yet fully understood. Most patients with high blood pressure can be helped by modern treatment. Such treatment often reduces some of the effects of cerebral vascular disease and may help prevent strokes.

Strokes among young people are most frequently caused by rupture of a congenital defect in a blood vessel, known as an aneurysm. Under favorable circumstances surgical treatment of such aneurysms may prevent further strokes. Strokes among young persons may also be caused by small blood clots (emboli) formed in the heart and pumped into a blood vessel in the brain. These emboli usually form as a result of rheumatic heart disease or a bacterial infection of the lining of the heart. Both of these conditions can usually be prevented or treated successfully, and possible strokes can thus be prevented.

Several conditions associated with blood-clot formation that often result in strokes can be effectively controlled in many patients by the use of anti-clotting drugs. In some cases warnings in the form of brief attacks of numbness, weakness, or visual difficulty precede the onset of a stroke. Immediate treatment may prevent the stroke.

LITTLE STROKES

Little stroke, minor stroke, and small stroke are names that are used to indicate a stroke that does not seriously handicap the patient. A little stroke may have a fleeting effect on a limited area of the brain or it may produce a permanent but slight effect. A name for this is transient ischemic attacks, or its initials, TIA's. Transient means temporary; ischemic indicates a lack of normal blood supply; attack dramatizes the effect on the brain.

A little stroke might show itself only by a dropping at the corner of the mouth for as short a time as twenty minutes. The patient's speech may be temporarily disturbed. Sometimes a brief tingling may occur in an arm or leg.

stroke volume — the amount of blood that is pumped out of the heart at each contraction of the heart.

strychnine — a substance obtained from the *Strychnos nux-vomica* tree found in India. Strychnine is no longer considered to be a useful drug.
See strychnine poisoning.

strychnine poisoning — poisoning from strychnine, a substance extracted from the *Strychnos nux vomica* tree. Strychnine is sometimes used as a rodent poison. When taken by humans, it acts as a central nervous system stimulant.

SYMPTOMS
The symptoms of strychnine poisoning progress very rapidly. There is a feeling of suffocation, and the face becomes blue. The muscles of the neck become rigid, and the neck itself becomes stiff. Convulsions occur, during which the body of the patient arches upward so that it rests on only the back of the head and the heels of the feet. The patient usually remains conscious until respiration ceases.

TREATMENT
Because strychnine acts so swiftly, prompt medical attention or first aid is needed to save the patient's life. One of the most important parts of immediate treatment is to promote vomiting in order to rid the patient's body of all strychnine that has not yet been absorbed. The faster this can be done, the less strychnine the body can absorb, and therefore the better are the chances for recovery.

sty — an inflammation of one of the sebaceous glands located in the eyelid. They are usually caused by bacteria.

stye — *See sty.*

subclavian arteries — two large arteries that are located beneath the clavicle or shoulder bone. There are a right and a left subclavian artery.

The right subclavian artery is a division of the innominate artery (one of the three branches arising from the arch of the aorta). The left subclavian is a direct branch from the arch of the aorta. These arteries supply blood to the arms and have branches leading to the shoulder, chest wall, and neck.

subcutaneous tissue — tissue located beneath the skin.

sucrose — a complex sugar.

sudden infant death — the sudden, unexpected and unexplained death of an apparently healthy baby. This syndrome attacks infants between the ages of two weeks and two years, but most of these deaths occur when a baby is two to three months old. It is estimated that each year a minimum of 10,000 infants die from sudden infant death. This figure is probably considerably smaller than the actual total, because the nature of the disease or syndrome makes it impossible to list the actual cause of death.

The most constant factor in these unexplained crib deaths (as sudden infant death is sometimes called) is that a healthy child is put to bed and dies while sleeping. In these cases, no evidence is found that the child suffocated.

There are few, if any, symptoms and because the death occurs so suddenly and there is no known cause, there is no treatment or prevention. Researchers are working on different theories related to possible causes. Some of the possible causes are vitamin or enzyme deficiencies and failure of the infant to develop a functioning immunological system.

suffocation — *See asphyxiation.*

sugar — *See carbohydrate.*

suicide — killing oneself. Suicide has ranked among the first ten causes of adult deaths in the United States for most of the past half century. Each year approximately 20,000 people take their own lives.

Of any ten people who kill themselves, eight

have given definite warnings of their suicidal intentions. Most suicidal people are undecided about living or dying, and they gamble with death — leaving it to others to save them. Almost no one commits suicide without letting others know how he is feeling. This cry for help is often given in code. Although a suicidal person is extremely unhappy, he is not necessarily mentally ill.

CRISIS

There are times when the pressures of life seem so intolerable to some people that suicide is seriously considered. This is known as a suicidal crisis. It passes when the pressures are gone or when the person is somehow able to carry on, but the period of crisis is painful and dangerous. Expert help and reassurance are often needed desperately during such a period. There are four main types of suicidal crisis.

1. *Impulsive suicidal behavior*

In the heat of anger, disappointment, or frustration, some people react with impulsive suicidal behavior. For example, a person who has been disappointed in love may walk out in front of a moving car, or young people who are angry with their parents may swallow a number of sleeping pills or cut their wrists. This kind of emotional state usually subsides quickly. Most impulsive people learn to control their actions.

2. *The feeling that life is no longer worth living*

A serious suicidal potential exists in the person who has come to feel (over a period of time) that life no longer has any meaning, or that he is no longer wanted or needed, or that he simply cannot go on in the face of what may seem like insurmountable difficulties. If these feelings are severe or last for some time, they may indicate a serious psychological condition called depression. The individual may not realize this. He may find it difficult to believe that such feelings do go away and that when the depression is gone he will once again feel that life is worth living. The key fact is that depressions typically "run their course" and disappear.

3. *Very serious illness*

The person who is in constant pain or who believes he has an incurable illness may think of suicide as an escape from suffering. Some, although willing to endure pain, do not want to impose the burden of a long and expensive illness on their loved ones.

4. *Communication suicide attempts*

Sometimes the motive behind a suicide attempt is to communicate some message to another person or to change the behavior of other people, rather than to commit suicide. This may also be an angry effort to strike back at someone, or to persuade him not to take an unwanted action, such as divorce or separation. The individual whose private life is so unhappy that he thinks of suicide as a way out does not usually recognize that such behavior increases his difficulties by arousing guilt and hostile feelings in those closest to him.

A person making an apparent suicide attempt (but not really planning to die) is gambling with death. Something may go wrong with his plans for being rescued. In many cases of "accidental" suicide, the person making the attempt could not reach his would-be rescuer by phone; someone did not come home at the proper time; the trip to the hospital was delayed; or some other unforeseen event occurred. There are also cases where a "mild" dosage of sleeping pills or other medication proved fatal because of some unusual physical reaction. What was meant to be merely a communication became, instead, an actual suicidal death.

PREVENTION

The person who is seriously thinking of suicide is undergoing a crisis in which he is not his normal self. During this crisis such an individual needs help to protect him from himself. This is an unnatural experience in his life, and he needs help just as surely as though he were fighting a severe physical illness. Even a mild suicide attempt indicates a desperate need for sympathy and understanding. More serious suicidal activity may follow if help is not forthcoming. Every effort should be made to get at the cause of the unhappiness and to remedy the situation in a truly satisfactory manner. In addition, the individual should be watched carefully for at least ninety days after the suicidal crisis, since other attempts often occur in that period.

sulfonamides — a class of drugs used to treat infections that are caused by bacteria. The sulfonamides were the first effective drugs to be used this way. These drugs were used extensively during World War II while research scientists were testing penicillin and other antibiotics. The great advantage the sulfonamides had were the relative ease with which they were produced and the small cost involved.

The use of sulfonamides has been greatly reduced by the discovery of drugs that are more effective and that have less-toxic side effects. However, the sulfonamides are still used in conjunction with antibiotics.

sulfones — a class of drugs used in the treatment of leprosy. The sulfone drugs have proved to be so effective that they are now the first choice of most physicians for treating leprosy. However, the sulfone drugs can have a number of unpleasant and sometimes serious side effects. Consequently, patients being treated with these drugs are always watched very carefully.

Included in this class of drugs are dapsone, cimedone, promizole, etc.

sulfur — a pale-yellow, naturally occurring element. Sulfur has been used for centuries as a medicine. Today it is used to treat infections or problems caused by fungus or by parasites. Additionally, sulfur is used for skin diseases and disorders such as psoriasis and seborrhea.

summer hay fever — *See hay fever.*

sunburn — a burn inflicted by sunlight. Skins differ in their sensitivity to sunlight. Children burn more quickly than adults. People with fair skins are quicker to burn than are people with darker skins. Some people never develop a tan and burn every time they stay out in the sun. Extreme sunburn can be as serious as other types of burns.
See burn.

sunstroke — *See heatstroke.*

superinfection — an occasional complication that follows the use of antibiotics for the treatment of infections. A superinfection occurs when the antibiotic upsets the natural balance of microorganisms that normally live in the body. These microorganisms cause no harm until the balance is changed, then they can multiply sufficiently to cause a serious infection.
See antibiotic.

suppository — a medicine in a solid form that can be inserted into the rectum, vagina, or urethra. The medicine dissolves once it enters the body. Rectal suppositories are sometimes used as laxatives.

Additionally, they are used when a patient has a severe upset stomach and cannot take any medication by mouth.

suppuration — the formation and discharge of pus in or from the body.

suprarenal gland — *See adrenal gland.*

surgery — any procedure that involves opening or cutting a body part or organ. Surgery is divided into two types of operations: minor surgery and major surgery.

Minor surgery can often be performed in a physician's office. Minor surgery includes such simple procedures as removing a mole, opening a boil, and removing an impacted tooth (usually a molar).

Major surgery is more serious. It is almost always performed in an operating room, and usually the patient must be given a general anesthetic. Major operations include repairing an ulcer, heart surgery, etc.

suture — the closing of a wound by artificial means and the material used to do so. Sutures may be divided into two classes: absorbable and nonabsorbable.

Absorbable sutures are absorbed by the tissue fluids. They are usually used in the deeper layers of the wound. Plain catgut is an example of the type of material used as an absorbable suture. Nonabsorbable sutures are not absorbed by body tissues. They are usually used to close the skin. They consist chiefly of silk, cotton, synthetic material, and rust-proof wire (stainless steel).

Needles used in suturing are either round or cutting, straight or curved. They vary in length, thickness, and shape, depending on the type of suturing used. In suturing the skin, the cutting type is often preferred; a round type is usually used for deep sutures or when suturing is necessary near blood vessels.

swallowing — the process by which food and liquids pass from the mouth, down the digestive tract, and into the esophagus. The material is pushed to the back of the mouth and down the throat. As this happens, the epiglottis (the flap at the top of the trachea, or windpipe) covers the entrance into the trachea, thus forcing the material to enter the esophagus.

sweat — a colorless liquid excreted by the sweat glands. Sweat consists of water, salts, and small amounts of nitrogenous wastes. It has a salty taste and may have a distinct rancid odor, or it may have no odor at all.

See sweat gland.

sweat gland — a coiled, tubular gland embedded in the dermis. Sweat glands are surrounded by small tufts of capillaries. These glands, located partly in the subcutaneous tissue, open by ducts to the surface of the skin. The sweat glands excrete sweat, also called perspiration. Sweat is a clear, colorless, slightly acidic liquid.

The sweat glands are constantly excreting sweat. However, this takes place so gradually that it evaporates as fast as it is formed. This is called insensible perspiration, meaning perspiration that cannot be sensed or felt. When the outside temperature is high, body temperature rises as it does when the body is exercising. The sweat glands then excrete excessive amounts in order to cool the body through evaporation of sweat. When evaporation cannot handle all that has been excreted, the sweat collects in beads on the surface of the skin. This is called sensible perspiration.

Normally, the sweat glands excrete about one liter of sweat a day.

See sweat.

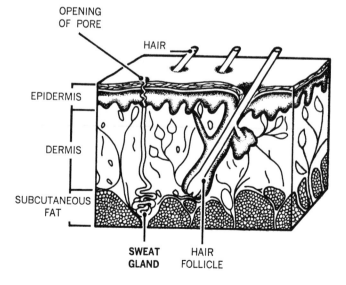

OPENING
OF PORE

HAIR

EPIDERMIS

DERMIS

SUBCUTANEOUS
FAT

SWEAT
GLAND

HAIR
FOLLICLE

SWEAT GLAND

Sydenham's disease — *See St. Vitus' dance.*

symbiosis — a relationship between two organisms in which one organism harbors or nourishes another organism. There are two types of symbiotic relationships. The relationship may be mutually beneficial to the two partners, in which case it is called mutualism. However one organism may injure, destroy, or live at the expense of the other. This type of relationship is called parasitism. Communicable diseases are manifestations of parasitism.

sympathectomy — an operation that interrupts some part of the sympathetic nervous system. (The sympathetic nervous system is part of the autonomic or involuntary nervous system and normally regulates tissues not under voluntary control.) Sometimes the interruption is accomplished by drugs. This is called a chemical sympathectomy.

See sympathetic nervous system.

sympathetic nervous system — one of two parts of the autonomic nervous system. With the parasympathetic nervous system, the sympathetic nervous system regulates tissues not under voluntary control, such as the glands, the heart, and the smooth muscles.

One function of the sympathetic system is to increase the activity of the body to enable it to meet danger or undergo physical activity. Consequently, it is sometimes called the "fight or flight" nervous system.

The sympathetic system, in general, acts in opposition to the parasympathetic system. The two opposing functions tend to keep the body in delicate balance.

symptom — any subjective evidence of a patient's condition. A symptom is something a patient feels. It differs from a sign in that it usually cannot be measured accurately. For example, a sign might be an elevated temperature, while a symptom might be a pain in the abdomen.

synapse — the small space between two nerves. The nerve impulse from one nerve jumps across the synapse to reach the next nerve.

syncope — a faint. A frequent cause for syncope is an insufficient supply of blood to the brain.

syndrome — a set of symptoms that occur together and are therefore given a name to indicate that particular combination.

synergists — drugs that work together. The combined effect of the drugs is greater than the normal effects of the separate drugs.

synovial membranes — membranes that serve as linings for joints. These membranes secrete a very small amount of fluid.

syphilis — a venereal disease. Syphilis is caused by the *Spirochaeta* or the *Treponema pallidum* microorganism. With the exception of transmission from mothers to babies, syphilis is transmitted by intimate body-to-body, skin-to-skin contact. The syphilis germ usually enters the body through the skin in or around the sex parts. The incubation period is variable: from ten to ninety days; but the average is about three weeks.

SYMPTOMS
The first sore or primary lesion of early syphilis usually appears at the site of the entrance of the microorganism into the body; however, it may appear on another part of the body, such as the fingers or the lips. This sore is called a chancre. It may look like a pimple, a blister, or an open sore. The chancre may last from one to six weeks and will heal with or without treatment. Generally, it causes no pain or itch and may even go unnoticed because of its location or size. This phase of syphilis is known as the primary stage.

Secondary syphilis may appear in the form of a spotty skin rash (often faint copper in color) and is usually accompanied by enlarged lymph nodes. This rash appears three to eight weeks or longer after the appearance of the chancre. There may also be papules (raised bumps), sore throat with patches in the mouth, and partial loss of hair. Other symptoms such as headache, general weakness, fever, and joint pains may appear. These secondary signs usually disappear within about three weeks after appearance. If untreated, they may reappear one or more times as relapses.

Latent syphilis is that stage of the disease in which clinical signs and symptoms of infection are absent. Latent syphilis is subdivided into early or late latent syphilis at a point four years after the onset of infection.

Late syphilis (formerly called tertiary syphilis) follows secondary syphilis after a latent period of from one to twenty years. Among the infinite variety of manifestations of this stage may be blindness, insanity, vascular disease (disease of the heart or blood vessels), loss of balance, atropic arthritis, and destructive ulcers of the skin or mucous membranes.

TREATMENT
Syphilis can be treated with penicillin when it is diagnosed and treated early enough.

CONGENITAL SYPHILIS
In the pregnant woman, syphilis can be passed on to the child. The syphilis germ can pass through the placenta and infect the baby. This may cause the death of the baby either before or after birth. A baby that is born with congenital syphilis may have severe physical or mental defects.

systemic circulation — the circulation of the blood through all parts of the body except the lungs. The flow is from the left lower chamber of the heart (left ventricle), through the body, and back to the right upper chamber of the heart (right atrium).
See pulmonary circulation.

systemic poisons — poisons that affect the body as a whole through their action on various systems, organs, or tissues. The systemic poisons are divided into two general groups: depressants and convulsants.

The depressant poisons have the general action of a narcotic drug: they produce sleep, with progressive lowering of the vital functions of the circulation and of respiration. The convulsant poisons produce spasms or convulsions, with rapid paralysis of the vital functions of the circulation, the respiration, or both.

systole — the period during each heartbeat when the heart contracts. Atrial systole is the period of the contraction of the atria or upper chambers of the heart. Ventricular systole is the period of the contraction of the lower chambers of the heart, the ventricles.

t

tablets — a form of medicinal dosage. Tablets are made by molding or compressing medicinal substances into disks. This is one of the most popular ways of administering drugs.

tachycardia — an abnormally fast heart rate. Generally, anything over one hundred beats per minute is considered tachycardia.

tachypnea — an excessive rate of respiration.

talipes — a birth defect of the foot in which the foot is misshapen or not in the proper position. Talipes is sometimes referred to as clubfoot.

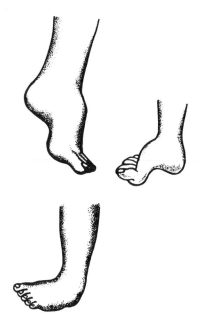

TALIPES

talus — one of the bones of the ankle. The talus (or astragalus) joins with the lower end of the tibia (one of the two bones of the lower leg).

tannic acid — one of the most valuable astringents (drugs that have the power to contract tissue). It is derived from vegetables.

Tannic acid is used externally in the form of an ointment or spray of a weak solution. It checks secretion in weeping ulcers, bedsores, and similar conditions. It is also used in the treatment of local hemorrhage, in ointment or suppository form in the treatment of hemorrhoids, and occasionally as a chemical antidote in alkaloidal or heavy-metal poisonings.

At one time, tannic acid was used extensively in the treatment of burns. However, it has now been replaced by chemicals that are as effective (or more so) and that do not cause a crust to form.

tapeworm — a flat, ribbonlike parasite sometimes found in the intestines of human beings. About twenty-six different species have been identified in man, but many of these are very rare. The three chief forms that infect people in the United States are beef and fish tapeworms (acquired by eating infected beef or fish that has not been cooked long enough) and dwarf tapeworms, which are spread by unsanitary handling of food.

Although these more common tapeworms seldom produce much physical disturbance, in a few cases the worms do cause abdominal pain, nausea, or diarrhea. Simply knowing that the worms are in the intestine is cause for worry and sometimes brings on mental depression.

The head of a tapeworm has muscular suckers

or hooklets that fasten to the intestines of the host (the person or animal that provides food and lodging for the parasite). Its body is a chain of oblong segments. In most species, segments filled with eggs continually separate from the chain and pass in the feces. Other egg-filled segments develop until a tapeworm may have as many as 4,000 units and be fifteen to thirty feet long.

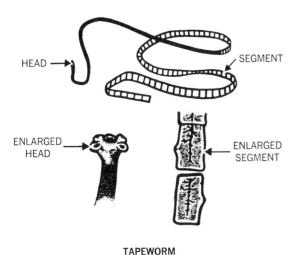

HEAD

SEGMENT

ENLARGED HEAD

ENLARGED SEGMENT

TAPEWORM

TYPES

Although there are many different types of tapeworms, only three are fairly common in the United States.

1. Beef tapeworm

This large tapeworm infects people of all ages in various parts of the United States. It is especially common among people who often eat infected raw beef that has not been inspected. The beef tapeworm is from twelve to twenty-five feet long and sometimes has enough segments to fill a two-quart container. Its head is small, with four cuplike suckers.

Cattle pick up the eggs of this worm while grazing on moist pasture contaminated with infected human feces or with sewage containing tapeworm eggs. The eggs hatch into larvae in the animal's small bowel. The larvae bore through the intestinal wall, enter the bloodstream, and lodge in the muscle tissues, where they develop a protective capsule. They then appear as cysts about ¼ inch in diameter.

When people eat uncooked infected meat, the capsule is digested, and the head and neck of a new worm are set free. A tapeworm attached to the wall of the human intestine will mature and grow segments in two to three months. New segments will continue to grow and produce eggs as long as the head of the tapeworm is attached to the wall. The eggs passed in a person's feces must then go through the life cycle in cattle to be able to infect another human being.

2. Dwarf tapeworm

This is a small tapeworm, about an inch long, that needs no intermediate host as the beef tapeworm does. Dwarf tapeworm eggs are expelled in human feces. If they are swallowed by a human being, they hatch in the person's intestines and develop into mature worms. Tapeworm eggs from human feces can be deposited on foods by infected food handlers who neglect washing their hands after using the toilet.

Much more frequent in children than in adults, dwarf tapeworms often infect members of a single household or persons in an institution. These worms are common in the southern region of the United States.

3. Fish tapeworm

Fish tapeworms have been known to live sixteen years and grow up to thirty feet long. When infected human feces are discharged into fresh water, the eggs mature and six-hooked embryos escape into the water. These develop into their first stage after having been eaten by small shellfish. When freshwater fish eat infected shellfish, the tapeworms mature into their second larval stage in the flesh of the fish. People may get the infection by eating raw or insufficiently cooked fish.

Fish tapeworms are less common than beef and dwarf tapeworms in the United States, but they are found in Canada, northern Michigan, and Minnesota. Infected fish shipped from endemic areas may be the source of much of this infection.

DIAGNOSIS

The only definite indication of beef tapeworm is segments in the stools. Pork tapeworms, although rare in the United States, give off similar segments, and treatment for infection should be given at once, because this species may seriously menace health, especially when the larvae lodge in the eye, heart, and central nervous system.

The presence of dwarf tapeworm is seldom suspected. Diagnosis of infection may be made accidentally while stools are being examined for some other reason.

Diagnosis of fish tapeworm is similarly made, because the eggs can be seen only under a microscope. This parasite may cause anemia in some patients.

TREATMENT

The specific treatment depends on the type of tapeworm and on the individual patient. Frequently, drugs are used as part of the treatment.

tarsus — the ankle. There are seven tarsal bones that form the ankle.

taste — the sensation of food and liquids in the mouth. Taste buds are located in the tongue. The sense of taste is limited to sour, sweet, bitter, and salty. Many foods that are "tasted" are actually smelled, and their taste depends on their odor. This is obvious to the patient who is suffering from a cold and whose sense of smell is partially impaired.

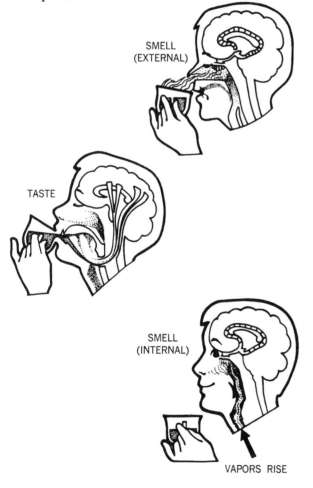

SMELL (EXTERNAL)

TASTE

SMELL (INTERNAL)

VAPORS RISE

TASTE

Tay-Sachs disease — an inherited disorder that destroys the nervous system and is always fatal. Tay-Sachs disease is caused by the absence of an enzyme (called hexosaminidase) that normally aids in the breakdown of fat. Because of the faulty metabolism, the fat accumulates and affects the tissues.

The disorder usually becomes apparent when the child is approximately six months old. After the first symptom appears, there is an increasing amount of deterioration, both mental and physical. Very few children with Tay-Sachs disease live to be five years old. By the time death occurs, there is profound mental retardation and an inability to perform even the simplest physical task.

This disorder is found most frequently in Jewish children. However, in order for the child to have Tay-Sachs disease, both parents must have the gene that causes the disorder. Because the gene is recessive (that is, the trait will not appear unless both parents are carriers), there are many more people who are carriers than there are children born with the disorder.

Since there is no treatment or cure for Tay-Sachs disease, scientists are trying to eliminate the disorder through genetic counseling. Thus, couples who are both carriers are made aware of the possibility of having a Tay-Sachs child. A technique known as amniocentesis is used to test the anmiotic fluid of a pregnant woman when the possibility of Tay-Sachs exists. If the test shows that the enzyme is lacking and that the child will have Tay-Sachs disease, an abortion can be performed.

teeth — the bone-like material located in the gums. Only about one third of a tooth (the crown) projects beyond the gums. The crown is covered with a layer of enamel, the hardest of all body tissues. Underneath this are layers of a softer substance, called dentin. The roots, which extend into the jawbone, are covered with cementum, a material that is harder than dentin but softer than enamel.

Inside the dentin is the pulp chamber, which contains tiny blood vessels and nerves that extend through a canal to the end of each root, where they join larger blood vessels and nerves. Front teeth have only one root and nerve. The bicuspids have one or two, and the molars have two, three, or four.

The dentin of the tooth, if exposed by decay or a

crack in the enamel, is likely to be sensitive to hot or cold foods, to pressure, or to sudden shock. The closer the decay approaches to the pulp chamber, the more pain there is.

The roots of the teeth are surrounded by a supportive membrane called the periodontal membrane. Between the roots and the crowns are the necks of the teeth, surrounded by the gingiva, or gums. The gums are, or should be, pink and firm. When irritated or diseased, they become tender and red and sometimes bleed.

PRIMARY TEETH

The baby teeth are formed long before birth. At about six months of age, the first baby teeth appear, usually the lower front ones. These are followed, at more or less regular intervals, by the upper front teeth, the back teeth, and the cuspids (also called eye teeth or canine teeth).

These first teeth are called primary, baby, or milk teeth. There are twenty of them, and their presence in the mouth is essential until the permanent teeth are ready to replace them. The health and proper placement of the baby teeth influence the formation of the child's jaws and his appearance.

With the cutting of the two-year molars or back baby teeth, usually by the age of thirty months, a child has all twenty of his primary teeth.

PERMANENT TEETH

The permanent teeth are formed under the primary teeth. They begin to form in the baby's jaw at about the time he is born.

The first permanent teeth to appear are the six-year molars, one on each side of the upper and lower jaws — a total of four molars. Because they appear at about the sixth year, behind the primary teeth, without interference and without replacing any of the first teeth, they are often mistaken for primary teeth.

However, these six-year molars are very important. They make it possible for the child to chew during the time the primary teeth are being replaced by permanent ones. The position of the six-year molars largely determines the position of the other permanent teeth, which in turn influence the shape of the jaws and the child's appearance. If the six-year molars are lost, the shape of the jaw may be changed, and correction and alignment may be required later.

Normally, permanent teeth that are to replace primary ones will grow beneath the first teeth.

The roots of the first teeth gradually disappear before the incoming second teeth emerge. Finally, only the crowns of the first teeth are left, and they drop out in time. Sometimes a permanent tooth may start to emerge inside or outside its proper place in the mouth. The root of the primary tooth then remains in place. It should be removed by the dentist before the second tooth has been forced out of line.

The permanent teeth erupt into the mouth in approximately this order: the first molars (at the age of six or seven); the central incisors (seven or eight); the lateral incisors (at about eight or nine); the bicuspids (between ten and twelve); the canines (eleven or twelve); the second molars (about twelve or thirteen); the third molars, also known as the wisdom teeth (between the seventeenth and twenty-first year).

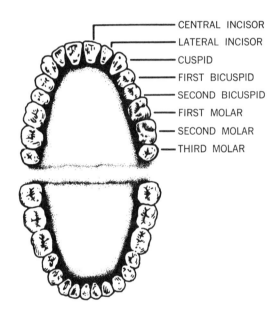

CENTRAL INCISOR
LATERAL INCISOR
CUSPID
FIRST BICUSPID
SECOND BICUSPID
FIRST MOLAR
SECOND MOLAR
THIRD MOLAR

TEETH

teething — the period of time that elapses between the first eruption of a new tooth and the time it is fully in position above the gums.

temperature — a measurement of the body's heat. Normal body temperature fluctuates between 98° F. and 100° F. The average normal temperature is considered to be 98.6° F. However, each individual has a slightly different "normal" temperature.

The center for the control of body temperature is located in the medulla oblongata of the brain.

Other body parts that play a role in regulating the temperature are the skin and the blood.

Essentially, the skin prevents body heat from escaping when the external temperature is below the body temperature, and it helps to release body heat when the external temperature rises and begins to influence the internal temperature. The release of body heat is accomplished through sweat.

Because of its fluid character, blood absorbs heat produced as a result of working muscles and other processes of metabolism. Because of its mobility, the blood distributes the heat throughout the body and to the skin for dissipation to the surrounding air. This function maintains a regular and uniform body temperature. In illness, this mechanism may be disturbed, and fever may result.

tendons — the thin but strong fibrous cords that attach muscles to bones. They are not elastic, but the power of contraction or extension of the muscles, to which they are attached, causes the bones forming joints to move. Tendons make it possible for muscles to apply their force at a considerable distance from their contracting part.

tennis elbow — pain located in the region of the elbow. Tennis elbow is thought by some to be a form of bursitis. Other authorities believe that tennis elbow actually involves some sort of tearing of tissues in the area. It is usually caused by wear and tear (such as occurs in tennis) over a period of time. Treatment may be restricted to avoiding strenuous use of the wrist and elbow or may necessitate some sort of surgery, depending upon the severity of the problem and the way it responds to the simpler forms of treatment.

testes — two oval male glands suspended by the spermatic cords in a cutaneous pouch called the scrotum. The testes perform two functions: the production of spermatozoa (sperm, or male sex cells); and the secretion of an endocrine substance, the male sex hormone. Lying close to each testis is a ductal system that collects and transmits sperm from the testis.

tetanus — a serious disease caused by the tetanus bacillus, a germ that produces a nerve toxin when it grows in deep wounds. The most common symptom of the disease is a painful spasm of the jaw muscles. This accounts for the common name, "lockjaw."

Human infection is most likely to result from wounds that carry the tetanus bacillus deep into the tissues. For example, a puncture wound, such as occurs from a gunshot or from stepping on a nail, is more likely to be followed by tetanus than is a surface abrasion. The germ is often found in and about stables and farmyards and in garden soil treated with animal manure, because the intestines of grass-eating animals harbor the bacillus.

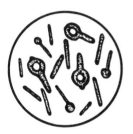

TETANUS BACILLI

SYMPTOMS

The first symptoms of tetanus usually appear from four days to three weeks after the wound becomes infected. The most common early symptoms are stiffness of the neck muscles and painful spasms (contractions) of the jaw muscles. Later in the course of the disease, spasms of other muscles may occur. The patient may be thrown into violent convulsions by any noise or by the slightest jarring.

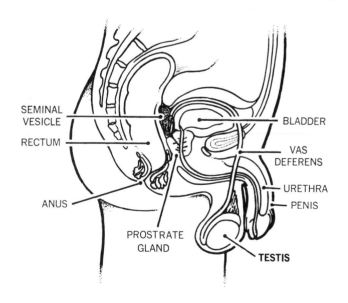

TESTIS

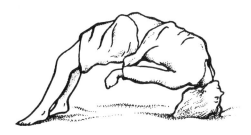

TETANUS SPASM

TREATMENT

Persons who develop symptoms of tetanus must have large doses of anti-tetanus serum as soon as possible after symptoms appear.

Because of the wide adoption of immunization for children and the introduction of new drugs, tetanus is not always fatal. But even today only one-half of its victims survive. Delay in the recognition and treatment of tetanus greatly lessens the chance of recovery. Most of the deaths take place before the tenth day.

tetracycline — a drug and a class of drugs that are antibiotics. This class of drugs was first used in 1948. Since that time, many additional tetracycline drugs have been developed.

The tetracycline drugs are considered to be broad-spectrum antibiotics because of the broad range of their effectiveness. These drugs are used to treat diseases such as syphilis, tularemia, Rocky Mountain spotted fever, as well as infections caused by streptococci and staphylococci.

See antibiotic.

tetralogy of Fallot — a congenital malformation of the heart involving four distinct defects (hence tetralogy). This problem is named for Etienne Fallot, the French physician who described the condition in 1888. The four defects are:

1. An abnormal opening in the wall between the lower chambers of the heart.

2. Misplacement of the aorta, "overriding" the abnormal opening, so that it receives blood from both the right and left lower chambers instead of only the left one.

3. Narrowing of the pulmonary artery.

4. Enlargement of the right lower chamber of the heart.

One of the earliest symptoms of this congenital defect is a blue tinge to the baby's skin, called cyanosis. This coloration is the reason for the term "blue baby." In some cases it is very pronounced; in mild cases, cyanosis may appear only in the lips and fingertips when the baby exerts himself.

In many patients, it is possible to correct the defect through open-heart surgery. In cases where this is not possible, closed-heart surgery may be able to relieve the condition even though the heart defect cannot be corrected.

thalamus — a part of the brain. The thalamus receives information from the sensory nerves and passes the information on to other areas of the brain. The thalamus is frequently compared to an electrical relay station, because it performs a similar function.

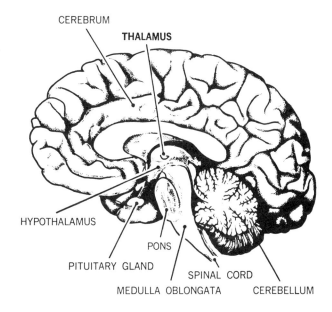

THALAMUS

thalassemia — a disease resembling sickle-cell anemia.

See sickle-cell anemia.

thalidomide — a sedative drug. During the late 1950's and early 1960's the drug was given to pregnant women. Use of the drug during early pregnancy caused severe birth defects. These usually took the form of limb defects, with the affected limb appearing to be more of a flipper than a limb. The drug (used primarily in Europe rather than in the United States) was withdrawn from the list of approved drugs, but not before thousands of children were born with deformed limbs.

therapeutic abortion — *See abortion.*

therapist — a person skilled in the treatment of disease. A physical therapist is a person skilled in the techniques of restoring use to body parts.

thermometer — an instrument for measuring body temperature. A thermometer (or fever thermometer) helps to detect illness, measure its severity, and charts the patient's progress.

It is a slender, hollow tube made of glass, sealed at the top and the bottom, with a bulb at the base that is filled with mercury. When the temperature of the bulb rises, the mercury expands and rises in the tube. The height of the column of mercury, measured on a graduated scale in or on the glass, gives an indication of the temperature.

Mercury is used because it is opaque and can be easily seen; has a low freezing point and is not damaged by normal cold weather; and expands uniformly with a rise in temperature, providing an accurate reading of temperature change.

TYPES
There are three types of fever thermometers. The oral thermometer has a long, thin bulb to fit under the tongue. It is the most sensitive type; it is also the most easily broken.

The rectal thermometer has a larger, pearl-shaped bulb that helps to keep it in place. It is somewhat sturdier than the oral type and is less easily damaged. Rectal readings are usually one degree higher than oral readings.

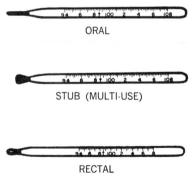

ORAL

STUB (MULTI-USE)

RECTAL

THERMOMETER

The multi-use or security thermometer can be used for either oral, rectal, or axillary (under the arm) readings. It has a short, stubby bulb and is considered to be the safest for use by children. It usually requires a longer time to record (approximately five minutes). Axillary readings are usually one degree lower than oral readings.

USE
To prepare a thermometer, it is necessary to "shake it down"; that is, centrifugal force must be exerted to drive or force the mercury column down to 96.0° F. or lower. This is necessary so that the mercury can rise to the actual temperature of the patient.

After shaking down the thermometer, for oral use the thermometer should be inserted under the tongue and rotated once or twice to ensure complete contact. The thermometer should remain in the mouth (with the lips closed around it) for three minutes. It should then be removed for reading.

thiamine — *See vitamin B.*

thigh — the area of the body between the lower end of the hip and the knee. The bone of the thigh is called the femur. The thigh is usually fairly fleshy and can be quite muscular.

thiocyanate — a chemical that causes the dilation of the blood vessels, thus lowering blood pressure. Thiocyanate is a vasodilator.

thiopental — *See sodium thiopental.*

thorax — a cone-shaped bony cage formed by the twelve thoracic vertebrae in the back, the ribs that terminate in cartilages, and the sternum or breastbone.

throat — the pharynx. The upper portion of the throat is an air passage. The lower portions serve both respiratory and digestive tracts as a common passageway. It is the corridor between the mouth and the esophagus and between the nasal passages and the larynx and trachea.
See pharynx.

thrombectomy — an operation to remove a blood clot from a blood vessel.

thrombocytes — blood platelets. They are round

bodies in the blood that contain no nucleus but contain only cytoplasm. They are smaller than red blood cells and average 250,000 per cubic milliliter of blood. Thrombocytes play an active but still incompletely defined role in the process of blood coagulation.

See blood.

thrombolytic agents — substances that dissolve blood clots.

thrombophlebitis — inflammation and blood clotting in a vein. This condition may be treated with drugs; however, it is sometimes necessary to operate to remove the clot or clots in order to restore proper circulation.

thrombosis — the formation or presence of a blood clot (called a thrombus) inside a blood vessel or in the cavity of the heart. Thrombosis can be very dangerous, depending on the size and location of the blood clot.

A clot of blood may form in a blood vessel (frequently in vessels located in or near a diseased heart) and may then be pumped to the brain, where it can reduce or even stop much of the blood flow to the brain.

A blood clot will often be carried by the blood flow away from its place of origin. The clot will continue to move with the flow until the blood vessel is smaller than the clot. If it becomes lodged in a blood vessel, it can cut off the flow of blood through that vessel. When the clot is a small one, it may not do too much damage. However, large blood clots tend to block large arteries or large veins, causing serious problems. The treatment for a thrombosis may range from drugs to dissolve the clot to an operation to remove it.

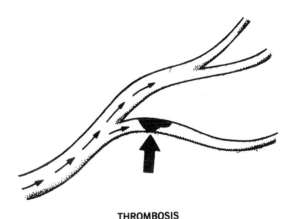

THROMBOSIS

thrombus — a blood clot that forms inside a blood vessel or within the cavity of the heart.

See thrombosis.

thrush — a common, mild infection that causes white spots (rather like milk curds that will not rub off) to appear on a baby's tongue. Occasionally, it will spread to the inside of the cheeks and the roof of the mouth or inner lips. The causative agent in thrush is the *Candida* fungus.

The fungus seems to grow more rapidly when there is a residue of milk left in the mouth. Thrush usually clears up without causing trouble. Frequently the only necessary treatment is to give the baby a drink of cool, boiled water to rinse out the mouth after feeding.

thumb — one of the digits of the hand. The thumb is composed of two bones (in contrast to the four fingers, each of which has three bones). Because of the way the thumb is joined to the hand, it has great freedom of movement. This freedom of movement allows the hand to grasp objects firmly and to perform a wide variety of manual jobs.

thymus — a gland that is now considered to be a part of the lymphatic system, although it formerly was thought to have some endocrine function. In childhood it is a conspicuous gland, lying beneath the sternum. It reaches its maximum development at the age of puberty and then undergoes some changes. At this time, thymic tissue is replaced by adipose (fatty) tissue. During its period of activity, the thymus manufactures lymphocytes, a type of white blood cell.

thyroid gland — a butterfly-shaped gland that is situated in the front part of the neck below the larynx. It consists of two lobes, one located on each side of the trachea, connected by a strip of tissue called the isthmus. The hormone secreted by the thyroid gland is known as thyroxin. This hormone controls the rate of metabolism of the body.

Excessive secretion of thyroxin raises the metabolic rate and causes a condition known as hyperthyroidism. This condition is characterized by a fast pulse rate, dizziness, increase in the basal metabolism, profuse sweating, and a tremendous appetite yet a loss of weight. The eyeballs may protrude (exophthalmos), and enlargement of the thyroid may develop. At first the enlargement can only be felt, but later it is plainly visible in the lower neck (exophthalmic goiter).

Hypothyroidism, the opposite of hyperthyroidism, is caused by an insufficient secretion of thyroxin. The patient exhibits a decrease in basal metabolism, and sweating is almost absent. There may be weight gain and a continually tired feeling. The heart rate may be slow. There may be an enlargement of the gland called simple goiter. To prevent simple goiter, iodine-containing foods such as vegetables, iodized salt, and sea food should be eaten.

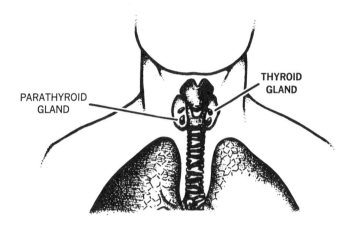

THYROID GLAND

thyrotoxic — pertaining to the overactivity or the abnormal activity of the thyroid gland.
See thyroid gland.

thyrotropic hormone — a hormone that influences the thyroid gland, stimulating the thyroid gland to secrete its hormone (thyroxin). Thyrotropic hormone is secreted by the anterior lobe of the pituitary gland, which is located at the base of the brain.
See pituitary gland, thyroid gland.

thyroxin — a hormone secreted by the thyroid gland. Thyroxin controls the rate of metabolism in the body.
See thyroid gland.

tibia — the larger of the two lower leg bones (the other is the fibula). The tibia is situated on the inner side of the leg; the fibula is on the outer side. The upper end of the tibia joins with the femur (the bone of the upper leg or thigh) and with the fibula. Its lower end joins with the talus (one of the bones of the ankle) and also with the fibula. A

prominence or bump that is easily felt on the inner side of the ankle is called the medial malleolus. This is part of the end of the tibia.

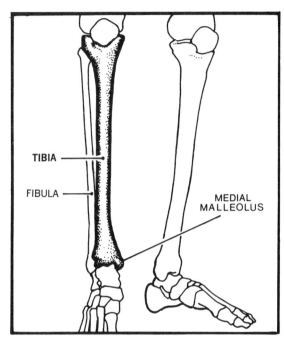

TIBIA

ticks — parasites that are closely related to insects. They are found in most areas of the world, chiefly along pathways in woods or uncleared land. They feed entirely on blood — usually that of animals but sometimes that of humans as well. Attaching themselves firmly to the skin by their barbed piercing organs, ticks suck blood for a period of from fifteen minutes to several days, until they are engorged. While the tick bite itself usually does not cause warning pain (indeed, people are often surprised to find ticks attached to their skin), the wounds caused by the bites of some species are severe. The bites can cause paralysis in young children and animals. Furthermore, ticks may carry Rocky Mountain spotted fever, tularemia, relapsing fever, and a number of other diseases. It is important to avoid tick bites if possible and to remove ticks at once if they do bite.

In removing ticks, great care should be taken to avoid breaking off mouth parts and leaving them embedded in the skin. If the tick is swollen from feeding, special care should be taken not to crush it so that the skin is smeared. A slow, steady pull with tweezers will usually remove the tick. Some people prefer to apply petroleum jelly or fingernail polish to the tick. This will cause it to withdraw its mouthparts, and it can then be removed easily. After removal, the wound should be painted with iodine or other antiseptic, and hands and tweezers should be washed with soap and water or rinsed with alcohol.

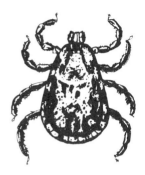

TICK

tidal air — *See respiration.*

tincture — an alcoholic or hydroalcoholic solution that is prepared from vegetable drugs or from chemical substances. Tinctures are used either for their therapeutic content or as flavoring agents or perfumes.

tinnitis — a term used to refer to a wide variety of noises in the ear. These sounds are usually described as buzzing, ringing, etc. Tinnitis can be caused by many problems, including infections, certain drugs, obstructions in the ear, and heart disease. The treatment for tinnitis depends on the exact cause.

tissue — a group of specialized cells that are similar in structure and function.

TYPES

Tissues are classified in five main groups. When these tissues are examined under a microscope, it is obvious that the cells of different tissues differ widely. Muscle cells are comparatively large and are shaped like long, slender rods; red blood cells are small, flat disks; and skin cells look like irregular blocks or scales.

1. Epithelial tissue

In this group are the free surface of the skin and linings of the digestive, respiratory and urinary tracts, of blood and lymph vessels, of serous cavities, and of the tubes of secreting glands such as the liver and kidneys.

2. Connective tissue

Connective tissue is the supporting tissue for the cellular layers of the body. This tissue, with its many varieites, is the most widespread tissue in the body. It surrounds cells, encases internal organs, sheathes muscles, wraps bones, encloses joints, composes the blood, and provides the supporting framework of the body.

Structures of connective tissue differ widely. Delicate, tissue-paper-thin membranes; strong, tough cords; rigid bones; and liquid blood are all made of connective tissue. Cells predominate in epithelial tissues with very little intercellular material; in connective tissues just the reverse is true. There is a large amount of intercellular substances, and comparatively few cells are found in connective tissues.

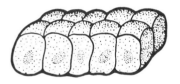

CUBOIDAL
EPITHELIAL TISSUE

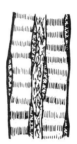

VOLUNTARY
MUSCLE
TISSUE

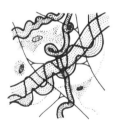

CONNECTIVE
TISSUE
(AREOLAR)

TISSUE

3. Muscular tissue

This type of tissue provides all movement of the body. Muscle tissue is divided into two categories: voluntary muscle fibers and involuntary muscle fibers. The voluntary muscle fibers are striated (or striped) and are under the control of the will. They move the skeleton the way the biceps muscle helps to move the arm. Involuntary muscle fibers are unstriated and are not under the control of the will. The muscles of the stomach are an example of involuntary muscle fibers. (Heart muscle, composed of a special, branched type of cell, is involuntary, although it is striated.)

4. Blood and lymph tissue

Although these are not fixed tissues, they may be considered as tissues consisting of free-flowing cells in body fluids or the bloodstream.

5. Nervous tissue

This tissue is found in the substance of the brain, spinal cord, and nerves that receive and transmit stimuli. Nerve tissue is composed of nerve cells, nerve fibers, and supporting tissue between the cells and fibers that keeps them in their proper position. This type of tissue is the most highly specialized tissue in the body and requires oxygen and nutrition to a higher degree than any other body tissue.

tissue culture — the technique of growing plant or animal cells in containers outside the body by using a medium that contains a variety of nutrients.

Tissue culture is a useful technique for studying cells. In this procedure (first introduced in 1907), a small fragment of tissue, usually from an embryo, is placed in blood plasma and maintained in a small flask under sterile, moist, warm conditions. The cells from the tissue will continue to grow and divide. They can be observed under the microscope and can be photographed. Cancer cells, too, can be grown in tissue culture. This is one way that research scientists study cancer cells.

tissue fluid — the fluid that continuously bathes all tissue cells of the body. This fluid is formed by leakage of blood plasma through minute pores in the capillaries. There is a continual interchange of fluids of the blood and tissue spaces with a free interchange of nutrients and other dissolved substances. Most of the tissue fluid returns to the circulation by means of venous capillaries that feed into the larger veins.

Large protein molecules that have escaped from the arterial capillaries cannot reenter the circulation through the small pores of the venous capillaries. However, these large molecules and, in addition, dead cells, bacterial debris, injected substances, and larger particulate matter can pass through the larger pores of the lymphatic capillaries and thus enter the lymphatic circulation with the remainder of the tissue fluid.

tocopherol — *See vitamin E.*

toe — one of the digits of the foot. The bones of the toes are similar in structure and arrangement to those of the fingers.

The toes are very important because they help the body to balance itself when standing.

toilet training — the method by which a child learns how to control his bowels and bladder. Control of these functions is more complicated than it might appear. Learning to control the bowel and bladder is a job that a baby cannot learn until his body develops sufficiently.

From birth on, the bladder and intestine empty automatically. To empty them is the natural thing to do. To hold back is somewhat harder, and it is even more complicated to empty them at precisely the right time and place.

There are many different methods used to help toilet train a child. The one thing most methods have in common is the use of applause for proper action and restraint from scolding or punishing improper action.

tolerance — a term used to indicate that the body no longer responds as strongly to a foreign substance as it did when the substance was first introduced into the body. Today the term is generally used in connection with drug abuse.

When certain drugs (such as narcotics or amphetamines) are taken over a period of time, the body adjusts to the drug or develops a tolerance for it. As a consequence, the person taking the drug needs to take increasingly larger doses to get the same effect. Many drug abusers build up a tolerance that allows (or forces) them to take an amount of the drug that could kill the average person who has developed no such tolerance.

The body does not develop a tolerance for all drugs. For example, the body will not develop a tolerance to aspirin. This means that under similar circumstances, aspirin will have the same effect even it if is used every day.

Once the use of a drug stops, the body begins to lose its tolerance for that drug, and, after an interval of time, the original dose is effective again.

tongue — a muscular organ attached to the lower jaw at the back of the mouth. The tongue is involved in taste, speech, mastication (chewing), and swallowing. Different areas in the tongue contain taste buds for specific taste sensations. However, the only tastes the tongue can perceive are sour, sweet, bitter, and salty.

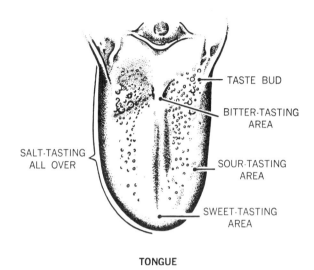

TONGUE

tonometer — an instrument for measuring eye pressure.

See glaucoma.

tonsillectomy — an operation that is performed to remove the tonsils.

tonsillitis — an inflammation of one or of both tonsils.

tonsils — two small, spongy masses of tissue at the back of the throat. Tonsils are composed of lymphatic tissue and are oval in shape. The function of the tonsils is similar to that of other lymphatic tissue: tonsils help to combat germs. They become involved whenever a patient has a cold or a throat infection. After repeated respiratory troubles, they may remain so swollen that they can interfere with breathing or swallowing. This occurs most frequently in childhood. If the situation becomes urgent, the physician may suggest that they be removed.

Until fairly recently the tonsils were removed in a general attempt to improve a child's health in some vague way. This is not the case today.

torticollis — *See wry neck.*

touch — a sensation received when the body comes in contact with itself or with a foreign object. Nerve endings for touch are widely distributed in the skin and mucous membranes. The receptors for touch are bare nerve endings juxtaposed to hairs and specialized encapsulated endings called Meisner's corpuscles. Some areas of the body are more sensitive (because they have more receptors) to touch than are other areas. For example, the skin of the back possesses relatively few touch receptors, while the fingertips have a great many touch receptors.

tourniquet — a constricting band that is used to cut off the supply of blood to an injured limb. Tourniquets are used when a person has been bitten by a poisonous snake or when the control of hemorrhage is difficult or impossible by any other means. (The proper use of a tourniquet in cases of snakebite is discussed under a separate entry.)

Basically, a tourniquet consists of a pad, a band, and a device for tightening the band so that the blood vessels will be compressed. A variety of materials can be used to improvise tourniquets. It is important, however, that the band be flat, because materials such as ropes, wires, or very narrow pieces of cloth will cut into the flesh. A short stick can be used to twist the band, thus tightening the tourniquet.

HEMORRHAGE

A tourniquet must always be applied above the wound, that is, toward the body, and it must be applied as close to the wound as possible. In order to be effective, a tourniquet must be tight enough to stop the arterial blood flow to the limb. If the pressure from the tourniquet is less than the arterial pressure, arterial bleeding will continue. Also, insufficient tourniquet pressure may actually increase the amount of bleeding from the veins. Although it is important to make it tight enough to stop the bleeding, it is also important not to make it any tighter than necessary.

The old technique of using a tourniquet required that it be loosened every fifteen or twenty minutes in order to allow some blood to circulate through the injured limb. It is true that a tourniquet is dangerous and that it can cause the loss of a limb if it is left on too long or if it is improperly applied. However, recent experience has shown that a tourniquet that is correctly applied may be allowed to remain in place for a considerable length of time, with very little risk to the limb. More important, it has been found that in any case where bleeding is severe enough to justify the application of a tourniquet, the danger to life involved in loosening the tourniquet is a much more urgent consideration than any possible risk to the limb. A tourniquet is never put on unless the hemorrhage is so severe that it cannot be controlled in any other way; by the time the tourniquet is applied, therefore, the victim has already lost a considerable amount of blood. The additional loss resulting from loosening the tourniquet may easily cause death. Once a tourniquet has been applied, therefore, it should be released only by medical personnel.

See snakebite.

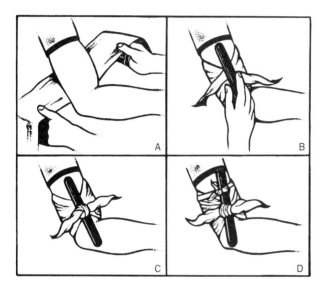

TOURNIQUET

toxemia — the condition caused by poisonous substances in the blood.

toxemia of pregnancy — a complicated disorder that may be associated (in advanced stages) with high blood pressure, marked swelling, marked weight gain, albumin in the urine, headaches, dizziness, blurred vision, nausea, vomiting, abdominal pain, and, in rare cases, convulsions and coma. Despite all these possibilities, no harm comes to the mother or child if the condition is properly treated in the early stages.

Certain conditions increase the likelihood of developing toxemia during pregnancy. Women with diabetes, kidney disease, or heart trouble are especially vulnerable. Additionally, high blood pressure and a previous case of toxemia are also predisposing factors.

The two most serious dangers in this type of toxemia are death of the baby before birth and the possibility of the mother's developing convulsions or eclampsia. These complications are much less common today than they used to be, because most patients now receive good prenatal care. They are more likely to develop in women who do not have the benefit of good prenatal care or who do not heed the advice of their doctors.

TREATMENT

For treatment in moderately advanced cases of toxemia, certain drugs are now available to lower the blood pressure and to ward off convulsions. Even these treatments are unnecessary if the earliest signs are noted and simple precautions are taken. The mother's circulation and kidney function usually return to normal after the birth of the baby.

toxic — pertaining to or referring to poison.

toxic shock — shock that may develop from two to five days after an injury. Toxic or bacterial shock results from the vasodilation of small blood vessels in the internal organs and muscles or after toxins or bacteria enter the bloodstream.

The treatment of toxic shock is directed toward controlling infection (identification of the organism and its sensitivity to various antibodies), increasing the urinary output, and treatment of symptoms as they appear. The prognosis in cases of toxic shock is often poor.

See shock.

toxin — a term used to describe the poisonous substances released by bacteria. The word toxin is usually limited to this usage. When a toxin is produced within the body, the body's defense mechanism tries to control or conquer the toxin. If the particular antibody (or antidote) is already available within the body, the toxin causes little or no harm. However, if the body is unprepared to defend itself against the specific toxin, it may be slightly damaged and the person will feel sick. The illness lasts until the body can manufacture the appropriate antibodies and the antibodies are in sufficient quantity to control or conquer the toxin. In some cases, the body requires outside help in the form of drugs (often antibiotics) to defend itself.

trachea — a long, cylindrical tube that begins at the lower end of the larynx and terminates by dividing into the right and left bronchi (bronchial tubes). The trachea or windpipe is a continuation of the respiratory tract.

It is composed of fibrous membrane in which cartilaginous rings (sixteen to twenty) are embedded.　These give firmness to the walls and prevent their collapse.

The trachea is lined with microscopic waving hairs (cilia) and mucous glands. The action of these parts aid in the entrapment of dust and foreign objects. The cilia also propel both healthy and diseased secretions and waste products from the lungs and bronchi to the pharynx and mouth, where they can be coughed up and spit out.

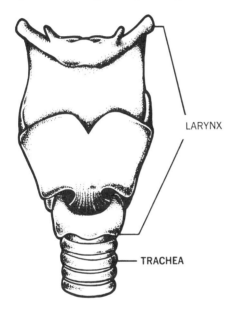

TRACHEA

tracheostomy — an emergency procedure to open the trachea and place a breathing tube through the opening down the trachea. This is a lifesaving procedure and is used only in those instances where an adequate airway must be provided to perserve life. It is performed for relief of asphyxia caused by obstructions of the airway, such as fractures of the trachea, spasm of the glottis caused by a foreign body in the larynx, edema of the larynx, and a prolapsed or swollen tongue, as well as for a number of other similar problems.

Despite the fact that the neck contains many important organs, a tracheostomy is a relatively simple operation. Because the operation is almost always performed in an emergency, the proper special instruments (such as a scalpel and a tracheostomy tube) are rarely available. In emergencies, tools such as sharp pocket knives and razor blades have been used in lieu of the scalpel, and rubber or plastic tubing has been used in place of the silver tracheostomy tube. When regular medical care becomes available (including sterile conditions), corrective work can then be performed.

tracheotomy — an incision into the trachea. *See trachea, tracheostomy.*

trachoma — an infectious disease of the conjunctiva and cornea of the eye. Trachoma produces sensitivity to light, as well as pain, the discharge of tears, and ulceration. This disease can lead to blindness when it is not treated promptly with the proper drugs (usually antibiotics).

traction — a term used to indicate any form of sustained pulling. Traction is used in several different ways. For example, when a leg bone is broken, the limb may be "placed in traction" to help aid in the healing process or to prevent further injury by helping to immobilize the affected area. Traction may also be used as a form of treatment for injuries or problems related to the spinal area. This treatment may help correct existing problems as well as provide relief from pain.

tranquilizers — a relatively new class of drugs. Tranquilizers allay or relieve anxiety and are used to treat mental and emotional disturbances. **Meprobamate** is one of the typical and frequently used tranquilizers. It acts on the central nervous system but has no effect on respiration, heart action, or other autonomic functions.

Tranquilizers differ from sedatives in that tranquilizers allow the patient to perform his normal duties. In fact, they often allow the patient to live a more normal life because they reduce anxiety that can be disruptive.

transfusion — a procedure used when an individual has lost so much blood that he must receive additional new blood to save his life. At other times, transfusions are given to treat anemia or other blood deficiencies. The actual technique used is very simple: blood is withdrawn (by a needle) from a healthy donor and is then injected into the patient (usually through the median cubital vein that crosses the surface of the inside of the elbow bend).

Blood may be classified into four major groups: A, B, O, and AB. Some of these types are mutually incompatible in blood transfusions; others are not. Blood group or type O can, in an emergency, be given to all types. For this reason, blood type O is sometimes referred to as the "universal donor."

Blood incompatibility occurs when the recipient has an immunity to some of the proteins of the red blood cells of the donor. This immunity causes agglutination (clumping of the red blood cells, which clogs the blood vessels in a relatively short amount of time). It also causes hemolysis of the injected red cells. Hemolysis involves the destruction of red blood cells, which allows the escape from the bloodstream of hemoglobin, the blood agent responsible for carrying oxygen. Blood incompatibility can cause severe problems and, in some cases, can be fatal.

Another very important factor in blood transfusions is the Rh factor. This is a protein factor that is a part of most people's red blood cells. It, too, can cause mismatching of blood. Approximately eighty-five per cent of the population has the Rh factor. These people are known as Rh positive. The fifteen per cent of the population who do not have this factor are referred to as Rh negative.

Rh positive blood can never be given to an Rh negative person, even though they both belong to the same blood group. The first transfusion may cause no trouble, but by the time a second transfusion is given, there may be enough antibodies against the Rh positive cells to cause a reaction. This reaction can be as severe as if the transfused blood belonged to a different blood group.

Tests have now been perfected that enable the laboratory technician to determine the suitability of blood for transfusion. These techniques involve crossmatching the blood of both the recipient and the donor.

transmission — a term used to describe the spread of a disease. There are many different ways that diseases may be transmitted. The method of transmission is frequently human contact. This classification includes the transfer of disease through touch, through intimate body-to-body contact, and the transmission of disease germs' through coughing, sneezing, etc.

Other modes of transmission include insects and animals, contaminated or infected food and water, the ground (when an individual walks on it without shoes, or when he handles it), and infected material objects.

Different diseases are transmitted in different ways. Many diseases are spread in only one particular way. For example, syphilis is transmitted only through intimate sexual contact, whereas malaria is transmitted only by the bite of an infected mosquito.

Another way of describing disease transmission involves the manner in which the foreign organism enters the body. For example, tetanus is almost always transmitted through an injury that causes a break in the skin. Pneumonia is transmitted through the respiratory system.

transplantation — the removal of a body organ or body tissue from one individual and placing that organ or tissue in another individual. A transplant is usually performed only to save a life. The dangers inherent in such a procedure are so great that transplant operations are not performed very frequently.

Thus far, the body organ that has been transplanted with the most success is the kidney. The kidney transplant can be extremely successful when it is performed on identical twins. The chances of success decrease when the transplant is performed on two close family members, but the odds are still very good.

The major difficulty in transplantation is the tendency on the part of the recipient's body to react to the transplanted organ as if it were an invading foreign organism. (When transplantation involves identical twins, this problem is very small because of the similarity of body tissues, blood, etc.) The recipient's body tries to defend itself by "attacking" the transplanted organ. When the body succeeds, the organ is "rejected." To counteract this natural body reaction, special drugs are given to the recipient. These drugs suppress the body's ability to react to foreign material and allow the body to accept the transplant as if it were the original body organ instead of a replacement.

During the initial recovery from the transplant operation, while the patient is taking the special drugs, he is very vulnerable to outside infection, because his entire system of immunity is thrown out of balance. For this reason, it is often necessary to keep the patient isolated to protect him.

trauma — any wound or injury. The term is also used to describe a severe mental or emotional shock.

travel sickness — *See motion sickness.*

tremor — an involuntary, uncontrollable movement of trembling or shaking. A tremor is a symptom rather than a disease.

Tremors are classified in several ways. They can be classified by cause: specific diseases, poisoning, and mental disturbance. Tremors are also classified according to when they occur. Some tremors occur only when the affected area is at rest; others occur only when the area is in motion or being used. The treatment for tremors depends on the cause. If the original cause can be cured, the tremors usually disappear.

trench mouth — *See Vincent's disease.*

triamcinolone — a drug used in treating psoriasis. *See psoriasis.*

triceps — a term meaning "three heads." However, the term is commonly used to refer to the triceps brachii, the large muscle located at the back of the upper part of the arm.

trichinosis — a disease caused by tiny worms called trichinae. Trichinosis is most often caused by eating raw or insufficiently cooked pork that is infested with trichinae. However, it can also be contracted by eating the flesh of other animals. It is a preventable disease, because thorough cooking of pork kills the worms or parasites and renders them harmless. The disease is not contagious. It is contracted only by swallowing living trichinae. The seriousness and the duration of a case of trichinosis depend on the number of trichinae that have been ingested and on the patient's resistance.

When a person eats raw or underdone pork or pork products that may contain trichinae, the digestive juices in his stomach dissolve the delicate covering that encases each worm. The liberated worms then travel down into the intestines, where they grow, mate, and bear young.

Each female parasite gives birth to hundreds of larvae. The parent worms eventually die and pass out of the intestinal tract. The tiny young parasites get into the bloodstream and are carried to the muscles. There, each one coils up and is encased in a covering exactly as its progenitors had been in the muscles of the hog. The larvae not only penetrate the muscles, but, during their migrating stage, sometimes get into the lungs,

heart, brain, spinal fluid, and other parts of the body.

SYMPTOMS

Irritation produced by the activity of the worms in the intestines causes nausea, vomiting, and diarrhea. The hundreds of parasites travelling through the body make the patient sick with fever, headache, and prostration — sometimes lasting for several months. These larvae can enter so many organs and cause such a variety of symptoms that mimic other diseases that diagnosis can be difficult.

Symptoms include swelling of the face and other parts of the body, soreness in the eyes, hemorrhages under the skin, pain in the muscles, and difficulty breathing. The patient may show symptoms of heart disease or of brain involvement such as delirium or coma. Fortunately, tests have been developed that aid greatly in making a correct diagnosis.

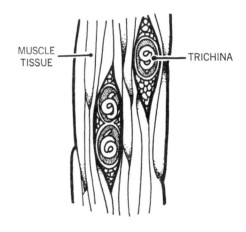

MUSCLE TISSUE — TRICHINA

TRICHINOSIS

TREATMENT

If the infection is recognized within the first few weeks, an attempt can be made to kill the adult worms in the intestine with an agent called a vermifuge. This removes the females before they have produced all their larvae and thus reduces the number of larvae that would get into the muscles. There is no known drug that will kill the larvae after they reach the muscles. Medical treatment is necessary, however, and is given to build up the patient's resistance, to treat symptoms as they arise, and to prevent complication. (Pneumonia sometimes follows the late stages of the disease.) Cortisone has been particularly effective in the alleviation of chronic symptoms, saving patients who might otherwise have died. The death rate from trichinosis is low, and even in severe cases the chance of recovery is good.

PREVENTION

Not all hogs are infested with trichinae, but because there is no way to judge by the appearance of the meat, it is necessary to cook all pork thoroughly — until it is white. When pork contains trichinae, the tiny encased worms are buried throughout the lean meat and are too small to be seen with the naked eye. (Worms, sometimes called "wigglers," which are occasionally found on the surface of hams, are not trichinae.)

Even infected pork cannot cause trichinosis if it is cooked properly. Thorough cooking is necessary for fresh, cured, or smoked pork; and for pork products such as sausages and frankfurters; and also for hamburgers if they contain pork. The amount of heat ordinarily used in smoking hams cannot kill trichinae.

In packing plants operating under Federal inspection, pork products that are usually eaten raw are treated to destroy parasites. When these foods, such as salami, cervelat, mettwurst, and Italian-style ham, have been made safe for eating raw, they are stamped in purple vegetable dye: federally inspected and passed.

Pork should always be cooked thoroughly (except when it has been specially treated as mentioned above). The least sign of pinkness means that a chop has not been cooked enough for safety.

tricuspid valve — a valve consisting of three cusps or

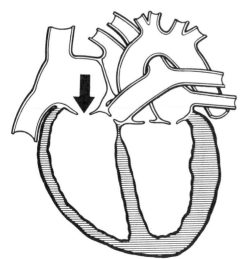

TRICUSPID VALVE

triangular segments; it is located between the upper and lower chamber in the right side of the heart. Its position corresponds to the bicuspid or mitral valve in the left side of the heart.

trigeminal nerve — one of the twelve pairs of cranial nerves. The trigeminal nerve is divided into three parts: ophthalmic, maxillary, and mandibular. It is sometimes referred to as the great sensory nerve of the head, because it supplies the sense of touch, pain, heat, and cold to the skin of the face and to the eyelids, cornea, conjunctiva, mucous membranes of the head, tongue, and teeth. A branch of the mandibular division also supplies motor fibers to the muscles that control chewing, or mastication.

triplets — the birth of three babies as a result of a single pregnancy.

troches — thin, flat disks (often called lozenges) that are placed in the mouth and allowed to dissolve or disintegrate. The medical ingredient (antiseptic, astringent, or anesthetic) in the troches is slowly released to medicate the throat and bronchial areas. Because of the method of administration, only tasteless or pleasant-tasting substances are used as a base.

trochlear nerve — one of the twelve pairs of cranial nerves. The trochlear nerve is a motor nerve. It controls the muscles that turn the eyeball down and to the side.

trophic nerves — specialized nerves that are concerned with the growth, nourishment, and repair of body tissues.

tropical diseases — diseases that occur primarily in tropical areas of the world. Most of these diseases are transmitted by insects or microorganisms that are found only in very warm climates.

trunk — the part of the body between the neck and the pelvis. The trunk is composed of fifty-six bones. It is the major part of the body; all of the extremities and the head are attached to it.

The major supports for the trunk are the spinal column in the back and the rib cage on the sides and in front. Many of the most important body organs, such as the heart, lungs, and liver, are located within the trunk.

truss — a band or similar device used to help support a hernia.

See hernia.

trypanosomiasis — any of several diseases caused by *Trypanosoma protozoa*. One of the diseases is African trypanosomiasis, which is also known as sleeping sickness or African sleeping sickness. This disease is transmitted by the tsetse fly. The term "sleeping sickness" refers to one of the symptoms of the disease, although the symptom is usually extreme apathy rather than actual sleeping.

All trypanosomiasis can be very serious. Fatalities can occur if the central nervous system becomes infected. A variety of drugs are used to treat these diseases, but when the disease is not treated and stopped before it reaches the central nervous system, the drugs are not totally effective.

trypsin — an enzyme produced by the pancreas. Trypsin helps reduce or partially digest proteins. It is secreted from the pancreas into the duodenum.

tsetse fly — a biting fly that ranks second only to the mosquito as a carrier of human disease. Tsetses are the essential carriers of several types of sleeping sickness. There are about twenty-five species of tsetse flies, but only a few of these are of primary importance in human disease.

These flies are usually found only in Africa, south of the Sahara Desert. They are dangerous bloodsucking flies that feed on both man and animals.

tubercle — a small, raised mass on the skin. Tubercle is also the term used to describe the small, round mass that is a symptom of tuberculosis.

tuberculin — an extract made from dead tubercle bacilli (the cause of tuberculosis). In 1890 Robert Koch produced tuberculin while doing research on tuberculosis. Originally, it was thought that tuberculin could both cure and prevent tuberculosis. This was later proved wrong. However, because tuberculin causes a reaction in those who have been infected with tubercle bacilli, it has proved to be a highly valuable testing agent.

The first tuberculin tests were done by injection into the tissues beneath the skin layers. This method sometimes caused severe reactions and scarring, and the reactions were difficult to measure and compare. A safer, more accurate test was introduced by the French physician Charles Mantoux in 1908. In this test, a precise amount of tuberculin is injected between the layers of the skin. If a swelling of a certain diameter or larger develops, the person is considered to be a reactor. This signifies that at some time he has been infected with the tubercle bacillus or one of its close relatives. This test, however, does not tell whether or not the infection was serious enough to cause tuberculosis. Various other methods of skin-testing have been used, but the Mantoux Test is the one used most widely.

See tuberculosis.

tuberculosis — a chronic bacterial infection. Tuberculosis of the lungs is the most frequently encountered form of the disease.

The reaction of some patients to the diagnosis of tuberculosis is one of shame and disgrace, since the disease is frequently associated with poverty, poor living conditions, jails, and homeless men. However, the disease does not recognize social or economic barriers. The death rate from TB (as it is often called) has dropped dramatically since 1900, when it was the leading cause of death. However, TB remains a serious, dangerous disease.

HISTORY

From ancient skeletons, drawings, and sculptures, it is known that the "White Plague" has existed for at least 6,500 years. Yet only in the last decades have there been effective means to control the disease. The accumulation of facts about the cause, nature, diagnosis, treatment, and prevention of tuberculosis has been a long process.

Through the centuries, many superstitions, mistaken theories, and assumptions about tuberculosis gained popularity before being discredited by facts. A commonly held belief among physicians from ancient times into the 18th century was that tuberculosis, like many other diseases, was caused by the imbalance of vital fluids, or "humors," of the body: blood, "yellow bile," "black bile," and phlegm. Many physicians thought of tuberculosis simply as a rapid degeneration, or using up, of the body (hence the old term "consumption" for the disease). Others saw it as a complication of other diseases, such as diabetes and measles. Because tuberculosis is communicable and therefore, unless checked, often develops in many members of the same family, the belief that it was inherited was widespread.

All sorts of substances were proposed as medicines for tuberculosis, including such curious items as elephant's blood, boiled mice, and sugar of roses. Patients were subjected to bleeding and inhalation of smoke or fumes during various periods. It has been said that if the disease did not kill the patients, these "cures" often did.

Modern understanding of tuberculosis began with the revival of the study of anatomy in the 17th century. In 1679 Franciscus Sylvius, a Dutch physician, concluded from a large number of autopsies that the disease, known then as "phthisis," was caused by the formation of small, round masses which he named "tubercles." His observation was a valuable step toward unearthing the cause of tuberculosis, although he was mistaken in his belief that the tubercles were diseased lymph glands.

The specific agent that, when transmitted, caused tuberculosis was still to be identified. However, largely because of the work of Louis Pasteur, the science of bacteriology and the germ theory of disease were attracting much interest and study. Of those who searched for the tuberculosis germ, Robert Koch of Germany was the first to discover the rod-shaped bacterium and to prove that it was the sole cause of tuberculosis. Koch demonstrated the presence of this bacillus in all types of tuberculous tissue. He grew pure cultures of it and by inoculating healthy animals with the cultures, he reproduced the specific disease.

In this research, Koch had enormous problems to overcome. The peculiar characteristics of the tubercle bacillus required a man with great ingenuity and insight to devise ways to strain and culture it. When Koch made known his findings in 1882, his discovery was, and still is, recognized as one of the greatest achievements in bacteriology and in medicine.

SPREAD

A person with active tuberculosis coughs or sneezes into the air tiny, moist droplets — each containing one or more tubercle bacilli. These droplets dry out and become small flecks called "droplet nuclei" — light enough to remain floating about in the air.

The typical setting for infection is a closed room with poor ventilation. If the germs float out into the sunlight, they are quickly killed. In a closed room, another person can easily breathe in these tiny droplet nuclei. However, the body has many natural traps for catching such foreign elements. To infect a person, a droplet nucleus must ride the air deep into the lungs without being stopped. There it becomes embedded, and the germ begins to multiply very slowly.

SYMPTOMS

Unfortunately, the symptoms of tuberculosis are mild and seldom noticed, at least during the early stages. This causes many problems, the most serious of which is postponing early detection and treatment. But the signs to look for are loss of weight, loss of strength and pep, irregular appetite, mild fever in normal circumstances, rapid pulse, cough, chest pains, and a large flow of thick mucus called "sputum" brought up from the lungs by coughing.

Germs such as those causing tonsillitis multiply in a matter of minutes. The TB germ requires about eighteen to twenty-four hours to reproduce itself just once. The tonsillitis germs cause disease rapidly but die out just as rapidly. The TB germ is never in a hurry — it grows slowly and dies slowly.

Even though the germ starts to multiply, the body immediately sets up a defense. It is usually strong enough to stop this growth. At this point, the person has a primary infection. After most primary infections, the disease is stopped for the rest of the person's life. This fact is possible because the germ is content just to infect and then to hibernate without ever developing into disease. Strangely enough, the damage that has been done seldom has any effect on the person's physical well-being.

Sometimes, though, either the body defenses are not strong enough or the germ is too strong, and what is known as "reinfection" results, with the germ causing actual disease. Also, in periods of stress caused by other illnesses or physical or emotional hardships, the sleeping germs of a primary infection from years earlier may suddenly spurt into action, causing disease.

Tuberculosis is usually an insidious disease, with a long dormant period. Some patients have been without symptoms for as long as forty years after being initially infected. Early symptoms of reactivation are often vague. They include tiredness, weight loss, a slight dry cough, slight elevation of temperature, and night sweats. There may be chest pains and a flow of thick mucus.

In about ninety percent of the cases, tuberculosis is found only in the lungs. But occasionally the germ makes its way into the bloodstream to other parts of the body.

DIAGNOSIS

A series of tests are useful for detecting tuberculosis. One of the best is a simple skin test, called the Mantoux Tuberculin Test, which shows whether or not a person has been infected. A positive reaction does not indicate that the person has an active case. A second step, sometimes used as a primary detection technique, is a chest X-ray, which may reveal disease in the lungs. If signs of disease are found on the X-ray, a sputum sample is taken and examined in the laboratory to see if TB bacilli are present.

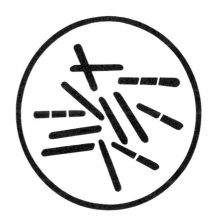

TUBERCULOSIS BACILLI

TREATMENT

Until recent times the treatment of tuberculosis consisted essentially of rest, often in a sanatorium. However, with the development in 1947 of the first drug effective against the tubercle bacillus, the treatment picture has changed. There are now several such drugs, and their use has dramatically shortened hospital stay. Active tuberculosis can be cured in about ninety-five percent of cases with these drugs, but the patient must take these medicines long after he leaves the hospital, usually from eighteen to twenty-four months. One of these drugs (INH) is now used to prevent dormant tuberculous infection from developing into active disease. Drugs also reduce the period of communicability and lessen the risk of reactivation.

Setting up the proper drug regimen is very important and requires extreme care. The patient's particular TB germ may be resistant to one or more of the drugs. Sputum samples containing the live germ are tested against a number of drugs to see how effective each drug is against the patient's germ. Although many antituberculosis drugs are available, the three most important are: INH (isoniazid), PAS (para-aminosalicylic acid), and streptomycin. These drugs are frequently used together in different combinations.

The remarkable and dramatic decline in the death rate from tuberculosis leads many to believe that the disease is no longer a problem and will soon be eradicated. However, many authorities believe that the decline in incidence of the disease is not solely the result of eliminating sources of infection, but rather is brought about by increased resistance through a higher standard of living in the population and early diagnosis and treatment.

tularemia — an animal disease that infects human beings. Named for Tulare County, California, where it was first studied in 1911, tularemia has stricken people throughout the United States and in many foreign countries. The disease is sometimes called rabbit fever.

Tularemia is rarely, if ever, carried from one person to another. It is most commonly acquired by handling the carcass or eating the undercooked flesh of infected animals. The bites of sick animals, or of insects that have bitten sick animals, also spread the disease. People have been infected by drinking water from streams inhabited by diseased animals such as beavers and muskrats.

The most common animal victims of the disease are rabbits. However, a variety of other animals (including dogs and cats) sometimes become infected. Insects and birds are also known to contract the infection. A biting fly, called the deer fly, and certain kinds of ticks are common carriers. A special risk lies in the fact that rabbits and other animals are more easily shot and killed when they are sick than when they are healthy.

CAUSE

Tularemia is caused by the germ *Pasteurella tularensis*. It needs no wound for entry into the body but is able to go through apparently healthy skin. Infection can result from rubbing the eyes with contaminated fingers.

SYMPTOMS

A fairly large ulcer usually develops at the place where the germs enter the body — on the hands, around the eyes, or at the site of the insect or animal bite. Lymph glands in the neck, armpit, or groin, closest to the part of the body that has been infected, become enlarged and are sometimes abscessed. The patient has chills and fever, often accompanied by extreme exhaustion.

DIAGNOSIS

A number of tests are useful in diagnosing tularemia. Some of these are made on samples of the patient's blood; others are made by inoculating a guinea pig with material from the patient's ulcers or sputum and observing the effects on the animal; another is a skin test. The incubation period of tularemia is usually about three days, and, if ten days have passed without symptoms since suspected exposure, there is little chance that the disease will develop.

TREATMENT

Some of the antibiotics, used as soon as diagnosis is made, provide a highly effective means of treating tularemia. Although patients are usually sick for several weeks, modern methods of treatment lead to recovery for most of them. Recovery results in permanent immunity from further attacks of tularemia.

PREVENTION

Prevention of tularemia is almost entirely a matter of personal precaution in the handling of sick or dead wild animals. Butchers and meat handlers, by the nature of their work, have a higher risk of infection, particularly if they handle wild game. It is best to wear rubber gloves while skinning or dressing wild game, especially rabbits. Any peculiar whitish spots found on the dark organs, such as the liver or spleen, should be a warning to bury or burn the carcass. If hands have been soiled, they should immediately be washed and disinfected.

tumor — an abnormal mass of tissue. Tumors can be benign or malignant. Benign tumors usually are not recurrent. They cause serious trouble only when they are pushing against vital body parts. When benign tumors are removed, the chances for complete recovery are almost always very favorable.

Malignant tumors are abnormal growths that threaten life. These tumors must be removed or death will result. Even if a malignant tumor has been removed, a new malignant growth may appear. Cancer is the growth of one or more malignant tumors.

See cancer.

twins — the birth of two children at the same time. Physicians refer to the birth of twins (or to any pregnancy that yields more than one child) as a multiple birth. The chances of having twins is only fairly good — about one pregnancy in ninety results in twins. Multiple births are more frequent in some races than in others and tend to run in families.

In earlier times, parents were usually taken by surprise when two babies were born instead of one. Today, however, doctors have several ways of knowing in advance when this is going to happen. The doctor may hear two distinct fetal heartbeats, or he may even feel two separate babies as he examines the mother's abdomen. An X-ray anytime after the fifth month will usually determine the fact.

TYPES

There are two kinds of twins: fraternal and identical.

Fraternal twins are different babies from the beginning. They come from two separate cells, each of which was separately fertilized. Each baby has its own placenta and its own bag of waters. Two such separate babies may develop either because both ovaries released a cell at the same time or because one ovary discharged two cells at once. These babies are just as different from each other as any two brothers and sisters. Boy and girl twins are always fraternal twins, although fraternal twins may also be of the same sex.

Identical twins form in another way. They begin, as all babies do, with the fertilization of a single ovum. However, when the new single cell begins to divide, the two halves separate. Each of the two new cells thus formed has all the powers of life and growth. The two babies resulting from these cells are usually attached to the same placenta, but in about thirty percent of the cases each has his own. They always have separate umbilical cords and separate bags of waters. Identical twins are always of the same sex and usually look so much alike that even the parents sometimes have trouble telling them apart.

Premature birth occurs more frequently in

twin pregnancies than in single births. However, these babies are usually relatively mature physically in spite of their small size and may be expected to do better than a single baby of the same size.

tympanic membrane — a tightly stretched membrane that separates the auditory canal from the middle ear. Sound waves are conveyed through the auditory canal to the tympanic membrane (or eardrum, as it is often called). The sound waves cause the membrane to vibrate. These vibrations are picked up by the small bones of the middle ear and are transmitted to the inner ear.

A rupture or perforation of the eardrum can have a variety of causes, including extreme air-pressure changes in the auditory canal, pressure from accumulated middle ear fluid against the eardrum, and accidental injury. Rupture of the eardrum can produce a hearing loss.

A torn eardrum can heal naturally, but if it leaves a thickened scar, a mild hearing loss may result. A substantial rupture may require surgery. After surgery, hearing is improved in many cases. A totally missing eardrum may cause a significant hearing loss. Reconstruction of the eardrum may improve hearing and prevent infection.

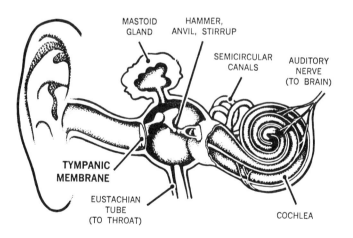

TYMPANIC MEMBRANE

typhoid fever — a communicable disease that is caused by the typhoid bacillus *Salmonella typhosa*. Body discharges (feces and urine) of persons who have the disease contain typhoid bacilli. If water, milk, or food becomes contaminated with such discharges, persons who drink the water or milk or eat the food are likely to contract the disease.

SYMPTOMS

Typhoid fever usually begins gradually, with a feeling of being tired and "out of sorts," a little fever, cough, headache, or dullness. Over about a ten-day period, the fever increases. The patient may have some abdominal pain and tenderness, either constipation or diarrhea, weakness, and mental confusion. He may have chills and severe headache. Rose-colored spots may appear on the body in the second week of illness, although they sometimes appear earlier or later. Patients usually have a high fever for about ten days. When the fever begins to subside, the patient begins to feel better and to regain his appetite, although he is likely to feel weak for some time.

During the first week after symptoms appear, physicians can usually confirm the diagnosis of typhoid by laboratory tests that show whether typhoid bacilli are in the blood, feces, and urine. They nearly always recommend that the patient be cared for in a hospital, since all his body discharges must be disinfected in order to prevent spread of the disease. The effectiveness of treatment for typhoid fever has been increased by the use of antibiotics.

CARRIERS

Some people who have recovered from typhoid fever, and a few who have picked up typhoid bacilli but have never been ill from them, are typhoid carriers. That is, they carry the bacilli in their bodies while apparently in good health and usually without knowing they are carrying them. Typhoid carriers are an important problem to physicians and public health officials, because typhoid bacilli can pass from their bodies and contaminate water, milk, or food.

In the typhoid carrier, the germs often lodge in the gallbladder. Removal of the gallbladder may eliminate the bacilli. Even without having such an operation, however, people who know they are typhoid carriers can, by cooperating with public health officials, learn to take special precautions that will prevent their infecting other people. Two of the most important procedures are washing the hands after using the toilet and avoiding the handling of food, drink, or dishes that are to be used by others. Typhoid carriers should not work as food handlers.

PREVENTION

Typhoid fever can be controlled through good community and home health practices. Improvements in sanitation in the past fifty years have reduced the number of cases that occur in the United States to less than 1,000 annually.

Properly protected public systems of water supply and sewage under the supervision of public health authorities are of the utmost importance. Whenever possible, water is obtained from sources where the likelihood of contamination is at a minimum. When community sewage is treated by modern methods, disease organisms are killed before the sewage is emptied into rivers and streams that may be the water supply for communities downstream.

In most cities and towns in the United States, chlorine is added to the public water supply to kill harmful microorganisms, including typhoid bacilli. In rural areas, the examination of water sources by local public health authorities and the use of sanitary systems for drawing and storing water protect the population against typhoid and other water-borne diseases. Privies or cesspools, properly built and located well away from the water supply and, if possible, at a considerably lower level, are equally important.

Milk and milk products, if they have not been pasteurized, can carry typhoid fever germs. Many cities and towns have regulations requiring the pasteurization of all milk that is sold. Anyone who is not sure of the purity of milk can make it pure by boiling it.

Typhoid germs can be carried in shellfish that have been grown in contaminated water. Federal and state governments have regulations controlling the sale of shellfish. Individuals are wise to insist that shellfish come from government-approved sources, and that food supplies and food service in public eating places are supervised by public health authorities.

Flies can serve as a "rapid transit" for typhoid bacilli and other disease organisms between the privy and the pantry. Food supplies should be protected from flies, and every effort should be made to get rid of them.

Because typhoid fever is very rare in the United States, many people forget that it is still possible to contract it when they are vacationing or traveling in other countries. A person who is going to travel to an area where he may be exposed to typhoid fever can give himself and his family a measure of protection by vaccination. The effect of a series of three injections lasts for a year, and this protection can be renewed with booster shots.

typhus — a term indicating any one of a group of diseases and infections caused by rickettsia (a type of microorganism).

Typhus fever is either epidemic or endemic. When it is epidemic, typhus fever is spread or transmitted through the bite of infected lice or through the feces of infected lice that is introduced into a bite or a wound. Endemic typhus fever is transmitted through the bite of an infected flea. Typhus fever cannot be transmitted from man to man.

SYMPTOMS

The incubation period is from six to fifteen days. The major symptoms are high fever and chills, severe headache, and severe back and generalized body aches and pains. About the fifth day after the symptoms begin, a rash appears that covers the trunk but usually does not appear on the hands, feet, or face. The patient may develop a cough or bronchitis. At times, the patient may become delirious. Complications from typhus fever include bronchopneumonia, otitis media, etc.

Typhus fever is usually treated with tetracycline, a broad-spectrum antibiotic.

u

ulcer — a sore or erosion that begins on the surface of the skin or a body organ and erodes into deeper tissue. Ulcers can be caused by disease, digestive juices, etc.

See peptic ulcer.

ulcerative colitis — an inflamed condition of the colon and rectum, which are the lowermost portions of the bowel. In this condition, many small ulcers develop in the colon. Psychological stress can make the condition worse.

See colitis.

ulna — one of the two bones of the lower arm (the other is the radius). When the arm is in an anatomical position with the palm facing forward, the ulna is on the little finger side, that is, closest to the body. When the hand is moved in the palm down position, the ulna and radius ro-

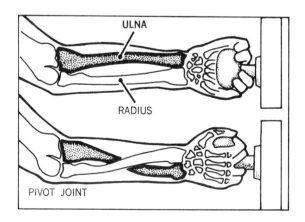

ULNA

tate on each other and cross in the middle. This makes it possible to turn the wrist and hand and to perform such tasks as turning a doorknob.

The ulna is joined with the humerus (the bone of the upper arm) at the top, with some of the carpal (wrist) bones at the bottom, and with the radius at both ends.

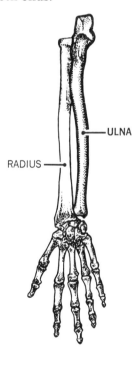

ULNA

ultraviolet rays — invisible rays that are beyond the violet end of the spectrum. Excessive exposure to sunlight (which contains ultraviolet rays) is related to cancer. However, the cancer-producing effects of the ultraviolet rays of sunlight appear to be limited to the skin. It has been observed that the incidence of skin cancer is highest in the southern and western parts of the United States and lowest in the north and is related to the amount of sunshine in the area.

umbilical cord — the cord that connects the placenta at one end and the baby's navel at the other end. Blood from the fetus flows in and out through two arteries and a vein that are encased within the umbilical cord. The waste products of the fetus are carried through the arteries of the umbilical cord and into the placenta, where they are exchanged for oxygen and nutrients from the mother. The vein in the cord carries these materials back to the baby.

After the baby is born, the doctor cuts the umbilical cord several inches away from the body. Some doctors put a dressing on the small piece of cord that remains attached to the baby's navel; some do not. The remnant of cord dries up within a few days. As it dries it turns black. It usually drops off after about a week. Sometimes, however, it takes longer for this to happen. Once the cord is gone, a small scar forms.

unconsciousness — a condition in which a patient exhibits a lack of awareness and a lack of responsiveness. In deep states of unconsciousness, the patient cannot be aroused. In partial unconsciousness, the patient may show intermittent responsiveness but appear to be unaware of his surroundings.

Unconsciousness can be a symptom of many different illnesses and injuries, including head injuries, poisoning, severe hemorrhage, shock, heart attack, etc.

TREATMENT

The treatment for unconsciousness depends on the cause. If the patient has merely fainted, he will regain consciousness, without treatment, in a few minutes. However, most cases of unconsciousness require medical attention. If the patient is pale, he should be kept lying down with his head level to or slightly lower than his feet. If the patient appears flushed, he should be kept lying down with his head and shoulders slightly raised.

Patients who are unconscious should never be given liquids. A person who is unconscious can-

not swallow properly, and liquids may enter the lungs.

undulant fever — *See brucellosis.*

universal antidote — an antidote that has been devised for use when a patient has taken a poison but the exact nature or type of the poison is not known. The universal antidote is especially effective against irritants, excitants, and depressants. This antidote contains ingredients that cause the poison in solution to form solid particles; that combine with the poison to make it less harmful; or that change it into a harmless chemical compound.

It is prepared from activated charcoal (two parts), magnesium oxide (one part), and tannic acid (one part). It is usually given (one-half of an ounce) in half of a glass of water. The universal antidote is followed by an emetic (a substance that causes vomiting), except when the poison is a corrosive. When these ingredients are not available, substitutions can be made. Burned toast or charred wood can be used in place of activated charcoal; milk of magnesia can be substituted for magnesium oxide; and strong tea can be used for tannic acid.

See poison.

urea — one of the waste products of the body's metabolic processes. Urea is excreted from the body in urine.

uremia — a disease state that permits an excess of certain waste substances (normally excreted by the kidneys) to remain in the blood. This condition results from kidney malfunction of various causes. When the kidneys are not functioning properly, nitrogenous products in the bloodstream are not removed and can accumulate in high concentrations. Uremia is a symptom, not a separate disease. When the kidneys begin to function properly again, they can remove the waste products, and uremia subsides.

ureters — two tubes that transport urine from the kidneys to the bladder. They are about thirty centimeters long. The diameter of each ureter varies throughout its length from about one to ten millimeters. The ureters extend from the kidney pelvis, down the gutter formed by the vertebral column and ribs, to the urinary bladder. Peristaltic contractions of the ureters aid in transporting the urine to the bladder.

See bladder, kidney.

urethra — the tube that carries urine from the bladder to the exterior. Its size and position differ in the two sexes. In the male, the urethra forms a part of the excretory system and a part of the reproductive system. In the female, the urethra belongs only to the excretory system.

The female urethra is about four centimeters long and is firmly joined with the wall of the vagina. The male urethra is about twenty centimeters long. It is divided into three parts: the prostatic, membranous, and penile portions. The prostatic portion is surrounded by the prostate gland and contains the openings of the prostatic and ejaculatory ducts. The penile urethra is the longest portion of the male urethra (about 15 centimeters in length) and lies in the front part of the penis, extending to its external opening, the urinary meatus.

uric acid — an organic substance that is a solid waste product contained in urine. When there is an excess of uric acid in the body, a condition known as gout develops. The excess of uric acid may be caused by a problem in the kidneys that reduces the normal excretion of uric acid, or it may be caused by an excess production of uric acid.

See gout.

urinalysis — a test or group of tests designed to examine a patient's urine. The results of a urinalysis are often very important aids in the diagnosis and treatment of diseases and conditions.

During the course of a urinalysis, the amount of urine is measured (this requires a twenty-four hour specimen), and the color, transparency, and odor are checked. Additionally, the urine is tested to determine the amount of alkali and acid. Other tests include the amount of albumin and the amount of glucose (sugar). Microscopic examination reveals the presence of pus cells, red blood cells, crystals, and other formed substances.

See urine.

urinary meatus — the external opening of the male urethra located in the penis.

See urethra.

urinary system — the system that excretes liquid wastes and regulates the composition of the blood. The urinary system conserves substances that are present in normal or subnormal concentrations. It removes excess water and excess normal chemical components to maintain optimum concentration, while at the same time totally removing harmful waste products.

The urinary system consists of two glands (the kidneys) that produce the urine; two tubes (the ureters) that drain the urine from the kidneys; a large reservoir (the bladder), where the urine is temporarily stored prior to discharge from the body; and a tube (the urethra) that carries the urine from the bladder to an external opening. All these parts are the same in both sexes, with the exception of the urethra.

See bladder, kidney, ureter, urethra, urine.

urination — the act of expelling urine from the body. Although urination is essentially reflex in nature, it is usually initiated by an effort of the will. Thus, it can be voluntarily inhibited or interrupted at any stage. The one essential limiting factor is the capacity of the bladder. When it has reached its full capacity, it will begin to empty, much as a lake will begin to overflow when the water level rises above its banks.

Urination is also called micturition.

urine — the fluid that contains waste products. It is filtered from the blood in the kidneys. From each kidney a tube called a ureter carries the urine to the bladder, where it is stored until it is discharged through another tube, the urethra.

The amount of urine excreted by a normal adult is from thirty-four to sixty fluid ounces per day. However, a person may excrete as little as seventeen fluid ounces per day. The amount of urine varies greatly with environmental body temperature; the amount may be markedly decreased with increased water loss through the sweat glands. Other factors that influence the production and excretion of urine are water intake, medicinal substances, and states of health or disease.

In the normal, healthy person, urine is transparent. The color varies from pale yellow to dark amber and can be influenced by certain foods, drugs, and diseases. Urine has a distinct odor similar to ammonia.

Water makes up ninety-five percent of urine. The other five percent consists of total solids.

Urea constitutes one half of this amount. The solids in urine consist of organic and inorganic substances. The chief organic substances are urea, uric acid, and ammonium salts; inorganic substances are sodium chloride, potassium, magnesium, and calcium. In addition to waste products found in the blood, the kidneys can also remove substances such as barbituric acid, mercury, and alcohol from the blood. These substances are then excreted in the urine.

uterus — a hollow, pear-shaped organ that is part of the female reproductive system. It has thick muscular walls but is fairly small — normally about three inches long and weighing about two ounces.

At the lower end the uterus (also called the womb) narrows into a neck-like portion called the cervix, which in turn leads into the vagina. Towards the top of the uterus two tubes, the fallopian tubes, join the uterus.

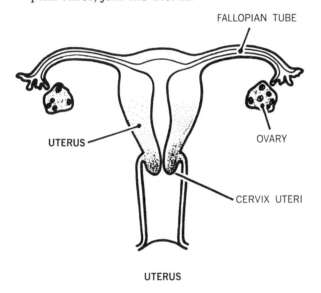

FALLOPIAN TUBE

UTERUS

OVARY

CERVIX UTERI

UTERUS

The uterus provides a place where a fertilized ovum can be protected and nourished while it is developing into a fetus (an unborn child). In pre-paring to receive and nourish an ovum, the lining of the uterus becomes swollen and soft and has much more blood in it than usual. If the ovum is not fertilized and the blood is not needed for its nourishment, the lining of the uterus gradually stops growing and comes loose. The excess blood and part of the swollen membrane (the unused top layer of the lining of the uterus) is sloughed off and discharged from the uterus through the vagina. This discharge ordinarily occurs every twenty-eight days and is called menstruation.

As soon as this first menstrual period ends, preparations for another one begin within the uterus. This cycle repeats itself, except during pregnancies, until the menopause, when the childbearing part of a woman's life comes to an end.

PREGNANCY

During pregnancy the uterus stretches to accommodate the size of the growing child. In the first stage of labor the uterus begins to contract. As the contractions continue, the cervix is stretched to permit the baby to pass into the birth canal. Finally, the contractions help push the baby out of the uterus through the cervix. After the baby is born, the uterus forces the placenta and membranes that have nourished the baby out of the body.

As soon as the baby is born, the uterus starts to shrink. It usually takes about six weeks for the uterus to shrink gradually from about two pounds to about two ounces.

utricle — one of two small sacs located next to the cochlea of the inner ear. The utricles are concerned with balance. When the body shifts position, material within the utricle also moves. The movement in the utricle touches off nerve impulses to the brain that indicate the new position of the body.

See semicircular canal.

vaccination — the injection of a substance containing dead or weakened bacteria or viruses. The purpose of a vaccination is to force the body to produce antibodies. These antibodies will provide immunity to the disease that the living or stronger forms of the microorganisms can cause.

Originally, the term was used with reference to smallpox vaccination. Today, the term is used to describe many different types of vaccination.

vaccine — a substance containing dead or weakened bacteria or viruses. This substance is introduced into the body. The body reacts to the vaccine by forming antibodies that provide immunity to any disease caused by those particular bacteria or viruses. The process of introducing the substance into the body is called vaccination when it requires the use of a needle. However, some vaccines, such as the Sabin oral vaccine for polio, do not require injection by needle.

vagina — a muscular canal lined with mucous membrane. It extends from the cervix of the uterus to the external opening of the female reproductive system. The vagina forms the last part of the birth canal, and during delivery it stretches to allow the baby to pass through it.

vaginitis — an inflammation of the vagina, which is the opening into the female reproductive system. The symptoms of vaginitis are pain and a discharge that may vary from mild and brief to mild yet persistent or to thick and profuse. The urine may appear clouded or bloody if it becomes mixed with the discharge. Vaginitis may be a fairly mild problem, but it may also be a serious infection. Drugs are usually used to relieve the condition.

vagus nerves — one of the twelve pairs of cranial nerves. The vagus nerves form part of the parasympathetic system. They extend from the brain, through the neck and thorax, and into the abdomen. These nerves, known as the inhibitory nerves of the heart, slow the heart when they are stimulated. The vagus nerves are composed of motor fibers (some of which are parasympathetic) and sensory fibers.

valve — membrane that is located within a body tube or organ and is responsible for preventing the backward flow of fluid from passing through it. Valves consist of two or three cusps or triangular segments that allow the free flow of fluid in only one direction. There are valves located in the heart, lymph vessels, and veins.

valvular insufficiency — a term applied to valves that close improperly and admit a backflow of blood in the wrong direction.

valvular stenosis — *See congenital heart defects.*

vaporizer — a small piece of equipment that heats water and releases it into the air. The air becomes warm and heavily laden with moisture. This moist, warm air can be very soothing for patients with congestion in some parts of the respiratory tract.

varicella — *See chickenpox.*

varicose veins — swollen, enlarged veins. They are found most frequently on the inner side and back of the calf and on the inner side of the thigh. Bluish in color, they are visible through the skin when they are close to the surface. Varicose veins look something like a map drawing of a river and the streams that flow into it.

The superficial veins, those lying just under the skin, are most commonly affected. The deep veins, which run inside the muscles of the leg and thigh, are seldom seriously involved, because they are surrounded and supported by the muscles.

Varicose veins are widespread throughout the population and affect almost all ages. However, they are most common in people over forty and affect one out of every two women and one out of every four men in this age group.

CAUSE

Veins contain valves that permit the blood to flow only in the direction of the heart. One of the main causes of varicose veins seems to be valves that leak, allowing blood to flow backward into the vessel rather than continuing on its way to the heart.

This increases blood pressure in the section of the vein below the faulty valve. Veins are low-pressure vessels. Their walls are thinner and have less muscle in them than do the walls of arteries. When continually subjected to abnormally high pressures, the veins become stretched and swollen.

Inherited weaknesses in the structure of the veins greatly increases the individual's susceptibility to varicose veins. Other contributing factors are diseases, such as phlebitis, that weaken or damage the walls and valves of the veins. Abdominal pressure from the stomach muscles (such as that caused by heavy lifting, coughing, and straining) may also contribute to the development of varicose veins.

Obesity and increasing age are other factors in causing this condition. Extra, useless weight may overwork the veins. With increasing age there is a loss of tone of the skin and of tissues that surround and support the veins.

Persons in occupations that require a great deal of standing seem more prone to varicose veins than people with desk jobs. To illustrate this point, it has been found that pressure in the leg veins is increased five times when a person stands erect from a lying-down position. How-ever, people in jobs requiring sitting in one place for long periods of time also have a problem. Unless they walk around or elevate their feet from time to time there will be an excessive pooling of blood in the veins of the lower leg.

Women frequently develop varicose veins during pregnancy because of the increased abdominal pressure that results from the enlarging uterus and the increased blood flow to and from the lower abdominal and pelvic areas. Both factors act indirectly to hinder return flow from the leg veins, thus increasing blood pressure in these vessels.

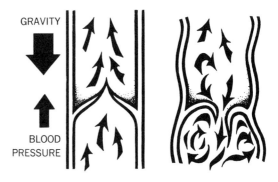

GRAVITY

BLOOD PRESSURE

VARICOSE VEINS

SYMPTOMS

Varicose veins usually produce a combination of many symptoms. Among these are changes in the appearance of the leg; increased tendency to fatigue of the leg muscles; a sensation of fullness and congestion; soreness in the region of the veins after standing for a long period of time; muscular cramps (particularly at night); and itching, burning sensations in the region of the varicose veins.

DIAGNOSIS

Although a doctor, by inspecting and manipulating areas of the leg, can usually establish their presence, various other tests have been developed to aid in diagnosing varicose veins. One of these procedures is called venography. In this test a radiopaque substance is injected into the veins. After this the blood flow and the working of the valves in the vessels are checked by means of X-rays.

TREATMENT

In medical terms, there are several kinds of varicose veins. Some can be helped by surgery, some by injection therapy, and some by simpler measures.

1. Conservative therapy

In mild cases of varicose veins it may be possible to relieve much of the discomfort and to prevent the veins from becoming worse by wearing support hosiery. This hosiery helps provide additional support to offset excessive blood pressure within the veins. Support hosiery, available in stockings for women and socks for men, should be carefully fitted on the basis of precise leg measurements.

The person with mild varicose veins should also get adequate periods of rest with his feet and legs elevated. Prolonged periods of standing should be avoided. However, if this is unavoidable because of occupational or other factors, elastic bandages may provide better support than can usually be obtained with support hosiery.

"Bicycling" exercises while lying on the back, swimming, and walking are often recommended forms of exercise for persons with mild varicose veins.

2. Injection

Varicose veins can be injected with a sclerosing (hardening) solution to block off the swollen part of the vein. The blood normally carried by that vessel is re-routed through other veins. For a time after injection the injected vein may be swollen and tender, but this subsides within a few hours or days. Thereafter, the injected section usually withers and gradually disappears over a period of weeks to months. This process may be hastened by removing some of the coagulated blood from the blocked section through a small incision. Injection is frequently reserved for the treatment of the small varicose veins lying very near the surface of the skin.

Injection treatment has some drawbacks. Permanent results cannot be guaranteed; numerous injections may be necessary; and elastic pressure bandages must be worn for the duration of the treatment.

3. Surgery

Surgery for tying off or removing the vein is quicker than injection treatment, and the results are more likely to be permanent. If the patient is in otherwise good health, the surgical risk is slight. However, surgery requires a hospital stay and is relatively expensive. In answer to the question of how well a patient can get along with-

out the veins that are being tied off or removed: he can do far better without them than he could with them. Varicose veins are inefficient in carrying out their function of returning blood "uphill" to the heart. In fact, in a severely affected vein, blood flow may be in the opposite direction. Thus, removing that vein actually improves the overall performance of the system of veins.
See veins.

varicosities — an alternate term for varicose veins. *See varicose veins.*

variola — *See smallpox.*

varioloid — a mild version of smallpox. Varioloid usually occurs as a reinfection of smallpox or as a mild form of smallpox occurring in people who have previously been vaccinated against the stronger form. In contrast with smallpox, varioloid seldom leaves the patient with scars.
See smallpox.

vascular — of or pertaining to vessels. The term is usually used with reference to blood vessels.

vas deferens — a small tube that connects the ductal system of the testes with the ejaculatory duct in the male reproductive system. It continues the transmission of sperm to the ejaculatory system. The vas deferens is also called the ductus deferens.

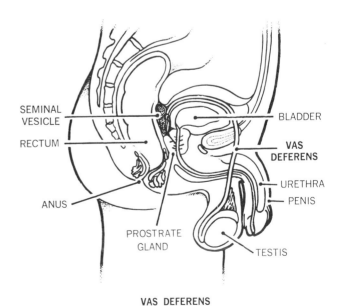

VAS DEFERENS

vasectomy — an operation that ties off, cuts, or removes part or all of the vas deferens. A vasectomy is usually performed to sterilize a male. It is a relatively simple operation, because the vas deferens is located very close to the skin. The vas deferens carries the sperm from the testes (where it is made) to the ejaculatory system. When the vas deferens is tied off or removed, no sperm can enter the ejaculatory system, and consequently no sperm is ejaculated. In recent years, vasectomies have become more popular as a means of birth control.

See vas deferens.

vasoconstrictor — an agent or substance that causes the blood vessels to contract. The vasoconstrictor nerves are one part of the involuntary nervous system. When these nerves are stimulated, they cause the muscles of the arterioles to contract, thus narrowing the arteriole passage, increasing the resistance to the flow of blood, and raising the blood pressure. Chemical substances that stimulate the muscles of the aterioles to contract are called vasoconstrictor agents or vasopressors. An example is epinephrine, which the body produces naturally but which can also be given in the form of a drug.

vasodilator — an agent or substance that causes the blood vessels to relax. Vasodilator nerves are certain nerve fibers of the involuntary nervous system that cause the muscles of the arterioles to relax, thus enlarging the arteriole passage, reducing the resistance to the flow of blood, and lowering the blood pressure.

Vasodilator agents are chemical compounds that cause a relaxation of the muscles of the arterioles. Examples of this type of drug are nitroglycerine, nitrites, and thiocyanate, among others.

vasoinhibitor — an agent or drug that inhibits the action of the vasomotor nerves. When these involuntary nerves are inhibited, the muscles of the arterioles relax; the passage inside the arteriole is enlarged; and the blood pressure is lowered. Compounds of nitrite are examples of vasoinhibitor drugs.

vasopressor — a chemical substance that causes the muscles of the arterioles to contract, thus narrowing the arteriole passage and raising the blood pressure. Such substances are also called vasoconstrictor agents.

vector — a term used to describe a disease carrier. Vectors can be insects, animals, or other human beings.

See carriers, transmission.

vectorcardiography — a method used to determine the direction and magnitude of the electrical forces of the heart.

vein — any one of a series of vessels that carry blood from various parts of the body back to the heart. All veins in the body, except the pulmonary veins, conduct unoxygenated blood.

Together, the veins comprise a system of vessels that collect the blood from the capillaries and carry it back to the heart. The structure of the veins is similar to that of the arteries except that the walls of the veins are thinner and have less muscular tissue. Veins begin as tiny venules that are formed from capillaries joining together much as tiny riverlets connect and form a small stream. These venules join and form larger veins, which in turn join, until the very largest veins are formed. These empty into the heart.

The force of muscles contracting next to veins aids in the forward propulsion of blood on its return trip to the heart. Valves, spaced frequently along the larger veins, prevent the backflow of blood.

There are three principal venous (vein) systems in the body: pulmonary, systemic, and portal.

1. Pulmonary

The pulmonary venous system is comprised of four vessels (two from each lung) that empty into the left atrium of the heart. These are the only veins in the body that carry freshly oxygenated blood.

2. Systemic

The systemic venous system is divided into deep and superficial groups. The superficial veins lie immediately under the skin and drain the skin and superficial structures. The deep veins, usually located in the muscle or deeper layers, drain the large muscle masses and various other organs. They usually lie close to the large arteries that supply the various organs of the body.

The superficial veins of the head unite to form

the external jugular veins. They drain blood from the scalp, face, and neck. The veins that drain the brain and the internal facial structures are known as the internal jugular veins.

The superficial veins of the upper extremity begin at the hand. One of these veins, the median cubital, crosses the inside surface of the elbow. This is the vein most commonly used for intravenous injections and infusions. In the lower extremity the saphenous vein (a superficial vein) originates in the foot and extends up the inside of the leg and thigh to join the femoral vein in the upper thigh. The saphenous vein is sometimes used at the ankle for intravenous injections.

3. Portal

The portal system is comprised of those veins that drain venous blood from the abdominal part of the digestive tract (except the lower rectum), spleen, pancreas, and gallbladder. This blood is then delivered to the liver. There it is distributed within the liver by a set of venous capillaries. The blood in the portal system conveys absorbed substances from the intestinal tract to the liver for storage, alteration, or detoxification.

vena cava — two large veins that empty into the heart. The superior vena cava conducts blood from the upper part of the body (head, neck, and thorax) to the right upper chamber of the heart. The inferior vena cava conducts blood from the lower part of the body to the right upper chamber.

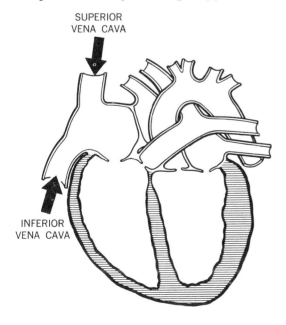

SUPERIOR
VENA CAVA

INFERIOR
VENA CAVA

VENA CAVA

venereal disease — any infectious disease that is transmitted almost exclusively from person to person through sexual intercourse. The two most common venereal diseases in this country are syphilis and gonorrhea. They are both serious communicable diseases.

Since 1957 venereal disease has been on the increase. Young people under the age of twenty are responsible for a large proportion of this increase. Despite the lack of reliable statistics, many authorities feel that the incidence of venereal disease has grown to almost epidemic dimensions.

For many patients, being informed of the diagnosis is a shocking experience, and the request to identify sex partners is even more disturbing. However, the necessity of having all sex partners treated must be recognized in order to protect the health of infected contacts and to protect the patient from reinfection.

Although syphilis is transmitted primarily by heterosexual relationships, it is now recognized that homosexual transmission is also an important factor in the spread of this disease.

Control of venereal disease is based on immediate treatment of the infected person, as well as his or her sexual contacts. The immediacy is important in order to stop the spread. Both syphilis and gonorrhea can be cured with some form of penicillin or other antibiotic when treated early. However, serious complications can arise when cases of venereal disease remain untreated.

See gonorrhea, syphilis.

venipuncture — the process of inserting a needle into a vein. Venipuncture is used in transfusions and in the injection of some types of fluids. This technique is also used when it is necessary to remove a sizable quantity of blood for tests or when a person is donating blood for a transfusion.

The skin at the inner bend of the elbow is cleaned with alcohol. When blood is being withdrawn, a tourniquet is then placed around the upper arm. The patient extends his arm fully and opens and closes the fist a few times to distend the veins. A sterile needle is then inserted into any prominent vein. After the required amount of blood has been removed, the tourniquet is removed, and the needle is withdrawn. A similar procedure is followed when an injection is given.

When necessary, venipuncture can be performed on a vein in the ankle.

venom — the poisonous substance injected by a snake. Different snakes have different types of venom.
See snakebite.

venous blood — unoxygenated blood. Venous blood, with hemoglobin in the reduced state, is carried by the veins from all parts of the body back to the heart. It is then pumped by the right side of the heart to the lungs, where it is oxygenated. Venous blood is dark red in color.

ventricle — a small cavity or hollow space that is within or is part of a body organ. There are ventricles in the heart and in the brain.

1. Heart
There are two ventricles in the heart. They are also called the lower chambers. The left ventricle pumps oxygenated blood through arteries to the body. The right ventricle pumps unoxygenated blood through the pulmonary artery to the lungs.

The walls of the ventricles, which actually comprise the bulk of the heart, are thick and muscular. Muscle fibers of the ventricles spiral and intertwine with each other so that when the heart contracts, it does so with a wringing motion as it squeezes the blood into the arterial system. The wall of the left ventricle is considerably thicker than that of the right, because more force is required to pump the blood into the circulation than is required to pump the blood into the lungs, which lie only a short distance from the heart.

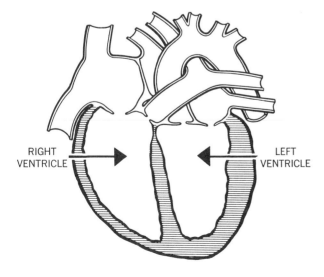

RIGHT VENTRICLE   LEFT VENTRICLE

VENTRICLES OF THE HEART

2. Brain
Inside the brain there are four ventricles that contain cerebrospinal fluid. This fluid is formed in the central ventricles of the brain. It is constantly being produced and reabsorbed. Cerebrospinal fluid circulates over the surface of the brain and spinal cord and serves as a protective cushion as well as a means of the exchange of food and waste materials.

ventricular septum — the muscular wall that divides the left and right lower chambers of the heart (the ventricles). The ventricular septum is thinner at the top than at the bottom. It is sometimes called the interventricular septum.

venule — a very small vein.
See vein.

veratrum — a drug that lowers the blood pressure and decreases the heart rate. Veratrum is an antihypertensive agent.

veriform appendix — the technical term for the appendix.
See appendix.

vermicide — a drug that kills or paralyzes an intestinal worm.

vermifuge — a drug that causes the expulsion of an intestinal worm from the body.

vermis — a part of the cerebellum of the brain.
See cerebellum.

Vernes' test — a test for syphilis.
See syphilis.

vernix — a white, creamy substance that forms on the body of a fetus at about the seventh month. The vernix, which protects the fetus, may remain on the baby until after birth.

vertebra — a term used to denote any one of the twenty-four movable segments that, together with the sacrum and the coccyx, form the spinal column.

The vertebrae are designed to support and provide motion to the body and extremities and to serve as a bony protection for the spinal cord and the nerves that arise from the spinal cord.

Each vertebra has an anterior (or front) portion, called the body, that is the large, solid segment of the bone. This body is for support, not only for the spinal cord but for the other organs in the body as well. Many of the main muscles are attached to the vertebrae. The hollow space or hole directly behind the body of each vertebra contributes to the formation of the spinal canal, which contains the spinal cord. The various facets and bony projections (called processes) enable the vertebrae to move one on the other and provide for the attachment of spinal muscles.

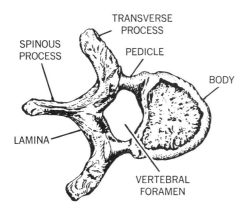

SPINOUS PROCESS

TRANSVERSE PROCESS

PEDICLE

BODY

LAMINA

VERTEBRAL FORAMEN

VERTEBRA

There are seven vertebrae in the neck. They are collectively referred to as the cervical vertebrae. The first of these is called the atlas, because it supports the head. The second vertebra is known as the axis, because it is the one upon which the head turns. These are the only named vertebrae; all the others are numbered. The seventh cervical vertebra presents an especially prominent projection that can easily be felt at the nape of the neck. This provides a landmark for counting and identifying vertebrae above and below it.

There are twelve vertebrae in the chest region. These are known as the thoracic vertebrae. They join with the twelve pairs of ribs and with the rear portions of the ribs from the back wall of the thoracic (chest) cage.

There are five lumbar (or lower back) vertebrae. The last of these joins with the sacrum.

vertigo — a sensation of motion or movement when no such movement or motion exists. The patient can feel as if he is moving (while, in fact, he is motionless) or that the area around him is moving (although it is entirely still). However, ver-

tigo is not simple dizziness. Vertigo is often caused by a problem within the inner ear that is interfering with the organs of balance (semicircular canals, saccules, and utricles). However, it may also be caused by brain damage, eye problems, and certain diseases.

Vesalius, Andreas — the Belgian anatomist (1514-1564) who questioned many of the theories of the circulatory system as taught by Galen. He chiefly questioned the existence of openings in the wall dividing the left from the right side of the heart, through which blood was believed to pass.

vesicant — a term used to describe a drug or agent that causes blisters to form.

Vibrio — a class of bacteria. One type of Vibrio causes cholera. These bacteria occur singly and in spiral chains. The cells may be long, thin and delicate, or they may be short and thick. Vibrio are shaped like slightly curved rods.
    See cholera.

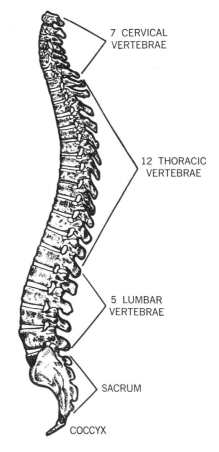

7 CERVICAL VERTEBRAE

12 THORACIC VERTEBRAE

5 LUMBAR VERTEBRAE

SACRUM

COCCYX

VERTEBRAE

369

villi — the minute, hairlike projections that cover the mucous membrane lining of the small intestine. The chief function of the villi appears to be the presentation of a large absorptive area through which digested food materials can be transferred to the lymph system or to tributaries of the venous (vein) system.

vinblastine — a drug extracted from the periwinkle plant. Vinblastine is used in the treatment of Hodgkin's disease and some types of cancer. This drug can have strong side effects involving the blood.

Vincent's angina — *See Vincent's disease.*

Vincent's disease — an acute or chronic infection of the gums. This disease is also known as trench mouth and as necrotizing ulcerating gingivitis. Vincent's disease is thought to be infectious but not contagious. However, it can occur in epidemics and can be transmitted from person to person where there is a lack of good oral hygiene.

SYMPTOMS
During the acute stages this disease is characterized by redness, swelling, pain, and bleeding of the gums. There is usually a film of white or grayish tissue around the teeth. This film may be wiped off, leaving a raw, bleeding base. The ulceration of the gum tissue results in a characteristic punched-out appearance. There is usually a very disagreeable odor and a foul taste in the mouth. The gums bleed easily when touched, and the patient may not be able to brush his teeth or eat very well because of the pain. The acute stage may be accompanied by a moderately high fever.

TREATMENT
The infection may be treated with antibiotics or by the frequent use of a mouthwash of salt water, sodium bicarbonate, or hydrogen peroxide. Physicians often recommend bed rest, especially in cases involving fever.

virus — a microscopic organism that causes disease in man and animals. Viruses differ from bacteria in several ways. Viruses are considerably smaller than bacteria and cannot multiply unless they are within another living organism or host. Viruses cause diseases such as smallpox, rabies, poliomyelitis, and yellow fever.

visceral pericardium — the outer layer of the heart wall. The visceral pericardium is also called the epicardium.

vision — *See eye, sight.*

visual field — the total area perceived when the eyes are focused straight ahead. This comprises both the small area on which the eyes are focused for sharp impression, called central vision, and the large area that is seen "out of the corner of the eye," called indirect or peripheral vision. Defects in the visual field may be regular or irregular in pattern, but the closer the defect is to the center of the field, the more serious it is.

vital signs — the temperature, pulse, and respiration of a patient. Blood pressure is sometimes included in this group. They are called vital signs because they give vital indications of the patient's condition. The measurement of these signs and their relationship to each other aid the doctor in making a diagnosis and prescribing treatment.

TEMPERATURE
Temperature is the degree of heat in the body. It is the balance between heat produced and heat lost by the body. When the balance is disturbed, deviations of body temperature result. Deviations above the normal range are called eleva-

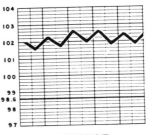
CONSTANT

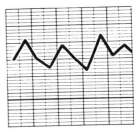
REMITTENT

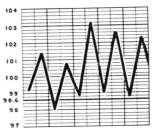
INTERMITTENT-SPIKING

VITAL SIGNS (FEVER)

tions, or fever; those below the normal range are called subnormal. Fever may begin suddenly or gradually, and its course may be constant, remittent, or intermittent.

1. A constant fever is one in which the temperature remains elevated at about the same level during a period of twenty-four hours or longer.

2. A remittent fever is one in which the patient's temperature rises and falls in a moderate range but does not approach normal.

3. An intermittent fever is one in which the temperature rises and falls in a great range, approaching normal or below in a twenty-four hour period.

Fever may subside by crisis, in which there is an abrupt drop to normal, with dramatic improvement in the patient; or the fever may drop gradually over a period of days or weeks.

PULSE

Pulse is the alternate contraction and dilation of the arteries created by the pumping of the blood by the heart. Changes in the character of the pulse may be caused by any factor that interferes with the function of the heart, the volume of the blood, and the elasticity of the blood vessels. Therefore, the measurement of the pulse is a valuable means of learning the condition of the heart, blood vessels, and general condition of the patient.

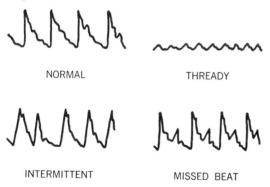

NORMAL   THREADY

INTERMITTENT   MISSED BEAT

VITAL SIGNS (PULSE)

The normal pulse is firm and smooth. Variations of the pulse include a missed beat, an intermittent pulse, and a thready pulse.

1. When the pulse is said to be missing a beat, it is regularly irregular in rhythm and rate. It may also be irregular in force and volume.

2. An intermittent pulse is irregular in rhythm and rate. It may also be irregular in force and volume.

3. A thready pulse is rapid, running, and difficult to count or to determine quality.

In general, the pulse rate will increase ten beats for each degree of rise in temperature.

RESPIRATION

Respiration is the act of breathing in air and breathing out carbon dioxide and other waste products. Normal respiration is regular in rate, rhythm, and depth and is performed without pain, strain, or difficulty. Respiration usually increases one to two in rate with every ten-beat rise in pulse and each degree rise in temperature. Some of the variations in respiration are dyspnea, Cheney-Stokes, stertorous, and edematous.

1. Dyspnea is a fairly general term for painful, difficult breathing.

2. Cheney-Stokes is a cycle or pattern of breathing difficulty. There is a gradual increase in the depth of respirations until dyspnea is reached. This is followed by a decrease in depth until breathing ceases for a few moments. The cycle then begins again with a gradual increase.

3. Stertorous respiration is defined as loud, snorting breathing.

4. Edematous respiration produces moist sounds, as if the air were passing through water.

vitamins — compounds that are essential in very small amounts for the proper utilization of foods and for healthy functioning of the human body. The various vitamins differ greatly in their composition, and each one has specific, separate, vital functions. Because the body cannot manufacture vitamins, they must be supplied preformed in food.

Vitamins play a dynamic role in body processes. They take part in the release of energy from foods, promote normal growth of different kinds of tissue, and are essential to the proper functioning of nerves and muscles.

Vitamins are found in varying quantities in different foods. For example, one-half cup of orange juice contains more than twice as much vitamin C as an equal portion of tomato juice. Most foods contain more than one vitamin, but no one food contains all of them in sufficient quantity to satisfy the body's requirements. Ordinarily, a well-balanced diet will provide enough of all the needed vitamins.

Vitamins are involved in the most basic, vital, life processes. Severe deficiencies in specific vitamins over prolonged periods may result in a variety of symptoms, such as night blindness and certain skin lesions or even full-blown deficiency diseases, such as rickets, scurvy, and others.

1. Vitamin A

Vitamin A is needed for normal growth and for normal vision in dim and night light. It also helps to keep the skin and inner linings of the body healthy and resistant to infection.

Vitamin A occurs only in foods of animal origin. However, many vegetables and fruits, particularly the green and yellow ones, contain a substance called carotene that the body can change into vitamin A. Liver is outstanding for its vitamin A content. Important amounts are also found in eggs, butter, margarine, whole milk, and cheese made with whole milk. Carotene is found in largest amounts in dark-green and deep-yellow vegetables and in deep-yellow fruits.

2. Vitamin B

Vitamin B is actually a complex of relatively similar vitamins. There are at least twelve known B vitamins.

Three of the B vitamins — thiamine, riboflavin, and niacin — play a central role in the release of energy from food. They also help with proper functioning of nerves, normal appetite, good digestion, and healthy skin.

Generally, foods in the meat group are leading sources of these vitamins. Whole-grain and enriched breads and cereals supply smaller but important amounts. A few foods are outstanding sources — milk for riboflavin, lean pork for thiamine, and organ meats for all three.

Getting enough niacin is not a problem if a good amount of protein is included in daily meals. An essential amino acid — tryptophan — that is present in the protein can be changed into niacin by the body.

Other B vitamins, — B_6 and particularly B_{12} and folacin (folic acid) — help prevent anemia. Vitamin B_{12} is found only in foods of animal origin. B_6 and folacin are widely distributed in foods. Folacin occurs in largest amounts in organ meats and dark-green, leafy vegetables. Good sources of vitamin B_6 include meats in general; whole-grain cereals; dry beans; potatoes; and dark-green, leafy vegetables.

3. Vitamin C

Vitamin C, also called ascorbic acid, helps form and maintain cementing material that holds body cells together and strengthens the walls of blood vessels. It also assists in normal tooth and bone formation and aids in healing wounds.

Citrus fruits — oranges, grapefruit, tangerines, lemons, and their juices — and fresh strawberries are rich in ascorbic acid. Other important sources include tomatoes and tomato juice; broccoli; brussels sprouts; cabbage; green peppers; some dark-green, leafy vegetables, such as collards, kale, mustard greens, spinach, and turnip greens; and potatoes and sweet potatoes, especially when cooked in the jackets.

4. Vitamin D

Vitamin D is important in building strong bones and teeth, because it enables the body to use the calcium and phosphorus supplied by food.

Few foods contain much vitamin D naturally. Milk with vitamin D added is a practical source. Small amounts of vitamin D are present in egg yolk, butter, and liver; larger amounts occur in sardines, salmon, and tuna.

Vitamin D is often referred to as the sunshine vitamin, because it is produced by the action of direct sunlight on the skin. Because vitamin D does not occur naturally in a sufficient amount in food, and because most children in the United States do not get enough sunshine (because of the weather, the clothing they wear, etc.), many physicians prescribe vitamin D preparations for infants and young children. This may be in the form of drops, capsules, tablets, or milk to which vitamin D has been added.

5. Other vitamins

There are many other vitamins. The most important of these is vitamin K. Vitamin K is an essential component of the body's blood-clotting mechanism, which prevents continuous bleeding after an injury to blood vessels.

Other vitamins are just as necessary, but the quantities in which they are present in many foods have not yet been determined fully. As a rule, the body is less dependent on outside foods for the supply of these vitamins, because they are also produced by bacteria in the intestines and absorbed directly into the body.

vitiligo — a condition in which patches of the skin lose their color or pigmentation. The skin appears to be perfectly healthy but becomes extremely white. The tendency is for the size of the patches to increase. No known treatment is effective against this condition. The patches of white skin will occasionally spread to the point where they cover most (if not all) of the body.

vitreous body — the semifluid, transparent substance that lies between the retina and the lens of the eye.

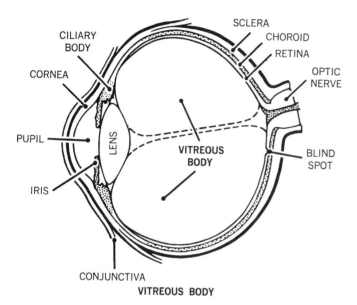

CILIARY BODY
CORNEA
PUPIL
IRIS
LENS
CONJUNCTIVA
SCLERA
CHOROID
RETINA
OPTIC NERVE
VITREOUS BODY
BLIND SPOT

VITREOUS BODY

vitreous humor — See *vitreous body*.

vocal cords — See *larynx*.

voice — the modified, refined sounds that emanate from the larynx. The quality of the voice depends on the size of the true vocal cords (located in the larynx) as well as on the presence or absence of any congestion in the upper respiratory tract.
See *larynx*.

Volkmann's contracture — a condition in which the fingers contract. This can be caused when a tourniquet or a plaster-of-paris cast is applied improperly.

voluntary muscles — muscles over which a person has conscious control.
See *muscle*.

vomiting — the reversal of the swallowing process. The esophagus is a muscular tube about ten inches long. It begins at the pharynx and continues to the stomach. By means of waves of muscular contractions, called peristalsis, food is pushed along this tube to the stomach. When peristalsis is reversed, vomiting occurs. Vomiting may be the result of overloading the stomach, disease of the intestinal tract, abnormalities of the brain, or a toxic reaction to certain drugs.

Vomiting is sometimes induced when a person has swallowed a poison. However, when corrosives have been swallowed, vomiting should not be induced, because the corrosive can damage the mouth, esophagus, etc. as it is being vomited from the stomach.

In general, vomiting is a symptom rather than a separate disease. However, vomiting itself can cause severe problems because of the amount of fluids and salts that are lost during prolonged spells of vomiting. The treatment will depend on the cause of the vomiting. When vomiting is severe and the patient cannot keep down the oral form of a drug, it is sometimes necessary to use a drug in the form of a rectal suppository in order to introduce the proper medicine into the body.

vulva — the entrance to the vagina.

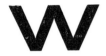

walleye — a form of strabismus. Walleye is a condition in which one or both eyes turn out (as opposed to crossed eyes, in which the eyes turn in). The technical name for walleye is exotropia.

See strabismus.

Wangensteen tube — a tube that is inserted into the stomach through the nostrils and pharynx to provide constant drainage of the gastrointestinal tract. The tube is connected to one or more drainage bottles. Because the pressure in the drainage bottle is lower than the pressure in the stomach, the stomach contents are siphoned into the drainage bottles.

The Wangensteen tube is used to relieve or prevent abdominal distention, to remove gas or fluids from the gastrointestinal tract, to relieve intestinal obstruction, or to relieve postoperative nausea or vomiting.

wart — a small tumor caused by a virus infection. Warts usually appear on the outer layer of the skin — most frequently on the hands and feet. Warts that occur on the bottoms or soles of the feet are called plantar warts. These can be quite painful because of the constant friction and pressure to which they are subjected.

Some warts will disappear by themselves. However, many warts must be artificially removed. The treatment may include drugs, freezing, burning, or surgery. Because warts are caused by a virus, it is possible for them to reappear.

Wasserman reaction — a test for syphilis.

See syphilis.

waste products — substances that have entered the body (usually as food or beverages) but which cannot be used by the body and are excreted in the form of feces, urine, and sweat. Other waste products (such as carbon dioxide) are expelled from the body through the respiratory system.

water — an essential body fluid. The normal life processes cannot take place without water. Over fifty percent of the body is composed of water, and over ninety percent of blood plasma (the liquid portion of the blood) is composed of water. The blood furnishes water to the cellular elements of the body to provide proper maintenance of the total water content of body tissues.

There must be a constant flow of water into and out of the body in order for the body to maintain itself. The body will begin to develop problems whenever this flow is interrupted.

Water enters the body in the form of beverages of all kinds. However, many of the so-called "solid" foods also contain a high percentage of water. (For example, a boiled potato is almost eighty percent water.) The body's water requirements depend to a large extent on the environmental temperature and on physical activity. As the level of outside temperature and the level of physical activity increase, so does the amount of water loss (in the form of sweat). This water loss must be replaced, but under normal circumstances the sensation of thirst will serve as a reliable guide for the necessary water intake.

Water leaves the body in the form of either urine or sweat. During an average day the adult body will lose more than a pint and a half through sweat. Ninety-five percent of urine is made up of water. The amount of urine excreted by a normal adult ranges from thirty-four to sixty fluid ounces per day. This amount (like the amount of sweat) can vary greatly, depending on factors such as environmental body temperature, water intake, and states of health or disease.

A large water intake does not put a strain on the kidneys. Rather, it eases the load of concentration placed on the kidneys. However, no matter how much water is taken into the body, the blood always remains at a relatively constant concentration as long as the kidneys are functioning properly. When the kidneys begin to fail, as may happen with congestive heart failure, excess sodium is retained in the body. The sodium holds excess water with it and causes an accumulation of fluids known as edema.

The relationship between sodium (salt) and water is very important. If the body lacks sodium, it cannot retain sufficient amounts of water. If, however, there is an excess of sodium, too much water is retained. In order for the body to remain healthy, a balance must be achieved and maintained. This balance can be greatly upset when there is severe vomiting or diarrhea, because the body loses so much water and sodium. It is not possible for the body to stay alive without replacing all lost water. The body cannot remain alive for more than a few days without water.

See edema, kidneys.

water on the brain — *See hydrocephalus.*

water on the knee — a condition in which there is an inflammation of the membrane in the knees. Fluid collects in the area as part of the inflammation process. This condition is usually the result of some kind of accident or injury. Water on the knee can be very painful. The treatment may include withdrawal of the fluid through a needle. It is usually necessary to reduce the stress and strain applied to the knee by restricting the amount of exercise. An elastic bandage is often used to provide additional support for the area.

weight — the size of the body expressed in ounces and pounds. The weight of the body influences health. Excessive body weight (obesity) puts an undue strain on the heart, and in predisposed individuals it encourages the emergence of latent diabetes. Obesity also increases the liability to a number of conditions such as high blood pressure and hardening of the arteries. Conversely, a person who is very underweight will often lack energy, may have little resistance to diseases, and may be suffering from nutritional deficiencies.

The weight of the body can be influenced by various diseases and conditions. Each individual's weight is partially determined by height and body frame. However, other important factors are the quantity and the quality of the food an individual consumes, the amount of physical activity, and the general health of the individual.

See obesity.

Weil's disease — *See leptospirosis.*

wen — a cyst or abnormal growth. Wens (also called sebaceous cysts) are formed when a duct from a sebaceous gland becomes blocked. The cyst contains sebum, the oily substance secreted by the sebaceous glands. Treatment for a wen usually involves surgical removal of the cyst. However, unless the entire cyst is removed, there is a tendency for it to reappear.

Wernicke's center — an area of the cerebral cortex of the brain. Wernicke's center is responsible for the ability to understand words that are spoken.

wheal — a slightly raised patch of skin. Wheals (sometimes called hives) can be either red or very pale. They are usually an allergic reaction to a foreign substance. The appearance of a wheal is considered to be a positive reaction during tests for allergies. In most cases, the wheal (or wheals) will disappear within a few days.

See allergy.

white blood cells — cells that allow the body to defend itself against disease.

See blood.

whitlow — an inflammation and/or infection of the skin and tissues surrounding the nail of one or more fingers. People whose hands are frequently exposed to water are the most prone to whitlow.

whooping cough — a childhood disease. Although it can occur at any age, whooping cough (also called pertussis) usually strikes those under seven. Fatal cases are usually babies. The disease is particularly dangerous because of the violent cough, which sometimes even ruptures blood ves-

WEIGHT

MEN
Age 25 and over

Weight in pounds according to frame (In indoor clothing)

Height (with shoes on) 1-inch heels		Small frame	Medium frame	Large frame
Feet	Inches			
5	2	112–120	118–129	126–141
5	3	115–123	121–133	129–144
5	4	118–126	124–136	132–148
5	5	121–129	127–139	135–152
5	6	124–133	130–143	138–156
5	7	128–137	134–147	142–161
5	8	132–141	138–152	147–166
5	9	136–145	142–156	151–170
5	10	140–150	146–160	155–174
5	11	144–154	150–165	159–179
6	0	148–158	154–170	164–184
6	1	152–162	158–175	168–189
6	2	156–167	162–180	173–194
6	3	160–171	167–185	178–199
6	4	164–175	172–190	182–204

WOMEN
Age 25 and over

For girls between 18 and 25, subtract 1 pound for each year under 25

Weight in pounds according to frame (In indoor clothing)

Height (with shoes on) 2-inch heels		Small frame	Medium frame	Large frame
Feet	Inches			
4	10	92–98	96–107	104–119
4	11	94–101	98–110	106–122
5	0	96–104	101–113	109–125
5	1	99–107	104–116	112–128
5	2	102–110	107–119	115–131
5	3	105–113	110–122	118–134
5	4	108–116	113–126	121–138
5	5	111–119	116–130	125–142
5	6	114–123	120–135	129–146
5	7	118–127	124–139	133–150
5	8	122–131	128–143	137–154
5	9	126–135	132–147	141–158
5	10	130–140	136–151	145–163
5	11	134–144	140–155	149–168
6	0	138–148	144–159	153–173

sels in the eyes. Whooping cough also lowers resistance to other illnesses, such as bronchopneumonia. Even when the worst stage has passed, recovery takes a long while, and patients have difficulty getting proper nutrition and rest. Before whooping cough vaccine was used extensively in the United States, nearly all children contracted the disease at some time or other, and thousands of deaths were reported every year. Now, with vaccinations and more prompt medical care, only a few hundred deaths are reported annually.

SYMPTOMS

At first whooping cough often resembles an ordinary cold, with a running nose and a slight, hacking cough. These signs usually develop about seven to ten days after exposure. Within two weeks, and sometimes in a few days, the cough develops into a series of coughs that prevent the patient from catching his breath. This is followed by the well-known whooping sound and oftens ends with vomiting. During the coughing attack the face gets red and the eyes are watery and bloodshot. The violence of these spasms is necessary to expel the sticky mucus from the air passages and throat. A child with whooping cough will generally awaken from a deep sleep in order to cough and get his breath. Very young infants and adults who have mild cases are sometimes spared the whoop.

The whooping stage lasts from four to six weeks, passing gradually into a declining stage, when attacks of coughing are less frequent. The final stage usually takes another two or three weeks, but some children cough for many months. The disease is generally easy to recognize by the coughing spasms, but mild cases sometimes can be detected only through laboratory tests.

SPREAD

Whooping cough germs are found in the discharge of the nose and throat. Talking, sneezing, and coughing spray these germs into the air. The disease can be caught by inhaling the germs, by drinking from an infected glass, or by handling things that have touched the patient's nose or mouth. Whooping cough is most infectious in its early stages and can be considered not communicable three weeks after onset.

TREATMENT

While the disease is running its course, the patient should be kept away from susceptible children and kept out of school and other public places. This isolation is also for the patient's own good because it protects him from catching other diseases to which he may be particularly susceptible at this time.

It is important to call a physician even in suspected cases of whooping cough, since there are medicines which, if given early, will speed recovery. There are also medicines that will help make the patient more comfortable. Afternoon naps help to rest the patient who suffers from coughing seizures at night. Proper diet is important. Foods such as nuts, crackers, toast, highly seasoned dishes, and very hot or very cold foods should be avoided, since they may start a coughing spell.

PREVENTION

Almost everyone can be protected against whooping cough by prescribed doses of whooping cough vaccine. Health authorities usually recommend that three doses of vaccine be given at four-week intervals beginning at two to six months of age. "Booster" shots to reinforce these early vaccinations are generally given when the child is one or two years old and again at four or five years of age. Whooping cough vaccine is usually combined with diphtheria, tetanus toxoid, and polio vaccine, so that protection against all four diseases is given at the same time.

Wilson's disease — an inherited defect that, if untreated, causes severe mental retardation. Wilson's disease (also known as hepatolenticular degeneration) is caused by the body's inability to use copper or protein. It usually begins between the ages of ten to twenty-five years (ranging from four to fifty years). If the desease is recognized in time, it can be effectively controlled by medicine and diet.

windpipe — *See trachea.*

wintergreen oil — a salve or liniment used in the treatment of strained muscles and for relief of rheumatoid conditions. Wintergreen oil (also called methyl salicylate) may be diluted with mineral oil before application to the skin. It produces rubefacient, counterirritant, and penetrating effects.

Wintergreen oil is never used internally because of its acute toxicity. One fluid ounce may cause death when taken internally.

wisdom teeth — a common term given to the third molars. These teeth appear between the ages of seventeen and twenty-one years. They are often the cause of extreme discomfort during their eruption. The soft tissues surrounding the molar may become acutely inflamed. This inflammation may be caused by infection resulting from the inability of the individual to keep the area clean or by infection from oral disease-forming organisms that have gained access to the tissues by way of the opening created by a projecting part of the tooth. Constant irritation from an opposing upper or lower third molar may cause inflammation and then allow an infection to begin.

An impacted wisdom tooth is one that is not growing straight and whose path is blocked so that it cannot erupt properly. Infection may be a complication of impaction. Treatment for an impacted wisdom tooth requires the removal of the tooth.
See teeth.

withdrawal sickness — a term used to describe the various symptoms a drug or narcotics addict experiences when the use of the addicting substance is stopped abruptly. Addiction is a physical dependence on a drug. When the drug is withdrawn, the body reacts to the absence of the substance. Symptoms of withdrawal sickness include diarrhea, vomiting, cramps, and convulsions.

Withering, William — an eminent English clinician (1741-1799) who discovered the use and proper dosage of digitalis in the treatment of heart disease. By analyzing the effective herbal mixture used by an old woman in Shropshire, he identified foxglove leaves as the active ingredient that influenced the function of the heart and kidneys.
See digitalis.

womb — a common term for the uterus.
See uterus.

woolsorter's disease — *See anthrax.*

work classification unit — a community facility involving a team approach to assessing the ability of a cardiac patient to work in terms of the energy requirements of the job.

worms — *See ringworm, tapeworm, etc.*

wound — any injury to the body. There are two major types of wounds: open and closed wounds. An injury that causes a break in the skin or other body membranes or in the underlying tissues is called an open wound. An injury that does not break the skin but does damage to the deeper tissues is called a closed wound.

CLOSED WOUNDS
Several types of injuries are classed as closed wounds.

1. Bruise
The bruise (also called a contusion) occurs most frequently. Bruises are responsible for the discoloration that almost always accompanies injuries to bones, joints, and muscles. They are caused by blows that damage bones, muscles, tendons, blood vessels, nerves, and other body tissues, although the skin is not necessarily broken. The symptoms are pain, swelling, and discoloration. The swelling occurs because blood from the broken blood vessels oozes into the soft tissues under the skin. At first the injured place is reddened by local skin irritation from the blow; later the characteristic "black and blue" marks appear; and, finally, perhaps several days later, the skin is yellowish or greenish in color.

2. Dislocation
A dislocation occurs when one or more of the bones forming a joint slips out of normal position. The ligaments holding the bones in proper position are stretched and sometimes are torn loose. Dislocations result from force applied at or near the joints, from sudden muscular contractions, from twisting strains on joint ligaments, or from falls where the force of the landing is transferred to a joint. The general symptoms of dislocations are rigidity and loss of function, deformity, pain, and swelling. The joints most frequently dislocated are those of the shoulder, hip, finger, and jaw.

3. Strain
A strain occurs when a muscle or a tendon of a muscle is overstretched. In severe strains the fibers forming the muscle or tendon may be torn. Strains are caused by sudden movements or by violent exertion in lifting or moving heavy weights. The symptoms of a strain are a sharp pain or cramp immediately. Any attempt to use the muscle is difficult and painful.

4. Sprain

Sprains are injuries that follow stretching or tearing of the ligaments or other tissues around a joint. They are caused by a sudden twist or wrench. Sprains range from minor injuries, causing pain or discomfort for only a few hours, to severe cases, where tearing of the tissues requires weeks of medical care before normal use of the joint is restored. The symptoms of a sprain are pain around the joint and inability to use it. Swelling is usually rapid and marked and is followed by discoloration.

5. Crush

Crush wounds are caused by a heavy physical force or blow that severely damages deep tissues. Crushed wounds are serious because they destroy tissues and often permit the spread of infections.

OPEN WOUNDS

Open wounds can be classified according to their general location, size, and the agent that caused the wound. However, open wounds are most frequently classified according to the manner in which the skin or tissue is broken.

In general, large wounds are more serious than small ones, because they usually involve more severe bleeding, more damage to the underlying organs or tissues, and a greater degree of shock. However, small wounds are sometimes more dangerous than large ones, because they may become infected more easily.

Since a wound may involve serious damage to the deeper structures, as well as to the skin and the tissues immediately below it, the location of the wound is an important consideration. For example, a knife wound in the chest is likely to puncture a lung and cause serious interference with breathing. The same type of wound in the abdomen might cause peritonitis (a dangerous infection in the abdominal cavity), or it might actually puncture the intestines, the liver, the kidneys, or other vital organs. A knife wound to the head might cause brain damage. The same kind of a wound in a less vital spot (as, perhaps, an arm or a leg) might be relatively unimportant.

Any break in the skin or other body membrane (such as the mucous membrane that lines the nasal passages) is dangerous, because it allows microorganisms (germs) to enter the wound. Although infection may occur in any wound, it is a particular danger in wounds that do not bleed freely, wounds in which torn tissue or skin falls back into place and so prevents the entrance of

air, and wounds that involve crushing of the tissues. Incisions, in which there is a free flow of blood and relatively little crushing of the tissues, are least likely to become infected.

When considered from the point of view of the manner in which the skin or tissue is broken, there are four general types of open wounds: abrasions, incisions, lacerations, and punctures. Many wounds are combinations of two or more of these basic types.

1. Abrasions

Abrasions are wounds of the skin that result from scraping or friction. Although abrasions are usually relatively minor wounds, they can become quite serious because of the possibilities of infection. Abrasions are easily infected, because dirt and germs are frequently rubbed into the underskin surface at the time of the injury. The bleeding in most abrasions is only from the capillaries, so the amount of bleeding is not as serious as in other types of wounds.

2. Incisions

Incisions are wounds caused by sharp materials that cut across the skin, sometimes cutting into deeper tissue. The edges of such wounds are smoothly divided without bruising or tearing. Incised wounds bleed freely, because they cut straight through the blood vessels. However, since there is such a free flow of blood, incised wounds are not as liable to infection as are other types of wounds, because the escaping blood washes out most of the dirt and germs that may have entered the wound.

3. Lacerations

Lacerations are wounds with ragged edges. They have been torn or mashed by blunt instruments, machinery, or rough surfaces. Because the blood vessels are torn or mashed, they do not bleed as freely as incised wounds. However, the ragged and torn tissues, with the foreign matter that is often forced or ground into the wound, make the danger of infection greater than in incised wounds.

4. Punctures

Punctures are wounds that are caused by pointed instruments. Such wounds usually are small but may be very deep. Most of the articles causing puncture wounds (nails, wire, etc.) are soiled and carry infection-causing microorganisms. Thus, puncture wounds are easily infected. Additionally, there is little bleeding to help wash the foreign matter out of the tissues.

wrist — the joint between the lower arm and the hand. Eight carpal bones arranged in two rows form the wrist. This arrangement allows great flexibility. The wrist will bend up and down, but it will not bend to either side. The wrist itself does not turn sideways. Rather, the bones of the lower arm turn and move the wrist.

wry neck — a condition that causes the head to turn to one side in spasms. Wry neck can be caused by many conditions and diseases, such as rheumatism, poliomyelitis, and syphilis. The treatment depends on the cause, but wry neck (also known as torticollis) is often very difficult to cure.

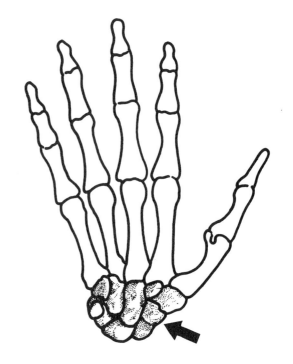

WRIST

X

xanthines — a class of drugs. Xanthines have many different types of therapeutic uses. They are used in the treatment of congestive heart failure and asthma. Many of these drugs are diuretics; that is, they increase the excretion of urine. Additionally, xanthines stimulate the central nervous system and help relieve headaches.

The best known of the xanthines is caffeine. This substance is used as a drug, but it is also found in coffee, tea, and other beverages that are extracted from plants. The presence of caffeine in popular beverages means that many people are taking more caffeine than they realize. Many people find that they are unable to sleep if they have had too much coffee during the day or if they drink coffee before going to bed. The reason for this is that the caffeine in the coffee is acting as a central nervous system stimulant.

xanthocyanopsia — a form of color blindness in which the patient cannot tell the difference between green and red colors.
See color blindness.

xanthoma — a condition in which yellow patches appear on the skin. The patch is actually a small collection of fat or fatlike substances.

xanthopsia — a condition in which all vision is slightly tinted with a yellow color. Xanthopsia is a complication of jaundice.
See jaundice.

X chromosome — one of the two sex chromosomes. When an ovum is fertilized by a sperm, the fertilized egg has two sex chromosomes, one from the mother and one from the father. All ova have the X chromosome. A sperm may have an X chromosome or a Y chromosome. When the sperm carries an X chromosome, the fertilized ovum has two X chromosomes and the child will be a female.
See genetics, Y chromosome.

xeroderma — *See ichthyosis.*

xerophthalmia — a condition in which the cornea becomes dry and painful. Xerophthalmia is caused by a lack or deficiency of vitamin A in the diet. The condition is treated by increasing or supplementing the amount of vitamin A in the patient's diet with vitamin A in pill or liquid form.

xerosis — a general term indicating unusual or abnormal dryness.

xerostomia — dryness of the mouth. The direct cause of xerostomia is a lack of saliva. However, the indirect cause may vary greatly. Many drugs can cause this condition as a side effect. Xerostomia is also a disease symptom. The treatment varies according to the cause. When a drug is the cause, the condition will usually correct itself when the patient stops taking the drug. In other cases some drug may be used to increase the amount of saliva.

xiphoid — the term given to the lowest portion of the sternum or breastbone. The xiphoid (also called the xiphoid process) is narrower than the rest of the sternum and ends in a tip.

See sternum.

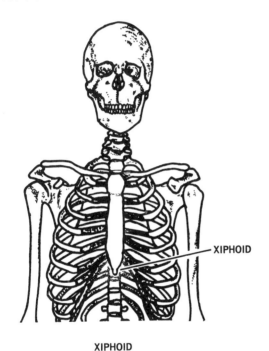

XIPHOID

xiphoid process — *See xiphoid.*

X-rays — any radiations of the same general nature as light but of an extremely short wave length. These rays are capable of passing through the body and acting on a photographic plate. The result of this is an X-ray picture. This picture is actually a negative. Because some areas of the body are much thicker, or more dense, than others, the X-rays will pass through them with different results. Thus, when an X-ray passes through a very solid part of the body, such as a bone, the image on the negative will be white.

Conversely, soft tissues show up as black or gray on the X-ray.

X-rays were discovered in 1895 by Wilhelm Konrad Roentgen, a physics professor at a German university. He discovered this process during the course of some experiments in electronics. Although he recognized the powers of penetration of X-rays, Roentgen was not sure what kind of rays or radiation were being produced. Consequently, he called them "X" rays. For his discovery, Roentgen was awarded the Nobel Prize for physics in 1901.

These rays are produced by passing a current of electricity through a sealed tube. The tube contains two electrodes. When the electric current hits the electrodes, it causes electrons to pass through the tube. The electrons hit the wall of the tube and produce X-rays.

USES

Soon after Roentgen discovered X-rays, they were used for the examination of inner parts of the body. Today, X-rays are used in two major areas of medicine: diagnosis and treatment.

1. Diagnosis

With the discovery of X-rays, it became possible to examine organs of the body without surgery. This technique is used for examining fractures, to discover the location of foreign objects in the body, and to discover or confirm the presence of tumors. Additionally, dentists use X-rays to locate cavities and to determine the size and location of teeth below the surface of the gums.

When a soft internal organ (such as the stomach) is to be X-rayed, it is necessary for the patient to swallow or to be injected with some opaque material. This material (often special forms of barium or iodine) helps outline the body organ on the X-ray.

In the past, extensive use has been made of X-rays to detect tuberculosis. Chest X-ray surveys of large numbers of people for signs of tuberculosis were begun in 1936. By 1956, the peak year for the mass X-ray screening programs in this country, some 18 million people (nearly eleven percent of the total population) were examined.

2. Treatment

Radiation from X-rays is used to treat cancer. This treatment may be used in conjunction with surgery or by itself. Properly controlled X-ray treatment destroys or retards the growth of cancer cells. However, when the cancer is widespread, X-ray treatment is not effective.

DANGERS

Despite the fact that X-rays are used in the treatment of cancer, they can also cause cancer. This discovery was actually made on human beings. Pioneer radiologists developed dryness, ulcers, and eventually, cancer on their hands.

Today, X-ray machines used in medical and dental work have been greatly improved to require less exposure time and lower total radiation dosage. While controlled X-rays are now safe for the patient, radiologists and others who work with X-ray machines are cautioned to shield themselves (usually behind lead doors). Additionally, the use of X-ray machines for fitting shoes has been discouraged because of the danger of frequent and excessive exposure.

xylometazoline — a drug used as a nasal decongestant.

yawn — an involuntary deep inspiration of air. Yawning is an attempt on the part of the body to increase the amount of oxygen in the body. It occurs most frequently when the body is tired and the rate of breathing has decreased. However, yawning can be contagious. Most people are susceptible to yawning when they see another person yawn.

yaws — a disease found primarily in tropical areas of the world. The disease can be spread from person to person and is caused by a microorganism called a spirochete. The major symptom of yaws is the appearance of lesions that become covered with a crusty yellow substance. Fever, headache, and pain in the area of joints are also present.

If untreated, yaws can cause deformity. However, when treated promptly (usually with penicillin), yaws can be cured.

Y chromosome — one of the two sex chromosomes. A fertilized ovum has two sex chromosomes, one from the mother and one from the father. The female ovum always contains the X chromosome (the other of the two sex chromosomes). The male sperm can contain either an X or a Y chromosome. When the sperm carries an X chromosome, the fertilized ovum will have two X chromosomes and will be a female child. When the sperm carries a Y chromosome, the fertilized ovum has an X and a Y chromosome and will be a male child.
See genetics, X chromosome.

yellow bone marrow — ordinary bone marrow in which fat cells predominate.
See marrow.

yellow fever — a virus disease transmitted by the bite of the *Aedes aegypti* mosquito. The virus that causes yellow fever multiplies in the body of the mosquito. In areas such as the United States, where this type of mosquito is only rarely found, yellow fever is not a problem. However, in tropical areas (especially in Africa) yellow fever remains a dangerous disease.

The symptoms of yellow fever are high fever, vomiting ("black" vomit), and jaundice. There is no specific cure for yellow fever; treatment is aimed at relieving the major symptoms. The fatality rate for yellow fever is fairly high, especially when it occurs as an epidemic.

yellow mecuric oxide — an ointment used as an antiseptic in the treatment of eye infections and in certain other skin infections where antibiotics cannot be used because of sensitivity.

zinc — a metal. Zinc is used in many medical compounds. Zinc chloride is an antiseptic and astringent that is used in irrigating washes for the eyes, mouth, urethra, and vagina. Zinc oxide has mildly astringent and antiseptic properties. It is used in the treatment of various skin diseases. Zinc sulfate is used internally as an emetic. It is one of the most valuable emetics in various poisonings. It is also used as an antiseptic and astringent.

Despite the fact that zinc compounds are used medically, they are also poisons that corrode the gastrointestinal tract. Symptoms of zinc poisoning include salivation, difficulty in swallowing, a metallic taste in the mouth, bloody vomiting, and, finally, collapse and death.

zona — *See herpes zoster.*

zoonoses — diseases of animals that accidentally affect man. Man is not a natural host for the infective agent in most cases. Zoonoses diseases include rabies, leptospirosis, and psittacosis.

zoxazolamine — a drug that is used as a skeletal muscle relaxant. It acts on parts of the brain and the spinal cord. It does not act directly on the skeletal muscles. This drug is used for disorders such as sprains, contusions, muscle strains, back disorders, bursitis, etc. It provides prompt relief from muscle-spasm discomfort. The most frequent side effects are headache, skin rash, and drowsiness.

zwieback — a hard, toasted bread that is given to babies when they are cutting teeth.

zygote — a fertilized ovum, formed by the union of a sperm and an ovum. The original, single cell soon divides into two cells that stay together. Each of these two divide, again into two, and this process continues. The enlarging cluster of cells is at first called a zygote, then an embryo, and then a fetus.